THIRD EDITION

NUTRITION EDUCATION

Linking Research, Theory, and Practice

Isobel R. Contento

Mary Swartz Rose Professor of Nutrition and Education
Teachers College
Columbia University

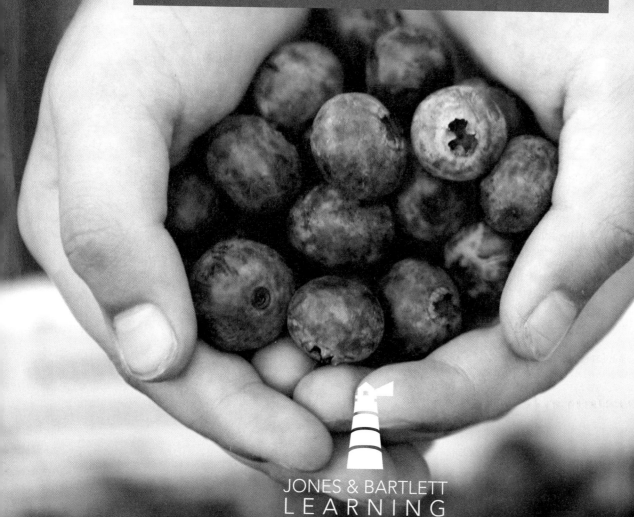

JONES & BARTLETT
LEARNING

World Headquarters
Jones & Bartlett Learning
5 Wall Street
Burlington, MA 01803
978-443-5000
info@jblearning.com
www.jblearning.com

Jones & Bartlett Learning books and products are available through most bookstores and online booksellers. To contact Jones & Bartlett Learning directly, call 800-832-0034, fax 978-443-8000, or visit our website, www.jblearning.com.

Substantial discounts on bulk quantities of Jones & Bartlett Learning publications are available to corporations, professional associations, and other qualified organizations. For details and specific discount information, contact the special sales department at Jones & Bartlett Learning via the above contact information or send an email to specialsales@jblearning.com.

08319-4

Production Credits

Chief Executive Officer: Ty Field
President: James Homer
Chief Product Officer: Eduardo Moura
VP, Executive Publisher: David D. Cella
Publisher: Cathy L. Esperti
Associate Acquisitions Editor: Sean Fabery
Production Editor: Leah Corrigan
Senior Marketing Manager: Andrea DeFronzo
VP, Manufacturing and Inventory Control: Therese Connell

Composition: CAE Solutions Corp.
Cover Design: Kristin E. Parker
Interior Design: Publishers' Design and Production Services, Inc.
Rights & Media Research Coordinator: Jamey O'Quinn
Media Development Editor: Shannon Sheehan
Cover Image: © ARENA Creative/Shutterstock
Printing and Binding: RR Donnelley
Cover Printing: RR Donnelley

Library of Congress Cataloging-in-Publication Data

Contento, Isobel R., author.
    Nutrition education : linking research, theory, and practice / Isobel R. Contento. -- Third edition.
        p. ; cm.
    Includes bibliographical references and index.
    ISBN 978-1-284-07800-8 (alk. paper)
    I. Title.
    [DNLM: 1.   Dietetics--education. 2.   Health Education--methods. 3.   Food Habits. 4.   Health Behavior.   WB 18]
    TX364
    613.2--dc23
6048   2015020543

Printed in the United States of America
19   18   17   16   15   10   9   8   7   6   5   4   3   2   1

BRIEF CONTENTS

CONTENTS

PART II   USING RESEARCH AND THEORY IN PRACTICE: A STEPWISE PROCEDURE FOR DESIGNING THEORY-BASED NUTRITION EDUCATION   213

PART III   RESEARCH AND THEORY IN ACTION: DELIVERING NUTRITION EDUCATION IN PRACTICE   485

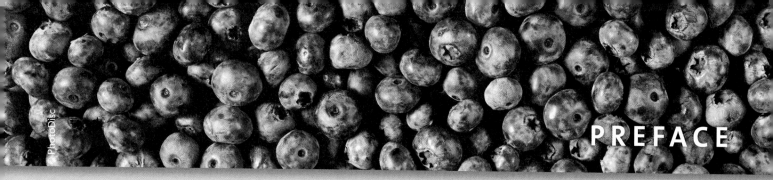

With the rates of diet-related diseases and obesity continuing to rise worldwide—alongside malnutrition in some countries—nutrition education is needed now more than ever. Fortunately, the important role played by nutrition education in reducing the risk of these conditions is increasingly recognized for schools, worksites, and communities, and consequently food and nutrition-related policy initiatives in institutions and government have increased over the past few years. This means that nutrition educators have an opportunity to make a genuine difference in the world.

Approach of This Text

This text seeks to assist nutrition educators by focusing on how to design, deliver, and evaluate the types of educational interventions and programs that the vast majority of nutrition educators conduct on an ongoing basis in their places of work, such as community programs, clinics, food banks, family programs, or schools.

Nutrition education is defined in this text as any combination of educational strategies, accompanied by environmental supports, designed to facilitate the voluntary adoption of food choices and other food- and nutrition-related behaviors conducive to health and well-being. It is delivered through multiple venues and involves activities at the individual, institutional, community, and policy levels.

Nutrition educators are usually very expert at creating sessions with interesting activities for their audiences. Research evidence suggests that these sessions can be more effective if the activities are clearly designed to address specific behavior change goals, along with the motivators, facilitators, and supports for change for their audiences. Research in behavioral nutrition and nutrition education has also generated conceptual models or theories that can help us understand how people make food choices and what may motivate and facilitate change. Consequently, the text focuses on how to use the key theories or models as tools to help nutrition educators design interventions, programs, or sessions that indeed address the identified motivators, facilitators, and supports for diet-related behavioral change for their audiences.

This text has been designed for upper-level undergraduate and graduate nutrition students who are taking their first course in nutrition education, as well as for practitioners and managers already working in nutrition education who want a comprehensive resource for planning and delivering effective programs to their audiences.

Organization of This Text

This text is divided into three parts.

Part I describes the complexity of influences on food choices and the key elements of success for nutrition education. Later chapters in this part provide a clearly organized description of each of the major theories that can be used in nutrition education interventions to address potential motivators and facilitators of change, referred to here as determinants (or mediators) of action and behavior change as well as evidence for their usefulness. For each theory, a leader orients the student to the theory, and a take-home message summarizes it. Each theory is followed by a description of how to translate the theory into practical nutrition education activities, along with a case example of its use.

There is an increased appreciation that our food choices are influenced by social and environmental contexts. Nutrition education needs to address the numerous personal, environmental, and policy influences on food choices and dietary behaviors in order to assist individuals and communities in practicing healthy behaviors. A larger scope for nutrition education thus has evolved.

While group sessions remain primary, nutrition educators also work in collaboration with others on activities such as school and community gardens, cooking with children and adults, farm-to-school programs, school and community wellness policies, and initiatives to improve policy, systems, and environments. Consequently, Chapter 6 describes how to design environmental supports for action using a social ecological model.

Part II features the centerpiece of this text: A stepwise procedure intended to make it easier for students and practitioners to design effective nutrition education. This procedure, called DESIGN, shows how behavioral theory is translated into theory-based strategies and educational objectives, and then how these strategies and objectives can be practically implemented. These activities are then organized into educational plans for program components directed at groups. The DESIGN procedure integrates theory, research, and practice at every step, providing guidance on designing, implementing, and evaluating theory-based nutrition education. Part II also provides guidance on how to develop environmental support plans for changes in policy, social structures, and environments to increase opportunities for action. It also explores how to link evaluation to theory and intervention objectives. At the end of each chapter in Part II, the DESIGN procedure is illustrated by a case study. A set of blank worksheets are included at the end of Chapter 13.

Part III describes the nuts and bolts of implementing nutrition education with diverse groups ranging from preschool children to older adults, as well as addressing low-literacy audiences and diverse cultural groups through a variety of venues, including group sessions, written and visual materials, new technologies, and social marketing.

Features and Benefits

Nutrition Education: Linking Research, Theory, and Practice, Third Edition, includes a variety of features to prepare students and others to provide effective nutrition education to specific groups and to foster environmental supports for action:

- At the beginning of each chapter, an *Overview* and *Chapter Outline* help students anticipate what will be covered. *Learning Objectives* improve retention of the material presented.
- *Nutrition Education in Action* features highlight concepts discussed in the chapter through examples of best practices and research culled from current education programs.
- *Boxes* draw out important information for the reader, particularly about specific theories in practice.
- A logic model approach is used in the DESIGN stepwise procedure, with the tasks and products of each step clearly stated.
- The *Worksheets* in Part II allow students and nutrition educators to develop their own programs using the DESIGN stepwise procedure.
- *Case examples* included throughout the text illustrate the use of each specific theory in practice. Furthermore, a case study introduced in Chapter 7 and followed throughout Part II illustrates each step of the DESIGN procedure for designing nutrition education.
- At the end of each chapter, *Questions and Activities* reinforce key concepts and references provide an opportunity for further study.

Instructor Resources

Qualified instructors can receive the full suite of Instructor Resources, including the following:

- Test Bank, containing more than 800 questions
- Slides in PowerPoint format, featuring more than 400 slides
- Instructor's Manual, providing Chapter Outlines and Teaching Suggestions
- Sample Syllabus, showing how a course can be structured around this text

The public needs and wants what nutrition education can offer. This text is designed to help students and nutrition educators gain the knowledge and skills needed to provide that nutrition education effectively.

Isobel R. Contento

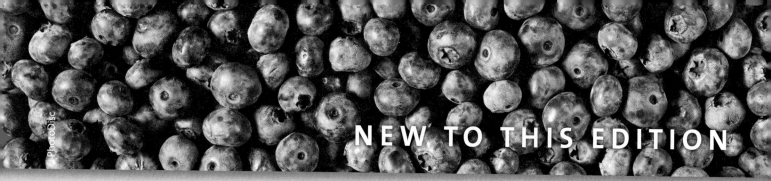

The basic structure of the text remains the same because it seems to work. However, just about every page has been extensively revised based on feedback from both faculty members and students who have used this text, as well as on ongoing research in the field. The chapters have been streamlined, shortened, and rewritten to make them easier to read and use. The addition of a full color presentation for this edition also enhances readability, clarifying both the illustrations and heading structure. Additional diagrams have been added. The *Nutrition Education in Action* examples have been updated throughout, as have all the references. Greater emphasis has been placed on the cultural context of nutrition education.

A key change in Part I is that the case examples have been greatly expanded to clarify how the theories are used in practice.

The chapters in Part II, meanwhile, have been rearranged to flow more logically. Chapters 7 through 13 lead the reader through the 6-step DESIGN Procedure for developing group sessions, cumulatively resulting in one or more educational plans (lesson plans) for use with groups, along with an evaluation plan. Chapter 14 leads the reader through the entire 6-step DESIGN procedure in one chapter, but this time resulting in an environmental support plan that includes an evaluation plan. In addition, the DESIGN Procedure worksheets have been completely reformatted and simplified to make them much easier for all to use.

Part III, focusing on how to effectively deliver nutrition education, has also been extensively edited to link it more closely to the design DESIGN activities in Part II.

Additional specific changes for each chapter are described in the following pages.

Chapter 1: Nutrition Education: Important, Exciting, and Necessary for Today's Complex World

- The chapter as a whole has been shortened, particularly the sections describing the effectiveness of nutrition education and viewpoints on its aims.
- A section has been added on the impact of our food choices on the planet.
- A table showing the conceptual framework for the text has been added to help orient the reader.
- The relationship between food and nutrition education *topics* and *behavior change* in nutrition education has been clarified.
- The behavior change approach has been clarified.

Chapter 2: Determinants of Food Choice and Dietary Change: Implications for Nutrition Education

- Box 2-1, "Assessing Our Audiences: A Checklist," has been added to provide guidance in determining whether nutrition education has been appropriately tailored to an audience.

Chapter 3: An Overview of Nutrition Education: Facilitating Motivation, Ability, and Support for Behavior Change

- Chapter 3 is key to understanding important concepts central to this text, and as a result it has been extensively rewritten to make these concepts easier to understand, particularly the terms *theory* and *beliefs* and their role in *behavior change*.

- In order to help the reader better understand psychosocial theory, a section has been added in which the experiences of case study subjects are examined through behavioral science. The words used by the subjects in the interviews are matched with the labels psychologists give to these very same words.
- In many other places in the chapter, a concept is first introduced in lay language terms and then the psychosocial term for it is given.
- The differences among *motivating knowledge, facilitating knowledge, nutrition literacy, and food literacy* have been clarified, along with their relationship to *beliefs* and *behavior change*.
- The overview of nutrition education has been reframed in terms of elements of success.

Chapter 4: Increasing Awareness and Enhancing Motivation and Empowerment for Behavior Change and Taking Action

- Two major additions have been made to the case studies of Alicia and Maria: (1) a diagram for each based on different theory models and (2) full educational plans based on their respective theory models.
- Blank diagrams for the health belief model, the theory of planned behavior, and self-determination theory have been added.
- The model of goal-directed behavior has been added.

Chapter 5: Facilitating the Ability to Change Behavior and Take Action

- Two major additions have been made to the case study centered on Ray: (1) a theory model diagram based on social cognitive theory and (2) full educational plans based on the theory model.
- A blank diagram for social cognitive theory has been added.

Chapter 6: Promoting Environmental Supports for Behavior Change

- This chapter has been extensively edited with new examples of the social ecological model, most notably the new Community Nutrition Education Logic Model used by the United States Department of Agriculture.

Chapter 7: Step 1: Deciding Behavior Change Goals of the Intervention Based on Assessing Issues and Behaviors of Audience

- This chapter introduces the new name for the stepwise procedure used to design nutrition education: DESIGN.
- The worksheets for all steps have been completely rewritten, reformatted, and simplified.
- The worksheet for the case study appears at the end of the chapter, while blank worksheets for all steps now appear at the end of Chapter 13.

Chapter 8: Step 2: Exploring Determinants of Intervention Behavior Change Goals

- This chapter has been edited to reflect the new arrangement of chapters so that only determinants of individual behavior change are assessed: motivational determinants and facilitators of change.

Chapter 9: Step 3: Selecting Theory and Clarifying Intervention Philosophy

- The description indicating how to choose various components for the intervention has been deleted and moved to Chapter 14.

Chapter 10: Step 4: Indicating Objectives: Translating Behavioral Theory into Educational Objectives

- All objectives described in this chapter are for group sessions only (and indirect nutrition education if used). All text describing objectives directed at an environmental support component has been deleted and moved to Chapter 14.
- For the cognitive domain, the more recent wording and arrangement of objective levels has been used: Remember, understand, apply, analyze, evaluate, and synthesize.
- An extensive example of objectives from a curriculum has been added to help the reader write appropriate nutrition education objectives.

Chapter 11: Step 5: Generating Educational Plans: A Focus on Enhancing Motivation for Behavior Change and Taking Action

- This chapter is at the heart of writing educational or lesson plans for direct group nutrition education and has been streamlined for ease of reading.
- The relationships among determinants, educational objectives, behavioral change strategies, and practical educational activities have been clarified.
- The list of behavior change strategies for enhancing motivation has been revised to reflect new research.
- An extensive example from a curriculum has been added to help the reader clearly state strategies and educational objectives for determinants and guide the development of practical activities for strategies and objectives.
- The section on sequencing activities to generate educational plans has been re-written, and the sequence is now referred to as the 4 *Es*: excite, explain, expand, and exit.

Chapter 12: Step 5: Generating Educational Plans: A Focus on Facilitating the Ability to Change Behavior and Take Action

- The description of behavior change strategies for facilitating behavior change has been revised to reflect new research.
- More examples of goal setting are provided.

Chapter 13: Step 6: Nail Down the Evaluation Plan

- This chapter, which appeared in the previous edition as Chapter 14, has been completely rewritten to focus on designing the evaluation plan for group nutrition education sessions only (and indirect education if used). All references to evaluation of environmental supports has been deleted and moved to Chapter 14.
- Many more examples of evaluation instruments are included.
- Increased attention is given to design principles for measurement instruments that are appropriate for low-literacy clients.
- The discussion of process evaluation has been expanded, and a conceptual model is presented showing how process evaluation components are related to outcome evaluation components.
- Blank worksheets for steps 1 through 6 of the DESIGN procedure are now collected at the end of this chapter. They have been simplified and totally reformatted.

Chapter 14: Using the DESIGN Procedure to Promote Environmental Supports for Behavior Change and Taking Action

- This new chapter takes the reader through all six steps of the DESIGN procedure to design interpersonal and policy, system, and environment support (PSE) components based on a social ecological model that uses the categories of the *Dietary Guidelines for Americans, 2010*.
- Chapter 14 describes the types of theories or conceptual models that are appropriate for each level.
- This chapter provides more examples of social ecological approaches, including one that uses social cognitive theory to link activities at various levels.
- Worksheets for all six steps to promote environmental supports are placed together at the end of the chapter.

Chapter 15: Delivering Nutrition Education Effectively in Group Settings

- The chapter has been extensively rewritten to link the content conceptually to the DESIGN procedure.
- Sections on learning theory and instructional theory have been added.
- The section on communications has been expanded.
- A graphic organizer has been created to show the relationships among behavior change goals, determinants, behavior change strategies, instructional design theory, and communication principles.
- A lesson plan has been added to show how to integrate all the above considerations into one session.

Chapter 16: Media Supports and Other Channels for Nutrition Education

- The section on social marketing has been revised to include more recent views.
- The section on using new technologies has been totally rewritten and expanded.

Chapter 17: Working with Diverse Age, Cultural, and Literacy Population Groups

- The section on working with diverse cultural groups has been greatly expanded.
- A section on appropriate design principles and delivery methods for culturally sensitive nutrition education for culturally diverse audiences has been expanded.
- Sections on strategies for developing and delivering culturally sensitive interventions for African-American and Hispanic/Latino audiences have been added.
- The section on developing nutrition education materials and working with low-literacy audiences has been expanded considerably with more examples.
- A short section has been added about targeting subgroups that differ by food-related lifestyle factors based on differences in behaviors, attitudes, personal and social norms, values, and other factors.

Chapter 18: Nutrition Educators as Change Agents in the Environment

- Information on professional associations, public policy activities, and legislation has been updated.
- Sponsorship policies for professional societies have been updated.
- The text still ends with the challenge put out by Margaret Mead: Never doubt that a small group of thoughtful people can change the world. Indeed it is the only thing that ever has. And the quote from nutritionist Fern Estrow, "You can't do everything but you can do something."

ACKNOWLEDGMENTS

The field of nutrition education has grown rapidly over the past few years, and I have had the privilege of being a part of this exciting development. Many people have influenced my thinking and contributed to my understanding of the field, and I thank them all. They include colleagues across the country and the world, members of the Society for Nutrition Education and Behavior, behavioral nutrition and nutrition education researchers, presenters at professional meetings, members of committees I have been on, practitioners in community sites, and many others with whom I have worked.

In particular, I want to thank a few I have worked with more closely. Joan Gussow first introduced me to the field of nutrition education, and her insights and forward thinking have always challenged me to dig deeper. She encouraged me to write this book and has been supportive throughout. Pamela Koch, with whom I have worked for the past two decades, has been an important contributor to this effort. Additionally, she created the DESIGN acronym for the stepwise procedure and the 4 Es for this edition. Marissa Burgermaster, an experienced and thoughtful educator, contributed substantially to the Nutrition Education in Action feature of the text, the DESIGN worksheets, and the Instructor's Manual. Rachel Paul has provided valuable assistance with the ancillary materials for this edition.

The many reviewers of the manuscript across all editions provided extremely valuable feedback from their vantage points as faculty members who teach nutrition education or community nutrition courses in a wide variety of colleges and universities. This text has benefited from their insights. A special thank you to the following reviewers who either provided feedback as I planned this revision or provided comments about draft chapters:

- Jennifer O. Barr, MPH, RD, LDN, West Chester University
- Leslie D. Cunningham-Sabo, PhD, RDN, Colorado State University
- Erika Deshmukh, MS, RD, San Jose State University
- Grace Falciglia, EdD, MPH, RD, University of Cincinnati
- Mary Beth Gilboy, PhD, MPH, RD, West Chester University
- Deborah A. Hutcheon, MS, RD, LD, Bob Jones University
- Deborah Kennedy, PhD, University of New Haven
- Lisa A. Kessler, DrPH, RD, California State Polytechnic University, Pomona
- Linda Knol, PhD, RD, The University of Alabama
- Katie R. Miner, MS, RD, LD, University of Idaho
- Cynthia Warren, PhD, Texas Woman's University

Equally important are the numerous students who road-tested the many versions of this book in more than a decade of my nutrition education courses. Their reactions, feedback, and suggestions have provided reality checks on using this text in the classroom and in the field.

I also want to thank the people at Jones & Bartlett Learning for their support for this project: Sean Fabery, the associate acquisitions editor; Leah Corrigan, the production editor; Shannon Sheehan, the media development editor; Jamey O'Quinn, the rights and media research coordinator; and Rhonda Dearborn, who was involved in the early stages of this edition.

And last, but definitely not least, I thank my husband Robert Clark for his many years of unwavering support. Having worked in the textbook business himself, he understands the effort that writing a textbook requires.

© PhotoDisc

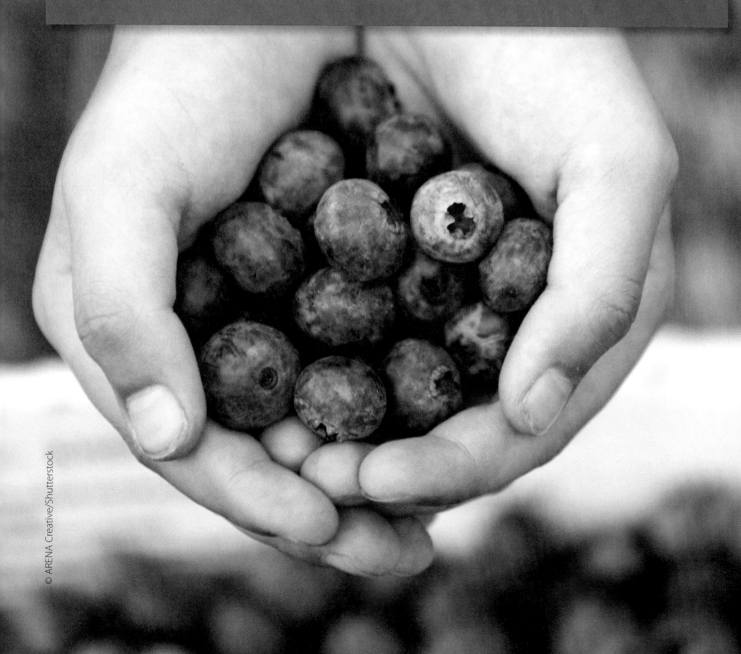

PART I

Linking Research, Theory, and Practice: The Foundations

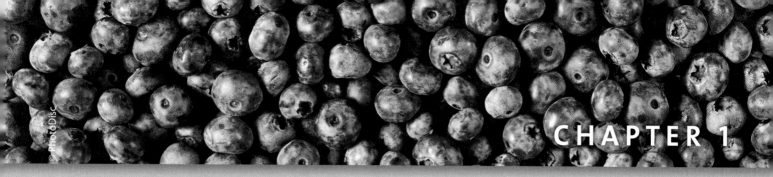

Nutrition Education: Important, Exciting, and Necessary for Today's Complex World

OVERVIEW

This chapter introduces the reader to the exciting field of nutrition education, why it is needed, and its aims, scope, and effectiveness. It introduces a contemporary definition of nutrition education and provides an overview of the book.

CHAPTER OUTLINE

- Introduction
- Why is nutrition education needed?
- The challenge of educating people about eating well
- Viewpoints on the aims of nutrition education
- A contemporary definition of nutrition education

- Nutrition education effectiveness
- What do nutrition educators do? Settings, audiences, and scope for nutrition education
- Nutrition education, public health nutrition, and health promotion: the roles and context of nutrition education
- Purpose and overview of this book

LEARNING OBJECTIVES

At the end of the chapter, you should be able to:

- State why nutrition education is both important and challenging to do
- Evaluate differing points of view about the purposes and scope of nutrition education

- Define nutrition education
- Describe whether nutrition education is effective
- Describe what nutrition educators do

Introduction

This is an exciting time for the field of **nutrition education**. Everyone seems to be interested in food and nutrition. Most newspapers have weekly sections on food. Restaurant guides have proliferated in print and online, and chefs are now celebrities. Cooking shows are popular on television, and in some areas entire television channels are devoted to food. The cookbook and food sections of bookstores have grown, and diet books and cooking magazines abound. Nutrition and health issues are discussed on the nightly news, and the Internet has exploded with information—websites, blogs, videos, and more. Annual surveys of supermarket shoppers show that nutrition is increasingly important as a factor in people's shopping decisions (Food Marketing Institute, 2012). School gardens have been enthusiastically embraced and urban community gardens have sprouted in many cities.

Food companies and food service providers, recognizing that *nutrition* is a buzzword that sells products, are also getting in on the act. They have created fat-free baked goods, low-fat yogurt, and a host of other products to satisfy one set of consumers, as well as low-carbohydrate products in response to another set of consumers. Reduced-sodium products sit side by side with their original, higher-salt versions. The fruits and vegetables sections of many supermarkets have doubled and tripled in size. Farmers' markets and farm stands are mushrooming and buying "local" or "organic" has gone mainstream, with even large supermarkets identifying such items for consumers. Although "sustainable food systems" is not yet a household phrase, more people understand what that means and belonging to a CSA (community supported agriculture) no longer seems esoteric. Many communities are requiring that fast food chains provide calorie information on their menu boards.

Food is also an important topic of conversation. As you have probably experienced, mentioning that you are in the field of nutrition means that people immediately have questions for you. In addition, food is not just a necessity but also, of course, one of life's great pleasures. While some eaters may be in and out of a fast-food restaurant in 10 minutes, others can spend hours discussing or eating a meal. Almost 200 years ago, Brillat-Savarin pointed out in a book on the physiology of taste that "the pleasure of eating . . . occurs necessarily at least once a day, and may be repeated without inconvenience two or three times in this space of time; . . . it can be combined with all our other pleasures, and even console us for their absence" (Brillant-Savarin 1825).

Why Is Nutrition Education Needed?

It would appear, then, that eating well should be getting easier for everyone. If the news media provide information and healthful foods abound in supermarkets, why is nutrition education needed?

THE ULTIMATE GOAL IS TO IMPROVE HEALTH AND WELL-BEING

Current eating patterns are associated with 4 of the 10 leading causes of death in developed countries such as the United States and increasingly in developing countries as well: coronary heart disease, some types of cancer, stroke, and type 2 diabetes. Obesity is on the rise in the United States and globally, carrying with it an increased risk of these chronic diseases (Flegal et al. 2012; Flint et al. 2010; Stevens et al. 2012). Indeed, a document from the Food and Agriculture Organization (FAO) of the United Nations points out that "many developing nations are now dealing with severe health issues at both ends of the nutritional spectrum. Countries still struggling to feed their people face the costs of preventing obesity and treating diet-related noncommunicable illness. This is called the 'double burden' of malnutrition" (McNulty 2013).

Within the United States, the rate of obesity has jumped in every state (see **FIGURE 1-1**). In 1990, obesity rates in most states were below 14%; now most states have an obesity rate of 20% or more. Indeed, it has been estimated that diet and other social and behavioral factors such as smoking, sedentary lifestyles, alcohol use, and accidents account for about half of all the causes of death in the U.S. (Institute of Medicine 2000).

The good news is that the fact that individual and social patterns of behavior are related to many chronic diseases means that positive changes in individual dietary and physical activity behaviors, community conditions of living, and social structures can play major roles in reducing risk of chronic disease and enhancing health. Better health provides people a better quality of life and enhanced functioning so that they are able to do the many things in life they value. By exercising control

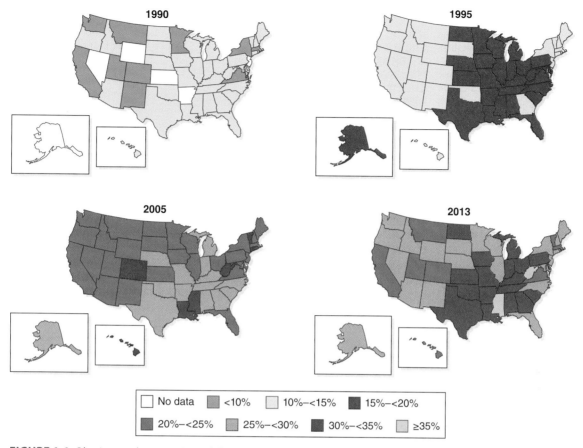

FIGURE 1-1 Obesity trends among U.S. adults, 1990, 1995, 2005, and 2013.

Reproduced from Centers for Disease Control and Prevention. Behavioral Risk Factor Surveillance Systems (BRFSS). http://www.cdc.gov/obesity/data/prevalence-maps.html

over modifiable behavioral and socio-environmental factors that affect health, people can live more healthfully as well as longer, representing a health-promoting, or "salutogenic," approach to well-being (Lindstrom and Eriksson 2005). Consequently, recommendations have been made for implementing national strategies to improve health and reduce disease (White House Task Force 2010; U.S. Department of Health and Human Services [HHS] 2010a). In the United States these are the *Dietary Guidelines for Americans* (HHS 2010b) and *Physical Activity Guidelines for Americans* (HHS 2008). A summary of the dietary guidelines worldwide by country is provided by the FAO (2014).

DIETARY AND PHYSICAL ACTIVITY PATTERNS ARE NOT OPTIMAL

Despite the abundance of food and food products, dietary intakes for many are not optimal (Krebs-Smith et al. 2010; Guthrie et al. 2013). For example, Americans today consume a little over half the recommended servings of fruits and vegetables each day and are especially short on dark green and orange vegetables (NHANES 2005–2008; HHS 2010b). Among children the situation is worse—only about 20% meet the recommendations for fruit and 4% for total vegetables, including potatoes, with only 0.2% meeting the recommendations for dark green vegetables and 1.2% for orange vegetables, eating only about 0.1 servings each. Americans eat the recommended total amount of grain products, but only a fraction of these are whole grains; thus, only 1% of people meet the whole grain recommendations. Average milk intakes have declined in the past 50 years and intakes of soda have increased over the same period, from 10 gallons to about 55 gallons per person per year. Meat consumption is high, and the quantity of total added fats and sugars is two to three times the recommended upper limits. Finally, based on the Healthy Eating Index, Americans on average score only 50% on the different components of a healthy diet (Center for Nutrition Policy and Promotion 2013). Food intake data

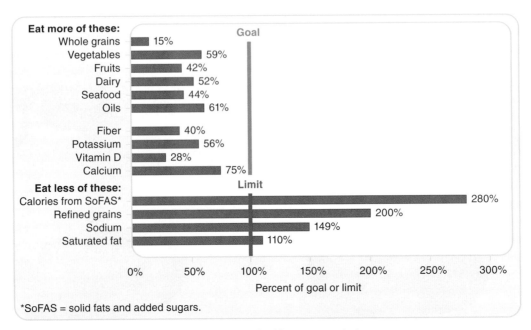

FIGURE 1-2 Americans are not eating according to health recommendations.

Reproduced from *Dietary Guidelines for Americans 2010*. U.S. Department of Agriculture and U.S. Department of Health and Human Services. www.dietaryguidelines.gov

in **FIGURE 1-2** clearly show that American eating patterns are not optimal, with most Americans eating too few of the more healthful foods and too much of the less healthful food components (HHS 2010b). Similar trends have been found in other countries, such as the United Kingdom, Netherlands, and Mexico, and indeed, increasingly worldwide, leading to global disease burden (Lock et al. 2005; Whitten et al. 2011; Van Rossum et al. 2011; Flores et al. 2010; Kearney 2010; Popkin 2009, 2010; McNulty 2013).

Physical activity patterns are likewise far from optimal. Regular physical activity reduces the risk of many health conditions and promotes health. The percentage of Americans who are meeting physical activity guidelines has increased somewhat in the past few years, but still only about half of the adult U.S. population engages in recommended levels of aerobic physical activity and only 20% met all the recommendations (Centers for Disease Control and Prevention 2013).

OUR FOOD CHOICES ARE NOT ALWAYS GOOD FOR THE PLANET

There has been increasing recognition that the kinds of diets we eat have an impact not only on our personal health, but also on our planet. This is because the foods we buy at the grocery store carry a cost not just in terms

money and impact on personal health, but also in terms of the "price" the environment pays for them. The diets that are most likely to contribute to risk of obesity and chronic disease tend also to be those that require considerable resources such as fertilizers, pesticides, fossil fuels, and packaging materials to produce and get to us (this is called the ecological footprint from our foods). These diets also cause excessive greenhouse gas emissions from the fossil fuels used throughout the system that delivers foods to us (this is called the carbon footprint). Considerable amounts of water are used to get the food to us as well (this is called the water footprint). To show you how much food can vary let's compare the footprints of beef versus fruits and vegetables. For the ecological footprint, beef takes an average 54 square meters per pound compared to 1–2 for fruits and vegetables. In terms of carbon footprint, beef creates a mean of 10,000 grams of carbon dioxide equivalent compared to 220–400 for fruits and vegetables. For the water footprint, beef takes about 7,500 gallons per pound compared to 100–400 for fruits and vegetables (Barilla Center 2015). Those are enormous differences, especially considering each person eats about 1,500 pounds of food a year. In addition, our eating patterns create tons of waste in terms of the paper plates and plastic utensils we use so freely as well as the millions of plastic bottles from our drinks that we use once and throw away (Pacific Institute 2013).

COMPLEX FOOD CHOICE ENVIRONMENT

Clearly people need help making dietary choices. One challenge is that the food environment has become increasingly complex. People in previous centuries lived on several hundred different foods, mostly locally grown. In 1928, large supermarkets in the United States stocked about 900 items. By the 1980s, a typical supermarket stocked approximately 12,000 food items, taken from an available supply of about 60,000 items (Moliter 1980). Today, 40,000–50,000 different brand-name processed food items perch on many supermarket shelves, from an available supply of 320,000 in the marketplace (Food Marketing Institute 2012). In addition, about 40% of all food is eaten away from home. Even food that is eaten in the home has often been prepared, purchased, and brought in from elsewhere. Indeed, 92% of individuals consume some form of "ready-to-eat" foods in the home on a daily basis (Okrent and Alston 2012). This is increasingly the case in many parts of the world. Consumers must make choices among these options and do not always choose well, as surveys suggest (see **FIGURE 1-3**).

The criteria for food choice have also expanded. As noted earlier, the way most food is grown, processed, packaged, distributed, and consumed has serious consequences for the planet. Many consumers and professionals believe that it is important to consider these consequences in making food choices (Gussow 2006, 1999; Gussow and Clancy 1986; Clancy 1999; Pollan 2008). Others are interested in social justice concerns and want to choose foods that were produced using fair labor practices. For all these reasons, individual and community food choices have become very complex.

COMPLEX INFORMATION ENVIRONMENT

The complexity of the foods available in the marketplace makes wise selection even harder. Our ancestors readily knew the foods they were eating just by looking at them, or could learn about them from family or cultural traditions. Most of the 40,000–50,000 items in today's supermarkets bear little resemblance to the simple foodstuffs previously eaten by humans. Foods with artificial sweeteners in them are being joined by foods made with artificial fats. Some 9,000 "new" food-related items are being introduced by food processors in the United States every year (about 30 per day). Knowledge about these items cannot possibly be derived from simply looking at them, and

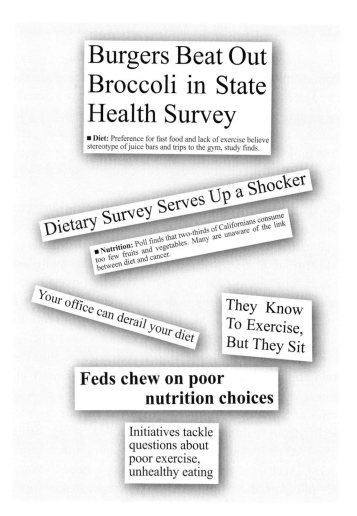

FIGURE 1-3 Newspaper headlines highlight United States eating patterns are not all they could be.

neither can their composition and effects on the body be learned by stories and attitudes passed down through the generations.

This complex food environment demands consumers who are nutritionally literate. Yet nutritional literacy does not come easily. For packaged foods, nutrition labels are very important. Although about 50% of consumers report that they read food labels always or most of the time and another 30% do sometimes, many admit that they don't always understand what they mean (Levy et al. 2000; Ollberding, Wolf, and Contento 2010; Supermarket Nutrition 2013). Some labels on products are actually misleading—lean frozen dinners labeled as "95% fat free" can contain 30% of calories as fat; 2% "low-fat" milk also has 30% of its calories as fat. Moreover, diet books highlight low-fat diets as the ideal one year and low-carbohydrate diets the next year.

CONSUMER BEWILDERMENT AND CONCERN

No wonder consumers are bewildered. Although many Americans are concerned about their health and are indeed eating more healthful foods than they were a decade or so ago, the average person's diet is getting better and worse at the same time. For instance, mothers may buy fat-free milk for their families along with high-fat premium "home-style" ice cream, the latter because of its perceived superior quality.

These contradictory behaviors often derive from genuine confusion about what is good to eat. Although food manufacturers have responded to consumer concern about healthful food, they have introduced at least as many less healthful items as they have more healthful ones. There is considerable confusion in developing countries as well: many people exchange locally grown whole foods for imported, processed items, believing the latter to be better for health. Well-off people in such countries are thus developing the same chronic diseases as people in more affluent countries and are experiencing increased obesity rates at the same time that those who are poor are suffering from malnutrition (Popkin 2009; Kearney 2010). The FAO points out that to avoid the major economic and social burdens of these conditions, people need to know about eating the *right* foods not just more or less food. Making good food choices is important for all consumers (McNulty 2013).

All these facts suggest that people need education about food and nutrition.

The Challenge of Educating People About Eating Well

Our analysis so far seems to suggest that what consumers need is information on the nutrients in food, label reading skills, and skills in preparing foods in a healthy fashion. However, research provides evidence there is more to good nutrition than knowing which foods to eat and having those foods available. Information about nutrients is not enough. The potent influences of biological factors, cultural and social preferences, and emotional and psychological factors make the job of assisting people to eat well a demanding one. Understanding these influences and addressing them are the major tasks of nutrition education. This makes nutrition education exciting but also challenging (see **FIGURE 1-4**).

BIOLOGICAL INFLUENCES: DO WE HAVE BODY WISDOM?

Some have argued that we have an innate "**body wisdom**" that guides us to select healthful foods naturally, intuitive eating if you will, thus implying that nutrition education is not needed beyond paying attention to our body signals or mindful eating. Much of this line of thought grew out of the work of Clara Davis (1928), who studied the spontaneous food choices of infants. The infants, aged 6 to 11 months, were weaned by allowing them to self-select their entire diets from a total of 34 foods, none of which contained added salt or sugar, which were rotated—a few

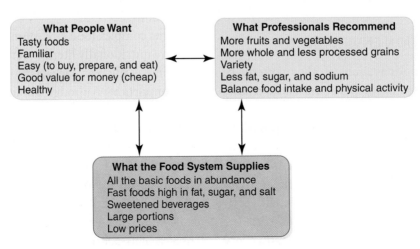

What People Want
Tasty foods
Familiar
Easy (to buy, prepare, and eat)
Good value for money (cheap)
Healthy

What Professionals Recommend
More fruits and vegetables
More whole and less processed grains
Variety
Less fat, sugar, and sodium
Balance food intake and physical activity

What the Food System Supplies
All the basic foods in abundance
Fast foods high in fat, sugar, and salt
Sweetened beverages
Large portions
Low prices

FIGURE 1-4 Nutrition education is exciting and challenging.

at a time—at each meal. Davis reported that after several months of such "spontaneous" food selection, the children's nutritional status and health were excellent. However, one should note that the 34 foods were all simply prepared, minimally processed, and nutritious whole foods, such as steamed vegetables, fruit juice, milk, meat, and oatmeal. In addition, the food items were offered by caretakers who were trained to provide no encouragements or discouragements while the children ate. Whether infants would demonstrate a similar "instinct" if they were offered tasty, energy-dense, low-nutrient food items has not been examined, but such an outcome seems unlikely given experiments in which rats exposed to such diets became obese. Neither do conditions of freedom from all outside influences exist in real-world settings. There appears to be no "safety net" biological mechanism that ensures that we will eat healthful food. Eating well needs to be learned.

Specific Tastes or "Sensory-Specific Satiety"

However, we appear to have a built-in mechanism that helps ensure that we eat a *variety* of foods, called sensory-specific satiety. As we eat more of a particular food in the course of a short time period such as a meal, we decrease our liking for the food, but our desire for other foods offered remains relatively unchanged (Rolls 2000). We know this phenomenon well: when we are too full to eat another mouthful of the entrée, we find ourselves quite able to eat dessert. Although the experience of hunger ensures that we will eat, our enjoyment of tasty foods combined with this liking for variety in tastes or *sensory-specific satiety* mechanism ensured that humans—in a "primitive" environment—would move from one food to another and thus select a balanced diet over the long term. Through the centuries, people obtained their needed nutrients mostly by getting enough calories. The key was in getting a varied diet. Yudkin (1978) argued that in the past, people could get the *nutrients* they *needed* simply by eating a variety of the *foods* they *wanted*. Today this mechanism works to our disadvantage because variety makes us eat more but variety in today's food system consists of the many, many highly processed food products that are high in calories but low in nutrients.

Our Bodies and Today's Food

Today, technology has made it possible to manipulate foods' taste or sensory properties to make them sweeter or saltier or richer tasting or more colorful at will. Processed food products are deliberately engineered to make them addictive by the addition of fat, salt, and sugar, and the array of such engineered items is vast (Schlosser 2001; Moss 2013; Lowe, Hall, and Staines 2014). Thus, technology has fully separated the tastiness of foods from their nutritional worth. In addition, current technology creates notorious hazards for energy perception. The fat content of many processed foods is not clearly evident from either the appearance of the food, its feel and taste, or the packaging and shape of the item. The energy content of a variety of similar-tasting foods can vary considerably. This means that by following our food preferences—eating a wide variety of tasty foods—we are no longer assured that we will get a nutritionally adequate diet. Indeed, such behavior increases the likelihood of overconsumption of high-fat, low-fiber diets that may place us at greater risk for a number of chronic diseases. There appears to be no biological set point for the amount of fat or sugar we will eat. Taken together, our desire to eat foods that are tasty and marketers' desire to put into the marketplace foods that cater to people's biological attraction to sugar, fat, and salt make the task of educating for a healthful diet a difficult one.

CULTURAL AND SOCIAL PREFERENCES

Cultural Context

Whatever biological predispositions humans possess operate in the context of food availability, and as Rozin (1982) notes, what is available to eat is determined not only by what is available geographically and economically, but also by what a culture dictates is appropriate to eat. Although humans worldwide eat just about everything edible, any particular group of people eats what is culturally available.

Anthropologist Margaret Mead years ago argued that traditionally, in all known societies, it was not biological mechanisms but transmission of culturally imposed eating patterns, derived from the group's experience with foods that kept humans alive. These traditional food patterns were not necessarily optimal but were nutritionally viable and enabled people to survive at least through the reproductive years (Gussow and Contento 1984). Biological preference and cultural influences are thus intertwined. What is made available by a culture comes to taste good: *people may eat what they like, but they also come to like what they eat.* Consequently, cultural context is highly important.

Social Preferences

Today, what is available to eat in the United States is determined largely by what is mass produced by food companies and available in the supermarket. These products are highly promoted by the communication instruments of mass culture (television, advertising, Internet, and so forth), leading to consumer demand.

Studies show that taste and availability are closely followed by convenience in influencing food selection. Modern culture emphasizes convenience or quickness in preparing or obtaining foods, to fit in with today's hectic lifestyles. Many people today think of a food as available only if it can be purchased already prepared or can be prepared quickly without much effort. People have thus lost many culturally transmitted cooking skills (Gussow 1993; Cunningham-Sabo and Simons 2012). Away-from-home foods account for 32% of calories (up from 18% in the 1970s) and about half of total food expenditures (Stewart, Blisard, and Jolliffe 2006). Yet quick and convenient foods that are readily available commercially are not always the most healthful, and neither are they produced, transported, or packaged in the most environmentally sustainable manner. All these cultural and social influences can make educating about foods, nutrition, and dietary change difficult.

FAMILY AND PSYCHOLOGICAL FACTORS

People have many expectations about the food they eat: it should taste good, it should look good, it should impress friends when they serve it to them, it should be healthful, it should help them stay thin, and it should remind them of the warmth of family. The opinions of family or important others as well as moral and religious values also influence food choices.

Within the constraints of biology and culture, as people grow up they also develop individual food preferences and patterns of eating because any given individual gains a unique set of experiences with respect to food (Rozin 1982). This uniqueness stems partly from the fact that an individual's exposure to the culture is filtered through the family's interpretation of culture. For example, there is evidence that one of the major influences on the acquisition of eating patterns by children is familiarity with given foods (Savage, Fisher, and Birch 2007). Such familiarity is determined by what the family serves, which in turn reflects the family's cultural and other beliefs about food. Thus, eating patterns and dietary behaviors are influenced by many familial and psychological factors, as well as by cultural and social ones.

Eating is clearly deeply embedded in the early development of individuals and continues to be tied in with many other aspects of life. Consequently, any changes in eating behaviors may involve many other changes as well, such as family traditions, social and professional occasions that involve food, making time in busy schedules for eating well, or changing how a person handles stress. A person must be motivated to make changes and to maintain them.

SENSE OF EMPOWERMENT: INDIVIDUAL AND COMMUNITY

Even if a person is motivated, the sheer number of food products available makes decision making a daunting task for the consumer. It is also a daunting task for the nutrition educator because the consumer needs a great deal of complex information, yet in an information-overloaded society, the consumer wants or can handle only simple messages. So, the challenge for the nutrition educator is how to convert complex information into simple but accurate messages that consumers will attend to and act on.

At the same time, to understand some of the choices they have to make, people need to be able to analyze and evaluate complex information in the midst of conflicting claims. For example, are calories the most important item on a food label? Is a breakfast cereal that is high in sugar but low in fat a better choice for children? Does it make a difference whether one chooses organically produced foods or foods produced by more conventional agriculture? And what is the difference based on—impact of food on personal health, or impact of food production methods on the long-term sustainability of the food system? Thus, eaters need critical thinking skills. In addition, they need affective skills such as assertiveness, self-management, and negotiation skills that enhance their sense of competence and control over their own food choices. People also need skills in preparing healthful foods quickly and conveniently. Finally, for community as well as personal empowerment, people need to have the skills and opportunity to identify food- and nutrition-related issues facing their communities and work with others to address these issues collectively.

MATERIAL RESOURCES AND THE ENVIRONMENTAL CONTEXT

Motivation and skills alone may not be enough. Material resources such as money and time also present challenges. Affordability of healthful food, as well as food availability, is crucial, particularly for low-income audiences. Having in one's neighborhood only convenience stores that charge high prices and carry limited supplies of healthful foods makes eating well extremely difficult. Whole grain products and fruits and vegetables are not as available as are more highly processed food items in fast food outlets, workplace cafeterias, or other places convenient to people's out-of-home activities. Some whole food items often cost more (such as fruits and vegetables) although others cost less (such as beans and grains) (Drewnowski 2012).

MARKETING, SOCIAL STRUCTURES, AND POLICY

Even the best of intentions are difficult to implement and behaviors difficult to maintain if social structures, food marketing practices, food policies, and other aspects of the food (and physical activity) environment are not conducive to health. Fast foods, made tasty and addictive by their high content of fat, sugar, and salt, are everywhere—convenient, tasty, and inexpensive—and their portion sizes are often large. Surveys have found that more than 90% of Americans are consuming food each day that was prepared away from home and are thus exposed to such foods (Okrent and Alston 2012).

In addition, the dietary pattern emphasized by marketers, shown in **FIGURE 1-5**, is very different from the dietary pattern recommended by the U.S. Dietary Guidelines (and food policy documents of international agencies such as the FAO) as likely to enhance nutritional health—one high in whole grains, fruits, and vegetables; adequate in dairy and meat; and sparing in foods that are high in fat and sugar. More marketing and advertising dollars are spent by far on promoting restaurant/fast foods (about 31%), soft drinks and other beverages (37%), and snack foods (14%) than are spent on foods in the basic food

groups such as fruits and vegetables (about 0.7%), resulting in increased consumption of and demand for these items. In terms of dollars, the U.S. food industry spent about $9.65 billion in 2009 on marketing and promotions, with about $1.8 billion directed at children (Federal Trade Commission 2012). It spent $3.5 billion on beverages, of which about $520 million was directed at children, along with about $200 million on candy bars and snack foods. About $3 billion was spent on marketing restaurants/fast food. In contrast, government health-related campaigns in most countries may amount to only a few million dollars a year. U.S. children see about 13–16 food advertisements every day all year but perhaps only one advertisement per week for healthy foods, such as fruits and vegetables and bottled water (Yale Rudd Center 2013). Most people may never have the opportunity to see a nutritionist during their entire lives. Such a situation cannot result in genuinely free, informed choice.

Finally, people of all ages, particularly children, have become more sedentary in the last 30 years. People use more labor-saving devices and cars, and spend more time watching TV and using computers. People have hectic jobs and work long hours, leaving less time for physical activity. Thus, people cannot eat as many calories as they once could to meet their other nutrient needs. The issues that demand attention from nutrition educators, then, are

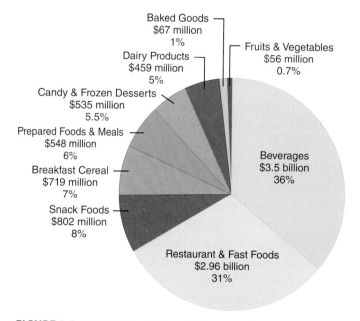

FIGURE 1-5 United States total marketing expenditures by food category.

Data from Federal Trade Commission. 2012. A review of food marketing to children and adolescents: A follow up report.

not only individual food-related behaviors and personal choice, but also external environmental factors such as material resources, social structures, food policies, and marketing practices.

Viewpoints on the Aims of Nutrition Education

We have seen that nutrition education is both necessary in today's world and challenging to accomplish. What exactly is nutrition education today and what are its aims? What impacts should it seek to achieve? Most nutrition education involves communication of food and nutrition information in some form. It is *why* and *how* information is communicated that makes a world of difference in terms of its impact on audiences and there are different viewpoints on just why and how such information should be communicated:

- Food and nutrition information is communicated in ways solely to inform.
- Food and nutrition information is communicated in ways to enhance motivation and facilitate the adoption or maintenance of individual behaviors and community practices that are conducive to health and well-being.
- Food and nutrition information is communicated to decision-makers and policymakers in order to engage them to work with us collaboratively on food and nutrition issues that are important.

INFORMATION COMMUNICATED SOLELY TO INFORM

In this viewpoint, food and nutrition information is communicated in such a way as to solely provide consumers with the information needed to make decisions about what to eat (e.g., how many grams of fiber in a product, reading food labels), rejecting the notion that nutrition professionals should also *actively promote* healthful choices. Consumers are viewed as being savvy and disliking being told what to do, lacking only in knowledge of what to eat and tips on how to do so. We are "information dispatchers."

However, most Americans believe that they are well informed about nutrition, with 73% saying they are confident that they know how to shop for healthy foods (Supermarket Nutrition 2013). The finding that despite believing themselves to be well informed they are not eating according to recommendations argues that communication of this kind of information alone is clearly not enough.

INFORMATION COMMUNICATED TO MOTIVATE AND FACILITATE BEHAVIORS CONDUCIVE TO HEALTH AND WELL-BEING

In this viewpoint, food and nutrition information is communicated in such a way that it is motivating and useful for facilitating change as well as being informative. Given that a major and urgent aim of nutrition education is to improve the health of a nation's people, and that people's health conditions are to some extent the result of individual and social patterns of behavior, nutrition education is designed to communicate science-based information in such a way that it motivates and facilitates the adoption or maintenance of individual behaviors and community practices that are conducive to the long-term health of individuals, communities, or the planet. For example, communicating science-based information on risk to individuals or communities of a health or food system condition and on the benefits of taking action can be very motivating. In addition, communicating the food- and nutrition-related skills needed by people to act on their motivations can facilitate behavior change. In this approach, the role of the nutrition educator moves from that of an "information dispatcher" to a "facilitator of change" for individuals and communities. This seems justified given the many forces in society that are not conducive to healthy eating.

COMMUNICATIONS TO INFLUENCE POLICYMAKERS

Many policymakers, government agencies, and international organizations argue that nutrition education is not effective and that policy and environmental change are needed (McKinley 1974; Dorfman and Wallack 2007; HHS, 2015). Changes include regulations and incentives for increasing accessibility and opportunities for action, for example by making foods offered in school meal programs healthier, nudging people toward healthier choices through behavioral economics principles (Hanks et al. 2012), increasing food security through agricultural policy, or increasing the number of supermarkets offering healthy foods in low-income communities. In this case nutrition educators focus their communications on educating policymakers about the importance of policy and environmental change in order to engage them to work with nutrition educators collaboratively to improve people's health and well-being.

> Nutrition education most often involves communication of food and nutrition information in some form. It is *what* and *how* information is communicated that make a world of difference as to whether it will be effective in motivating and facilitating change.

A Contemporary Definition of Nutrition Education

Taking into account these various viewpoints on nutrition education and health promotion, a contemporary definition is needed. For the purposes of this book, *nutrition education* is defined as any combination of educational strategies, accompanied by environmental supports, designed to facilitate voluntary adoption of food choices and other food- and nutrition-related behaviors conducive to health and well-being and delivered through multiple venues, involving activities at the individual, institutional, community, and policy levels.

Combination of educational strategies. Because many factors influence behavior, nutrition education needs to employ a variety of strategies and learning experiences that are appropriately directed at these multiple influences on, or determinants of, food choice and dietary behavior to motivate and facilitate dietary change. Nutrition education focuses on enhancing health and facilitating solutions.

Education is *not* synonymous with information dissemination, although the public and many in the nutrition science, biomedical, public health, and policy fields think it is. The word comes from the Latin *educare*, meaning to bring up or lead out, and can be seen as a process that not only provides information and skills, but also fosters motivation, growth, and change. In short, nutrition education uses strategies that seek to help people learn to eat well by enhancing people's motivation through effective communication as well as by improving their ability and opportunities to do so.

Designed means that nutrition education is a systematically planned set of activities. Such systematically planned nutrition education can occur through multiple venues, such as schools, communities, workplaces, and clinics, and through the mass media. A step-wise procedure for systematically designing nutrition education, called the Nutrition Education DESIGN Procedure, is described later in this book. Note that *informal*, often powerful, "nutrition education" is carried out by other institutions in society such as families, businesses, newspapers, magazines, radio and television stations, and the Internet, where the information is of varying degrees of reliability.

Facilitate is used to emphasize the fact that educators can only *assist* people to make diet-related changes: people make changes when they themselves see the need and want to do so. Motivation ultimately comes from within individuals, and actions with respect to food are voluntarily chosen in the light of individuals' values and larger life goals and situations. Education about foods and nutrition, and, where appropriate, physical activity, is about using strategies that enhance people's motivations involving effective communication and encouraging self-understanding and deliberation. Motivation is key. It is also about using strategies to facilitate people's ability to take action through increased food and nutrition knowledge and skills and critical thinking and reflection, and through an increased sense of personal agency or empowerment. Finally, it is building on assets that people bring to the issue, such as personal and cultural practices that are already health-promoting or community structures that are supportive of sustainable eating patterns.

Voluntary means recognizing and respecting that human beings have agency and free will and make choices in light of their own personal goals and values (Bandura 1997, 2001; Deci and Ryan 2000; Buchanan 2000). It means the program is conducted without coercion and with the full understanding of the participants about the purpose of the nutrition education activities. Individuals are both "the changers" and "the changed." *Voluntary* does not mean that nutrition education is limited to dissemination of information solely to inform. Health psychologist Leventhal (1973) noted that "the decision to avoid coercion does not free (health professionals) of the obligation to state facts, warn, and argue skillfully."

Indeed, it can be said that truly informed and voluntary choice can be made by consumers *only* when they have the benefit of understanding arguments from all sides. Without the benefit of health communications from nutrition educators, consumers would receive only the arguments of the other forces in society, such as food advertising and promotion, that are providing messages persuading people to choose foods for reasons other than nutrition and health (Gussow and Contento 1984; Dawson 2014). In other words, nutrition education strategies can be designed in such a way as to integrate the health-promoting role of nutrition educators with the notion of free will and personal agency and empowerment on the part of individuals.

Behaviors are the observable food choices and other food- and nutrition-related actions that people undertake to achieve an intended effect of their own choosing and are the direct focus of nutrition education. Eating fruits and vegetables, whole grain foods, sustainably produced foods, or breastfeeding can be referred to as behaviors. Sometimes behaviors are defined broadly, such as "healthy eating and active living." The terms practices, behaviors, and actions are often used interchangeably. *Actions* generally refer to specific actions or sub-behaviors that constitute *behaviors*. Thus, the behavior of eating more fruits and vegetables may involve the specific actions of shopping for fruits and vegetables, adding orange juice at breakfast, including a vegetable at lunch, and so forth. The word *practices* is also used interchangeably with *behaviors* and *actions*, although the term *practices* tends to refer to more general and continuing patterns of behavior, such as food-related parenting practices, eating balanced meals, and being physically active.

The emphasis on actionable behaviors is at the heart of the MyPlate dietary guidance system of the United States government. Here the public is recommended to eat according to a meal pattern where half the plate is made up of fruits and vegetables, about a quarter grains, of which half should be whole grains, and about a quarter high-protein foods, accompanied by milk or other dairy (see **FIGURE 1-6**). Similar food behavior-based guidelines have been produced in other countries (Food and Agricultural Organization [FAO] 2014).

Environmental supports refer to the food, physical, social, informational, and policy environments external to a person that are relevant to the behavior or practices at issue. Taking action and maintaining a behavioral change is much more likely if the relevant environment is supportive. Promoting supportive environments

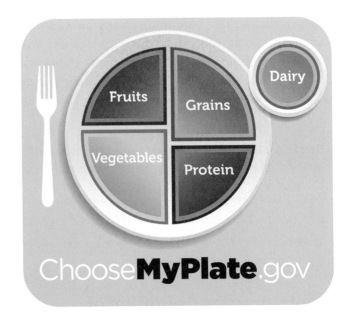

FIGURE 1-6 The United States food guide features a plate showing the recommended proportions of food groups to eat.

Reproduced from ChooseMyPlate.gov. United States Department of Agriculture. http://www.choosemyplate.gov

usually requires nutrition educators to educate a different audience—providers of food and services, key decision makers, and others with influence—and to work in **collaboration** with them to achieve food and nutrition goals (and physical activity goals, where relevant). These individuals and organizations might include community leaders and organizations, food service personnel, school principals, workplace managers, and policymakers at local, state, and national levels, as well as the media, government agencies, and nongovernmental or private voluntary organizations.

The terms **health** and **well-being** refer to both the nutritional health of individuals and an overall sense of well-being, both absence of disease and possession of positive attributes of being healthy, such as optimal functioning or high-level wellness. The concept of health and well-being can extend to include the health of the environment and sustainability of the food systems on which people depend for their food.

Multiple venues refers to the fact that systematically planned nutrition education can be delivered through multiple channels, such as group sessions and other in-person activities and through indirect activities involving newsletters, printed materials, emails, visuals, and social media in formal settings such as schools and colleges or in nonformal settings such as community centers, food banks, workplaces, supermarkets, Supplemental Nutrition Assistance Program (SNAP) offices, Women, Infants, and Children (WIC) clinics, or outpatient clinics, and through mass media, billboards, the Internet, smartphones, and social marketing approaches.

Activities at the institutional, community, and policy levels can enact policies and system changes that promote physical and social environments supportive of healthful food choices and diet- and physical activity–related behaviors.

IS "NUTRITION EDUCATION" AN ACCURATE TERM?

The term *nutrition education* is widely used in the United States, although not in other parts of the world. The term is problematic. *Nutrition* is the word used to describe the way people are nourished by the nutrients in food. Nutrition education can be seen as education about nutrients. However, people eat foods, not nutrients. So people need education about food. So at the very least, the term should be *food and nutrition education*. In addition, however, it is hard for nutrition professionals to let go of the meaning of the word *education* as being solely about teaching or disseminating some set of information, even though even in the context of schooling, the word means much more than that, as noted previously. Thus the term *nutrition education* is inadequate, and indeed misleading. As we have seen, contemporary nutrition education goes considerably beyond these two words and involves enhancing people's *motivation, abilities,* and *opportunities* to take action. To capture this larger meaning of the term, many countries and international agencies such as the FAO use the terms *social and behavior change communication (SBCC)* or *food and nutrition communication and education (FNCE)* (McNulty 2013; Hawkes 2013*)*. Some in the United States have used the terms *food and nutrition education* and *nutrition education and promotion* (Briggs, Fleischhacker, and Mueller 2010). For the purposes of this book we will continue to use the term nutrition education, despite its considerable limitations, because it is so familiar in the United States, but we will be mindful at all times that the term refers to a contemporary view of nutrition education as an enterprise much larger than suggested by these two words, and is similar to the international term *social and behavioral change communication.*

Behaviors Versus Topics for Nutrition Education

Research in nutrition science, food studies, and food systems and related areas generates information that forms the basis of all nutrition education content. It is how the information is communicated that is crucial to its impact on people. When nutrition educators think of planning programs or individual sessions, they tend to immediately organize them in their heads in terms of "topics," such as diabetes risk reduction, malnutrition, sports supplementation, the science of energy balance, food security, or organic farming. How do these *topics* relate to *behaviors* as defined here?

When we examine these "topics," we see that many are descriptions of *issues* that are of national or local concern or of potential interest to the audience. If you choose an issue, remember that your audience will want to know what to do about the issue. So, what behaviors or practices are you going to recommend in order to address the particular issue of concern? These *behaviors* become the focus of your program or session(s). Note that some behaviors can serve more than one purpose or can address more than one issue of concern. For example, consuming fewer highly processed snacks or sweetened drinks may be good not only for personal health, but also for reducing people's carbon footprint on the planet.

Other "topics" may fall into the *general information* category—what foods are in which food groups and what vitamins and minerals they contain. Think carefully about what purpose this information serves. As an update for professionals, general information may be quite appropriate and important under the assumption that the professionals will use the information in their work with their audiences to assist them to enhance their behaviors. But for the general public, given the finding that knowledge by itself has not been shown to be effective for behavior change and given that most people do not have much time, is this the best use of their time? What will they do with this information? If your unspoken hope is that they will eat better, then your goal is really behavior change after all. It is important to lay out your unstated behavioral goals.

Behavior Change Versus Critical Thinking: Opening Doors

Often there is a concern that nutrition education that is behavior focused does not encourage critical thinking and careful reflection. However, this is not at all the case. Indeed, nutrition education can and should open doors. Critical thinking skills and careful reflection are necessary for our audiences in identifying which behaviors or actions to undertake in the context of their values and larger life goals and situations and in their being able to carry out the actions they choose. We can help our audiences develop conceptual frameworks to understand the complexities of issues related to food and nutrition. For young children, where critical thinking skills are not yet well developed, opening doors may involve other values, such as the appreciation of new foods, becoming taste literate, and becoming ready to adopt health-promoting behaviors.

SUMMARY OF A CONTEMPORARY DEFINITION OF NUTRITION EDUCATION

In summary, our definition suggests that nutrition education focuses on effective communication and activities to facilitate the voluntary enactment of specific observable *behaviors or actions* that are conducive to health and well-being. This summary is shown visually in **FIGURE 1-7**. The situations of individuals are very different from each other and so are their social and cultural contexts. Nutrition education is more likely to be effective when it takes these differences into account and designs activities to be appropriate to the needs and cultures of their audiences.

Enhancing Motivation and Empowerment to Change: "Why-To" Take Action

Increasing awareness is an important first step toward making behavior changes or taking action but it is not sufficient. Motivation is central in diet-related behavioral

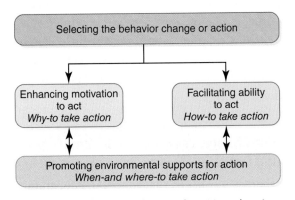

FIGURE 1-7 A contemporary definition of nutrition education.

change, so its role in nutrition education must be specifically recognized and addressed. Food and nutrition information can be very motivating and empowering when it is communicated in such a way that it helps individuals understand and value *why* to take action. For example, reasons why to take action may include science-based information on the impact of diet (and physical activity) on health, or the impact of people's food choices in the food system on the environment. Reasons can also include personal health concerns, self-identities, concern for the social impact on communities, and so forth. Nutrition education thus focuses on enhancing people's motivations by providing science-based information on the benefits of action and emphasizing self-understanding and deliberation of reasons and values to take action, particularly in light of their own larger life goals and of cultural expectations.

Facilitating the Ability to Change: "How-To" Take Action

Individuals also need to feel empowered to take action on the desired behavior or practice, once motivated. Individuals are more likely to feel empowered if they have the specific how-to knowledge and skills they need and self-confidence in their ability to bring about change in themselves and their environment. Here nutrition education communicates information in such a way as to focus on building appropriate food and nutrition skills and strengthening people's ability to initiate and guide their own behavior.

Promoting Environmental Supports for Action: "When- and Where-To" Take Action

Nutrition education can also help to make the healthy choice the easy choice by working with institutions, communities, or government to promote more supportive food and physical activity environments and policy.

VISION OF PROFESSIONAL ASSOCIATIONS

The view of nutrition education described here is in keeping with the vision of the foremost nutrition education professional organization, the Society of Nutrition Education and Behavior (SNEB), which states that its *vision* is "healthy communities, food systems, and behaviors" and its *mission* is to "promote effective nutrition education and healthy behavior through research,

---

BOX 1-1 Society for Nutrition Education and Behavior—Mission and Identity Statements

Vision

Healthy communities, food systems and behaviors.

Mission

To promote effective nutrition education and healthy behavior through research, policy and practice.

Identity Statements

The Society for Nutrition Education and Behavior (SNEB) represents the unique professional interests of nutrition educators in the United States and worldwide. SNEB is dedicated to promoting effective nutrition education and healthy behavior through research, policy and practice and has a vision of healthy communities, food systems and behaviors.

SNEB is an international community of professionals actively involved in nutrition education and **health promotion**. Their work takes place in colleges, universities and schools, government agencies, cooperative extension, communications and public relations firms, the food industry, voluntary and service organizations and with other reliable places of nutrition and health education information.

The *Journal of Nutrition Education and Behavior*, the official journal of the society, is a refereed, scientific periodical that serves as a resource for all professionals with an interest in nutrition education and dietary/ physical activity behaviors. The purpose of *JNEB* is to document and disseminate original research, emerging issues, and practices relevant to nutrition education and behavior worldwide.

Reproduced from Society for Nutrition Education and Behavior. What is SNEB? http://www.sneb.org/about/mission.html. Accessed 4/2/15.

---

policy and practice" (Society for Nutrition Education and Behavior 2015) (**BOX 1-1**). SNEB uses the contemporary definition of nutrition education. This view is also in keeping with the *vision* of the Academy of Nutrition and Dietetics (AND) to "optimize the nation's health through food and nutrition," and its *mission* to "empower members to be the nation's food and nutrition leaders" (Academy of Nutrition and Dietetics 2015), as well as with the mission of the International Society of Behavioral Nutrition and Physical Activity, which is to "stimulate, promote, and advocate for innovative research and policy in the area of behavioral nutrition and physical activity toward the betterment of human health worldwide" (International Society of Behavioral Nutrition and Physical Activity 2015).

Nutrition Education Effectiveness

Nutrition education is exciting but also challenging. How effective is it? A number of reviews have been conducted to examine the question of whether nutrition education is effective. One such review used meta-analysis to examine

303 studies conducted over a 74-year period from 1910 to 1984 that included a total of 4,108 separate findings (Johnson and Johnson 1985). Meta-analysis is a sophisticated statistical method that involves combining data from all relevant studies and calculating significant change based on the combined data. This meta-analysis found that, overall, nutrition education increased knowledge by 33 percentiles, attitudes by 14 percentiles, and behaviors by 19 percentiles. Comprehensive reviews and meta-analyses of more recent studies have found that behavior change interventions were able to bring about statistically significant though moderate improvement in eating and physical activity behaviors and weight status (Johnson, Scott-Sheldon, and Carey 2010; Khambalia et al. 2012; Wang and Stewart 2013).

More specifically, studies have shown nutrition education to be effective in improving dietary intakes:

- Increasing fruit and vegetable intake in children and adults through educational activities in studies worldwide (Pomerleau et al. 2005; Thompson and Ravia 2011; Evans et al. 2012), by adding salad bars to school meals (Harris et al. 2012) and through the use of gardens in schools and communities, which has been gaining in popularity in the United States (Langellotto and Gupta 2012), Britain, Australia, Mexico, and elsewhere (Gibbs et al. 2013), and is part of recommendations by the FAO.

- Reducing risk of childhood obesity (da Silveira et al. 2013; Khambalia et al. 2012, Wang et al. 2013).
- Food security for infants and toddlers in the United States and other countries (Colman et al. 2012; Thompson and Amoroso 2011).
- Breastfeeding (Schlicka and Wilson 2005; Dyson, McCormick, and Renfrew 2008; Hill 2009).
- Healthy eating in low-income audiences, in particular increased intake of fruits and vegetables and fat-free or low-fat milk (Long et al. 2013).

Cost-benefit and cost-effectiveness analyses have also been conducted for nutrition education programs. Cost-benefit analysis compares the economic benefits of a nutrition education program for participants to the actual costs of delivering the program and cost-effectiveness analysis compares the health benefits of the program for participants with the cost of delivering the program. Several such analyses have shown nutrition education to be cost-beneficial and cost-effective (Rajopal et al. 2003; Schuster et al. 2003; Dollahite, Kenkel, and Thompson 2008; Roux et al. 2008; Gustafson et al. 2009).

Thus, the evidence from these reviews and cost analyses of intervention studies demonstrates that nutrition education programs can make a moderate but significant contribution to improving dietary practices when they use appropriate messages and strategies.

What Do Nutrition Educators Do? Settings, Audiences, and Scope for Nutrition Education

As we have noted, this is an exciting time to be in the field of nutrition education. Everyone seems to be interested in food and nutrition, which is good news for nutrition educators who want to help the public eat well. Because nutrition can be seen as the link between agriculture and health, behavior change communication and education about food and nutrition covers a wide range of issues and takes place in a variety of settings, with different audiences. This means that nutrition educators are involved in a wide scope of activities.

SETTINGS: WHERE IS NUTRITION EDUCATION PROVIDED?

Nutrition educators work in many settings; some are well known and others quite unusual. Some of them are described in the following sections. Some examples are shown in **NUTRITION EDUCATION IN ACTION 1-1**. More examples are given throughout this book.

Communities

Much nutrition education for the public at large occurs in communities through programs sponsored in the United States by the U.S. Department of Agriculture (USDA), such as Cooperative Extension programs that provide nutrition education activities to adults, families, and children to assist them to eat healthfully. Most states have developed extensive nutrition education programs for Supplemental Nutrition Assistance Program participants (called SNAP-Ed). The USDA's Special Supplemental Program for Women, Infants, and Children (WIC) program provides nutrition education to its participants in addition to providing food. The Head Start program provides both food and nutrition education to preschool children. The HHS Administration for Community Living's Administration on Aging provides meals to low-resources older adults in a group setting and serves most communities in the nation. Nutrition education is a required component of the program. Most countries have similar programs.

Many other agencies and private volunteer and nonprofit organizations, such as heart associations, cancer societies, and food banks, also provide nutrition education. Social marketing campaigns focusing on nutrition and physical activity have become more common within communities.

Food- and Food System–Related Community and Advocacy Organizations

Community nutritionists work in emergency food organizations such as food pantries and soup kitchens, providing needed education to low-resources audiences. Community nutritionists also work in organizations that seek to enhance the availability and accessibility of affordable, nutritious—and often local, sustainably produced—food to individuals and communities by linking food producers to consumers through such programs as farmers' markets, community-supported agriculture, and farm-to-institution programs. Most of these programs include

NUTRITION EDUCATION IN ACTION 1-1 Nutrition Education Programs in Different Settings

Small Steps Big Rewards

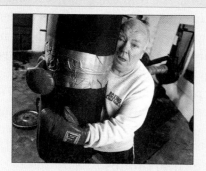

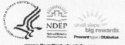

Get Real!
National Diabetes Educator.

"Live well. Eat healthy. Be active. *It's not easy, but it's worth it,"* announces the National Diabetes Education Program's website. This federally-funded program, sponsored by the National Institutes of Health and the Centers for Disease Control and Prevention, is based on findings from several landmark studies of diabetes control and prevention that showed modest weight loss and regular physical activity can prevent type 2 diabetes (T2DM) in those at risk and improve treatment outcomes for those who have T2DM. A national, multicultural campaign that aims to "Identify, disseminate, and support the adoption of evidence-based, culturally and linguistically appropriate tools and resources that support behavior change, improved quality of life, and better diabetes outcomes," targets children and adults with diabetes or at risk for T2DM as well as their families and caregivers, particularly populations disproportionately burdened by diabetes and its complications. Included in this campaign are healthcare professionals, community health workers, community and healthcare-focused organizations, media, businesses, schools, and other groups concerned about diabetes. For more information visit http://ndep.nih.gov.

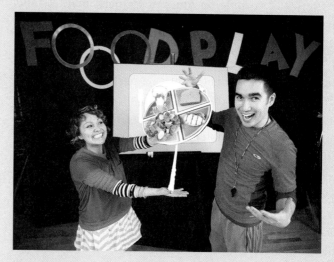

Nutrition education using live theater performances.
Courtesy of FoodPlay Productions, www.foodplay.com

FOODPLAY: Theater for Kids

FOODPLAY, a live theater performance for school assemblies, conferences, and special events, was developed by a nutrition educator and has been presented all over the United States. *FOODPLAY* performances feature captivating characters, motivating health messages, juggling, music, magic, and audience participation to help kids take charge of growing up healthy, happy, and fit. The program uses the power of live theater to motivate kids to say "yes!" to healthy eating and exercise habits, seeing through media messages, and building self-esteem from the inside out. *FOODPLAY* performances come with extensive Follow-Up School Resource Kits providing materials for students, teachers, school food service, and health staff so that they can continue nutrition education lessons in the classroom, integrate nutrition into core curriculum areas, and help schools improve their health environments and wellness policies. It has won an Emmy Award and has been shown to be effective. The website is http://www.foodplay.com.

Stellar Farmers' Markets

New York City's Department of Health uses Stellar Farmers' Markets to provide community-based nutrition education and resources. At select markets, nutritionists use the *Just Say Yes to Fruits and Vegetables* curriculum to provide free nutrition education for market shoppers about locally grown, seasonal produce; food safety; healthy eating; food resource management; and cooking. The website is http://www.nyc.gov/html/doh/html/living/cdp-farmersmarkets.shtml.

special outreach efforts to low-income communities. Nutrition educators provide educational sessions in these settings, take people on tours of farmers' markets and farms, and work with community policymakers.

Schools

Nutrition education is taught as a part of school health education in many states in the United States. In these instances, classroom teachers deliver the nutrition education. The role of the nutrition educator is to develop good curricular materials, provide professional development to teachers, and help teachers provide nutrition education, usually through specific projects externally funded by nonprofit organizations. In addition, school food service personnel often provide informal nutrition education through posters and food-related activities in the lunchroom. Nutrition educators also work in numerous school-based nutrition education research interventions that have been conducted in schools in recent decades with funding from federal agencies such the National Institutes of Health and the USDA.

Workplaces

In recent decades, workplace health promotion has grown considerably, usually incorporating nutrition education, weight control, and physical activity along with other health education efforts to reduce the risk of chronic diseases, such as cardiovascular disease and cancer. These efforts have been directed at both the general population of employees and high-risk individuals. Nutrition educators often assist in designing the programs and delivering them.

Healthcare Settings

Although one-on-one nutrition counseling is the norm in healthcare settings, many medical centers provide outpatient nutrition education to at-risk individuals served by the center. Health maintenance organizations and health insurance plans often provide nutrition education to their membership. Nutrition educators also work in physician practices, weight control programs, and eating disorders clinics.

AUDIENCES FOR NUTRITION EDUCATION

Nutrition education is provided to a wide range of audiences who differ on many counts, including age, life stage, socioeconomic status, cultural background, and other characteristics.

Life Stage Groups

Nutrition education programs have been developed and delivered to people throughout the entire life span: preschool children and their caregivers; school-aged children through school curricula, after-school activities, or family-based programs; college students through nutrition or health courses, cafeteria interventions, and student health center activities; adults through community or workplace programs; pregnant and lactating women and their infants and toddlers through WIC and other programs; and older adults through a variety of specifically targeted programs.

Diverse Cultural Groups

The United States is becoming increasingly diverse ethnically and culturally. Some nutrition education programs are developed specifically for different cultural groups, such as programs for African Americans, Latino/Latina groups, Asian Americans, or recent immigrants who speak a variety of languages. Many other countries have become similarly diverse. Nutrition educators need to become culturally competent as they work with such diversity.

Socioeconomic Background

Socioeconomic status (SES) has been linked to health status, with those of low SES experiencing more health problems and greater premature death than those of higher SES. Many government programs are designed to reduce these health disparities through food assistance activities such as the SNAP and WIC programs or public health programs. Head Start seeks to reduce educational inequities by providing free schooling to eligible preschoolers. Nutrition education is an important component of all these programs, assisting low-income participants to eat more healthfully.

Athletes and Exercising Individuals

Athletes and other exercising individuals are often specially interested in, and in need of, nutrition education. Nutrition educators with additional training in sports nutrition work with such groups as college and professional athletic teams and exercising individuals in fitness centers, worksites, and community programs.

Gatekeepers: Policymakers, Media, and the Food Industry

Traditionally, the term *gatekeepers* referred to those in the family (usually the mother) who purchased and prepared the food because such people controlled what the family ate. However, the term can be used more broadly. Today individuals receive food from a variety of sources. Gatekeepers include individuals or organizations that provide food or services or have some policymaking role in the accessibility and availability of food- or nutrition-related services in organizations, communities, and local and national government. Gatekeepers may also be those who influence social and informational environments, such as the mass media. Nutrition educators can educate these gatekeepers about current food and nutrition conditions (e.g., anemia, food insecurity, unhealthy eating patterns, chronic disease risk, or obesity) and make the case for the relevance of nutrition education and policy alternatives in order to encourage policymakers to take actions that are more supportive of healthful eating, active living, and sustainable food systems.

SCOPE OF NUTRITION EDUCATION

The major function of nutrition education activities is to assist people to eat and enjoy healthful food by increasing awareness, enhancing people's motivations, facilitating the ability to take action, and improving environmental supports for action. However, nutrition education can expand its scope not only in terms of appropriate audiences, but also in terms of the content to be addressed and the nature of the strategies to be used.

Wide Range of Content: Health and Beyond

Nutrition education can address an extremely wide range of content issues related to food and nutrition. The primary content issues are, of course, related to personal health, such as the relationship between diet and health, healthful eating as recommended by the *Dietary Guidelines* and MyPlate, how to get the best nutrition within one's budget, food safety, breastfeeding, how to get one's children to eat more healthfully, eating breakfast, balancing eating and physical activity, reducing diet-related chronic disease, and so forth. However, any given nutrition education program can address any issue of concern or interest.

Food Systems Issues

In recent years, there has been an increase in interest among consumers and nutrition professionals in issues related to how and where food is produced, because eating fresh and local food is good for personal health, for farmers, and

for the environment (Gussow 2006). Some programs have focused on these issues of eating locally (Englberger et al. 2010) and farm to school linkages (Feenstra and Ohmart 2012). Farmers' markets have emerged in many communities. To increase the accessibility and affordability of local foods to low-resources individuals, the USDA has made it possible for such individuals to use SNAP electronic benefits transfer (EBT) cards at farmers' markets. Various community organizations have also worked to link food banks and soup kitchens to local farmers. Nutrition professional organizations have suggested that nutrition education in schools be linked with working in school gardens and other strategies to help children develop a deeper appreciation for the environment and food systems (Briggs, Fleischhacker, and Mueller 2010).

Gardening and Cooking

Gardening and cooking have long been considered part of nutrition education in developing countries. Their importance for people of all ages has also become increasingly recognized in developed countries. These activities provide important skills and also help to connect people to food in a way that is engaging, motivating, and health promoting.

Social Justice and Sustainability

Some consumers are interested in what are called social justice and sustainability issues related to food. Indeed, some surveys suggest that about one-third of consumers are motivated in their purchases by concern for the environment as well as for their health, and mainstream food producers are beginning to cater to this segment (Burros 2006; McLaughlin 2004). One study found that worldwide, an average of 38% agreed or strongly agreed that "fair trade food and beverages are worth paying a little extra for" (Agriculture and Agri-Food Canada 2012). Consequently, the scope of nutrition education can be expanded to address these content issues as well. Numerous other issues of interest and concern will no doubt emerge that can be addressed by nutrition educators.

Physical Activity and Nutrition

Given the increasing recognition that being less sedentary and more physically active decreases the risk of chronic disease and obesity and improves health, many nutrition education programs now address physical activity in tandem with individual and community nutrition education–related behaviors and practices.

A Variety of Approaches: Beyond the Traditional

Nutrition educators can embark on a wider variety of activities beyond mass media campaigns, lectures, group discussions, workshops, health fairs, newsletters, videos, brochures, and other print and audiovisual materials.

Empowerment Approaches

Nutrition education can use a critical consciousness–raising approach, originally proposed by Freire (1970), in which people participate in a process involving a careful analysis of the causes of the food or health issue facing the group and of the structure of power in their communities, and then plan ways to organize to take action. This approach has been used in nutrition education to assist low-resources groups identify the causes of their problems of access to food and to take political and economic actions to reduce nutritional inequities (Travers 1997).

Nutrition educators can also use a growth-centered educational approach, which seeks to foster self-reliance by building on the abilities and assets of the participants, providing opportunities for self-directed learning and activities, and building social support (Abusabha, Peacock, and Achterberg 1999; Arnold et al. 2001; WIC Works Resource System 2013). These approaches are related to an empowerment process through which individuals, communities, and organizations gain mastery over their lives (Israel et al. 1994; Rody 1988; Minkler, Wallerstein, and Wilson 2008). And indeed, an aim of nutrition education is for nutrition programs to assist individuals to become more able to take control of their own food choices and practices and to take collective action regarding their environments to make them more supportive—in short, to become more empowered.

Collaboration

Nutrition educators can also work in collaboration with other professionals, organizations, and governmental agencies to increase the accessibility and affordability of foods for low-income audiences; promote environments at the institutional and community levels that foster attitudes and behaviors conducive to health; encourage the development of social networks and social support; build food and nutrition programs that involve genuine community participation and control; and promote policies at local, state, and national levels that are supportive of food- and nutrition-related health.

Nutrition Education, Public Health Nutrition, and Health Promotion: The Roles and Context of Nutrition Education

Nutrition education that addresses both environmental and personal motivating and facilitating factors and includes expanded audiences and strategies begins to overlap public health nutrition and health promotion efforts. To make the situation even more complex, we should note that dietary interventions are often integrated with interventions directed at other health-related behaviors, such as smoking cessation, blood pressure control, and increased physical activity. Within the context of today's emphasis on health promotion and disease prevention, the roles of nutrition education, public health nutrition, health education, and health promotion are indeed overlapping and intertwined.

At the same time, the scope of nutrition education is broader than educating about nutrition in relation to personal health. Nutrition has often been defined as the link between agriculture and health. Some nutrition educators are concerned about the agriculture-to-nutrition component of the link as well as the nutrition-to-health component. Thus, nutrition education can address such concerns as food safety and how to ensure the availability and accessibility of nutritious and wholesome food for all, poor and rich alike. As we have seen, for many nutrition educators and consumers, considerations about how and where food is produced are also important. Nutrition education can thus be visualized as including the overlapping portion of several intersecting circles, as shown in **FIGURE 1-8**.

Clearly, nutrition education by itself cannot accomplish everything needed for improved nutritional well-being for all people. It must be conducted in conjunction with many other related strategies, some not educational in nature. Facilitating individual behavior change and bringing about change in the environment are both important and interactive. Nutrition education is directed primarily at individual and group behaviors through direct and indirect activities that enhance motivations,

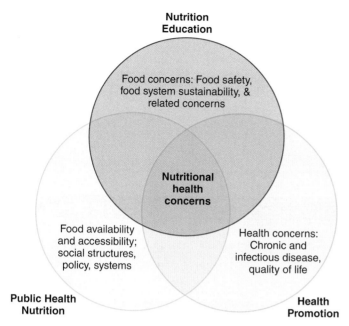

FIGURE 1-8 The overlapping roles of nutrition education, public health nutrition, and health promotion.

knowledge and skills, and social support. However, it also includes nutrition education activities conducted in collaboration with decision-makers and policymakers in order to promote specific policy, systems, and environmental supports that make it easier for the public to engage in healthy behaviors (Story et al. 2008). Public health nutrition efforts and food assistance programs, on the other hand, are directed primarily at environmental, systemic, and policy factors such as the availability and accessibility of food, access to nutritional services within the healthcare system, community structures that enable active living, policy, and legislation, and secondarily at personal and behavioral factors. In addition, those in nutrition education, public health nutrition, and health promotion share an interest in fostering collective efficacy and capacity building in communities so that communities can become empowered to act on their own food, nutrition, and physical activity issues for the long term.

Purpose and Overview of this Book

Nutrition educators have the opportunity to make a real difference in the lives of the people with whom they work. This book is intended to be a *guide* to designing, implementing, and evaluating effective, evidence-based nutrition education intervention programs and dietary change

strategies. Effective interventions and strategies are those that enhance people's motivation, ability, and opportunities to eat well and live actively and are grounded in the integration of theory, research, and practice. We first explore the research and theoretical foundations of nutrition education and then examine a systematic and practical procedure for conducting it, called the DESIGN Procedure.

We have seen that nutrition education and promotion can be delivered through multiple venues and that its scope can be broad. One book cannot cover all aspects. Consequently, this text focuses on designing, implementing, and evaluating the types of educational interventions and programs that the vast majority of nutrition educators offer on an ongoing basis in their places of work:

- *Providing direct, site-based, in-person educational activities with groups* in a variety of settings, such as communities, outpatient clinics, health maintenance organizations, fitness centers, schools, workplaces, or private nonprofit organizations
- *Developing and implementing indirect activities and accompanying materials,* such as activities involving the Internet and emerging technologies, mass media campaigns, and social marketing activities, or health fairs and printed materials and visual media
- *Engaging in activities and coalitions with others* to promote environments, social structures, and policies that are supportive of the public's ability to eat healthfully

Many factors in the larger society, such as public policy, systems, and social structures, have important impacts on food- and nutrition-related behaviors and practices. Designing interventions to change directly these larger environmental forces operating at the community and national levels is the subject of many available health promotion planning and community nutrition books, and discussion of such design in detail is beyond the scope of this book. The focus of this book is thus on how to design and implement real-world educational programs that can stand alone or be conducted within, or in collaboration with, these larger programs. Specifically, this book provides a systematic stepwise procedure for translating theory and research evidence into exciting, effective direct and indirect educational activities for a variety of audiences and also policy, system and environmental supports for these activities. Working with individuals one on one, as in nutrition counseling, is also very important but is the

Table 1-1 Conceptual Framework of This Book

Designing and conducting direct and indirect nutrition education with various audiences using many channels and including environmental and policy supports:

	Children	Teens	Adults/Families	Cultural Groups	Low Literacy
The Foundations (Chapters 1–6)					
Introduction to contemporary definition of nutrition education				•	
Determinants of food choice and dietary change				•	
Foundation for successful nutrition education				•	
Enhancing motivation and facilitating behavior change and action				•	
Promoting policy, system, and environmental supports for action				•	
Design of Direct and Indirect Nutrition Education (Chapters 7–13)					
Deciding on behavior change goals of nutrition education programs				•	
Identifying determinants of behaviors				•	
Creating strategies and education plans to deliver nutrition education				•	
Planning the evaluation				•	
Delivery of Nutrition Education (Chapters 15–18)			**Audiences**		
Understanding learning theory and audience learning styles	•	•	•	•	•
Understanding instructional design for teaching sessions/working with groups	•	•	•	•	•
Materials/visuals, Internet/social media	•	•	•	•	•
Mass media campaigns and social marketing	•	•	•	•	•
Design and Delivery of Strategies for Environmental and Policy Supports (Chapter 14)					
Family/social networks	•	•	•	•	•
Institutional/community strategies	•	•	•	•	•
Policy, systems and environmental change actions	•	•	•	•	•

subject of other available texts and will not be addressed in this book.

A *conceptual* outline of the book is shown in **TABLE 1-1**.

LEARNING A NEW VOCABULARY

You will encounter many new terms and ideas. Indeed, you will learn a new vocabulary. Just as when you took your first course in biochemistry or nutrition you had to learn new terms such as *metabolism*, *Kreb's cycle*, *lipogenesis*, *glycemic index*, and *electrolyte balance*, so you will learn new terms such as *outcome expectations* (beliefs about desired outcomes of behavior), *self-efficacy* (confidence in being able to perform a behavior), *attitudes*, *perceived social norms*, *personal agency*, and so forth. The terms are explained as you encounter them in this book. They are labels or terms used by health behavior professionals and psychologists to describe people's common perceptions and experiences. You will soon be comfortable using this new vocabulary and speaking the language of behavioral nutrition and nutrition education.

OVERVIEW OF THE BOOK

Nutrition education is challenging but also highly rewarding for those who work in the field. The public is interested in food and nutrition. Research is very active, drawing investigators from a variety of fields so that there is rich cross-fertilization of ideas. Such research has generated evidence about effective approaches to nutrition education and has produced usable conceptual frameworks and theories as tools to guide practice. The remainder of this book is devoted to discussing relevant theories, emerging nutrition education research evidence, and practical techniques for increasing awareness and enhancing motivation for *why* to take action, facilitating the ability for *how* to take action, and promoting *supportive* environments in order to assist people to adopt and maintain food- and nutrition-related practices conducive to long-term health.

- Part I of this book provides the background in behavioral nutrition and nutrition education research and theory for understanding the determinants of food choices and the processes of dietary behavior change in order to provide you with guidelines

and tools to make nutrition education practice more successful.

- Part II presents a six-step Nutrition Education DESIGN Procedure for designing effective practical nutrition education strategies that use theory and evidence as a tool or guide.
- Part III describes the nuts and bolts of implementing the direct and indirect nutrition education activities planned in Part II and making theory and research practical in real-world settings, including working successfully in group settings, using other channels and media effectively, social marketing, and working with diverse age, cultural, and literacy groups.

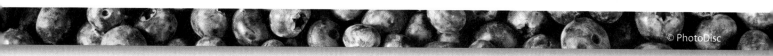

© PhotoDisc

Questions and Activities

1. Why is nutrition education for the public needed?
2. Describe some reasons why it is difficult for people to eat healthfully, despite the abundance of choices and extensive media coverage of diet and health.
3. Social and behavioral factors contribute to a broad range of health outcomes for people and ecological conditions for the planet. What are the implications for nutrition education?
4. Although food and nutrition information is used in nutrition education in some form, why and how the information is communicated makes a difference in outcomes for people. Describe different ways that the information can be presented and indicate the

implications for outcomes for each way of communicating the information.

5. Think carefully about the contemporary definition of nutrition education presented in this chapter. How does it differ from a definition you may have had previously? How do you think it will impact your work as a nutrition educator?
6. If someone now asks you to explain what nutrition education is, what would you say, using your own words?
7. As you review the audiences and settings for nutrition education, where you do see yourself as a nutrition educator? What would you like to do?

References

Abusabha R., J. Peacock, and C. Achterberg. 1999. How to make nutrition education more meaningful through facilitated group discussions. *Journal of the American Dietetic Association* 99:72–76.

Academy of Nutrition and Dietetics [AND]. 2015. AND: Who we are, what we do. http://www.eatright.org/About/Content.aspx?id=7530 Accessed 3/5/15.

Agriculture and Agri-Food Canada 2012. Socially conscious consumer trends: Fair trade. Market analysis report, International Markets Bureau, Ministry of Agriculture and Agri-Canada. http://www5.agr.gc.ca/resources/prod/Internet-Internet/MISB-DGSIM/ATS-SEA/PDF/6153-eng.pdf Accessed 3/6/15.

Arnold, C. G., P. Ladipo, C. H. Nguyen, P. Nkinda-Chaiban, and M. Olson. 2001. New concepts for nutrition education in an era of welfare reform. *Journal of Nutrition Education* 33:341–346.

Bandura, A. 1997. *Self efficacy: The exercise of control.* New York: WH Freeman.

———. 2001. Social cognitive theory: An agentic perspective. *Annual Review of Psychology* 51:1–26.

Barilla Center for Food & Nutrition (2015). Food and the environment: Diets that are healthy for people and the planet. http://www.BarillaCFN.com Accessed 2/1/15.

Briggs M., S. Fleischhacker, and C. G. Mueller. 2010. Position of the American Dietetic Association, School

Nutrition Association, and Society for Nutrition Education: Comprehensive school nutrition services. *Journal of Nutrition Education and Behavior.* 42:360–371.

Brillant-Savarin, A. S. 1825. *The physiology of taste: Meditations on transcendental gastronomy,* translated by M. F. K. Fisher. Reprint. Washington, DC: Counterpoint Press, 2000.

Buchanan, D. R. 2000. *An ethic for health promotion: Rethinking the sources of human well-being.* New York: Oxford University Press.

Burros, M. 2006. Idealism for breakfast: Serving good intentions by the bowl full. *The New York Times,* January 11.

Center for Nutrition Policy and Promotion, U.S. Department of Agriculture. 2013. Diet quality of Americans in 2001–02 and 2007–08 as measured by the Healthy Eating Index. *Nutrition Insights* 51. *www.cnpp.usda.gov/healthyeatingindex. htm* Accessed 8/15/14.

Centers for Disease Control and Prevention. 2013. Adult participation in aerobic and muscle-strengthening physical activities—United States, 2011. *Morbidity and Mortality Weekly Report.* 62(17):326–330. http://www.cdc.gov/media/releases/2013/p0502-physical-activity.html Accessed 7/17/13.

Clancy, K. 1999. Reclaiming the social and environmental roots of nutrition education. *Journal of Nutrition Education* 31(4):190–193.

Colman, S., I. P. Nichols-Barrer, J. E. Redline, B. L. Devaney, S. V. Ansell, and T. Joyce. 2012. *Effects of the Special Supplemental Nutrition Program for Women, Infants, and Children (WIC): A Review of Recent Research.* http://www.fns.usda.gov/ora/MENU/Published/WIC/WIC.htm Accessed 4/2/15.

Cunningham-Sabo, L. and A. Simons. 2012. Home economics: An old-fashioned answer to a modern-day dilemma? *Nutrition Today* 47:128–132.

da Silveira, J., J. Taddei, P. Guerra, and M. Nobre. 2013. The effect of participation in school-based nutrition education interventions on body mass index: A meta-analysis of randomized controlled community trials. *Preventive Medicine* 56(3–4):237–243.

Davis, C. M. 1928. Self selection of diet by newly weaned infants. *American Journal of Diseases of Children* 36: 651–679.

Dawson, A. 2014. Information, choice, and the ends of health promotion. *Monash Bioethics Review* 32: 106–120.

Deci, E. L., and E. M. Ryan. 2000. The "what" and "why" of goal pursuits: Human needs and the self-determination of behavior. *Psychological Inquiry* 11(4):227–268.

Dollahite, J., D. Kenkel, and C. S. Thompson. 2008. An economic evaluation of the Expanded Food and Nutrition Education Program. *Journal of Nutrition Education and Behavior* 40(3):134–143.

Dorfman, L., and L. Wallack. 2007. Moving nutrition upstream: The case for reframing obesity. *Journal of Nutrition Education and Behavior* 39(2 Suppl):S45–S50.

Drewnowski, A. 2012. The cost of U.S. foods as related to their nutritive value. *American Journal of Clinical Nutrition* 92(5):1181–1188.

Dyson, L., F. McCormick, and M. J. Renfrew. 2008. Interventions for promoting the initiation of breastfeeding. *Cochrane Database of Systematic Reviews* (2):CD001688.

Englberger, L., A. Lorens, M. E. Pretrick, R. Spegal, and I. Falcam. 2010. "Go local" island food network: Using email networking to promote island foods for their health, biodiversity, and other "CHEEF" benefits. *Pacific Health Dialog* 16(1):41–47.

Evans, C. E., M. S. Christian, C. L. Cleghorn, D. C. Greenwood, and J. E. Cade. 2012. Systematic review and meta-analysis of school-based interventions to improve daily fruit and vegetable intake in children aged 5 to 12 y. *American Journal of Clinical Nutrition* 96(4):889–901.

Federal Trade Commission. 2012. A review of food marketing to children and adolescents. http://ftc.gov/os/2012/12/121221foodmarketingreport.pdf Accessed 8/14/13.

Feenstra G., and J. Ohmart. 2012. The evolution of the school food and farm to school movement in the United States: Connecting childhood health, farms, and communities. *Child Obesity* 8(4):280–289.

Flegal, K. M., M. D. Carroll, B. K. Kit, and C. L. Ogden. 2012. Prevalence of obesity and trends in the distribution of body mass index among US adults, 1999-2010. *Journal of the American Medical Association* 307:491–497.

Flint, A. J., F. B. Hu , R. J. Glynn, H. Caspard, J. E. Manson, W. C. Willett, and E. B. Rimm. 2010. Excess weight and the risk of incident coronary heart disease among men and women. *Obesity* 18:377–383.

Flores, M., N. Macia, M. Rivera, A. Lozada, S. Barquera, and J. Rivera-Dommarco. 2010. Dietary patterns in Mexican adults are associated with risk of being overweight or obese. *Journal of Nutrition* 140:1869–1873.

Food and Agricultural Organization. 2014. Food-based dietary guidelines by country. http://www.fao.org/ag/humannutrition/nutritioneducation/fbdg/en/ Accessed 2/15/15.

Food Marketing Institute. 2012. Supermarket facts 2011–2012. http://www.fmi.org/research-resources/supermarket-facts Accessed 8/15/13.

Freire, P. 1970. *Pedagogy of the oppressed.* New York: Continuum.

Gibbs, L., P. K. Staiger, B. Johnson, K. Block, S. Macfarlane, L. Gold, et al. 2013. Expanding children's food experiences: The impact of a school-based kitchen garden program. *Journal of Nutrition Education and Behavior* 45(2): 137–145.

Gussow, J. D. 1993. Why Cook? *Journal of Gastronomy* 7(1):79–87.

———. 1999. Dietary guidelines for sustainability: Twelve years later. *Journal of Nutrition Education* 31(4):194–200.

———. 2006. Reflections on nutritional health and the environment: The journey to sustainability. *Journal of Hunger and Environmental Nutrition* 1(1):3–25.

Gussow, J. D., and I. Contento. 1984. Nutrition education in a changing world: A conceptualization and selective review. *World Review of Nutrition and Dietetics* 44:1–56.

Gussow, J. D., and K. Clancy. 1986. Dietary guidelines for sustainability. *Journal of Nutrition Education* 18(1):1–4.

Gustafson A., O. Khavjou, S. C. Stearns, T. C. Keyserling, Z. Gizlice, S. Lindsley, et al. 2009. Cost-effectiveness of a behavioral weight loss intervention for low-income women: The Weight-Wise Program. *Preventive Medicine* 49(5):390–395.

Guthrie, J., B. H. Lin, A. Okrent, and R. Volpe. 2013. Americans' food choices at home and away: How do they compare with recommendations? *Amber Waves*. U.S. Department of Agriculture, Economic Research Service. http://www.ers.usda.gov/amber-waves/2013-february/americans-food-choices-at-home-and-away.aspx#.Uf035WRgZOF Accessed 12/4/14.

Hanks, A. S., D. R. Just, L. E. Smith, and B. Wansink. 2012. Healthy convenience: Nudging students toward healthier choices in the lunchroom. *Journal of Public Health (Oxf)* 34(3):370–376.

Harris, D. M., J. Seymour, L. Grummer-Strawn, A. Cooper, B. Collins, L. DiSogra, et al. 2012. Let's move salad bars to schools: A public-private partnership to increase student fruit and vegetable consumption. *Child Obesity* 8(4):294–297.

Hawkes, C. 2013. *Promoting healthy diets through nutrition education and changes in the food environment: An international review of actions and their effectiveness.* Rome: Nutrition Education and Consumer Awareness Group, Food and Agriculture Organization of the United Nations. http://www.fao.org/docrep/017/i3235e/i3235e.pdf Accessed 5/15/15.

Hill, J. A. 2009. Evidence for excellence: Systematic review of breastfeeding education benefits. *American Journal of Nursing* 109(4):26–27.

Institute of Medicine. 2000. *Promoting health: Intervention strategies from social and behavioral research*, edited by B. D. Smedley and S. L. Syme. Washington, DC: Division of Health Promotion and Disease Prevention, Institute of Medicine.

International Society of Behavioral Nutrition and Physical Activity. 2015. About us. http://www.isbnpa.org/index.php?r=about/index. Accessed 3/6/15.

Israel, B. A., B. Checkoway, A. Schulz, and M. Zimmerman. 1994. Health education and community empowerment: Conceptualizing and measuring perceptions of individual, organizational, and community control. *Health Education Quarterly* 21(2):149–170.

Johnson, B. T., L. A. J. Scott-Sheldon, and M. P. Carey. 2010. Meta-synthesis of health behavior change meta-analyses. *American Journal of Public Health* 100:2193–2198.

Johnson, D. W., and R. T. Johnson. 1985. Nutrition education: A model for effectiveness, a synthesis of research. *Journal of Nutrition Education* 17(Suppl):S1–S44.

Kearney, J. 2010. Food consumption trends and drivers. *Philosophical Transactions of the Royal Society* 365:2793–2807.

Khambalia, A. Z., S. Dickinson, L. L. Hardy, T. Gill, and L. A. Baur. 2012. A synthesis of existing systematic reviews and meta-analyses of school-based behavioral interventions for controlling and preventing obesity. *Obesity Reviews* 13:214–233.

Krebs-Smith, S. M., P. M. Guenther, A. F. Subar, S. I. Kirkpatrick, and K. W. Dodd. 2010. Americans do not meet federal dietary recommendations. *Journal of Nutrition* 140:1832–1838.

Langellotto, G. A., and A. Gupta. 2012. Gardening increases vegetable consumptions in school-aged children: A meta-analytical synthesis. *Fort-Technology* 22(4): 430–445.

Leventhal, H. 1973. Changing attitudes and habits to reduce risk factors in chronic disease. *American Journal of Cardiology* 31(5):571–580.

Levy, L., R. E. Patterson, A. R. Kristal, and S. S. Li. 2000. How well do consumers understand percentage daily value on food labels? *American Journal of Health Promotion* 14(3):157–160, ii.

Lindstrom, B., and M. Eriksson. 2005. Salutogenesis. *Journal of Epidemiology and Community Health.* 59:440–448

Lock, K., J. Pomerleau, L. Causer, D. R. Altmann, and M. McKee. 2005. The global burden of disease attributable to low consumption of fruit and vegetables: Implications for the global strategy on diet. *Bulletin of the World Health Organization* 83(2):100–108.

Long, V., S. Cates, J. Blitstein, K. Deehy, P. Williams, R. Morgan, et al. 2013. Supplemental Nutrition Assistance Program Education and Evaluation Study (Wave II). Prepared by Altarum Institute for the U.S. Department of Agriculture, Food and Nutrition Service.

Lowe, C. F., P. A. Hall, and W. R. Staines. 2014. The effect of continuous theta burst stimulations to the left dorsolateral prefrontal cortex on executive function, food cravings, and snack food consumption. *Psychosomatic Medicine* 76(7):503–511.

McKinley, J. B. 1974. A case for refocusing upstream—the political economy of illness. In *Applying behavioral science to cardiovascular risk*, edited by A. J. Enelow and J. B. Henderson. Seattle, WA: American Heart Association.

McLaughlin, K. 2004. Food world's new buzzword is "sustainable" products; fair trade certified mangos. *The Wall Street Journal*, February 17, D1–2.

McNulty, J. 2013. *Challenges and issues in nutrition education.* Rome: Nutrition Education and Consumer Awareness Group, Food and Agriculture Organization of the United Nations. http://www.fao.org/docrep/017/i3234e/i3234e.pdf Accessed 5/15/15.

Minkler, M., N. B. Wallerstein, and N. Wilson. 2008. Improving health through community organization and community building. In *Health education and health behavior: Theory research and practice*, 4th edition, K. Glanz, B. K. Rimer, and K. Viswanath, editors. San Francisco: Jossey-Bass.

Moliter, G. T. T. 1980. The food system in the 1980s. *Journal of Nutrition Education* 12(suppl):103–111.

Moss, M. 2013. *Salt, fat, sugar*. New York: Random House.

National Health and Nutrition Examination Survey. 2005–2008. Two-day averages for individuals age 2 and older who are not pregnant or lactating. http://www.ers.usda.gov/Briefing/DietQuality/Data/ Accessed 7/20/13.

Okrent, A. and J. M. Alston. 2012. The demand for disaggregated food-away-from-home and food-at-home products in the United States. *Economic Research Service* Report No. (ERR-139).

Ollberding, N., R. Wolf, and I. R. Contento. 2010. Food label use and its relation to dietary intake among U.S. adults. *Journal of the American Dietetic Association* 110:1233–1237.

Pacific Institute. 2013. Bottled water and energy facts. www.pacinst.org Accessed 12/4/13.

Pollan, M. 2008. *In defense of food: An eater's manifesto*. New York: Penguin.

Pomerleau, J., K. Lock, C. Knai, and M. McKee. 2005. Interventions designed to increase adult fruit and vegetable intake can be effective: A systematic review of the literature. *Journal of Nutrition* 135(10):2486–2495.

Popkin, B. M. 2009. Global nutrition dynamics: The world is shifting rapidly toward a diet linked with non-communicable diseases. *American Journal of Clinical Nutrition* 84: 289–298.

———. 2010. Patterns of beverage use across the lifecycle. *Physiology and Behavior* 100:4–9.

Rajopal, R., R. H. Cox, M. Lambur, and E. C. Lewis. 2003. Cost-benefit analysis indicates the positive economic benefits of the Expanded Food and Nutrition Education Program related to chronic disease prevention. *Journal of Nutrition Education and Behavior* 34:26–37.

Rody, N. 1988. Empowerment as organizational policy in nutrition intervention programs: A case study from the Pacific Islands. *Journal of Nutrition Education* 20: 133–141.

Rolls, B. 2000. Sensory-specific satiety and variety in the meal. In *Dimensions of the meal: The science, culture, business, and art of eating*, edited by H. L. Meiselman. Gaithersburg, MD: Aspen Publishers.

Roux, L., M. Pratt, T. O. Tengs, M. M. Yore, T. L. Yanagawa, J. Van Den Bos, et al. 2008. Cost effectiveness of community-based physical activity interventions. *American Journal of Preventive Medicine* 35(6):578–588.

Rozin, P. 1982. Human food selection: The interaction of biology, culture, and individual experience. In *The psychobiology of human food selection*, edited by L. M. Barker. Westport, CT: Avi Publishing Company.

Savage, J. S., J. O. Fisher, and L. L. Birch. 2007. Parental influence on eating behavior. *Journal of Law and Medical Ethics* 35(1):22–34.

Schlicka J. M., and M. E. Wilson. 2005. Breastfeeding as health-promoting behaviour for Hispanic women: Literature review. *Journal of Advanced Nursing* 52(2):200–210.

Schlosser, E. 2001. *Fast Food Nation*. Boston: Houghton Mifflin.

Schuster, E., Z. L. Zimmerman, M. Engle, J. Smiley, E. Syversen, and J. Murray. 2003. Investing in Oregon's expanded food and nutrition education program (EFNEP): Documenting costs and benefits. *Journal of Nutrition Education and Behavior* 35(4):200–206.

Society for Nutrition Education and Behavior. 2015. Society for Nutrition Education mission and identity statements. http://www.sneb.org Accessed 3/2/15.

Stevens, G. A., G. M. Singh, Y. Lu, G. Danaei, J. K. Lin, M. M. Finucane, et al. 2012. National, regional, and global trends in adult overweight and obesity prevalences. *Population Metrics* 10:22.

Stewart, H., N. Blisard, and D. Jolliffe. 2006. Let's eat out: Americans weigh taste, convenience, and nutrition. *Economic Information Bulletin* No. EIB-19.

Story, M., K. M. Kaphingst, R. Robinson-O'Brien, K. Glanz. 2008. Creating healthy food and eating environments: Policy and environmental approaches. *Annual Review of Public Health* 9:253–272.

Supermarket Nutrition. 2013. How grocery retailers and supermarket dietitians can impact consumer health, in-store & online. http://supermarketnutrition.com/how-grocery-retailers-and-supermarket-dietitians-can-impact-consumer-health-in-store-online/ Accessed 5/15/15.

Thompson B., and L. Amoroso, eds. 2011. *Combating micronutrient deficiencies: Food-based approaches*. Rome: Food and Agricultural Organization.

Thompson, C. A., and J. Ravia. 2011. A systematic review of behavioral interventions to promote intake of fruit and vegetables. *Journal of the American Dietetic Association* 111(10):1523–1535.

Travers, K. D. 1997. Reducing inequities through participatory research and community empowerment. *Health Education and Behavior* 24(3):344–356.

U.S. Department of Health and Human Services. 2008. Physical activity guidelines for Americans. www.health.gov/paguidelines Accessed 8/14/13.

———. 2010a. *Healthy People 2020: Improving the Health of Americans*. Washington, DC: Government Printing Office. http://www.healthypeople.gov/2020/topicsobjectives2020/objectiveslist.aspx?topicId=29 Accessed 3/2/15.

———. 2010b. *Dietary Guidelines for Americans*. www.health.gov/dietaryguidelines/ Accessed 8/14/13.

———. 2015. *Dietary Guidelines for Americans*. www.health.gov/dietaryguidelines/ Accessed 3/2/15.

Van Rossum, C. T. M., H. P. Fransen, J. Verkaik-Kloosterman, E. J. M. Buuma-Rethans, and C. Ocke. 2011. *Dutch national food consumption survey 2007–2010: Diet of children and adults aged 7 to 69 years*. Netherlands: National Institute for Public Health and the Environment, Ministry of Health, Welfare and Sports. http://www.rivm.nl/bibliotheek/rapporten/350050006.pdf Accessed 5/5/15.

Wang, D, and D. Stewart. 2013. The implementation and effectiveness of school-based nutrition promotion programmes using a health-promoting schools approach: A systematic review. *Public Health Nutrition* 16(6):1082–1100.

Wang Y, Y. Wu, R. F. Wilson, S. Bleich, L. Cheskin, C. Weston, et al. 2013. Childhood obesity prevention programs: Comparative effectiveness review and meta-analysis. *Agency for Healthcare Research and Quality: Comparative Effectiveness Reviews.* June;13-EHC081-EF.

White House Task Force on Childhood Obesity. 2010. *Solving the problem of childhood obesity within one generation.* Washington, DC: White House Task Force on Childhood Obesity, Policy Domestic Council. http://www.letsmove.gov/sites/letsmove.gov/files/TaskForce_on_Childhood_Obesity_May2010_FullReport.pdf Accessed 3/6/15.

Whitten, C., S. K. Nicholson, C. Roberts, C. J. Prynne, G. Pot, A. Olson et al. 2011. National Diet and Nutrition Survey: UK food consumption and nutrient intakes from the first year of the rolling programme and comparisons with previous surveys. *British Journal of Nutrition* 106(12):1899–1914.

WIC Works Resource System. 2013. Revitalizing Quality Nutrition Services (RQNS) http://www.fns.usda.gov/wic/benefitsandservices/rqns.htm Accessed 7/15/13.

Yale Rudd Center for Food Policy & Obesity. 2013. Food marketing to youth. http://www.yaleruddcenter.org/what_we_do.aspx?id=4 Accessed 8/15/13.

Yudkin, J. 1978. *The diet of man: Needs and wants.* London: Elsevier Science.

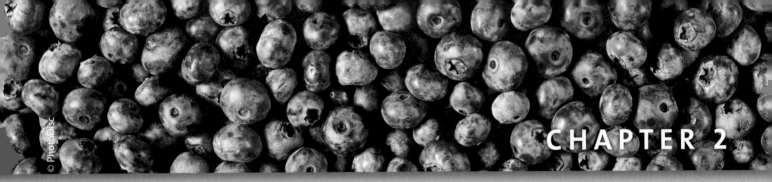

CHAPTER 2

Determinants of Food Choice and Dietary Change: Implications for Nutrition Education

OVERVIEW

This chapter provides readers with an overview of the numerous influences on food choice and dietary practices. Understanding these influences will help nutrition educators design appropriate and relevant nutrition education. These influences are called determinants. The chapter also provides a description of the desired competencies outlined by professional nutrition societies for nutrition educators.

CHAPTER OUTLINE

- Determinants of food choice and diet-related behavior: an overview
- Food-related determinants: biology and experience
- Person-related determinants

- Social and environmental determinants
- What does all this mean for nutrition educators?
- Implications for competencies and skills needed by nutrition educators
- Summary

LEARNING OBJECTIVES

At the end of the chapter, you should be able to:

- Describe the research evidence for the influences of biological predispositions, experience with food, personal factors, and environmental factors on human food choice and dietary behaviors
- Understand the key role of intra- and interpersonal processes in food choice and dietary behaviors

- Appreciate the importance of these understandings for designing effective nutrition education
- State the competencies needed to be an effective nutrition educator

Determinants of Food Choice and Diet-Related Behavior: An Overview

You have known a person like Alicia: she knows a lot about nutrition, and, in particular, she knows that she should eat more fruits and vegetables. She just can't seem to do it. Or Ray, who wants to lose weight and knows what he is supposed to do, but just can't seem to get to it. Or maybe it is yourself—there is some eating habit you want to change but don't.

Nutrition education is often seen as the process of translating the findings of nutrition science to various audiences using methods from the fields of education and communication. If only the public knew all that we did, nutrition educators think, surely they would eat better. Thus, we believe that our task as nutrition educators is solely to provide the public with the information needed to eat well. We plan sessions on our government's food guide such as the United States' MyPlate and food label reading. We provide lists of high-fat or high-fiber foods, or food sources of nutrients such as calcium or vitamins. We discuss managing food budgets. However, studies show that simply communicating this kind of information is not enough. It is not motivating. People often know how to eat well but do not—just like Alicia and Ray.

This is because eating is about more than health. Eating is a source of pleasure and is related to many of life's social functions. Brillat-Savarin enthusiastically wrote an entire book on taste 200 years ago in which he noted that, "Taste, such as Nature has given to us, is yet one of our senses . . . that, all things considered, procures to us the greatest of enjoyment, because: the pleasure of eating is the only one that, taken in moderation, is never followed by fatigue; it can be combined with all our other pleasures, and even console us for their absence . . ." (Brillat-Savarin 1825). Eating behaviors are acquired over a lifetime, and are embedded in so many aspects of our lives. Unlike other health-related behaviors such as smoking, eating is not optional. We have to eat, and any changes we make are undertaken with a great deal of ambivalence. We want to eat to satisfy physical hunger and psychological desires and yet also want to be healthy, which may require adopting eating patterns that conflict with these desires.

We make decisions about food several times a day: when to eat, what to eat, with whom, and how much. Whether the act of eating is a meal or a snack, at home or at work, the decisions are complex and the influences many. Biologically determined behavioral predispositions such as liking of specific tastes are, of course, important influences. However, these can be modified by experience with food as well as by various intrapersonal and interpersonal factors. In addition, the environment either facilitates or impedes our ability to act on our biological predispositions, preferences, or personal imperatives. The influences are so numerous that they become overwhelming to try to understand. Yet understand we must if we want to be effective nutrition educators or communicators. It is very important for us to understand people, their behaviors, and the various forces that influence an individual's or a community's decision to eat in a particular way. This chapter simplifies matters by examining these influences in three categories that are commonly used in studying food choice or food selection: factors related to food, to the individuals making the choices, and to the external physical and social environment—factors related to food, person, and environment (Shepherd 1999).

Many factors within each of these categories influence our eating. These influences on our food choices or decisions are explored in greater detail in the following sections. We will call these influences *determinants*.

Food-Related Determinants: Biology and Experience

When asked, most people say their food choices are largely determined by "taste" (Clark 1998; Food Marketing Institute [FMI] 2012). By taste, they mean flavor, which includes smell and the oral perception of food texture as well (Small and Prescott 2005). Our sensory and emotional responses to the taste, smell, sight, and texture of food are a major influence on food preferences and food choices. What are we born with and what is learned?

BIOLOGICALLY DETERMINED BEHAVIORAL PREDISPOSITIONS

The Basic Tastes

Humans are born with biological predispositions toward liking the sweet taste and rejecting sour and bitter tastes (Desor, Mahler, and Greene 1977; Beauchamp and Mennella 2011; Gravina, Yep, and Khan 2013). The liking for the sweet taste remains throughout life and appears to be universal to all cultures (Drewnowski et al. 2012).

The liking for salt seems to develop several months after birth, when infants have matured somewhat (Mattes 1997). It has been suggested that these predispositions may have had adaptive value: the liking for the sweet taste because it signals a safe carbohydrate source of calories and the rejection of bitterness because it may signal potential poisons.

A fifth taste has been identified: umami, a Japanese word for deliciousness, which is associated with a savory taste such as the brothiness of soup or the meatiness in mushrooms. It seems to be related to glutamate, an amino acid, and may capture the taste of protein in food (Beauchamp 2009). In addition, because some taste buds are surrounded by free nerve endings of the trigeminal nerve, people are able to experience the burn from hot peppers and the coolness of menthol (Breslin and Spector 2008).

Preference for fat may have a genetic basis as well (Mattes 2009; Gravina, Yep, and Khan 2013). Fat is less a flavor than a contributor to texture (Mattes 2009) although some genes are thought to be related to the fat taste (Breslin and Spector 2008; Tucker, Mattes, and Running, 2014). It imparts different textures to different foods: it makes dairy products such as ice cream seem creamy, meat juicy and tender, pastries flaky, and cakes moist. Many high-fat foods are those in which fat is paired with sugar (desserts) or salt (potato chips), enhancing their palatability. Foods containing fat are more varied, rich tasting, and higher in energy density than are nonfat foods and hence are more appealing.

Individual Differences: Nontasters and Supertasters

Some genetic differences in sensitivity to tastes exist between individuals. Research shows that people differ in their responses to two bitter compounds called phenylthiocarbamide (PTC) and 6-*n*-propylthiouracil (PROP). When given PTC-impregnated paper or PROP in liquid form, some people cannot taste it and are labeled nontasters, others are medium tasters, and still others are supertasters (Tepper 2008; Lipchock et al. 2013). Such differences between individuals may be related to differences in being able to discriminate between different foods and may contribute to some of the differences in liking for certain foods (Duffy and Bartoshuk 2000; Tepper 2008).

Hunger and Fullness or "Satiety"

Many genetic and biological mechanisms control our feelings of hunger and fullness (called satiety), ensuring that people will eat enough to meet their energy needs (de Castro 2010). Throughout most of human history, getting enough food was the primary challenge. The human body developed to function in an environment where food was scarce and high levels of physical activity were mandatory for survival. This situation resulted in the development of various physiological mechanisms that encourage the body to deposit energy (i.e., fat) and defend against energy loss (Konner and Eaton 2010; Chakravarthy and Booth 2004). Today's environment, however, is one in which for many countries in the world and increasingly for others, food is widely available, inexpensive, and often high in energy density, while little physical activity is required for daily living. Researchers have proposed that the "modern environment has taken body weight control from an unconscious process to one that requires substantial cognitive effort. In the current environment, people who are not devoting substantial conscious effort to managing body weight are probably gaining weight" (Peters et al. 2002). This means that nutrition education has an important role.

Specific Tastes or Sensory-Specific Satiety

Humans also appear to have a built-in biologically determined mechanism whereby we get tired of one taste and move on to another one over a short time span, such as while eating a meal (Rolls 2000). This mechanism is called *sensory-specific satiety*. Such a mechanism probably had adaptive value for humans because it ensures that people eat a variety of different-tasting foods and thus obtain

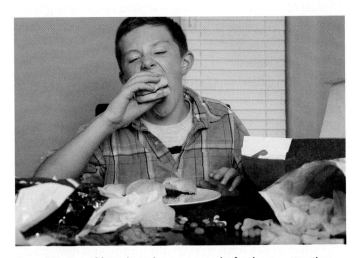

A combination of fat, salt, and sugar can make foods very attractive to eat in large quantities.

© StaffordStudios/iStock

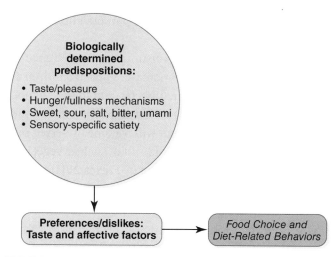

FIGURE 2-1 Our biologically determined behavioral predispositions influence food choices and dietary behaviors.

all the nutrients they need from these foods. Studies also reveal that for adults, the variety of foods available influences meal size, with greater variety stimulating greater intake. Again, this mechanism might have been very useful in a situation where food was scarce. However, in today's food environment, the variety possible in meals may contribute to overweight.

These biologically determined predispositions contribute to some degree to preference and to food choices or food selections and behavior, particularly in children, and are shown in **FIGURE 2-1**. In today's food marketplace, food products are being specially formulated to take advantage of these biological predispositions by manipulating their fat, salt, and sugar content to make them more desirable (Gearhardt et al. 2011; Moss 2013). However, as we see in the next section, these biological predispositions can be modified and most specific preferences are actually learned or conditioned—which is good news for nutrition educators because that means they can be modified.

EXPERIENCE WITH FOOD

Research in this area suggests that people's liking for specific foods and their food acceptance patterns are largely learned (Birch 1999, 2014; Birch and Anzman-Frasca 2011a; Mennella and Beauchamp 2005; Beauchamp and Mennella 2009). Thus, what humans seem to inherit primarily is the innate capacity to learn about the consequences of eating particular foods. Learning, in this context, does not mean cognitive learning, but rather *physiological learning* or *conditioning* arising from the positive or negative consequences

that people experience physically and emotionally from repeated exposure to a food.

Pre- and Postnatal Experience

Such learning begins early, even prenatally. Flavors such as garlic and alcohol have been detected in mothers' milk, possibly familiarizing infants with these flavors (Beauchamp and Mennella 2009, 2011). In one study, breastfed infants whose mothers were fed carrot juice during pregnancy or during lactation or breastfeeding showed increased acceptance of carrot flavor in their cereal at weaning (Mennella, Jagnow, and Beauchamp 2001). In another study, infants who were fed a formula made of an unpleasant-tasting, sour and bitter protein (hydrosylate) from birth (from necessity because they did not tolerate milk) drank it well when tested with the hydrosylate formula at 7 months, whereas those fed milk formula rejected it (Mennella, Griffin, and Beauchamp 2004). Infants fed hydrosylate liked sour tastes into early childhood (Liem and Mennella 2002). There appear to be sensitive periods during which early experience has more impact on flavor learning (Trabulsi and Mennella 2012).

Learning from the Physiological Consequences of Eating: Preferences and Aversions

How humans feel physiologically after eating a food can have a powerful impact on food preferences. If eating is followed by negative effects, such as a feeling of nausea, a conditioned aversion follows. Conditioned aversions can be quite powerful. A one-time experience of illness following eating a food can turn us off that food for decades. On the other hand, liking for foods usually develops more slowly through a process of learned or conditioned preference, whereby repeated eating of a food, or familiarity, is followed by pleasant consequences such as a feeling of fullness or satiety.

Conditioning of food preferences continues throughout our lives, but early experience with food and eating is especially crucial in the development of eating patterns, in terms of both the kinds of food we come to like and the amount we eat. Experience with food influences the development of eating patterns of children and adults in several ways.

Exposure, Familiarity, and Learning to Accept New Foods

Humans, like other omnivores, experience the "omnivore's dilemma": we need to seek variety in our diets to meet nutritional requirements, but ingesting new substances can be potentially dangerous (Rozin 1988). This dilemma can be resolved through familiarity and conditioning as described in the following sections.

Neophobia and Picky/Fussy Eating

Although food neophobia, or negative reactions to new foods, is minimal in infants, it increases through early childhood so that 2- to 5-year-olds, like other young omnivores, demonstrate neophobia (Birch 1999; Dovey et al. 2008). This would have adaptive value because infants are fed by adults, whereas toddlers are beginning to explore their world and have not learned yet what is safe to eat and what is not. However, neophobia can be reduced by repeated opportunities to sample new foods, sometimes requiring 6–12 or more exposures (Savage, Fisher, and Birch 2007; Anzman-Frasca et al. 2012), and probably through a "learned safety mechanism." That is, when eating a food is not followed by negative consequences, the child learns it is safe to eat and increased food acceptance results. Once the foods are familiar, the preferences tend to persist (Skinner et al. 2002). In addition, tasting or actual ingestion has been found to be necessary—not just looking at or smelling the food (Savage et al. 2007). Picky or fussy eating is somewhat different—it is the rejection of a large proportion of familiar (as well as new or novel) foods, tending to result in a diet that is lower in variety (Dovey et al. 2008). This quality tends to persist, even into adulthood, and may have a genetic component. Here, even more frequent food exposures may be necessary for acceptance

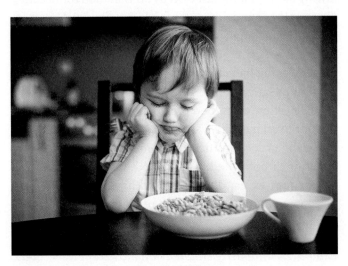

Neophobia increases through early childhood.

© djedzura/iStock/Thinkstock

to occur, presenting a challenge to parents and nutrition educators alike.

In sum, with repeated consumption, preference for initially novel foods tends to increase. Thus, if children are exposed to many high-sugar, high-fat, and high-salt foods at home, at school, and in other settings, then these foods will become more familiar and will become preferred over those that remain relatively unfamiliar, such as vegetables or whole grains (Birch and Anzman-Frasca 2011a).

Experience with Food and the Basic Tastes

Biologically determined behavioral propensities can be modified by experience in adults as well (Pliner, Pelchat, and Grabski 1993; Pelchat and Pliner 1995). For example, those who eat lower-salt diets come to like them more (Mattes 1997). The dislike for bitterness can be overcome, as shown by the study described earlier where infants, with experience, comfortably consumed the bitter protein hydrosylate and by the fact that people come to like a variety of bitter tastes, such as coffee, dark chocolate, or bitter vegetables such as broccoli. Sour tastes, such as vinegar and grapefruit, can also become liked. Likewise, the liking for dietary fat can be modified. Studies have found that those who switched from a high-fat diet to naturally low-fat foods such as grains and vegetables (Mattes 1993) or to reduced-fat foods (Ledikwe et al. 2007) came to like the fat taste less. Maintaining these changed preferences involved continuing to eat these new foods.

Learning What Fullness Means: Conditioned Satiety

Research shows that in both young children and adults, a feeling of fullness or satiety is also influenced by associative conditioning or learning (Birch et al. 1987; Birch and Fisher 1995). The ability of our bodies to learn about how full familiar foods can make us feel may explain how it is that we end meals most often before we have yet experienced the physiological cues that signal satiety. Thus, as a result of repeatedly consuming familiar foods, people's bodies recognize the "filling" and the "fattening" quality of familiar foods and normally make adjustments in what they eat in anticipation of the end of the meal (Stunkard 1975). This is supported by the repeated observations that portion size is influenced by outside events, such as serving size, size of plate, and so forth (Fisher and Kjal 2008; DiSantis et al. 2013).

Our Preference for Calorie-Dense Foods

Humans seem to prefer calorie-dense foods over calorie-dilute versions of the same foods (Birch 1992; Birch and Fisher 1995). The biological mechanism that assists us to like calorie-dense foods was very adaptive when food, and especially calorie-dense food, was scarce and probably explains the universal liking for calorie-dense foods in adults. The finding that tasty high-fat and high-sugar foods induce overeating and obesity in animals (Sclafani and Ackroff 2004, Birch and Anzman-Frasca 2011b) suggests that this feature is less adaptive for humans in today's environment, where calorie-dense foods are widely available.

LEARNING FROM SOCIAL-AFFECTIVE CONTEXT: SOCIAL CONDITIONING

The emotional context, called the social-affective context, of eating also has a powerful impact on food preferences and on the regulation of how much people eat. Food is eaten many times a day, providing opportunities for individuals' emotional responses to the social context of eating to become associated with the specific foods being eaten. This is particularly true in children.

Social Modeling

Children learn about food not only from the direct experience of eating, but also from observing the behaviors of peers and adults (Birch 1999). Familiar adults have been found to be more effective than unfamiliar ones, and having the adults themselves eat the same foods is more effective than when adults offer the foods without eating the foods themselves (Harper and Sanders 1975; Addessi et al. 2005). Food preferences also increase when adults offer the foods in a friendly way (Birch 1999).

Parenting Practices

Parents not only provide genes, but also create a home environment that plays a critical role in shaping children's food preferences, eating behaviors, and energy intake (Savage, Fisher, and Birch 2007; Frankel et al. 2012). Children learn what, when, and how much to eat based on the transmission of cultural and family beliefs, attitudes, and practices. Parenting practices are specific parental actions or behaviors that are designed to influence children's eating behaviors and nourishment. Parents shape children's eating behaviors by the foods they make accessible to children (as food providers), by their own eating styles (as role models), how they discipline their children around food issues, and their actual child feeding practices. These feeding practices may be carried out not only by parents, but also by family and other caregivers, and these practices can encourage healthful eating or modify and interfere with the child's ability to respond to food appropriately.

Parents as Providers of Food

Exposure and accessibility. Parents can shape their children's food preferences by frequently exposing them to healthy foods at home and making them more easily accessible. Putting fruits and vegetables in a place where the child can easily reach them (e.g., in a bowl on the table or on a lower shelf in the refrigerator) and preparing them into sizes that are easy to eat (e.g., fruit cut into bite-size pieces) may increase the child's intake of these foods (Baranowski, Cullen, and Baranowski 1999).

Portion sizes. While very young children seem to be able to adjust their intakes to some extent over time (Cecil et al. 2005), recent studies show that portion sizes influence the amount eaten by children as young as 2 years of age (Fisher 2007; Birch, Savage, and Fisher 2015). Many parents apparently are not concerned about portion sizes for their children (Croker, Sweetman, and Cooke 2009) and yet there are many studies of meals with energy-dense foods that show that the larger the portion size, the more is consumed (Fisher and Kjal 2008; Fisher et al. 2007). In addition, when children are allowed to serve themselves, they tend to eat more (Savage et al. 2012). Thus, parents need to learn more about age-appropriate serving sizes and offer these to children. The good news is that serving vegetables as a soup or first course at the beginning of a meal (Spill et al. 2010, 2011) or placing large amounts of fruits and vegetables on the dinner plate also increases consumption of these items (Mathias et al. 2012).

Parents as Role Models

Parents can indirectly influence their children's eating habits by modeling good eating behaviors. Evidence suggests that parents who eat fruits and vegetables and other healthy foods have children who eat more healthfully (Fisher et al. 2002). The impact of role modeling may be enhanced by positive comments that are tied to the food. Unfortunately, modeling of negative behaviors can have an equally strong, but opposite effect and has been associated with the development of emotional eating, excessive snacking, and body dissatisfaction (Brown and Ogden 2004). Thus, parents and caregivers who offer healthful foods in appropriate portion sizes and enjoy the foods themselves are likely to facilitate healthful eating in their children.

Prompting to Eat Healthful Food and Restricting Access to Less Healthful Food

Prompting or encouraging children to eat healthful foods and restricting less healthful foods are behaviors widely practiced by parents (Savage et al. 2007; O'Connor et al. 2009; Carnell et al. 2011). The relationship of these practices of parents and caregivers to children's preferences and intakes are quite complex (Blisset 2011). Often parents do not trust that their child will select the right kinds and amounts of food and feel that they need to help the child along (Savage et al. 2007). Some research suggests the excessive use of pressure to eat specific—usually healthy—foods is associated with lower intakes and more negative comments about those pressured foods. However, the middle ground of encouragement or prompts to try new foods, in particular vegetables, such as to take at least one bite, may be effective in increasing intake and preference (Blisset 2011). Likewise, very high levels of restriction of children's access or intake of specific foods, usually those that are most tasty because of their high sugar, fat, and/or salt content, may increase preference for and consumption of these items (Savage et al. 2007). Again, a middle ground of mealtime rules and limits on unhealthy snacks seems to be effective.

Interviews with parents suggest that they use a variety of practical strategies to encourage their children to eat healthfully (Carnell et al. 2011; Blisset 2011; O'Connor et al. 2010). These include presenting foods in an attractive way, verbal encouragement, playing games with the child, making eating healthful foods fun, use of teachable moments, involving the child, and flexible responses to individual differences shown by children.

Rewards

The use of rewards is another very common but controversial practice of parents (Ventura and Birch 2008). There is concern that rewards might reduce reasoned action and intrinsic motivation. And indeed, some studies suggested that using rewards did not increase liking for the foods and actually decreased liking. However, these items tended to be those that were initially moderately liked items such as fruits and sweet drinks. There is evidence that non-food tangible rewards (e.g., stickers) or non-tangible rewards (praise) can be highly effective in encouraging children to taste new or initially moderately disliked foods such as vegetables sufficiently often so that children become familiar with the foods and benefit from the familiarity effect (Cooke et al. 2011b).

For example, some studies found that exposure plus rewards increased the liking and intake for the targeted vegetables (Wardle et al. 2003; Remington et al. 2012). In a peer-modeling and reward-based intervention, children aged 4–11 years watched video adventures of heroic cartoon characters eating fruits and vegetables, and were given rewards for tasting the fruits and vegetables that the cartoon models ate. Liking for both fruits and vegetables increased significantly, as did consumption, both immediately after the intervention and at 4-month follow-up after gradual withdrawal of the rewards (Horne et al. 2004, 2011). Social rewards (praise) can be more effective than tangible rewards (Cooke et al. 2011a). Incentives offered in the school context have also increased intake of fruits and vegetables (Hendy, Williams, and Camise 2005). These findings suggest that judicious use of rewards can facilitate healthy eating by getting children to at least try new or initially disliked foods and hence become familiar with them (Cooke et al. 2011a).

Parental Feeding Styles

Parents influence their children's eating not only by their practices but also by their feeding styles. By *parenting feeding styles* we mean the attitudes and beliefs of parents that create the socio-emotional climate in which parenting practices are carried out (Rhee 2008; Blisset 2011). Parental feeding styles vary on the dimensions of responsiveness to the child (warmth and nurturance) versus control (expectations and demands) (Hughes et al. 2005; Blissett 2011). The *authoritarian* feeding style involves high demands and encourages eating using highly controlling behaviors or strict rules, threats, or bribes, with little regard for the child's needs (low in warmth and unresponsive to the child). The *authoritative* style is typified by high demands of the child's diet and eating behavior with a clear set of boundaries, but also by high warmth and sensitivity to child needs. It involves actively encouraging eating through non-directive and supportive behaviors, such as reasoning with the child or explaining why it is important to eat vegetables. By contrast, the *permissive parenting styles* impose little control or demands. There are two types, one where parents are overly *indulgent* (expressing warmth and responsiveness to child needs) and another where parents are *uninvolved/neglectful* (lacking warmth and responsiveness and indifferent to child needs).

There has been considerable concern that the *authoritarian* or controlling feeding style may be detrimental to child healthful eating. Indeed, it has been negatively associated with parents offering and children eating vegetables (Patrick et al. 2005). However, the relationship with child weight is mixed. Some studies have found an association with higher weights of children (Faith et al. 2004; Rhee 2008; Ventura and Birch 2008), and others found that authoritarian parents are equally likely to have normal weight children as overweight children (Robinson et al. 2001; Pai and Contento 2014). On the other hand, the authoritative feeding style, where there are clear boundaries and the child is encouraged to eat healthful foods, but where the child is also given some choice about eating options, all in a warm emotional atmosphere, has been shown to be associated with increased consumption of dairy and vegetables and decreased consumption of sweet drinks (Patrick et al. 2005; O'Connor et al. 2010; van der Horst et al. 2007).

The *permissive* parental feeding styles (both *indulgent* and *uninvolved*) appear to be the most problematic. They are related negatively to children's intake of fruits and vegetables (Blisset 2011) and nutrition-rich foods such as 100% juice, fruit, vegetables, and dairy foods (Hoerr et al.

2009). Permissive styles, in particular the indulgent style, are also most associated with higher levels of overweight in several cultural groups (Rhee 2008; Hughes et al. 2008; Pai and Contento 2014).

In reality, parents use a mixture of styles (although one or another style may dominate) and parenting styles and practices are closely interconnected (O'Connor et al. 2010; Carnell et al. 2011).

Clearly neither too much nor too little control is effective. Encouragement to eat healthy foods is desirable, as are clear boundaries. It is the emotional tone and the way these practices are carried out that is the issue. The authoritative style seems to work best. It is typified by non-controlling practices that encourage healthful eating but do not force consumption, accompanied by moderately restrictive practices about eating less healthful foods and snacks, all in a climate of emotional warmth and sensitivity to the child (Blisset 2011; O'Connor et al. 2010; Satter 2000).

SUMMARY OF OUR EXPERIENCE WITH FOOD

Biologically determined behavioral propensities, physiological mechanisms, and conditioning through experience with food all influence people's sensory experience of food and food preferences. These influences are summarized in **FIGURE 2-2**. Given that energy-dense, high-fat, high-sugar foods are widely available in the environment, tend to be used as rewards, are most often offered in positive social

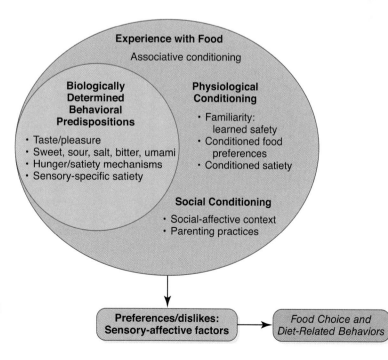

FIGURE 2-2 Our experiences with food influence our food choices and dietary behaviors.

contexts such as celebrations and holidays, are liked by other family members, satisfy biological predispositions, and produce positive feelings of being full, it is not surprising that they become highly preferred by adults and children alike. On the other hand, fewer opportunities are provided for people to learn to like whole grains, fruits, and vegetables in similar social contexts. When such opportunities are provided, children can develop liking for healthy foods such as vegetables (Anzman-Frasca et al. 2012). Practices that encourage healthful eating include making healthful foods available and accessible, offering encouragement to try them, setting boundaries but providing choices among them, and using strategies designed to facilitate acceptance but that are not excessively firm and controlling seem to work best for both children and adults.

Person-Related Determinants

Biology and personal experiences with food are not the only influences on individuals' food intake. Children tend to eat the foods they like and reject the foods they do not like in terms of taste, smell, or texture. However, as individuals become older, they also develop perceptions, expectations, and feelings about foods. These perceptions, attitudes, beliefs, values, emotions, and personal meanings are all powerful determinants of food choice and dietary behavior, as are individuals' interactions with others in their social environment. These influences or determinants are shown in **FIGURE 2-3**. They operate whether people are purchasing groceries at the store, choosing food when eating out, or making food at home.

INTRAPERSONAL DETERMINANTS

Perceptions, Beliefs, Attitudes, and Motivations

Our food choices and dietary practices are powerfully influenced by a variety of personal factors, such as our beliefs about what we will get from these choices. We want our foods to be tasty, convenient, affordable, filling, familiar, or comforting. Our food choices may be determined by the personal meanings we give to certain foods or practices, such as chicken soup when we are ill or chocolate when we feel self-indulgent. We may also be motivated by how the food will contribute to how we look, such as whether it will be fattening or, in contrast, good for our complexion. Our food- and nutrition-related behaviors are also determined

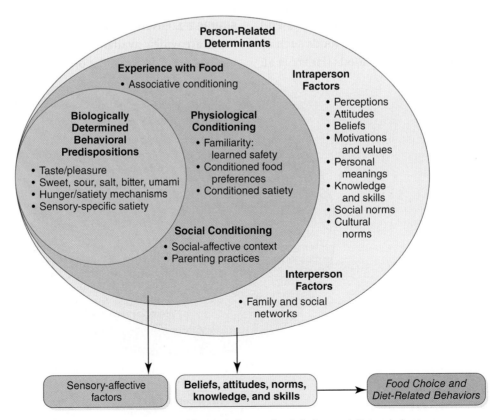

FIGURE 2-3 Intra- and interpersonal factors influence food choices and dietary behaviors.

by our attitudes toward them—for example, our attitudes toward breastfeeding or certain food safety practices.

Our identity in relation to food may also influence our behaviors. For example, some teenagers may see themselves as health conscious, but many others may see themselves as part of the junk-food-eating set. We may see that there are health benefits to eating more healthfully but may consider the barriers, such as high cost or the effort required to prepare the foods in healthful ways, just too great to take action. Or perhaps we lack confidence in preparing foods in ways that are tasty and healthful. Or again, we may have specific culturally related health beliefs that influence what we eat. For example, although the concepts of balance and moderation are common among many cultures, individuals may come from cultures in which foods are believed to have hot and cold qualities and must be eaten in such a way as to balance cold and hot body conditions. These cultural beliefs can have a major influence on food choices.

We come to value some aspects of food over others. In the United States, the major values in choosing foods are taste, convenience, and cost (Glanz et al. 1998; FMI 2012). In Europe, the major values are quality/freshness, price, nutritional value, and family preferences, in that order (Lennernas et al. 1997).

Food rejections are also highly influenced by psychological processes, based on both previous experience and beliefs. Rozin and Fallon (1987) place the motivations for rejecting foods into three main categories: (1) sensory-affective beliefs (e.g., the food will smell or taste bad) that lead to distaste; (2) anticipated consequences or beliefs about the possible harmful outcomes of eating certain foods (e.g., vomiting, disease, social disapproval), leading to danger; and (3) ideation or ideas about the origin or nature of foods, leading to disgust.

Knowledge regarding all these numerous person-related factors is crucial for nutrition educators so that we can better understand and assist our audiences to eat more healthfully (Krebs-Smith et al. 1995). Indeed the next three chapters are devoted to understanding these person-related influences on eating behavior and how we can use such understandings in nutrition education.

The Process of Choosing Foods

Response to Environmental Stimuli

Our thoughts and feelings interact with what we experience in the environment. For example, we may see a news story on the role of fruits and vegetables in reducing cancer risk, or a friend of ours develops colon cancer (external stimuli). We process such environmental stimuli or external events both cognitively and emotionally. These stimuli are filtered through a host of internal personal reactions of the kind listed previously, such as our perceptions, beliefs, values, expectations, or emotions, and together these filters determine what actions we will take. For example, we may process the idea of eating more fruits and vegetables in terms of taste, convenience, expected benefits, perceived barriers, or what our friends and relatives do, in addition to our concerns about getting cancer. Consequently, our decisions about whether to eat more fruits and vegetables to reduce cancer risk are based on our beliefs and knowledge about expected consequences (of eating fruits and vegetables), our motivations and values about desired consequences (reduced risk of cancer), and our personal meanings and values (with respect to developing cancer).

Trade-Offs

In the food choice process, most times we will also need to make trade-offs among various determinants or reasons for food choice, such as trade-offs among health considerations, taste, and cultural expectations. People may also trade off between items within a meal or between meals. For example, individuals may choose an item for its fillingness (e.g., a donut) but then balance it with something perceived as more healthful (e.g., orange juice). Individuals may choose a "healthy" dinner to balance what they consider to have been a less-than-healthful lunch (Contento et al. 2006).

Knowledge and Skills or Nutrition Literacy

People's nutrition literacy or food-related knowledge and skills also influence what they eat. For example, a national survey found that about one-third of individuals thought that the recommended number of servings of fruit and vegetables per day was two or three, and only about 20% thought it was five (National Cancer Institute 2007). Many consumers have difficulty judging the amounts of fat and number of calories in many common foods and in their own diets or knowing what an appropriate serving size should be (Brug, Glanz, and Kok 1997; Chandon and Wansink 2007). Health claims on product labels are hard to evaluate and the symbols used by different companies to indicate food ingredients in the package, such as fiber or sugar, are hard to decode. Lack of skills in preparing foods also influences what individuals eat.

Social, Cultural, and Religious Norms

Humans are social creatures. We all live in a social and cultural context and experience society-wide social norms and cultural expectations, which can be extraordinarily powerful. We feel compelled to subscribe to these norms and expectations to varying degrees. For example, teenagers may feel pressure to eat less-nutritious fast food items in a choice situation with peers (e.g., after school), or individuals may experience family members' expectations that they will eat in a certain way. Whether to breastfeed may be influenced very much by the desires of a woman's family or her husband's family, depending on the culture. Being "large" has positive value in some societies. In the United States there is a saying: "you can never be too rich or too thin," especially when it comes to women. But in some societies, "people share goods, so no one is too rich, and friends share food, so no one is too thin" (Sobo 1997). Indeed weight gain, good appetite, and large stature are signs of good health, good social relations, generosity, and many friends. By contrast, weight loss, a small appetite, and thinness are considered signs of poor health, poor social relations, lack of friends, and meanness (the person did not share food when the person had it and so now the person has no friends to share food with him or her) (Rittenbaugh 1982; Sobo 1997).

Our perceptions of our status and roles in our communities are also important. The food choices and eating patterns of celebrities create social expectations for us all. What others in our community think are appropriate foods to eat in various situations may also create social pressures. Thus, our choice of foods may be heavily influenced by our perceptions of the social and cultural expectations of those around us.

INTERPERSONAL DETERMINANTS

Within societies, we all participate in a network of social relationships, the extensiveness and density of which vary among individuals (Israel and Rounds 1987). These networks involve family, peers, coworkers, and those in various organizations to which we belong. For example, in one study, food choices were 94% similar between spouses, 76–87% similar between adolescents and their parents, and 19% similar between adolescents and their peers

(Feunekes et al. 1998). Food choices and eating patterns are also influenced by the need to negotiate with others in the family about what to buy or eat (Connors et al. 2001; Contento et al. 2006). Relationships with peers and those with whom we work also have an impact on our day-to-day choices (Devine et al. 2003).

Indeed, eating contexts and the management of social relationships in these numerous contexts play a major role in what people eat (Furst el al. 1996). For example, if a woman becomes motivated to reduce her fat intake by using nonfat milk instead of whole milk, she may find that other family members like whole milk and do not want to switch. She must decide whether to go along with family wishes or to buy low-fat milk separately for herself, which then becomes a barrier to change. Or the teenage son may have special food requests and the family needs to decide whether to accommodate the requests.

In addition to the impact of needing to manage social relationships within social networks, social support for healthy eating is also important, especially for those with long-term health conditions such as hypertension or diabetes where following special eating patterns has to be maintained indefinitely (Rosland et al. 2008).

Social and Environmental Determinants

Social and environmental factors are powerful influences on food choice and nutrition-related behaviors and must be considered by nutrition educators in planning programs.

PHYSICAL/BUILT ENVIRONMENT

The built environment includes all aspects of the environment that are modified by humans, including food outlets (e.g., grocery stores), homes, schools, workplaces, parks, industrial areas, and highways. There is a growing body of evidence that the built environments in relation to food and physical activity have important impacts on health (Sallis and Glanz 2009; Ding et al. 2013).

Food Availability, Accessibility, and Quality

In developed countries and increasingly in less developed countries, food and processed food products are available in an ever-widening array of choices. More than 40,000 food items are available in U.S. supermarkets, and about 9,000 new brand name processed food products are introduced each year (FMI 2012, 2013). The typical shopper averages 2.2 trips to the supermarket each week (FMI 2013). Overall availability may be described as the array of food options that are present in the food system that are acceptable and affordable. Accessibility may be thought of as "immediate" availability, referring to the readiness and convenience of a food—whether the food requires little or no cooking, is packaged in a convenient way so that it can be eaten anywhere, or whether it can be stored for some time without spoilage. Food quality has many meanings, but here is used to refer to whether the foods were produced in an environmentally sustainable manner and are wholesome (Gussow 2006). Availability of such foods influences the quality and healthfulness of the diet.

Markets

Studies have shown that the availability of more healthful options in neighborhood grocery stores, such as fruits and vegetables or low-fat milk, is correlated with these foods being more available in homes, which in turn is related to a higher quality of food choices and intakes (Morland, Wing, and Diez Roux 2002; Powell et al. 2007; Boone-Heinonen et al. 2011). Thus, what is available in the community influences what is purchased and consumed. The availability and accessibility of fruits and vegetables at home and school enable their consumption by children (Hearn et al. 1998). Many low-income and minority neighborhoods have fewer supermarket chains that have a wider range of foods and cheaper prices. There is now discussion of "food deserts" to describe the lack of healthy foods at affordable prices in neighborhoods (Ver Ploeg et al. 2009; United States Department of Agriculture [USDA] 2012a). Just as important, and maybe more so, is the notion of "food swamps" or the overabundance of less healthy foods in neighborhood (Rose et al. 2009; Boone-Heinonen et al. 2011). Certainly youth report this as a major temptation to eat high-calorie food products and beverages and a barrier to healthful eating (Koch et al. 2015).

Accessibility also is dependent on where sources of food are physically located. Supermarkets, where a wide range of foods is available, may require transportation to reach, limiting the accessibility of food for many people, such as older people who are no longer able to drive or lower-income people without cars. The types of foods that are readily available in the local grocery stores, small

corner stores, and restaurants within a given community depend on potential profits, consumer demand, and adequate storage and refrigeration facilities. The foods served or products stocked thus tend to be those that sell well, which are not always the most nutritious. Farmers' markets provide fresh, local foods but may require transportation to reach and are often only seasonal. Hence, some foods that are very important for health, such as fruits and vegetables, may not be readily accessible or are available only at a higher cost.

Workplaces, Schools, and Homes

Foods available at or near workplaces also tend to be those that are convenient, low in cost, and that sell well. In most schools, food is available and accessible. In the United States, the National School Lunch Program provides meals that conform to federal guidelines that specify nutritional standards. Participation in the program declines with age so that by high school two-thirds of students obtain their lunch from other sources. The majority of competitive foods in these other venues have been found to be high-fat and high-sugar items, including snack chips, candy, and soft drinks. In some countries commercial vendors provide meals for purchase. It has been shown that what is available in school environments affects the dietary behaviors of children (Briefel et al. 2009). Within the home, accessibility means that clean and safe water is easy to reach, a vegetable is not just available in the refrigerator but is already cut up and ready to eat, or fruit has been washed and is sitting on a table ready to eat. The limited accessibility of healthful, convenient foods in many settings may narrow good choices and make it difficult to eat healthfully.

Behavioral Economics and Environmental Change

In this context, nutrition educators can use behavioral economics principles in their work (Hanks, Just, and Wansink 2013; Wansink et al. 2012). Given that external cues can have a major effect on the food selected and the amount consumed, adjusting these factors can have a major impact on how much is eaten for a meal or snack. Here, we can implement changes to make the healthier options more attractive, convenient, and normative, which can nudge people to eat the healthier options. See Nutrition Education in Action 2-2, later in the chapter for how this approach is being used in school lunchrooms.

Built Environment and Physical Activity

The role of environmental determinants of physical activity has also been studied. The walkability of neighborhoods as well as the availability and accessibility of neighborhood safe parks, green spaces, and physical activity facilities have been shown to have some impact on physical activity or obesity of residents in those neighborhoods (Ferreira et al. 2007; Wendel-Vos et al. 2007).

Social and Cultural Environment

Social environments and cultural contexts are no less important than the physical environment. Social influences and cultural practices all influence food choice and dietary behavior (Rozin 1996).

Social Relations

Society has been described as a group of people interacting in a common territory who have shared institutions, characteristic relationships, and a common culture. Most eating occurs in the presence of other people. The effect can be positive or negative in terms of healthful eating, in part because family and friends serve as models as well as sources of peer pressure. For example, there is evidence that eating with others can lead to eating more food compared with eating alone, especially when the others are familiar people (de Castro 2000; Salvy et al. 2009). Spending more time at a meal eating with others also increases intake. Eating with others can result in pressure to eat higher-fat foods. On the other hand, eating with others can also result in pressure to try new foods that are healthy (MacIntosh 1996). Parents' own eating patterns likely influence those of their children (Fisher et al. 2002; Contento et al. 2006), and it has been shown that children and adolescents who eat with their families most days each week have better-quality diets than those who eat with their families less frequently (Gillman et al. 2000; Berge et al. 2013).

Cultural Practices and Family of Origin

Culture has been described as the knowledge, traditions, beliefs, values, and behavioral patterns that are developed, learned, shared, and transmitted by members of a group. It is a worldview that a group shares, and hence it influences perceptions about food and health. Cultural practices and family of origin have an important impact on food choices and eating practices even in modern, multiethnic societies where many different types of cuisine are available. Those from different regions of the country may have different practices. For example, for those from the American South a home-style meal is chicken-fried steak, mashed potatoes, corn bread, and bacon- and onion-laden green beans, with pie for dessert, whereas those who live in Texas may expect to eat barbecue or Tex-Mex foods that are hot and spicy. Those who have immigrated from different countries from around the world maintain some of their cultural practices in varying degrees, chief among them traditions that influence eating patterns. Religious practices also influence what is eaten (Satia-Abouta et al. 2002).

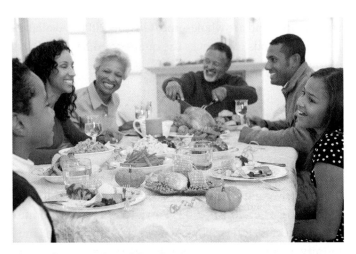

Most eating occurs in social settings.
© Monkey Business Images/ShutterStock, Inc.

Cultural rules often specify which foods are considered acceptable and preferable, and the amount and combination of various categories of foods that are appropriate for various occasions. The cultural practices of family and friends, especially at times of special celebrations and holidays, provide occasions to eat culturally or ethnically determined foods and reinforce the importance of these foods. If dietary recommendations based on health considerations conflict with family, cultural, and religious traditions, individuals who want to make dietary changes may find themselves having to think about and integrate their cultural expectations with their concern about their personal health. All of these considerations influence individuals' willingness and ability to make changes in their diets. These beliefs and practices must be carefully understood so that nutrition educators can become culturally competent and can design culturally sensitive nutrition education programs.

Social Structures and Policy

The organizations to which we belong can have a profound effect on our eating patterns. Some are voluntary organizations, such as religious, social, or community organizations; others include schools, our places of work, and professional associations to which we belong. The influence of these organizations comes from their social norms as well as their policies and practices. Local, state, and national government policy can govern and determine the availability and accessibility of opportunities for healthy eating and active living.

ECONOMIC ENVIRONMENT

Many factors in the economic environment influence food choices and dietary practices, among them the price of food, income, time, and formal education. Nutrition educators must consider these factors when designing nutrition education programs.

Price

Economic theory assumes that relative differences in prices can partially explain differences among individuals in terms of their food choices and dietary behaviors. The price of food as purchased is usually per item, by unit weight, or by volume. However, price can also be considered in terms of the amount of food energy obtained per dollar. Processed foods with added fats and sugar are cheaper to manufacture, transport, and store than are perishable meats, dairy products, and fresh produce. This is partly because sugar and fat on their own are both very inexpensive, which is in part a result of government agricultural policies. A diet made up of refined grains and processed foods with added sugar and fats can be quite

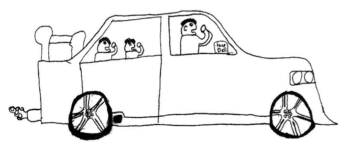

This child was asked to draw a picture of her family eating their favorite meal together.

Courtesy of Cooking with Kids.

inexpensive (a day's worth of calories for 2–3 dollars). Beans cost about the same, but animal protein sources may cost 5 to 10 times more per calorie, and fruits and vegetables (except potatoes and bananas) can cost some 50 to 100 times more per calorie than high-fat, high-sugar, mass-produced food products (Drewnowski 2012). Not surprisingly, low-income individuals eat fewer fruits and vegetables. These disparities in cost may also contribute to the higher prevalence of obesity in those of lower socioeconomic status.

Income and Resources

People in the United States and United Kingdom spend only about 8–10% of their income on food, compared with 15% in Europe and Japan, 35% in middle-income countries, and 45–50% in low-income countries (Muhammad et al. 2011; USDA 2012b; *Washington State Magazine* 2013). However, this is an average. The amount of money spent on food depends on income level within a country. Upper-income individuals in the United States spend more money on food, but it is a smaller proportion of their income—about 8%. Lower-income households economize by buying discounted items and generic brands and thus spend less on food; despite this, food accounts for 25–35% of their income (Thompson 2013; U.S. Department of Labor 2013b). Compared with other economic variables, income has the strongest marginal impact (i.e., additional effect) on diet behavior: those with higher incomes eat a higher-quality diet (Macino, Lin, and Ballenger 2004). Other material resources also influence diet—those below certain poverty levels in many countries qualify for government assistance—such as free or reduced price meals for children at school, food coupons in some form, or direct cash aid (U.S. Department of Labor 2013b). These may improve the quality of diets.

In this context, statistics show that about 14.5% of American households are food insecure, meaning that they have limited or uncertain availability of nutritionally adequate and safe foods or limited or uncertain ability to acquire acceptable foods in socially acceptable ways. Within this category, about 6% are very food insecure (USDA 2013).

Time Use and Household Structure

Surveys and time use diaries show that the amount of time people spend on food-related activity in the home depends on many factors, including whether men or women are employed outside the home and whether they have children (Robinson and Godbey 1999). In the United States, women spend an average of 8 hours per week and men 5 hours in food preparation and cleanup activities (U.S. Department of Labor 2013a).

Time is scarce for all households, regardless of income. Many people with whom nutrition educators work today say they are too busy to prepare healthful foods or to cook at all. This is particularly true of low-income families who often work long hours. For some households, time constraints may limit personal investments in healthier behaviors. For example, it has been found that men and women who are married with children have a higher-quality diet than single parents, probably because they can share child care duties and thus are better able to attend to their own health (Macino, Lin, and Ballenger 2004). Nutrition educators need to consider these time constraints in the development of nutrition education interventions. (However, it should be noted that Americans spend an average of 25 hours per week watching television and another 3 hours per week on computer use for leisure.)

Educational Level

In general, more highly educated individuals eat a higher-quality diet and are less sedentary partly because they watch less TV (Macino et al. 2004). People with more education may be better able to obtain, process, interpret, and apply information that can make them more able to eat healthfully. They also may be more forward looking and optimistic about their future and thus willing to seek

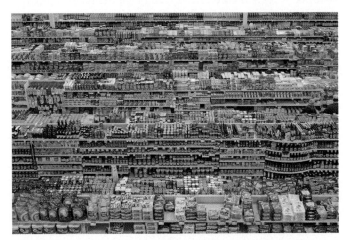

Consumers are inundated with food choices at the supermarket.

Photo by Lyza, https://www.flickr.com/photos/lyza/49545547/in/photolist-5nWaz-9Gd5xM. Used under Creative Commons Attribution-ShareAlike 2.0 Generic.

health information and make greater investments in their health (Macino et al. 2004).

Grocery Shopping Trends

The influences described earlier affect how people shop for food. Surveys of grocery shoppers have found that about one-third of shoppers are economizers, who are budget conscious and usually come from lower-income households. They plan weekly menus, check for sales, and use coupons. Another third are carefree spenders, who are the least price conscious and least likely to compare prices and use coupons. The final third are time-challenged shoppers who are obsessed with convenience because of their hectic, multitasking lifestyles. They have the largest households and are most likely to have preteen children (FMI 2012).

INFORMATION ENVIRONMENT

Knowing the information context of the audience is important for nutrition educators to design messages and programs that are appropriate (see **BOX 2-1**).

Media

The current media-saturated environment has undergone revolutionary changes in the past 2 decades, resulting in the availability to individuals and households of numerous television channels, radio stations, websites, and other emerging communication routes. Time spent on these various media is high: children aged 2–4 years are exposed to about 4 hours per day of various media. This increases to 8 hours per day in middle school, in consideration of the fact that adolescents often use several media simultaneously. Television viewing is dominant and increases to 25 hours per week through childhood and then declines somewhat in adolescence to 19 hours per week as music becomes more important. Adults spend about 15–17 hours per week on television viewing. The media are the main source of information about food and nutrition for many people, making them collectively a major source of informal nutrition education. Information about food and nutrition is now widely covered in newspaper articles, magazines, and television programs. Many magazines are devoted to health and nutrition, and entire channels on TV are devoted to food-related shows. As **NUTRITION EDUCATION IN ACTION 2-1** shows, media and other influences also affect the decisions mothers make with regard to their children.

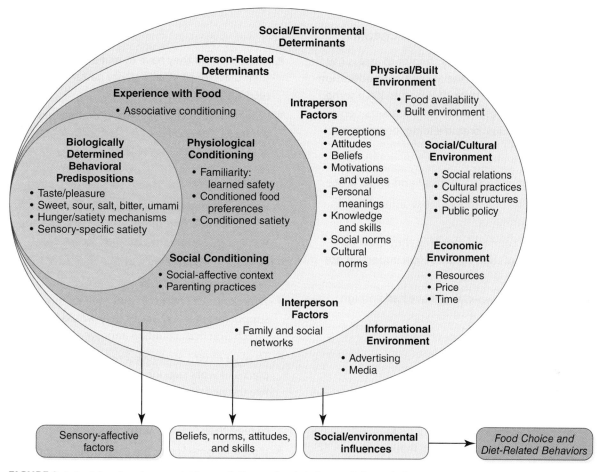

FIGURE 2-4 Social and environmental factors influence food choices and dietary behaviors.

Advertising

The media have demonstrated a powerful capacity to persuade. Today advertising occurs in a variety of venues such as magazines, the Internet, and video games as well as television. The U.S. food industry spends close to $10 billion per year on food marketing and advertising (Federal Trade Commission [FTC] 2012), with $1.8 billion aimed at children. Most of this is spent by companies that produce high-fat and high-sugar products that are highly processed and packaged; examples include $800 million for snack foods, $3.5 billion for beverages, and more than $3 billion for restaurants/fast foods (FTC 2012). Food advertising is strong in Europe and other countries as well (World Health Organization 2013). Information on the impact of marketing on sales of food products is not easily available because it is considered proprietary information. However, there is evidence that these marketing activities influence food choices (Story and French 2004; Institute of Medicine 2006). The ubiquity of advertising, together with

the amount of time people spend watching television and being exposed to marketing, makes these influences considerable. The environmental influences on food choice and dietary behavior are summarized in **FIGURE 2-4**.

What Does All This Mean for Nutrition Educators?

It is important for nutrition educators to realize that many factors influence eating behavior and that nutrition education needs to develop strategies to address these influences, often referred to as *determinants* of behavior.

In Figure 2-4, a series of concentric circles schematically represents the ways in which biological, experiential, personal, social, and environmental determinants influence food choice and diet-related practices. No factor is independent of any other, rather, they are all related, each larger circle encompassing the influences of the smaller

BOX 2-1 Assessing our Audiences: A Checklist

We can use the information in this chapter to assess our audiences in order to ensure that our nutrition education is appropriately tailored to them. It is best to have some specific behavior changes in mind for this assessment, such as eating vegetables, breastfeeding, or managing diabetes:

Food-related determinants: biology and experience

- What are their favorite foods? Most disliked foods? Why?
- What are some comfort foods that they grew up with or are part of their culture? How important are these to them?
- How do they judge when they have had enough to eat?
- How willing are they to try new foods?

Person-related determinants

- What does the term [healthy eating] [eating vegetables] [breastfeeding] [buying sustainably produced foods] mean to them?
- How important is [healthy eating] [eating vegetables] [breastfeeding] [buying sustainably produced foods] to them?
- What are some culturally expected behaviors in relation to diet (and physical activity)?
- What are some diet-related behaviors expected of them because of their role or status (e.g., mothers, managers)?
- How motivated are they to make the changes in their diets (or physical activity patterns) toward recommendations?

- What skills do they have to make the changes in their diets (or physical activity patterns) toward recommendations?
- What family or social networks do they have that would be supportive of the behavior (or physical activity) changes they wish to make?

Social and environmental determinants

- How easily can they get the foods they need from the stores near them? What kinds of stores are these (e.g., supermarkets, small stores, etc.)?
- How satisfied are they with the quality of these foods?
- What kinds of practices from their culture are supportive of the changes they would like to make? Which practices could be improved?
- To what extent are foods available at or near their places of work supportive of healthful eating? Are the policies at work supportive of breastfeeding?
- Do they feel they have enough healthful food to feed their families throughout the month?
- If their income is low, are they eligible for food assistance programs? Which ones? How helpful are these for making the behavior changes they would like to make?
- What media do they watch or use? How much time do they spend on these in a typical week?
- What are their major sources of information for food, nutrition, or physical activity?

These questions are the basis of the assessment described in Chapter 8.

---

circles. These concentric circles reflect levels of influence or overlapping spheres of influence.

KNOWLEDGE OR NUTRITION LITERACY IS NOT ENOUGH

Knowledge is needed for people to be able to make wise choices and to take action. But Figure 2-4 shows us that knowledge is only one of many, many influences on, or determinants of, food choice and diet-related behaviors.

In addition, consumers in the United States often say they already know enough. For example, one survey found that 7 of 10 consumers said their diet needed some improvement. Guilt, worry, fear, helplessness, and anger were the primary emotions expressed about their diets. However, they said they knew enough about nutrition: "Don't tell us more" (IFIC Foundation 1999). Another survey found that about 25% said they "always" felt comfortable selecting healthy foods when grocery shopping and another 50% said "most of the time" (Supermarket News 2013).

Clearly, although many Americans say their diets need improvement, they also indicate that they are knowledgeable about nutrition and are just unable to change or are uninterested in changing. Thus, many other factors besides knowledge must influence or determine their food choices and diet-related behaviors. To be successful, nutrition education also must address these other determinants, which are discussed below in the three categories of food-related determinants; person-related determinants; and social and environmental determinants.

NUTRITION EDUCATION ADDRESSING FOOD-RELATED DETERMINANTS

Addressing food-related determinants is very important in nutrition education. Food is a powerful primary reinforcer that produces instant gratification in taste and a sense of satisfaction and fullness. Because taste or preference is also shaped by repeated experience with foods and eating, nutrition educators working with any age group need to create opportunities to offer nutritious and healthy foods such as fruits and vegetables frequently in a positive social-affective context so that individuals will come to like nutritious foods. Cooking and gardening experiences can be particularly helpful strategies because they provide opportunities for people to become familiar with and enjoy healthful foods and to learn how to make healthy foods taste good. Similarly, interventions to decrease the intake of food components such as fat or salt should help people adopt eating plans that include foods naturally low in these components for a long enough time that people can become used to them and come to like them. Indeed, in a long-term nutrition education intervention with women, those who were able to stay with a low-fat diet for 2 years or more were those who came to dislike the taste of fat (Bowen et al. 1994).

NUTRITION EDUCATION IN ACTION 2-1 Multiple Influences on Breastfeeding: A Study of Low-Income Mothers

Media influences: TV shows and print media foster the perception that formula feeding is the norm whereas breastfeeding is not. Instead, women's breasts are used to advertise lingerie, perfume, or alcohol: these images influence personal beliefs.

Policy influences: There is legislation that supports breastfeeding in the work setting. Low income mothers receiving benefits need to work after a certain time, thus making breastfeeding difficult.

Community and organizational factors: Workplaces can be supportive or not. Baby-friendly hospitals can encourage breastfeeding, whereas free infant formula packages on discharge do not. Returning to work predicts quitting breastfeeding after having initiated it in the hospital.

Interpersonal factors: The father of the baby can be a major influence, followed by the mother's mother. Cultural beliefs are also a factor, such as the belief that women may not have enough milk, particularly when babies are "greedy."

Personal factors: Beliefs, knowledge, and skills. The study found that cultural beliefs positive to breastfeeding were often outweighed by personal beliefs or anticipation that breastfeeding would be painful. There also were concerns about the appropriateness of feeding in public settings because of sexual images in the media, or the disapproval of the baby's father.

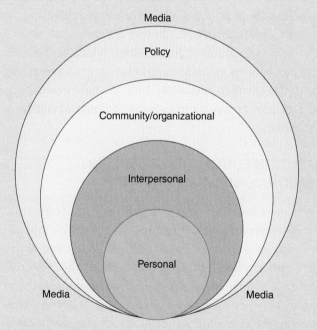

Modified from Bentley, M. E., D. L. Dee, and J. L. Jensen. 2003. Breastfeeding among low-income, African-American women: Power, beliefs and decision-making. *Journal of Nutrition* 133:305S–309S. Used with permission of the American Society for Nutrition and the authors.

As nutrition educators, we can also work with families and caregivers in preschool and school settings to assist them to adopt practices that encourage healthful eating, such as making healthful foods available and easily accessible, modeling the desired behavior, serving age-appropriate serving sizes, providing healthful options and allowing the child to choose among them, encouraging children to taste the desired foods, using rewards appropriately so children can acquire preferences for healthful food, moderately restricting unhealthful snack foods, using teachable moments, and giving flexible responses to individual differences shown by children. Most of these practices work with adults as well.

NUTRITION EDUCATION ADDRESSING PERSON-RELATED DETERMINANTS

Although biological mechanisms and food-related experiences influence eating behaviors directly, psychological processes can be perhaps even more powerful. Individuals develop attitudes toward foods, values, feelings, beliefs, and personal meanings, and these intra- and interpersonal determinants also influence food choices and eating patterns. In fact, it is clear that such factors play a central role in food-related behaviors. As Epictetus said many hundreds of years ago, "We are troubled not so much by events themselves but by the views we take of them." This is good news for nutrition educators because these perceptions, attitudes, and beliefs are to some extent modifiable through education. Indeed, these perceptions and attitudes form a central focus of much of nutrition education.

NUTRITION EDUCATION ADDRESSING ENVIRONMENTAL DETERMINANTS

Nutrition education needs to address environmental factors by promoting the increased availability and accessibility of wholesome and healthful foods and active living options, and by taking into account the resources people have, their social networks and relationships, and the influence of media and advertising. Nutrition education must also address social structures and policy. However, we need to recognize that these environmental determinants are also filtered by people's attitudes, beliefs, and values, which in turn influence food choices and dietary behavior.

Availability: Reality and Perception

Availability, for example, means different things to different people. Recent immigrants may consider familiar food products "available" even if a long car or subway ride is needed to get to stores where the food is stocked. For others, a food is not available if it cannot be cooked in the microwave and ready to eat in 5 minutes. Such differences in the interpretation of availability influence individuals' food choices.

Economic Environment: Reality and Perception

Likewise, the economic environment is based on the analyses, values, and interpretations of individuals, all of which have an impact on dietary choices. Economics is a behavioral science based on the fundamental notion that human wants are infinitely expansible, whereas the means to satisfy them are finite. Human wants always exceed the means to satisfy them, and there is, therefore, scarcity. (This has been simplified to the statement that human greed is infinite whereas the means to satisfy that greed are finite.) Economics is the study of people's reaction to the fact of scarcity—how people make choices when they must choose among alternatives to satisfy their wants. Economics is concerned with desired scarce goods, not free goods, such as air in natural settings, because free goods do not present a problem of choice. Cost can be seen as the sacrifice, or what needs to be exchanged, to obtain what is desired. In this context, the full price of a food or dietary practice is not just its monetary price but includes all the costs or sacrifices individuals make, such as travel costs, time, or child-care costs while shopping. For example, a person may be willing to exchange money for time by purchasing a food that is already prepared. As nutrition educators, we need to learn about the sacrifices individuals are willing to make to engage in a healthy behavior. How willing are they to sacrifice convenience for more healthful meals?

Time: Reality and Perception

In the same way, time is both an objective feature of life and a perception. The time for food-related tasks such as cooking or eating can be easily quantified in hours and minutes. However, the *perception* of time and its worth to individuals for different tasks varies considerably. For example, the time required to make decisions about food has increased because information has become more complex. As we noted before, there are about 40,000 items in a supermarket and about 9,000 new food items are introduced each year that people must learn about. No longer do people choose from three or four types of cold breakfast cereal, but instead from a whole supermarket aisle of cereals. This takes time.

In addition, people have become more avid consumers and consumption takes time: it takes time to use all the gadgets and objects that people have acquired, particularly electronic devices such as cell phones, music players, and televisions. To overcome the scarcity of time, people do more than one thing at once, multitasking. Add to that the economic necessity of two jobs for many and it is not surprising that the perception is that there is not just scarcity of time, but a time famine. This has

impacts that are important for nutrition educators. For example, low-wage employed parents find there is spillover from working long hours into family food-related tasks (Devine et al. 2006). There is stress and fatigue; parents reduce the time and effort spent on family meals, they make trade-offs with other family needs, and they have to develop various time management strategies to cope. Nutrition educators need to be mindful of people's real and perceived economic and time constraints and how they make choices in light of these constraints. **NUTRITION EDUCATION IN ACTION 2-2** showcases programs that were created to work with economic and time constraints, and to use behavioral economics to help people eat better.

NUTRITION EDUCATION IN ACTION 2-2 Programs to Address Economic and Time Restraints

Barbershop Nutrition Education

Prostate cancer is twice as high in African American men as in white men. Eating fruits and vegetables may help to reduce risk. A novel site for nutrition education was the barbershop. A program was delivered to African American men while they were waiting for service. A set of five true or false statements was developed about the rate of prostate cancer in men and the role of fruits and vegetables in cancer risk reduction. The men were asked to answer them, and then the nutrition educator went over the answers. The men could keep the statements and the answer sheet. This simple intervention increased awareness of both prostate cancer and ways to reduce risk.

People at Work: 5-a-Day Tailgate Sessions

Because many people working in factories and other similar locations do not have time to go to a different site for nutrition education sessions, the nutrition educator can go to them. At one sawmill, the workers ate their lunches from coolers in their cars. The nutrition educator therefore met them in the parking lot and provided monthly tailgate sessions over the course of a year (including through the Midwestern winter), providing a different food each time that involved interesting ways to use fruits and vegetables (such as baked apples, chili, or vegetable wraps). The focus was on how to incorporate fruits and vegetables into meals and snacks. The results showed that the workers' interest and motivation

were enhanced, as were skills in incorporating more fruits and vegetables in their diets.

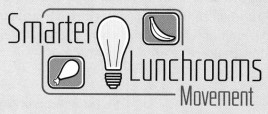

Smarter Lunchroom is a Trademark of the Cornell Center for Behavioral Economics In Child Nutrition Programs. Used by permission.

Smarter Lunchrooms Movement in U.S. Schools

Children in the United States are usually served lunches in school, with reduced price and free meals available for those with low incomes. External cues can have a major effect on the food selected and the amount consumed. Adjusting these factors can have a major impact on how much is eaten for a meal or snack. In a behavioral economics approach, changes are made to these environmental factors to nudge children to eat the healthier options. For example, making items more *attractive* by changing the names, such as "X-ray Vision Carrots" and displaying fresh fruit attractively in bowls or baskets increases consumption. When healthful items are made more *convenient* by placing them in the front of the food line, students will choose them more often (Wansink et al. 2012; Hanks, Just, and Wansink 2013).

http://smarterlunchrooms.org

Summary: Nutrition Education Addresses Determinants of Behavior

In summary, people's perceptions and attitudes form a central focus of much of nutrition education. Thus, nutrition education can be seen as the process of addressing all the major categories of determinants, as shown in **FIGURE 2-5**, with personal perception interacting with all of them. Building on the contemporary definition of nutrition education, Figure 2-5 shows that nutrition education is directed at:

- *Biology and food experiences* by providing food tasting and cooking experiences to increase familiarity and preferences for healthy foods.
- *Person-related determinants* by providing audiences with educational experiences on *why-to* take action on healthy food choices and diet-related behaviors (through addressing people's perceptions, attitudes, norms and self-efficacy) and *how-to* take action (through addressing knowledge and skills).
- *Social/environmental determinants* by providing environmental and policy supports through facilitating opportunities for when and where to take action on healthy choices.

Exactly how nutrition education activities can address these determinants of food choice and dietary behaviors is described in detail in the remaining chapters in this book.

Implications for Competencies and Skills Needed by Nutrition Educators

Nutritionists and dietitians are well grounded in nutrition science and medical nutrition therapy and are anxious to transmit what they know to a variety of audiences in exciting ways. They are less well grounded in the social sciences, particularly the behavioral sciences and the field of communications. Yet as we have seen, food choices and dietary behaviors are determined by a multitude of factors. Understanding behavior and its context is crucial for effective nutrition education. Consequently, what the field needs is nutritionists who are sufficiently conversant with the relevant fields of behavioral science and communications to be able to design effective nutrition education programs. This book aims to help nutritionists develop these competencies.

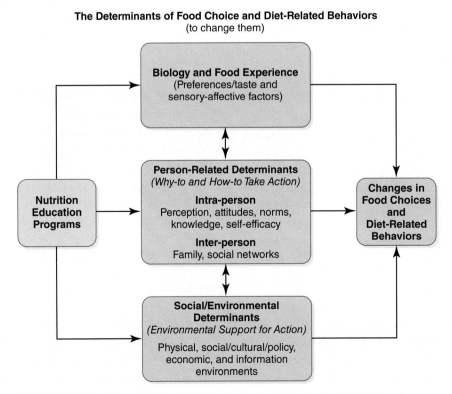

The Determinants of Food Choice and Diet-Related Behaviors
(to change them)

FIGURE 2-5 Nutrition education addresses the many determinants of behavior.

THE SOCIETY FOR NUTRITION EDUCATION AND BEHAVIOR'S COMPETENCIES FOR NUTRITION EDUCATION SPECIALISTS

The Society for Nutrition Education and Behavior is updating its list of competencies (SNEB 1987) that nutrition educators should have. The revised draft list is summarized below. Please check its website for the final updated list of competencies (www.sneb.org).

1. *Basic food and nutrition knowledge:* Describe the fundamentals of nutrition science, food groups and the dietary guidelines; ability to explain different types of nutrition-related study designs and accurately assess nutrition-related claims

2. *Nutrition across the life cycle:* Identify the primary dietary issues and challenges at different phases of the life cycle and use dietary guidelines to make recommendations

3. *Food science:* Identify the effects of food processing and culinary practices on food and best practices to address safe food handling

4. *Food policy:* Understanding the purpose, funding and implementation of various government food-related programs; the roles of government agencies in regulating food and dietary supplements

5. *Agriculture/food systems:* Describe the potential effects of differences in agricultural practices and various food processing, packaging, distribution, and marketing practices on food choices and food availability; explain effects of natural resources on the quantity and quality of the food and water supply

6. *Behavior and education: theory:* Describe the biological, psychological, social, cultural, political, and economic determinants of eating behavior; psychosocial theories of behavior and behavior change and apply them; and apply theory-based learning and instruction practices in nutrition education

7. *Nutrition education: implementation:* Assess population to design and evaluate nutrition education for all ages and diverse audiences using the following steps: determine the behavior change goals of the program; identify theory-based mediators and facilitators of behavior change, including social and environmental influences; select appropriate theoretical models; determine objectives to address mediators; select or design appropriate strategies/techniques; develop a budget; and design **evaluation** and assess progress

8. *Written, oral, and social media communication:* Communicate effectively with diverse audiences, both orally and in writing, and advocate effectively for nutrition education and healthy diets in various sectors

9. *Nutrition education research methods:* Analyze, evaluate, and interpret nutrition education research and apply it to practice

ACADEMY OF NUTRITION AND DIETETICS COMPETENCIES

The Academy of Nutrition and Dietetics' accreditation standards for the education of entry-level dietitians (Academy of Nutrition and Dietetics 2012) include some competencies that are related to nutrition education.

Core Knowledge for the Registered Dietitian

- The curriculum must include opportunities to develop a variety of communication skills sufficient for entry into pre-professional practice. (KRD 2.1)
  (Tip: Students must be able to demonstrate effective and professional oral and written communication and documentation.)

- The curriculum must include the role of environment, food, nutrition, and lifestyle choices in health promotion and disease prevention. (KRD 3.2)
  (Tip: Students must be able to develop interventions to affect change and enhance wellness in diverse individuals and groups.)

- The curriculum must include education and behavior change theories and techniques. (KRD 3.3)
  (Tip: Students must be able to develop an educational session or program/educational strategy for a target population.)

- The behavioral and social science foundation of the dietetics profession must be evident in the curriculum. Course content must include concepts of human behavior and diversity, such as psychology, sociology, or anthropology. (KRD 5.3)

Summary

People's food choices and nutrition-related practices are determined by many factors. This has consequences for nutrition education.

BIOLOGY AND PERSONAL EXPERIENCE WITH FOOD

Humans are born with biological predispositions toward liking the sweet, salty, and umami tastes and rejecting sour and bitter tastes. Some genetic differences exist between individuals in sensitivity to tastes, and these may influence food choices. However, individuals' preferences for specific foods and food acceptance patterns are largely learned from familiarity with these foods. People's liking for foods thus can be modified by repeated exposure to them. Sense of fullness is also learned.

- Check out the food preferences and prior experiences with food when you work with an audience. Provide food experiences to the extent that you can.

PERSON-RELATED DETERMINANTS

People acquire knowledge and develop perceptions, expectations, and feelings about foods. These perceptions, attitudes, beliefs, values, personal meanings, and perceived cultural norms are all powerful determinants of food choice and dietary behavior. Families, social networks, and cultural group also influence food choices.

- Conduct a thorough assessment of your audience before you design any nutrition education in terms of their beliefs, attitudes, values, cultural group membership, social networks, and food and nutrition-related knowledge and skills. Check out your own cultural competence.

SOCIAL/ENVIRONMENTAL DETERMINANTS

The physical/built environment influences the foods that are available and accessible as well as venues for active living such as walkable streets and attractive parks. Cultural practices, social structures, and social policies make it easier or harder to be healthy. The economic determinants of behavior include the price of food, income, time, and education. The information environment, including the media, is very powerful in influencing people's food choices.

- Understand fully the social, economic, and cultural settings of your audience so that the recommendations you provide are appropriate.

KNOWLEDGE AND SKILLS ARE NOT ENOUGH

Consequently, knowledge and skills are not enough for people to eat healthfully and live actively. Nutrition education must address these many other food, person, and environmental determinants of behavior if it is to be effective.

- Check that your sessions or intervention includes activities that address motivation as well as knowledge and skills and takes into account other influences on behavior.

CONSEQUENCES FOR THE SKILLS OF NUTRITION EDUCATORS

These considerations make it clear that nutrition educators need an additional set of skills beyond our knowledge of food and nutrition. We need to develop the skills to understand people, their behavior, and the context of their behavior in order to create programs to address these factors.

- Review your knowledge and skills as an educator and check what skills you still need to enhance.

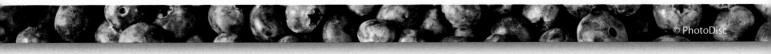

© PhotoDisc

Questions and Activities

1. Think about the influences on your eating and physical activity behaviors and list them. Compare them to the categories of influences described in this chapter. Into which categories do the items on your list fall? Are there some surprises? How would you describe the motivations for your eating patterns?

2. List at least five biological predispositions people are born with, and describe each in a sentence or so. Are they modifiable? If so, provide the evidence. How can the information be useful to nutrition educators?

3. One often hears parents say that their child will just not eat certain healthful foods, such as vegetables.

They believe that such dislikes cannot be changed. Based on the evidence, what would you say to such a parent?

4. How can nutrition educators help young children learn to self-regulate the amount of food they eat?

5. "You can have dessert if you eat your spinach." Is this a strategy you would recommend to parents and child-care personnel to use to get children to like spinach? Why or why not?

6. Influences on dietary behavior arising from within the person have been stated to be central to his or her food choices and dietary practices. Why is this so? Describe three of these influences in a sentence or two, and indicate why they are so important. How might understandings of these personal factors help people make dietary changes?

7. People live within social networks and may experience cultural expectations about how and what they eat. Because these can't be changed by nutrition education, why should nutrition educators be interested in such information about their intended audience?

8. Distinguish between food availability and food accessibility. How can they influence food choice? How might nutrition educators address these issues?

9. Describe four environmental factors that influence people's food choices and dietary practices. What can nutrition educators do with such information?

10. As stated earlier, in terms of healthy eating and active living, "knowledge is not enough." In your view, is that true? Why do you say so? Give evidence for your view.

11. In reviewing the competencies suggested by the Society for Nutrition Education and Behavior for a nutrition educator, which competencies do you believe that you already possess? Which ones would you like to develop further? Keep these in mind as you read the remainder of this book.

References

Academy of Nutrition and Dietetics. 2012. *ACEND Accreditation Standards for Didactic Programs in Nutrition & Dietetics.* Chicago: Academy of Nutrition and Dietetics, Accreditation Council for Education in Nutrition and Dietetics. www.eatright.org. Accessed 3/15/14.

Addessi, E., A. T. Galloway, E. Visalberghi, and L. L. Birch. 2005. Specific social influences on the acceptance of novel foods in 2–5-year-old children. *Appetite* 45(3):264–271.

Anzman-Frasca, S., J. S. Savage, M. Marini, J. O. Fisher, and L. L. Birch. 2012. Repeated exposure and associative conditioning promote preschool children's liking of vegetables. *Appetite* 58(2):543–553.

Baranowski, T., K. W. Cullen, and J. Baranowski. 1999. Psychosocial correlates of dietary intake: advancing dietary intervention. *Annual Review of Nutrition* 19:17–40.

Beauchamp, G. K. 2009. Sensory and receptor responses to umami: An overview of pioneering work. *American Journal of Clinical Nutrition* 90(3):723S–727S.

Beauchamp, G. K., and J. A. Mennella. 2009. Early flavor learning and its impact on later feeding behavior. *Journal of Pediatric Gastroenterology and Nutrition* 48(Suppl 1): S25–S30.

———. 2011. Flavor perception in human infants: Development and functional significance. *Digestion* 83(Suppl 1):1–6.

Berge, J. M., S. W. Jin, P. Hannan, D. Neumark-Sztainer. 2013. Structural and interpersonal characteristics of family meals: Associations with adolescent body mass index and dietary patterns. *Journal of the Academy of Nutrition and Dietetics* 113(6):816–822.

Birch, L. L. 1992. Children's preferences for high-fat foods. *Nutrition Reviews* 50(9):249–255.

Birch, L. L. 1999. Development of food preferences. *Annual Review of Nutrition* 19:41–62.

———. 2014. Learning to eat: Birth to two years. *American Journal of Clinical Nutrition* 99(3):723S–728S.

Birch, L. L., and S. Anzman-Frasca. 2011a. Learning to prefer the familiar in obesogenic environments. *Nestle Nutrition Workshop Series Pediatric Program.* 68:187–196.

———. 2011b. Promoting children's healthy eating in obesogenic environments: Lessons learned from the rat. *Physiology and Behavior* 104(4):641–645.

Birch, L. L., and J. A. Fisher. 1995. Appetite and eating behavior in children. *Pediatric Clinics of North America* 42(4): 931–953.

Birch, L. L., L. McPhee, B. C. Shoba, L. Steinberg, and R. Krehbiel. 1987. Clean up your plate: Effects of child feeding practices on the conditioning of meal size. *Learning and Motivation* 18:301–317.

Birch, L. L., J. S. Savage, and J. O. Fisher. 2015. Right sizing prevention: Food portion size effects on children's eating and weight. *Appetite* 88:11–16.

Blissett, J. (2011). Relationships between parenting style, feeding style and feeding practices and fruit and vegetable consumption in early childhood. *Appetite* 57(3):826–831.

Boone-Heinonen, J., P. Gordon-Larsen, C. I. K. M. Shikany, C. E. Lewis, and B. M. Popkin. 2011. Fast food restaurants and food stores longitudinal associations with diet in young to middle-aged adults: The CARDIA Study. *Archives of Internal Medicine* 171(13):1162–1170.

Bowen, D. J., M. M. Henderson, D. Iverson, E. Burrows, H. Henry, and J. Foreyt. 1994. Reducing dietary fat: Understanding the successes of the Women's Health Trial. *Cancer Prevention International* 1:21–30.

Breslin, P. A. S., and A. C. Spector. 2008. Mammalian taste perception. *Current Biology* 18(4):R148–R155.

Briefel, R. R., M. K. Crepinsek, C. Cabili, A. Wilson, and P. M. Gleason. 2009. School food environments and practices affect dietary behaviors of US public school children. *Journal of the American Dietetic Association* 109 (2 Suppl):S91–S107.

Brillat-Savarin, A. S. 1825. *The physiology of taste: Meditations on transcendental gastronomy.* Reprinted 1949. Translated by M. F. K. Fisher. New York: Heritage Press. Reprinted 2000. Washington, DC: Counterpoint Press.

Brown, R., and J. Ogden. 2004. Children's eating attitudes and behaviour: A study of the modelling and control theories of parental influence. *Health Education Research* 19:261–271.

Brug, J., K. Glanz, and G. Kok. 1997. The relationship between self-efficacy, attitudes, intake compared to others, consumption, and stages of change related to fruit and vegetables. *American Journal of Health Promotion* 12(1):25–30.

Carnell, S., L. Cooke, R. Cheng, A. Robbins, and J. Wardle. 2011. Parental feeding behaviours and motivations. A qualitative study in mothers of UK pre-schoolers. *Appetite* 57(3):665–673.

Cecil, J. E., N. A. Colin, W. Palmer, I. M. Wrieden, C. Bolton-Smith, P. Watt, et al. 2005. Energy intakes of children after preloads: Adjustment, not compensation. *American Journal of Clinical Nutrition* 82:302–308.

Chakravarthy, M. V., and F. W. Booth. 2004. Eating, exercise, and "thrifty" genotypes: Connecting the dots toward an evolutionary understanding of modern chronic diseases. *Journal of Applied Physiology* 96(1):3–10.

Chandon, P., and B. Wansink. 2007. Is obesity caused by calorie underestimation? A psychophysical model of meal size estimation. *Journal of Marketing Research* 44:84–99.

Clark, J. E. 1998. Taste and flavour: Their importance in food choice and acceptance. *Proceedings of the Nutrition Society* 57(4):639–643.

Connors, M., C. A. Bisogni, J. Sobal, and C. M. Devine. 2001. Managing values in personal food systems. *Appetite* 36(3):189–200.

Contento, I. R., S. S. Williams, J. L. Michela, and A. B. Franklin. 2006. Understanding the food choice process of adolescents in the context of family and friends. *Journal of Adolescent Health* 38(5):575–582.

Cooke, L. J., L. C. Chambers, E. V. Anez, H. A. Croker, D. Boniface, M. R. Yeomans, and J. Wardle. 2011. Eating for pleasure or profit: The effect of incentives on children's enjoyment of vegetables. *Psychological Science* 22(2):190–196.

Cooke L. J., L. C. Chambers, E. V. Anez, and L. Wardle. 2011. Facilitating or undermining? The effects of reward on food acceptance. A narrative review. *Appetite* 57(2):493–497.

Croker, H., C. Sweetman, and L. Cooke. 2009. Mothers' views on portion sizes for children. *Journal of Human Nutrition and Dietetics* 22(5):437–443.

de Castro, J. M. 2000. Eating behavior: Lessons learned from the real world of humans. *Nutrition* 16:800–813.

———. 2010. Control of food intake of free-living humans: Putting the pieces back together. *Physiology and Behavior* 100(5):446–453.

Desor, J. A., O. Mahler, and L. S. Greene. 1977. Preference for sweet in humans: Infants, children, and adults. In *Taste and the development of the genesis for the sweet preference*, edited by J. Weiffenback. Bethesda, MD: U.S. Department of Health, Education, and Welfare.

Devine, C. M., M. M. Connors, J. Sobal, and C. A. Bisogni. 2003. Sandwiching it in: Spillover of work onto food choices and family roles in low- and moderate-income urban households. *Social Science Medicine* 56(3):617–630.

Devine, C. M., M. Jastran, J. Jabs, E. Wethington, T. J. Farell, and C. A. Bisogni. 2006. "A lot of sacrifices": Work–family spillover and the food choice coping strategies of low-wage employed parents. *Social Science Medicine* 63(10):2591–2603.

Ding, D., M. A. Adams, J. F. Sallis, G. J. Norman, M. A. Hovell, C. D. Chambers et al. 2013. Perceived neighborhood environment and physical activity in 11 countries: Do associations differ by country? *International Journal of Behavioral Nutrition and Physical Activity* 10:57.

DiSantis, K. I., L. L. Birch, A. Davey, E. L. Serrano, L. Zhang, Y. Bruton, and J.O. Fisher. 2013. Plate size and children's appetite: Effects of larger dishware on self-served portions and intake. *Pediatrics* 131(5):e1451–e1458.

Dovey, T. M., P. A. Staples, E. L. Gibson, and J. C. Halford. 2008. Food neophobia and "picky/fussy" eating in children: A review. *Appetite* 50(2–3):181–193.

Drewnowski, A. 2012. The cost of U.S. foods as related to their nutritive value. *American Journal of Clinical Nutrition* 92(5):1181–1188.

Drewnowski, A., J. A. Mennella, S. L. Johnson, and F. Bellisle. 2012. Sweetness and food preference. *Journal of Nutrition* 142(6):1142S–1148S.

Duffy, V. B., and L. M. Bartoshuk. 2000. Food acceptance and genetic variation in taste. *Journal of the American Dietetic Association* 100(6):647–655.

Epictetus. *Discourses.* http://ancienthistory.about.com/od/stoicism/a/121510-Epictetus-Quotes.htm Accessed 3/10/15.

Faith, M. S., K. S. Scanlon, L. L. Birch, L. A. Francis, and B. Sherry. 2004. Parent–child feeding strategies and their relationships to child eating and weight status. *Obesity Research* 12(11):1711–1722.

Federal Trade Commission. 2012. *A review of food marketing to children and adolescents.* http://ftc.gov/os/2012/12/121221foodmarketingreport.pdf Accessed 8/14/13.

Ferreira, I., K. van der Horst, W. Wendel-Vos, S. Kremers, F. J. van Lenthe, and J. Brug. 2007. Environmental correlates of physical activity in youth—a review and update. *Obesity Reviews* 8(2):129–154.

Feunekes, G. I., C. de Graaf, S. Meyboom, and W. A. van Staveren. 1998. Food choice and fat intake of adolescents and adults: Associations of intakes within social networks. *Preventive Medicine* 27(5 Pt 1):645–656.

Fisher, J. O. 2007. Effects of age on children's intake of large and self-selected food portions. *Obesity (Silver Spring)* 15:403–412.

Fisher, J. O., A. Arreola, L. L. Birch, B. J. Rolls. 2007. Portion size effects on daily energy intake in low-income Hispanic and African-American children and their mothers. *American Journal of Clinical Nutrition* 86(6): 1709–1716.

Fisher, J.O., and T. V. E. Kjal. 2008. Supersize me: Portion size effects on young children's eating. *Physiology & Behavior* 94(1):39–47.

Fisher, J. O., D. C. Mitchell, H. Smiciklas-Wright, and L. L. Birch. 2002. Parental influences on young girls' fruit and vegetable, micronutrient, and fat intakes. *Journal of the American Dietetic Association* 102(1):58–64.

Food Marketing Institute. 2012. *U.S. grocery shopper trends 2012. Executive summary.* Washington, DC: Author. http://www.icn-net.com/docs/12086_FMIN_Trends2012_v5.pdf Accessed 5/15/15.

———. 2013. *Supermarket Facts 2011–2012.* Washington DC: Author. http://www.fmi.org/research-resources/supermarket-facts Accessed 9/15/13.

Frankel, L. A., S. O. Hughes, T. M. O'Connor, T. G. Power, J. O. Fisher, and N. L. Hazen. 2012. Parental influences on children's self-regulation of energy intake: Insights from development literature on emotion regulation. *Journal of Obesity* 2012:327259.

Furst, T., M. Connors, C. A. Bisogni, J. Sobal, and L. W. Falk. 1996. Food choice: A conceptual model of the process. *Appetite* 26:247–266.

Gearhardt, A. N., C. M. Grilo, R. J. DiLeone, K. D. Brownell, and M. N. Potenz. 2011. Can food be addictive? Public health and policy implications. *Addiction* 106(7): 1208–1212.

Gillman, M. W., S. L. Rifas-Shiman, A. L. Frazier, et al. 2000. Family dinner and diet quality among older children and adolescents. *Archives of Family Medicine* 9(3): 235–240.

Glanz, K, M. Basil, E. Maibach and D. Snyder. 1998. Why Americans eat what they do: taste, nutrition, cost, convenience, and weight concerns as influences on food consumption. *Journal of the American Dietetic Association* 98(10):1118–1126.

Gravina, S. A., G. L. Yep, and M. Khan. 2013. Human biology of taste. *Annals of Saudi Medicine* 33(3):217–222.

Gussow, J. D. 2006. Reflections on nutritional health and the environment: The journey to sustainability. *Journal of Hunger and Environmental Nutrition* 1(1):3–25.

Hanks, A. S., D. R. Just, B. Wansink. 2013. Smarter lunchrooms can address new school lunchroom guidelines and childhood obesity. *Journal of Pediatrics* 162:867–869.

Harper, L. V., and K. M. Sanders. 1975. The effects of adults' eating on young children's acceptance of unfamiliar foods. *Journal of Experimental Child Psychology* 20:206–214.

Hearn, M. D., T. Baranowski, J. Baranowski, C. Doyle, M. Smith, L. S. Lin, et al. 1998. Environmental influences on dietary behavior among children: Availability and accessibility of fruits and vegetables enable consumption. *Journal of Health Education* 29:26–32.

Hendy, H. M., K. E. Williams, and T. S. Camise. 2005. "Kids Choice" school lunch program increases children's fruit and vegetable acceptance. *Appetite* 45(3):250–263.

Hoerr S. L., S. O. Hughes, J. O. Fisher, T. A. Nicklas, Y. Liu, and R. M. Shewchuk. 2009. Associations among parental feeding styles and children's food intake in families with limited income. *International Journal of Behavior Nutrition and Physical Activity* 13(6):55.

Horne, P. J., J. Greenhalgh, M. Erjavec, C. Fergus, S. Victor, and C. J. Whitaker. 2011. Increasing pre-school children's consumption of fruits and vegetables: A modeling and rewards intervention. *Appetite* 56:375–385.

Horne, P. J., K. Tapper, C. F. Lowe, C. A. Hardman, M. C. Jackson, and J. Woolner. 2004. Increasing children's fruit and vegetable consumption: A peer-modeling and rewards-based intervention. *European Journal of Clinical Nutrition* 58(164):1649–1660.

Hughes, S. O., T. G. Power, J. Orlet Fisher, S. Mueller, and T. A. Nicklas, 2005. Revisiting a neglected construct: Parenting styles in a child-feeding context. *Appetite* 44(1):83–92.

Hughes, S. O., R. M. Shewchuk, M. L. Baskin, T. A. Nicklas, and H. Qu. 2008. Indulgent feeding style and children's weight status in preschool. *Journal of Developmental and Behavior Pediatrics* 29(5), 403–410.

Institute of Medicine. 2006. *Food marketing to children and youth: Threat or opportunity.* Washington, DC: National Academies Press.

International Food Information Council (IFIC) Foundation. 1999. Are you listening? What consumers tell us about dietary recommendations. *Food insight: Current topics in food safety and nutrition.* Washington, DC: Author.

Israel, B. A, and K. A. Rounds. 1987. Social networks and social support: A synthesis for health educators. *Health Education and Promotion* 2:311–351.

Koch, P. A., I. R. Contento, and A. Calarese-Barton. In preparation. A qualitative analysis with 7th grade students to understand if and how the Choice, Control & Change (*C3*) curriculum develops agency in making healthy food and physical activity choices.

Konner, M. J., and S. B. Eaton. 2010. Paleolithic nutrition: Twenty-five years later. *Nutrition in Clinical Practice* 25(6):594–602.

Krebs-Smith, S. M., J. Heimendinger, B. H. Patterson, A. F. Subar, R. Kessler, and E. Pivonka. 1995. Psychosocial factors associated with fruit and vegetable consumption. *American Journal of Health Promotion* 10(2):98–104.

Ledikwe, J. H., J. Ello-Martin, C. L. Pelkman, L. L. Birch, M. L. Mannino, and B. J. Rolls. 2007. A reliable, valid questionnaire indicates that preference for dietary fat declines when following a reduced-fat diet. *Appetite* 49(1):74–83.

Lennernas, M., C. Fjellstrom, W. Becker, I. Giachetti, A. Schmidt, A. Remaut de Winter, et al. 1997. Influences on food choice perceived to be important by nationally-representative samples of adults in the European Union. *European Journal of Clinical Nutrition* 51(Suppl 2):S8–S15.

Liem, D. G., and J. A. Mennella. 2002. Sweet and sour preferences during childhood: Role of early experiences. *Development Psychobiology* 41(4):388–395.

Lipchock, S. V., J. A. Mennella, A. I. Spielman, and D. R. Reed. 2013. Human bitter perception correlates with bitter receptor messenger RNA expression in taste cells. *American Journal of Clinical Nutrition* 98:1136–1143.

Macino, L., B. H. Lin, and N. Ballenger. 2004. The role of economics in eating choices and weight outcomes. In *Agricultural Information Bulletin No 791*. Washington, DC: U.S. Department of Agriculture, Economic Research Service.

MacIntosh, W. A. 1996. *Sociologies of food and nutrition*. New York: Plenum Press.

Mathias, K. C., B. J. Rolls, L. L Birch, T. V. Krajl, E. L. Hanna, A. Davry, and J. O. Fisher. 2012. Serving larger portions of fruits and vegetables together at dinner promotes intake of both foods among young children. *Journal of the Academy of Nutrition and Dietetics* 112(2):266–270.

Mattes, R. D. 1993. Fat preference and adherence to a reduced-fat diet. *American Journal of Clinical Nutrition* 57(3):373–381.

———. 1997. The taste for salt in humans. *American Journal of Clinical Nutrition* 65(2 Suppl):692S–697S.

———. 2009. Is there a fatty acid taste? *Annual Review of Nutrition* 29:305–327.

Mennella J. A., and G. K. Beauchamp. 2005. Understanding the origin of flavor preferences. *Chemical Senses* 30 Suppl 1:242–243.

Mennella, J. A., C. E. Griffin, and G. K. Beauchamp. 2004. Flavor programming during infancy. *Pediatrics* 113(4):840–845.

Mennella, J. A., C. P. Jagnow, and G. K. Beauchamp. 2001. Prenatal and postnatal flavor learning by human infants. *Pediatrics* 107(6):E88.

Morland, K., S. Wing, and A. Diez Roux. 2002. The contextual effect of the local food environment on residents' diets: The atherosclerosis risk in communities study. *American Journal of Public Health* 92(11):1761–1767.

Moss, M. 2013. *Salt, fat, sugar*. New York: Random House.

Muhammad, A., J. A. Seale, B. Meade, and B. Regmi. 2011. *International evidence on food consumption patterns (Technical Bulletin No 1929)*. Washington, DC: U.S. Department of Agriculture, Economic Research Service.

National Cancer Institute. 2007. *Health information national trends survey*. http://hints.cancer.gov/docs/HINTS2007FinalReport.pdf Accessed 5/19/15.

O'Connor, T. M., S. O. Hughes, K. B. Watson, T. Baranowski, T. A. Nicklas, J. O. Fisher, et al. 2010. Parenting practices associated with fruit and vegetable consumption in preschool children. *Public Health Nutrition* 13(1), 91–101.

Pai, H. L., and I. R. Contento. 2014. Parental perceptions, feeding practices, feeding styles, and level of acculturation of Chinese Americans in relation to their school-age child's weight status. *Appetite* 80:174–182.

Patrick, H., T. A. Nicklas, S. O. Hughes, and M. Morales 2005. The benefits of authoritative feeding style: Caregiver feeding styles and children's food consumption. *Appetite* 44:243–249.

Pelchat, M. L., and P. Pliner. 1995. "Try it. You'll like it." Effects of information on willingness to try novel foods. *Appetite* 24(2):153–165.

Peters, J. C., H. R. Wyatt, W. T. Donahoo, and J. O. Hill. 2002. From instinct to intellect: The challenge of maintaining healthy weight in the modern world. *Obesity Reviews* 3(2):69–74.

Pliner, P., M. Pelchat, and M. Grabski. 1993. Reduction of neophobia in humans by exposure to novel foods. *Appetite* 20(2):111–123.

Powell, L. M., S. Slater, D. Mirtcheva, Y. Bao, and F. J. Chaloupka. 2007. Food store availability and neighborhood characteristics in the United States. *Preventive Medicine* 44(3):189–195.

Remington, A., E. Anez, H. Croker, J. Wardle, and L. Cooke. 2012. Increasing food acceptance in the home setting: A randomized controlled trial of parent-administered taste exposure with incentives. *American Journal of Clinical Nutrition* 95:72–77.

Rhee, K. 2008. Childhood overweight and the relationship between parent behaviors, parenting style, and family functioning. *Annals of the American Academy of Political and Social Science* 615(1):11–37.

Rittenbaugh, C. 1982. Obesity as a culture-bound syndrome. *Culture and Medical Psychiatry* 6:347–361.

Robinson, J. P., and G. Godbey. 1999. *Time for life: The surprising ways Americans use their time*, 2nd ed. University Park, PA: Pennsylvania State University Press.

Robinson, T. N., M. Kiernan, D. M. Matheson, and K. F. Haydel. 2001. Is parental control over children's eating associated with childhood obesity? Results from a population-based sample of third graders. *Obesity Research* 9(5):306–312.

Rolls, B. 2000. Sensory-specific satiety and variety in the meal. In *Dimensions of the meal: The science, culture, business, and art of eating*, edited by H. L. Meiselman. Gaithersburg, MD: Aspen Publishers.

Rose, D., J. N. Bodor, C. M. Swalm, J. C. Rice, T. A Farley, and P. L. Hutchinson. 2009. Food deserts in New Orleans? Illustrations of urban food access and implications for policy. Presented at *Understanding the Economic Concepts and Characteristics of Food Access.* USDA, Washington, DC. January 23, 2009. University of Michigan National Poverty Center/USDA Economic Research Service. http://www.npc.umich.edu/news/events/food-access/index.php Accessed 10/1/10.

Rosland, A. M., E. Kieffer, B. Israel, M. Cofield, G. Palmisano, et al. 2008. When is social support important? The association of family support and professional support with specific diabetes self-management behaviors. *Journal of General Internal Medicine* 23(12):1992–1999.

Rozin, P. 1988. Social learning about food by humans. In *Social learning: Psychological and biological perspectives,* edited by T. R. Zengall and G. G. Bennett. Hillsdale, NJ: Lawrence Erlbaum.

———. 1996. Sociocultural influences on human food selection. In *Why we eat what we eat: The psychology of eating,* edited by E. D. Capaldi. Washington, DC: American Psychological Association.

Rozin, P., and A. E. Fallon. 1987. A perspective on disgust. *Psychology Review* 1:23–41.

Sallis, J. F., and K. Glanz. 2009. Physical activity and food environments: Solutions to the obesity epidemic. *Milbank Quarterly* 87(1):123–154.

Salvy, J. S., M. Howard, M. Read, and E. Mele, 2009. The presence of friends increases food intake in youth, *American Journal of Clinical Nutrition* 90(2):282–287.

Satia-Abouta, J., R. E. Patterson, M. L. Neuhouser, and J. Elder, 2002. Dietary acculturation: Applications to nutrition research and dietetics. *Journal of the American Dietetic Association* 102(8):1105–1118.

Satter, E. 2000. *Child of mine: Feeding with love and good sense.* 3rd ed. Boulder, CO: Bull Publishing.

Savage, J. S., J. O. Fisher, and L. L. Birch. 2007. Parental influence on eating behavior: Conception to adolescence. *Journal of Law and Medical Ethics* 35(1):22–34.

Savage, J. S., I. H. Halsfield, J. O. Fisher, M. Marini, and L. L. Birch. 2012. Do children eat less at meals when allowed to serve themselves? *American Journal of Clinical Nutrition* 96(1):36–43.

Sclafani, A., and K. Ackroff. 2004. The relationship between food reward and satiation revisited. *Physiology and Behavior* 82(1):89–95.

Shepherd, R. 1999. Social determinants of food choice. *Proceedings of the Nutrition Society* 58(4):807–812.

Skinner, J. D., B. R. Carruth, B. Wendy, and P. J. Ziegler. 2002. Children's food preferences: A longitudinal analysis. *Journal of the American Dietetic Association* 102(11):1638–1647.

Small, D. M., and J. Prescott. 2005. Odor/taste integration and the perception of flavor. *Experimental Brain Research* 166(3–4):345–357.

Sobo, E. 1997. The sweetness of fat: Health, procreation, and sociability in rural Jamaica. In *Food and culture: A reader,* edited by C. Counihan and P. Van Esterik. New York: Routledge, pp. 251–255.

Society for Nutrition Education. 1987. Recommendations for the Society for Nutrition Education on the academic preparation of nutrition education specialists. *Journal of Nutrition Education* 19(5):209–210.

Society for Nutrition Education and Behavior. 2015. Competencies for nutrition educators. SNEB.org. Accessed 4/27/15.

Spill, M. K., L. L. Birch, L. S. Roe, and B. J. Rolls. 2010. Eating vegetables first: The use of portion size to increase vegetable intake in preschool children. *American Journal of Clinical Nutrition* 91(5):1237–1243.

———. 2011. Serving large portions of vegetable soup at the start of a meal affected children's energy and vegetable intake. *Appetite* 57(1):213–219.

Story, M., and S. French. 2004. Food advertising and marketing directed at children and adolescents in the US. *International Journal of Behavioral Nutrition and Physical Activity* 1(1):3.

Stunkard, A. 1975. Satiety is a conditioned reflex. *Psychosomatic Medicine* 37(5):383–387.

Supermarket News. June 3, 2013. Study shows shoppers' digital, health trends. http://supermarketnews.com/datasheet/june-3-2013-study-shows-shoppers-digital-health-trends Accessed 5/7/15.

Tepper, B. J. 2008. Nutritional implications of genetic taste variation: The role of PROP sensitivity and other taste phenotypes. *Annual Review of Nutrition* 28:367–388.

Thompson, D. 2013. In America, food is getting cheaper—unless you're poor. *The Atlantic.* http://www.theatlanticcities.com/politics/2013/03/america-food-getting-cheaper-unless-youre-poor/4923/ Accessed 11/3/14.

Trabulsi, J. C., and J. A. Mennella. 2012. Diet, sensitive periods in flavor learning, and growth. *International Review of Psychiatry* 24:219–230.

Tucker R. M., Mattes R. D., Running CA. 2014 Mechanisms and effects of "fat taste" in humans. *Biofactors* 40(3): 313–326.

U.S. Department of Agriculture, 2012a. *Food Environment Atlas.* Washington, DC: USDA, Economic Research Service. http://www.ers.usda.gov/data-products/food-environment-atlas.aspx Accessed 9/15/13.

———. 2012b. *Food Expenditures.* Washington, DC: USDA Economic Research Service. http://www.ers.usda.gov/data-products/food-expenditures.aspx#26654 Accessed 1/15/14.

———. 2013. *Food security status of United States Households, 2012.* Washington, DC: USDA, Economic Research Service, http://www.ers.usda.gov/topics/food-nutrition-assistance/food-security-in-the-us/key-statistics-graphics.aspx. Accessed 5/19/15.

U.S. Department of Labor, 2013a. *American time use statistics, 2013.* Washington, DC: United States Department of Labor, Bureau of Labor Statistics, http://www.bls.gov/tus/ Accessed 5/19/15.

U.S. Department of Labor, 2013b. *Consumer Expenditure Survey,* Washington, DC: U.S. Department of Labor, Bureau of Labor Statistics. http://www.bls.gov/cex/ Accessed 5/19/15.

Van der Horst, K., S. Kremers, I. Ferreira, A. Singh, A. Oenema and J. Brug. 2007. Perceived parenting style and practices and the consumption of sugar-sweetened beverages by adolescents. *Health Education Research* 22(2) 295–304.

Ventura, A. K., and L. L. Birch. 2008. Does parenting affect children's eating and weight status? *International Journal of Behavioral Nutrition and Physical Activity* 5:15.

Ver Ploeg, M., V. Breneman, T. Farrigan, K. Hamrick, D. Hopkins, P. Kaufman, et al. 2009. Access to affordable and nutritious food—measuring and understanding food deserts and their consequences. *Report to Congress. United States Department of Agriculture*, Administrative Publication No. (AP-036).

Wansink B., D. R. Just, C. R. Payne, and M. Z. Klinger. 2012. Attractive names sustain increased vegetable intake in schools. *Preventive Medicine* 55(4):330–332.

Wardle, J., L. L. Cooke, E. L. Gibson, M. Sapochnik, A. Sheiham, and M. Lawson. 2003. Increasing children's acceptance of vegetables; a randomized trial of parent-led exposure. *Appetite* 40(15), 155–162.

Washington State Magazine. 2013. Annual income spent on food. [map]. Washington State University. http://wsm.wsu.edu/researcher/WSMaug11_billions.pdf Accessed 8/15/13.

Wendel-Vos, W., M. Droomers, S. Kremers, J. Brug, and F. van Lenthe. 2007. Potential environmental determinants of physical activity in adults: A systematic review. *Obesity Reviews* 8(5):425–440.

World Health Organization. 2013. *Marketing of food high in fat, salt and sugar to children: update 2012–2013.* Copenhagen, Denmark: WHO Regional Office for Europe.

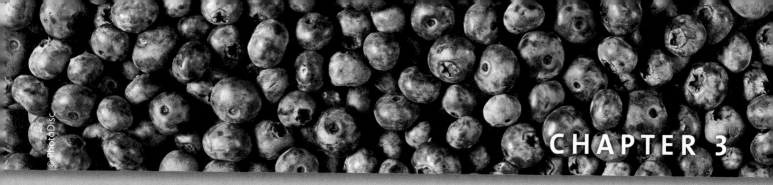

An Overview of Nutrition Education: Facilitating Motivation, Ability, and Support for Behavior Change

OVERVIEW

Given the many influences on behavior, how can nutrition education best assist people to eat better? This chapter provides an overview of how research from behavioral sciences and nutrition education can help nutrition educators understand these influences on behavior and can provide tools for how to increase nutrition education effectiveness. These tools help nutrition educators to enhance motivation, facilitate the ability to make behavior changes, and provide environmental and policy supports for behavior change and taking action by the audiences they serve.

CHAPTER OUTLINE

- Introduction: Elements contributing to nutrition education success
- Element of success 1: Focusing on behavior change and actions
- Element of success 2: Addressing the influences or determinants of behavior change and action
- Element of success 3: Using theory as the guide or tool for nutrition education

- Element of success 4: Addressing multiple influences on behavior change with sufficient duration and intensity—a social-ecological approach
- Element of success 5: Designing nutrition education using theory- and evidence-based strategies
- Putting it all together: Conceptual framework for nutrition education
- Summary

LEARNING OBJECTIVES

At the end of the chapter, you should be able to:

- Explain what is meant by a behavior change- or action-focused approach to nutrition education
- Appreciate that the primary role of nutrition education is to address the influences on or determinants of behavior change or action
- Discuss how nutrition behavior theory and nutrition education research can provide tools for how to design effective nutrition education

- Critique the importance of behavioral theory and research for nutrition education practice
- Describe the three components of nutrition education and the educational goal for each
- Describe a conceptual framework for theory-based nutrition education
- Describe the five elements of success in nutrition education

Introduction: Elements Contributing to Nutrition Education Success

There are numerous and often conflicting influences on people's eating patterns—no wonder it is difficult for people to eat healthfully. For example, Alicia is a 19-year-old high school graduate who works in a busy dentist's office as an administrative assistant. She knows she should eat fruits and vegetables, but she just can't seem to do it. Maria has a 4-year-old daughter who goes to a Head Start program in her community and loves sweet drinks. The parents are part of a close community who think children are healthier when they are a little heavier. Ray is in his mid-40s. His weight just crept up on him, a pound or two each year, and now he is about 40 pounds overweight, mostly in his mid-region, and is at risk for diabetes. His serum cholesterol count is also a bit high. He would like to lose the weight, but it seems so hard.

If a contemporary definition of nutrition education is that it is a combination of educational strategies and environmental supports to facilitate behaviors conducive to health, what can nutrition educators do to assist people like Alicia or Ray to eat more healthfully?

When health professionals first became interested in promoting health and facilitating change in health-related behavior, the emphasis was on providing information to patients and to the public. The assumption was that when individuals such as Alicia and Ray became well informed, they would take the necessary actions to avoid disease and improve their health, such as getting vaccinations, eating healthfully, attending health screenings, or stopping smoking. Consequently, much of health and nutrition education was knowledge-based. However, analyses of the results of health campaigns revealed that the kind of information provided was not sufficient to lead to the desired behavior. For most people, health is not an end in itself but a means to an end: the ability to do what they want to do in life and to achieve their goals; for example, to do well in school or work, be a good parent, have a good relationship, enjoy sports or a vacation, and so forth. Thus, taking actions related to health in the absence of symptoms is not a high priority for most, as is the case for Alicia. Even for those who are at risk for health conditions, such as Ray, motivations are complex and very mixed.

In the area of food especially, eating healthfully is not an end in itself for most people. Eating is about providing essential nourishment for life's many other activities. It is a source of pleasure and enjoyment, and for many, a means of family and cultural cohesion. Given that our food choices and behaviors are influenced by myriad factors, we can all agree that change is hard. The question then is: How can nutrition education programs best assist people to eat more healthfully?

ELEMENTS CONTRIBUTING TO NUTRITION EDUCATION SUCCESS

In a comprehensive review of nutrition education around the world between 1900 and 1970, Whitehead (1973) came to some very broad conclusions about what made nutrition education effective: nutrition education was a factor in improving dietary practices when changing behavior was clearly specified as a goal, when appropriate educational methods were used, when individuals themselves were actively involved in problem-solving, and when an integrated community approach was used.

Research in the area of diet and physical activity has been very active in the past several decades and has generated findings that are very useful for nutrition education practice (Contento et al. 1995; Ammerman et al. 2002; Lemmens et al. 2008; Johnson, Scott-Sheldon, and Carey 2010; Waters et al. 2011; Thompson and Ravia 2011; Hawkes 2013). These studies confirm and extend the earlier findings of Whitehead. They all agree that nutrition education is more likely to be successful when it does the following:

- *Element of Success 1: Focuses on behaviors, actions or practices.* Given that people's food choices and diet-related behaviors have important consequences for themselves, their communities, or the planet, nutrition education is more likely to be successful when it focuses on specific behaviors and actions people take. These specific behaviors may also serve larger goals valued by the individual, family, or community.

- *Element of Success 2: Addresses the influences on, or determinants of, behavior change and action.* Nutrition education is more likely to be successful when it clearly identifies the specific influences on behavior change and action in the intended audience. These influences are called *determinants* and they are the direct targets of nutrition education interventions. Nutrition education is about the *process* of addressing these **determinants of behavior change**. These determinants very often involve food and nutrition *content*, but depending on what content is communicated and how, the content may engage people and be effective in motivating behavior change or the content may not be motivating but can serve to facilitate change.

- *Element of Success 3: Uses theory and evidence.* Nutrition education is more likely to be successful when it uses relevant behavior change theory and research evidence as a map or tool to guide the design of nutrition education.
- *Element of Success 4: Includes multiple levels.* Nutrition education is more likely to be effective when it attends to the multiple levels of influences on food choice and eating behaviors, ranging from the individual level to policy, and uses multiple channels to convey messages with significant intensity over a sufficient duration of time. This is called a social ecological approach.
- *Element of Success 5: Uses appropriate behavior change strategies and education principles to deliver nutrition education.* Nutrition education is more likely to be successful when it uses appropriate theory- and evidence-based strategies to address the identified determinants of behavior change and action and uses instructional design principles to *deliver* it in practice.

These elements of success are explored in the following sections. They also form the foundation of this book.

Element of Success 1: Focusing on Behavior Change and Actions

Evidence suggests that nutrition education is more likely to be effective when the central focus of the program or activities is on addressing the *specific* food choice behaviors, nutrition-related actions, or community dietary practices that influence health and well-being rather than on simply disseminating food or nutrition information in a general manner about various *topics* (Contento et al. 1995; Baranowski, Cerin, and Baranowski 2009*)*. **Behavior** can be defined as an observable action of individuals. Behaviors may be more general involving *behavioral categories* (e.g., eating fruits and vegetables) or be *specific behaviors* involving individual foods (adding fruit to lunch). Other examples include shopping at a farmers' market, reading food labels, or breastfeeding. Thus, dietary actions or behavior change can include the following:

- *Observable food choices or behaviors related to health,* such as eating sufficient quantities of fruits

and vegetables each day, following a lower-fat diet, consuming smaller portions of food, or eating breakfast or healthy snacks.

- *Observable behaviors and actions related to food and food systems,* such as following food safety practices, practicing food preparation or cooking behaviors, managing food-related resources, using eating patterns that have a lower carbon footprint, or vegetable gardening.
- *Observable behaviors and actions related to other nutrition-related concerns,* such as breastfeeding.

The same considerations apply to physical activity, which can be defined as observable actions such as running, walking, bicycling, or playing baseball.

FOCUSING ON SPECIFIC BEHAVIORS OR ACTIONS IS CRUCIAL FOR SUCCESS

A behavior-focused approach means that the expected outcomes for nutrition education are actions taken, or changes in behaviors or patterns of behavior/practices. These behaviors may serve the desired long-term outcomes of improvements in health or in quality of life for individuals, communities, or the planet, or all of them. If our program or intervention seeks to reduce cardiovascular and cancer risk, it might focus on a pattern of behaviors that involves eating more fruits, vegetables, and whole grains and fewer foods high in saturated fat. If our program or intervention seeks to reduce excessive gain in weight, it can focus on these same behaviors along with the behaviors of controlling portions of energy-dense foods and increasing physical activity. If the intervention seeks to increase choice of local produce by low-income families, then one action or "behavior" could be for participants in the Supplemental Nutrition Assistance Program (SNAP) to use their electronic benefits transfer (EBT) cards at farmers' markets.

An example illustrates this approach. In collaboration with a community, researchers sought to design an intervention to "eat a healthier diet" (Reger et al. 1998; Booth-Butterfield and Reger 2004). The planning group soon realized that "eating a healthier diet" was in fact a very general behavioral category that was much too broad because their audience would not know what exactly to do. They narrowed the action to eating less fat, but that was still too broad. So given the data about sources of dietary fat, they decided to focus on getting people to *drink* low-fat milk, which they then honed to *purchasing* low-fat milk.

So the targeted behavior was for people to purchase low-fat (1%) milk, with the campaign message of "1% or less." To ensure it was easy to buy low-fat milk, the researchers made sure that the grocery stores in the community stocked low-fat or fat-free milk. The results showed that market share of low-fat milk rose from 18% to 41%. In a telephone survey, 38% of people reported switching from high-fat milk to low-fat milk.

For any given intervention, the specific behaviors nutrition educators choose to address are identified from the needs, perceptions, and desires of the intended audience, as well as from national nutrition and health goals and nutrition science–based research findings. Behaviors must of course be addressed and framed within their social and cultural context because behaviors both influence and are influenced by their cultural, social, and environmental contexts. A focus on behavior is important even in interventions designed to reduce malnutrition (Bonvecchio et al. 2007; Hawkes 2013).

The behaviors or actions recommended by the U.S. government are shown in **BOX 3-1**. Most governments in the world similarly have recommended dietary patterns for health (Hawkes 2013).

Food and Nutrition-Related Behaviors or Actions Can Be Part of Broader Goals

For example, teaching specific parenting skills may improve the eating patterns of their children. It may also serve the goal of building capacity and empowering parents. Another example is that schools may institute gardens to increase children's fruit and vegetable intakes (a specific behavior). However, school gardens can help children learn where food comes from and serve science education goals as well. A school garden can make the school grounds more attractive and help schoolchildren feel that the school cares. This may increase school attendance and hence academic achievement (Ozer 2007).

Critical Thinking Skills and Autonomy Are Still Important

A behavior-focused approach means that the food and nutrition information and skills provided by the intervention should be relevant to the behaviors and practices being targeted and should be designed to assist individuals and families in becoming motivated and able to take action. For many complex food and nutrition behaviors,

---

BOX 3-1 Dietary Guidelines 2010: Selected Messages for Consumers

Take action on the Dietary Guidelines by making changes in these three areas. Choose steps that work for you and start today. Download the Selected Messages as a PDF.

Balancing Calories
- Enjoy your food, but eat less.
- Avoid oversized portions.

Foods to Increase
- Make half your plate fruits and vegetables.
- Make at least half your grains whole grains.
- Switch to fat-free or low-fat (1%) milk.

Foods to Reduce
- Compare sodium in foods like soup, bread, and frozen meals and choose the foods with lower numbers.
- Drink water instead of sugary drinks.

Reproduced from "Selected Messages for Consumers," ChooseMyPlate.gov. U.S. Department of Agriculture. http://www.choosemyplate.gov/print-materials-ordering/selected-messages.html. Accessed 01/02/2015.

---

a good deal of nutrition-related information and skills may be needed, along with critical thinking skills. Developing a conceptual framework, often through discussion and dialogue, into which to place the behavior is also important. Thus, a behavior-focused approach does *not* mean that nutrition education should be directed at manipulating people's behaviors to make them more healthful in the old behaviorist sense. Individuals take action and change their behaviors only when they themselves see a need to do so and want to make a change. Nutrition education honors and fosters such autonomy and self-responsibility (Buchanan 2004).

Popular author John C. Maxwell (2000) puts it this way: "People change when they hurt enough that they have to, learn enough that they want to, and receive enough that they are able to."

Element of Success 2: Addressing the Influences or Determinants of Behavior Change and Action

The many influences on food choice and diet-related behaviors are shown in **FIGURE 3-1**. Our behavioral science colleagues usually call these influences "determinants" of behavior. In the context of nutrition education, this means modifiable personal determinants and even some environmental factors such as food availability and access, as opposed to non-modifiable factors such as socioeconomic status or educational level.

Nutritionists tend to think of nutrition knowledge and skills as the main areas to address in nutrition education. We talk about the importance of "educating" our clients. This approach is widely used in nutrition education, whether it is made explicit or not.

This seems logical because knowledge at some level is essential for making healthful choices. The importance

of information seems to be corroborated when millions can switch from eating "low-fat" diets to eating "low-carb" diets or the other way around in a matter of weeks, based on news reports that one approach is supposed to be better than the other for weight control. However, this phenomenon is really more about motivated people's interest in a quick fix rather than about changed behaviors resulting from new scientific evidence or information. Witness the difficulty of getting people to eat more fruits and vegetables, despite health campaigns. Indeed, many people in surveys believe they already know enough to make healthful food choices (American Dietetic Association 2002; Supermarket Nutrition 2013).

We can see from Figure 3-1 that "knowledge and skills" is one of the determinants of behavior, but only one. The strong belief of nutrition professionals that knowledge is primary in nutrition education may be due to the fact that the word "knowledge" has several meanings.

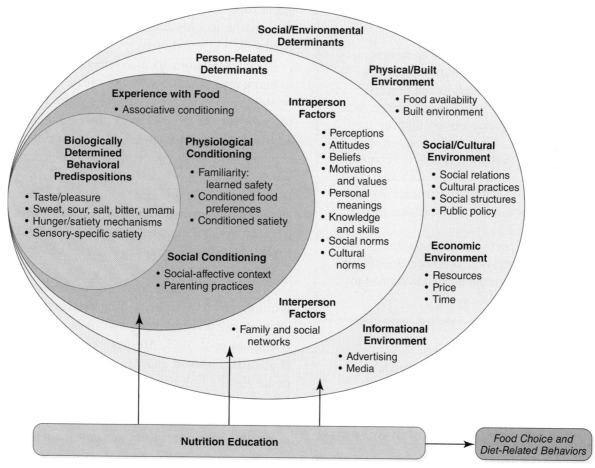

FIGURE 3-1 Factors influencing food choice and dietary behaviors and the role of nutrition education.

KNOWLEDGE IS A PROBLEMATIC TERM IN NUTRITION EDUCATION

The term *knowledge* is problematic probably because the term *nutrition education* itself is problematic. We noted in Chapter 1 that the term nutrition education seems to imply that the function of the field is to provide education, meaning *knowledge/information*, about nutrition. This is an inaccurate way to think of the field. Education is not just about providing information but about enhancing motivation and facilitating dietary change. Yes, nutrition education involves communicating information in some form throughout this process. However, what food and nutrition information we communicate and how we communicate it differs during the behavior change process. This makes all the difference in terms of its impacts on our audiences to achieve desired outcomes. It is essential that we realize that some kinds of information and how we communicate it are very motivating while other kinds of information are not motivating but crucial for facilitating change.

> Nutrition education is about the *process* of learning and behavioral change, focusing on enhancing motivation and empowerment, and on facilitating diet-related change. Food and nutrition content knowledge is essential throughout this process. However, it is important that we realize that some kinds of content knowledge are very motivating while other kinds are not motivating but are needed for facilitating change. We can call content knowledge that is used to motivate our audiences *motivating knowledge* or *why-to knowledge*. We can call knowledge that is essential to facilitate change **facilitating knowledge** or **how-to knowledge**. We need both kinds, of course, but usually at different times to serve these two different purposes. We need to keep this distinction in mind as we design nutrition education.

ROLE OF KNOWLEDGE AS DETERMINANT OF ACTION OR BEHAVIOR CHANGE

Food and Nutrition Content Knowledge as Facilitating Knowledge: Role of Nutrition Literacy

In most nutrition education programs, the term *knowledge* refers to communicating information about basic facts about food and nutrition, such as knowing the food groups in the nation's dietary guidance graphic (e.g., MyPlate), which foods have which nutrients, or how to read food labels. This kind of information is referred to as *factual knowledge*. Such knowledge is the basis of *nutrition literacy*, which has been defined, similarly to **health literacy**, as the degree to which people have the capacity to obtain, process, and understand the basic health (nutrition) information and services they need to make appropriate health (nutrition) decisions (Zoellner et al. 2009; Silk et al. 2008; Carbone 2012).

Nutrition literacy is particularly important for the low-literacy audiences with whom many of us work as they need the most help understanding basic food and nutrition guidance information (Silk et al. 2008; Carbone and Zoellner 2012). Such literacy is also very important for those at risk or those who have nutrition related health conditions and want or need to understand instructions in order to manage their conditions (Institute of Medicine 2002, 2004; Carbone and Zoellner 2012). In this context, it should be noted that misinformation and misconceptions about food and nutrition sometimes cause problems for those wishing or needing to eat healthfully and, of course, need to be addressed.

The term *knowledge* also refers to certain skills such as being able to follow a recipe, create a balanced meal, or store foods appropriately (see **FIGURE 3-2**). This kind of knowledge is referred to as *procedural knowledge*. In addition, the term *knowledge* can also refer to *critical thinking and decision-making skills* involved in shopping wisely, managing a food budget, and deciding whether to eat organically produced foods. It includes problem-solving skills for decision making. Such factual knowledge, procedural knowledge, and decision-making skills together constitute what can be described as *facilitating knowledge*.

Facilitating knowledge, though necessary for action, is unlikely by itself to lead to improved behaviors in those who are not already motivated or ready to take action (Contento et al. 1995, Atkinson and Nitzke 2001; Ajzen et al. 2011; Fishbein and Ajzen 2010). The scientific evidence for the link between this kind of knowledge and behavior is weak (Silver Wallace 2002; Baranowski et al. 2003) and surveys that show a link between nutrition literacy and behavior do not account for whether people were already motivated (Zoellner et al. 2011; Carbone and Zoellner 2012).

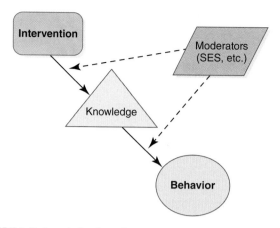

FIGURE 3-2 Knowledge-based programs: functional (or facilitating) knowledge as the determinant of behavior change.

Adapted from Baranowski, T., T. O'Connor, and J. Baranowski. 2010. Initiating change in children's eating behaviors. In *International handbook of behavior, diet, and nutrition.* edited by V. R. Preedy, R. R. Watston, and C. R. Martin. New York: Springer.

Food and Nutrition Content Knowledge as Motivator of Behavior Change

On the other hand, food and nutrition information can be communicated in such a way as to enhance motivation for behavior change. Take the following example. You conduct the following activity in a group: Have everyone stand up. If one blood relative has diabetes, sit. If the person sitting has a second blood relative that has a diagnosis of diabetes, the person can hold up a finger, and so forth through several chronic diseases. You can explain that those siting are at increased risk. Now tell them that if any of those sitting eat 4 ½ cups of fruit and vegetables, few energy dense snacks, and carry out 30 or more minutes of moderate to vigorous physical activity per day, they can stand up again, indicating that they have reduced their risk by their actions. You can note that chronic disease risk is partly genetic but also partly due to lifestyle and then lead the participants in a discussion of actions they can take to reduce their risk. Contrast this activity with providing the group with a list of government recommendations for healthy eating along with tips on how to follow them.

Which approach would the group find more motivating to take action?

In the first, you communicated science-based nutrition content knowledge/information in such a way that it increased people's perception of their personal risk. According to research in behavioral science, *perception of personal risk* has been shown to be a *motivating determinant* of behavior change. Thus this piece of information that nutritionists would label as *knowledge* engages people's affective or psychological side as well as their analytical side, and so social psychologists would describe it in terms of the psychological purpose of the information, which in this case is to arouse a *perception of risk*.

Likewise, understanding the *benefits* of eating healthfully (*nutrition content knowledge* derived from sound science) serves a psychological purpose as well as a cognitive, nutrition content purpose and can be considered a motivating *determinant*. There are many instances where science-based information is both what nutritionists would label as a piece of knowledge/information and what social psychologists would label as a motivator of change. We will refer to the kinds of knowledge that provide reasons for "why-to" change behavior as **motivational** or **why-to knowledge**.

In the second activity, the lecture, you also communicated to the group science-based knowledge/information, but it was the kind of information needed by those who are already motivated for how to take action, and not motivating in itself. Nutritionists would label this as functional knowledge or nutrition literacy, as described above, whereas our behavioral science colleagues would refer to it as *behavioral capability*—that is, it is the kind of information that makes people capable of taking on the behavior change. We will refer to this kind of information about "how-to" change behavior or take action as *facilitating*, or *how-to* knowledge.

You can see, then, that *food and nutrition content knowledge or information* serves different functions depending on how you communicate it: motivational or functional/facilitating. These relationships are summarized as follows:

Food and Nutrition Content Knowledge	Psychological Purpose of the Knowledge
Knowledge that motivates behavior change ("Why-to" change behavior)	
▪ Scientific information about the relationship between dietary behaviors and disease (e.g., sweetened beverages → overweight/type 2 diabetes; low-calcium foods → osteoporosis)	▪ Increases motivation by increasing perception of negative outcomes from the behavior (called *perceived risk*)

Food and Nutrition Content Knowledge	Psychological Purpose of the Knowledge
■ Scientific information about the relationship between dietary behaviors and health (e.g., high fruit and vegetable intake → improved eye, skin, and metabolic health; high whole grain food intake → improved digestive functions)	■ Increases motivation by increasing perception of positive outcomes from the behavior (called *perceived benefits*)
Knowledge that facilitates behavior change ("How-to" change behavior)	
■ Information on recommended number of servings of food to eat from each of the food groups based on MyPlate or other guidelines	■ Increases facilitating knowledge needed to carry out a targeted behavior, thus called *behavioral capability*: factual knowledge
■ Information on how to read a food label	■ Increases facilitating knowledge needed to carry out a targeted behavior, or *behavioral capability*: cognitive skills
■ Information on, and practice for, how to prepare food from a recipe	■ Increases facilitating knowledge needed to carry out a targeted behavior or *behavioral capability*: behavioral skills

The Scope of Nutrition Education

Jane Sherman summarizes the role of information in nutrition education well as follows: Clear, accurate information has a role of course. When an individual or community perceives a problem, believes that change is needed and urgent, is seeking a solution, has experience of success in changing practices, has the means to hand, sees that change is easy and attractive, is not tempted to other actions, can see the benefits (or at least believes in them), and feels social approval and support—then new information and knowhow can indeed help to precipitate a change. However, if the other conditions are lacking, then clear correct information is a valuable, but generally wholly insufficient part of the process. (Jane Sherman, personal communication, 2015)

Sisters Together

Why-to information and how-to information can be used in brochures or website venues as well. An example is shown in **NUTRITION EDUCATION IN ACTION 3-1** about the Sisters Together campaign, called Celebrate the Beauty of Youth. The flyer begins with motivational component nutrition education messages focusing on why-to information such as the positive outcomes or benefits to be expected from taking action. The flyer then continues with action component how-to information such as relevant functional physical activity and food- and nutrition-related knowledge and skills (some of this is not shown).

PSYCHOSOCIAL INFLUENCES AS DETERMINANTS OF ACTION AND BEHAVIOR CHANGE

In sum, the field of nutrition supplies the science-based food and nutrition content and the field of social psychology explains the purpose of that content being to serve as determinants—motivators and facilitators—of behavior and behavior change.

Our behavioral scientist and health educator colleagues refer to all such information as "**beliefs**." The term is often used in lay language to refer to some piece of information that a person holds that is not true. In the health literature, this is not at all the meaning. *Beliefs* is defined as the mental acceptance of a particular concept, arrived at by weighing external evidence, facts, and personal observation and experience. Social psychologists Fishbein and Ajzen (2010) define beliefs as the expectation that an object has a certain attribute, for example, that physical activity (the object) reduces the risk of diabetes (the attribute). These beliefs *have motivational power* because individuals come to believe, or find the scientific reasons convincing, for why to make a particular food choice or dietary change, such as eating more fruits and vegetables or foods produced more sustainably, or food behaviors related to diabetes management or breastfeeding.

Such information can be especially powerful when it is communicated in the form of a group activity as described above, or presented visually in a very motivational way that appeals to the emotional side in individuals as well as to their rational side and helps to stimulate thinking and develop convictions. All behavior change (indeed all learning) requires both affective (emotional) and cognitive engagement of people. The "Pouring on the Pounds" campaign is an example of accurate scientific information that is motivating because it portrays consequences of behavior in a way that engages the interest, emotions, and convictions of the public (see **FIGURE 3-3**). In this poster, a sweetened beverage becomes fat as it enters the glass. The online version shows a young man drinking

NUTRITION EDUCATION IN ACTION 3-1

Celebrate the Beauty of Youth's WIN program provides women "why-to" and "how-to" information to improve their health and nutrition.

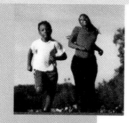
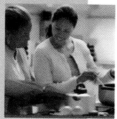

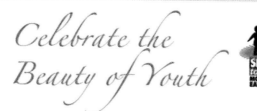

Celebrate the Beauty of Youth

You lead a busy life. Being young is exciting, but it can also be a bit hectic. So many things to take care of! Getting the little ones ready in the morning and tucked in bed at night, juggling work tasks, keeping in touch with your parents, and spending quality time with your partner may leave you with little time for yourself. This tip sheet, part of the Sisters Together Series, will give you ideas on how to stay active, healthy, and strong during this exciting phase of your life.

Why should I move more and eat better?

Being physically active and making smart food choices is good for your health. But moving more and eating better have lots of other benefits as well. They can help you do the following:

- Feel good about yourself and have more energy.
- Look good in the latest fashions.
- Prevent weight gain and related health problems like heart disease and diabetes.
- Reduce stress, boredom, or the blues.
- Tone your body (without losing your curves).

How can I move more?

Physical activity can be fun! Do things you enjoy, like

- dancing
- fast walking
- group fitness classes, such as dance or aerobics
- running

If you can, be physically active with a friend or a group. That way, you can cheer each other on, have a good time while being active, and feel safer when you are outdoors. Find a local school track or park where you can walk or run with your friends, or join a recreation center so you can work out or take a fun fitness class together.

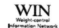
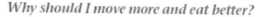

National Institute of Diabetes and Digestive and Kidney Diseases   **WIN** Weight-control Information Network

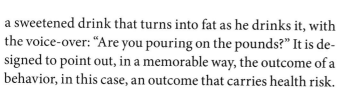

a sweetened drink that turns into fat as he drinks it, with the voice-over: "Are you pouring on the pounds?" It is designed to point out, in a memorable way, the outcome of a behavior, in this case, an outcome that carries health risk.

To organize and address the many psychosocial determinants of change, we are grateful that our colleagues in the behavioral sciences, such as psychology, anthropology, and economics, can provide some help. Anthropologists help us understand the shared meanings and values of a group and the cultural context in which people's food and nutrition motivations and practices are formed and enacted. Economists help us understand how people make choices in a world where wants are greater than the means to satisfy these wants. Psychologists help us understand people's mental functioning, emotions, personality, motivations, preferences, attitudes, behaviors, and

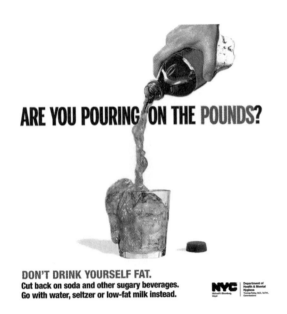

FIGURE 3-3 Pouring on the pounds.

Reproduced from "Pouring on the Pounds Ad Campaign Archive." New York City Department of Health and Mental Hygiene. http://www.nyc.gov/html/doh/html/living/sugarydrink-media-archive.shtml Accessed 1/2/2015.

interpersonal relationships—many are listed in Figure 3-1 and **FIGURE 3-4**. These perceptions and attitudes can be the targets of nutrition education.

An example may illustrate this point. A teenage girl develops type 2 diabetes. She learns about the disease and all the things she needs to do to take care of herself. This will require that she changes what she eats and drinks. But she does not make the changes. Why? You talk with her and realize it is because her priority at this point in her life is to be popular with her peers; eating and drinking the same food and beverages is much more important to her than her health. No amount of information of the facilitating knowledge kind will be helpful. Instead, we have to look for other

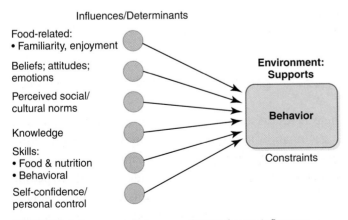

FIGURE 3-4 Common influences on dietary change. Influences = "determinants" and are shown as circles. The items listed next to the circles are the names of the "determinants."

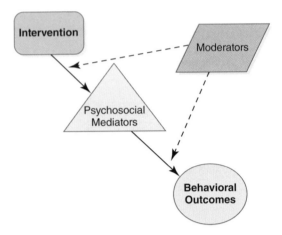

FIGURE 3-5 Theory-based programs: psychosocial factors as the determinants of behavior change.

Data from Baranowski, T., T. O'Connor, and J. Baranowski. 2010. Initiating change in children's eating behaviors. In V. R. Preedy, R. R. Watston, and C. R. Martin (eds.). International handbook of behavior, diet, and nutrition. New York: Springer.

reasons that may be relevant for her. These could include scientific, nutrition-related content information about potential outcomes of behavior, such as positive *benefits* of appropriate behaviors on her part, or *risks* from neglecting the appropriate behaviors, which might include loss of her feet or her eyesight. Or, the outcomes or reasons can be more immediate—the right foods and drinks at the right times will give her energy to do things with her peers. Once truly motivated by nutrition and health information communicated as why-to take action and by personally relevant reasons, she may be ready to follow nutritional guidance about her condition provided in the form of facilitating knowledge or nutrition literacy.

The most effective way to assist people to make changes in their dietary practices is to identify the influences on, or determinants of, their current diets as well as the influences or determinants that can potentially bring about behavior change and then develop strategies to address these determinants. These determinants operate in the context of family, community, and culture and identifying them is most desirable and effective when carried out in partnership with the intended audience.

An Analogy: The Rider and the Elephant

The importance of determinants in behavior change can be more dramatically illustrated using a metaphor from psychologist and author Jonathan Haidt (2006, 2012). He points out that all of us find it hard to change our behavior because we have both a reasoning or analytical side and an intuitive or emotional side to our being that often disagree.

We want to get up early to exercise but like the warmth of our beds; we want to cut down our portion sizes but find the food irresistible. Haidt proposes the metaphor of the Rider and Elephant to describe this dilemma of human action. Haidt says that our intuitive or emotional side is like an elephant and our analytical side a rider that sits perched on top of the elephant. The rider seems to be in control, but being so small relative to the size of the elephant, the rider cannot get to any destination without the willing cooperation of the elephant. The rider reflects the part of the human brain, the frontal cortex or gray matter, that makes possible the mental processes of thinking, planning and decision making. The elephant is the much more ancient and larger part of our brain, the limbic system, which involves the more automatic human activities and involves our gut feelings, visceral reactions, intuitions, and emotions. This part of the brain did not go away when humans developed more gray matter. The gray matter was just superimposed over our more automatic, intuitive, and emotional selves.

The elephant looks for more immediate gratification and pay-offs while the rider is able to think long term. In the area of nutrition and health, the immediate pay-offs are often pleasurable (such as eating tasty high-fat, high-sugar foods or being a couch potato), which the elephant in us likes, while the long-term outcomes are usually abstract (such as health), which is important to the rider. On the other hand, the elephant is the source of motivation and stamina, while the rider can often overanalyze and agonize over a decision. They are both needed for human functioning. For example, when our hand touches a hot flame, we do not need the rider to analyze the situation to decide what to do; we are grateful for the instant reaction of our elephant to remove our hand.

The rider in us needs very clear directions. Remember the "1% or less" intervention described earlier? "Healthy eating" was too broad a message, and even "eat less fat" was not specific enough. The rider in people would not know what to do. "Buy low fat milk," however, was a clear message.

A clear message by itself is not enough in nutrition education—we need to engage the elephant in people. In the case of the "1% or less" intervention, a punchy and specific media campaign was mounted using paid advertising, educational programs, and public relation efforts (Booth-Butterfield and Reger 2004). For example, one ad pointed out that one glass of whole milk has the same amount of saturated fat as five strips of bacon. At the news conference,

the researchers showed a glass tube full of fat and pointed out this was the amount in a half-gallon of whole milk. These vivid images were to engage the elephant's emotional response that this was gross. Haidt said that if you want to change people's mind, talk to the elephant in them first (Haidt 2012, p. 59). Shaping the path to make it easier for rider and elephant is also important.

Influences, Determinants, and Mediators: A Clarification of Terms

There are many terms that describe influences on our behaviors. The term **determinant** suggests that the specific influence has been demonstrated to be associated with or to cause the behavior or behavior change of interest. It *predicts* the change. **Mediators** refer to those influences that in intervention studies have been demonstrated statistically to be the mechanism by which the intervention has had an impact on the outcome. That is, these influences or mediators *explain* how the intervention causes the behavior change (Baranowksi et al. 1997; Conner and Armitage 2002). These two terms are thus very similar. Some researchers prefer one term and other researchers prefer the other. For the purposes of this book, we will use the term *determinants* to describe potential influences on behavior change and action.

BEHAVIORAL SCIENCE COLLEAGUES HELP US UNDERSTAND ALICIA AND RAY

To help us understand our friends Alicia and Ray, let's now examine their experiences in light of the work of behavioral scientists.

Let's say that you interview Alicia about why she is not eating fruits and vegetables. Perhaps she will tell you that at lunchtime she likes to eat food that is filling and can be picked up fast and eaten quickly. She is also not enthusiastic about the taste of most fresh fruit—she would much rather eat a slice of apple pie than an apple. In particular, she does not like vegetables other than cooked carrots and green beans, although she does not even eat these very often. Salads seem like a waste of money, because she soon gets hungry again. She tried cooking broccoli once but it came out mushy and smelled bad. She is not confident she would know how to make vegetables taste good. She does not know exactly how much she should eat each day (maybe once a day?) but because she seems to be doing fine in terms of health, she figures she is eating enough. Her family did not eat many vegetables so she is not used to them.

Let's analyze what she says in terms of her motivations and experiences, which are listed in the following table. She seems to want the following features from the food she eats: it should be filling, convenient, taste good, and not cost too much. Social psychologists would label these as "*beliefs about outcomes* for performing a behavior," in this case from eating a food. Her lack of experience with fruits and vegetables from her family background means she has not had the opportunity to develop what social psychologists would call *preferences* for them. She certainly lacks confidence in preparing vegetables. Lack of confidence may be labeled as a lack of *self-efficacy*. She does not have knowledge about how much to eat; such knowledge can be labeled *facilitating knowledge* to be able to perform a behavior. She does not

know how to cook vegetables properly, which can also be labeled as a lack of skills. Facilitating knowledge and skills are labeled as *behavioral capability* by social psychologists. This can also be labeled as *how-to* knowledge. If we compare her beliefs about the anticipated positive and negative outcomes she expects from eating fruits and vegetables, they all tilt towards the negative. Thus all of these influences or determinants are obstacles to her eating fruits and vegetables. Ultimately, she is not really concerned because she is in good health and does not believe she will get ill anytime soon. Taken together, her beliefs would predict that she will not make any changes. Another way of saying this is that her elephant is definitely not motivated to take action despite the clear direction provided by her rider.

Why Alicia does or does not eat fruits and vegetables	Psychological label = "determinants"
■ She wants her food to be filling at lunch and vegetables are not filling.	■ Beliefs about outcomes from eating vegetables (negative)*
■ She wants the food to be picked up fast and eaten quickly—that is, convenient.	■ Beliefs about outcomes from eating F&V (negative)*
■ She does not like the taste of most fresh fruit.	■ Taste or preference (negative)
■ She does not like vegetables.	■ Attitude towards vegetables (negative)
■ Salads are a waste of money, i.e., cost is a problem.	■ Beliefs about outcomes (negative)
■ She does not know how to cook vegetables.	■ Self-efficacy (lacking)
■ Cooking some vegetables can smell bad.	■ Beliefs about outcomes (negative)*
■ She does not know how much F&V to eat each day.	■ Food-related knowledge or how-to knowledge (lacking)
■ She is not used to eating vegetables as her family did not eat them regularly or in abundance.	■ Familiarity or preference (lacking)
■ Ultimately, she is not really concerned because she is in good health and does not believe she will get ill anytime soon.	■ Perceived risk (low)

*If this factor leads her to believe she would experience a positive outcome from eating fruits and vegetables (F&V), the "beliefs about outcomes" would be described as "positive"; that is, she would be motivated to eat F&V. If she anticipates a negative outcome, she would ***not*** be motivated to eat F&V.

Now you talk with Ray about his issues and concerns. He might say that his doctor tells him that losing weight will help to reduce his risk of diabetes, and that watching what he eats and being more active might reduce his cholesterol count and thus reduce his risk of heart disease. He really wants to take these actions, but it seems so hard. After a day at his job as a salesman in a store, where he is mostly on the phone or standing and talking to customers, he just wants to sit and watch TV when he comes home. Besides, he does not see how he would fit any exercise into his day. His wife is interested in cooking more healthful meals for both of them, but he likes a hearty meal with lots of meat and has a "sweet tooth."

Let's analyze what Ray says and give psychological labels to his motivations. He believes that there would be good health outcomes if he ate more healthfully and was more active. Social psychologists would label these as "*beliefs about outcomes* for performing the behavior." In this case, they are positive toward taking healthful action, so we would call them "beliefs about benefits" of taking action. However, he also believes that eating lots of meat expresses his manhood—which is also a belief about outcomes, this time *self-evaluative outcomes*. He likes desserts because they taste good. In this case, both sets of expected outcomes are barriers to healthful eating. Being physically active can lead to the anticipated long-term benefit of improvements in health and he participates in a game of basketball with friends from time to time. But the anticipated short-term outcomes of enjoying being a "couch potato" are considerably more appealing to Ray. Clearly humans have a bundle of conflicting motivations.

Ray has tried to lose weight a few times in the past and has not been very successful. Therefore he has little confidence he can do so this time. Thus he can be said to be lacking in "*self-efficacy.*" Ray has a number of positive beliefs about anticipated outcomes (or motivations) for taking action—he will be healthier if he eats a healthful diet and achieves a healthy weight—but he also has a number of negative beliefs about the same behaviors. He also has the support of his wife, who is eager to cook more healthy meals for both of them. In summary, Ray is clear on direction, and he has some motivation towards health, but sees many barriers and needs encouragement. His wife is willing to help shape his path.

Why Ray is having a hard time achieving a healthy weight	Psychological label = "determinants"
■ He understands that losing weight will help to reduce his risk of diabetes.	■ Belief about outcomes of losing weight (positive)*
■ Watching what he eats and being more active might reduce his cholesterol count and heart disease.	■ Belief about outcomes for healthful eating and physical activity (positive)*
■ It is enjoyable to sit and watch TV.	■ Attitude towards exercise (negative)
■ He does not have time to exercise.	■ Perceived barrier to exercise
■ He likes large and hearty meals.	■ Taste or preference (negative motivator of change)
■ He likes rich, high-calorie desserts.	■ Taste or preference (negative motivator of change)
■ He has tried unsuccessfully to lose weight before and lacks confidence he can do so now.	■ Self-efficacy (lacking)
■ His wife is supportive.	■ Social support (positive)
■ When he is honest with himself, he admits he is not really very concerned because he does not think he will have ill health*.	■ Perceived risk (low)

*If this factor leads him to believe he would experience a positive outcome from losing weight or performing the food or physical activity behavior, the "beliefs about outcomes" would be described as "positive." That is, he would be motivated to perform the behavior. If the outcome would not be perceived as contributing to his desired outcome, it would be described as "negative." He would not be likely to perform the behavior.

Our social psychologist colleagues would point out that there are several categories of motivations in common between the two individuals: "expectations about outcomes" are important to both Alicia and Ray, outcomes of their current behaviors as well as those from making changes. Taste or "preference" is important. "Self-efficacy" is a problem for both of them. "Barriers" certainly exist for both. Ultimately, neither of them feels real urgency to make changes or *perceived risk* is low.

We can see in the cases of Alicia and Ray, as for most people, that these beliefs, though unseen, can be powerful determinants of behavior and behavior change.

INTERACTIONS OF CULTURE AND SOCIAL PSYCHOLOGICAL FACTORS

Social psychological determinants of dietary behavior are embedded in culture. Children acquire their culture's beliefs and values both directly and indirectly (Spiro 1984).

Direct influence occurs when the child is told explicitly about "facts," norms, values, and so forth about the culture (e.g., "we don't eat pork"). Indirect acquisition occurs through observing what other people do (norms), whether in interpersonal settings or through media such as television, and making inferences from norms and cultural artifacts about the values of the culture. For example, if families within a culture typically spend a lot of time preparing healthful food (norms) and enjoying it, or if their kitchens are equipped for making healthful foods (artifacts), children growing up in that culture are likely also to value healthful food. Anthropologists suggest that this outcome is likely in part because there is a tendency for the descriptive understanding of one's culture—how things are—to become fused with a normative understanding—how things should be.

Given these definitions and observations, culture can be seen as connected intimately with the beliefs, attitudes, and values described by social psychological theories and

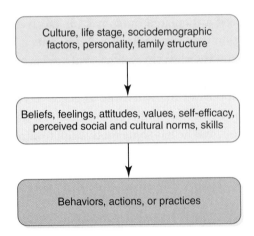

FIGURE 3-6 Relationship of culture and background factors to psychosocial factors in influencing behaviors and practices.

research; culture may be considered their primary source. These relationships are shown in **FIGURE 3-6**.

THE INFLUENCE OF CULTURAL CONTEXT

Consequently, consideration of cultural context is very important in planning nutrition education. Each country has many subcultures. Cross-country migrations world wide involve millions of people each year, people who bring with them various cultural traditions that add to the country's cultural diversity. Cultural knowledge and values develop over time for a group or society in ways that help

to promote its survival (LeVine 1984). Food, which is essential to survival, is, not surprisingly, very much part of culture. Culture defines what people should or should not eat and prescribes how to prepare food; defines where, when, and with whom it should be eaten; determines who does the shopping and cooking; and whose opinions are most important in the choice of family meals or of healthcare decisions (Rozin 1982; Sanjur 1982; D'Andrade 1984; Kittler, Sucher, and Nelms 2011).

Differences in cultural values about health in general can also influence dietary practices. For example, some cultures, such as mainstream American culture, emphasize personal responsibility or self-help in promoting individual health or preventing illness, whereas other cultures believe that chance or fate is more important. Although mainstream culture may emphasize personal choice and responsibility in matters of food and eating, other cultures emphasize the role of family in decisions related to food and health. Some view health from a biomedical viewpoint; others, experiential or psychosocial (Chesla et al. 2000; Stein 2010). Some of these differing cultural norms are shown in **TABLE 3-1**.

Immigrants from one culture to another maintain traditional eating patterns and acculturate to different degrees. Thus, nutrition educators will be more effective when they understand the degree of acculturation of their audience to mainstream cultural values (Satia-Abouta et al. 2002).

Table 3-1 Comparison of Some Common Cultural Values Relevant to Dietary Behavior	
Mainstream American Culture	**Other Cultural Groups**
Health and illness located in the person	Health and illness are long-term, fluid, and continuous expressions of relationships between an individual and others.
Illness caused by natural etiological agents such as genes, viruses, bacteria, and stress	Illness is caused by quasi-natural agents such as weather or various states of one's blood (e.g., thin, weak, or bad), or by violations of religious or moral expectations, emotions such as envy or jealousy, or punishment for misconduct.
Personal responsibility for health; importance of sense of control	Chance, fate, and God influence health, illness, and healing.
Nutritional health the result of deficiencies and imbalances in food components and nutrients in food	Health is the result of the balance of forces in the body, such as hot–cold; imbalances cause illness, and health can be restored by balancing hot and cold foods.
Self-help	Families are highly involved and there is a societal or community obligation to assist.
Emphasis on individualism/privacy	Welfare of the group and interpersonal harmony are important.
Time highly important	Personal interactions are highly important, sometimes more so than time considerations.
Future orientation	May have a past or present orientation; tradition is important.
Interactions emphasize directness and openness	Interactions emphasize indirectness, importance of "face."
Informality and egalitarianism	Status and formal relationships are important.

Cultural Sensitivity and Cultural Competence

All countries are increasingly ethnically and culturally diverse. Culture can be seen as "the values, norms, and traditions that affect how individuals of a particular group perceive, think, interact, behave, and make judgments about their world" (Chamberlain 2005, p. 197). Because social psychological determinants of behavior are strongly influenced by people's cultures, it is extremely important that nutrition educators truly understand and value the cultural contexts of their audiences (Chamberlain 2005; Stein 2009, 2010; Moule 2012). That is, nutrition educators need to be *culturally sensitive*, described as awareness of the educators' own cultural beliefs, customs, and practices as well as those of other cultural groups, and recognizing and accepting similarities and differences without judgment. Nutrition educators must also develop *cultural competence*, which is described as the skills needed to design programs that are culturally sensitive and that can work effectively in cross-cultural settings (e.g., Suarez-Balcazar et al. 2013). This involves awareness, respect, and acceptance of the cultural beliefs and practices of the audience and willingness to work within the traditions and customs of the culture. These issues are discussed in greater detail in Chapter 17.

Culture "Out There" and "In Here"

At the same time, researchers point out that culture "out there" is interpreted by the family and passed down to children as family cultural traditions (Triandis 1979; Ventura and Birch 2008). Children, in turn, filter these family cultural traditions through their own personal experience with food and with the world to develop their own interpretations of their culture (Rozin 1982). Likewise, traditional cultures of immigrants and subcultures are interpreted by communities and families to varying degrees. Individuals filter these family and community interpretations of traditional culture through their own experiences with food and mainstream culture to create their own personal or family interpretations of their traditions and cultures. These interpretations result in different degrees of acculturation to mainstream culture, which need to be considered in nutrition education (Satia et al. 2001). For example, some cultures believe that foods have "hot" and "cold" (or yin and yang) qualities and must be eaten to balance hot and cold body conditions to maintain health. However, individuals within a culture differ in how strongly they believe this interpretation of health and consequently on the extent to which these beliefs influence their health behaviors (Liou and Contento 2001, 2004). Likewise, in some cultures fate is an important determinant of health behaviors. Again, members of a culture may differ considerably on how strongly they personally believe this. In the case of breastfeeding, although cultural and family expectations are very important, individuals *still* differ in their opinions about these expectations (Bentley, Dee, and Jensen 2003). Knowing about the strength of these beliefs for a given audience can be useful to us in planning nutrition education (Kreuter et al. 2003, 2005).

All these considerations help us recognize that individuals internalize the beliefs, norms, and values of their culture, and it is these *personal interpretations* that are powerful in people's lives (Triandis 1979). They become part of people's psychosocial makeup and thus become the determinants of behavior that are captured in the psychosocial theories described here. This means that while nutrition educators need to be aware of the cultural contexts of their audiences they must also recognize the individual differences that exist because of family and personal interpretations of culture and they must design their interventions accordingly.

Element of Success 3: Using Theory as the Guide or Tool for Nutrition Education

Having a list of the determinants of behavior change such as those in Figure 3-1 and Figure 3-4 is a good beginning. However, we need more information in order to help us design more effective nutrition education strategies. Some determinants may be more important than others in truly bringing about behavior change for a given group or for a specific behavior, that is, in motivating the elephant and providing the critical moves or skills to the rider. How do we know which of the determinants are more important than others? Are these determinants related to each other? And if so, how do we know their relationships to each other? Are there some that enhance motivation and others that facilitate change? Fortunately, research in the behavioral sciences has investigated just such questions.

SOCIAL PSYCHOLOGICAL APPROACHES TO ACTION AND BEHAVIORAL CHANGE

Much of the work in the health behavior area is based on the pioneering thinking of Kurt Lewin, a leading social psychologist. In the 1940s, he and his graduate students (who went on to become noted social psychologists in their own rights) constituted a vibrant research group who were interested in public health problems facing the country—tuberculosis was rampant and vaccinations were free or very low cost, yet people were not getting these vaccinations. They wanted to find out why or why not. Later, during World War II, when food was short, they wanted to devise educational messages to encourage use of organ meats and whole wheat bread (not considered desirable at that time). They conducted studies to examine what seemed to motivate people to take action in the context of their social world (Lewin 1936; Lewin et al. 1944; Rosenstock 1960). They were researchers who wanted to use their science to solve very practical public health problems. Using their findings, they developed very effective strategies to motivate people to eat these foods.

Their line of research identified perceptions and inner experiences as major determinants of people's actions or behavior. The emphasis was on motivation—what perceptions or inner experiences would motivate people to go for vaccinations or eat organ meats? They found that a major determinant was people's beliefs about the expected outcomes of their behavior: if people thought that a vaccination would truly prevent them from getting tuberculosis or polio, they would go for vaccinations. We have noted that psychologists call this belief an "outcome expectation." The researchers found that people also had to value the outcome—in this case, freedom from tuberculosis or polio (which of course all did). For organ meat, the expected outcome was "support for the war effort" and the value was "supporting the war effort is important to me."

A BASIC "THEORY"

From many studies, the researchers found that together, the determinant "expectations (E) about the outcome of behavior" and the determinant "value (V) of the outcome" statistically predicted "behavior (B)." That is, $E \times V = B$.

This simple description of how the determinants, *expected outcomes* and *values* statistically predict *behavior* is called a **theory**, because it explains why people do what they do. Here are some other examples that illustrate this basic theory. Individuals will be likely to engage in the stated behavior if they believe the following:

I *expect* (E) that buying food at the farmers' market will help local farmers and I *value* (V) supporting local farmers.

I *expect* (E) that eating fruits and vegetables will reduce my risk of chronic diseases, give me good-looking skin, help me maintain a healthy weight, and contribute to a good ecological footprint; I *value* (V) all of these outcomes.

I *expect* (E) that if I model healthy eating practices, my children will also eat healthfully; I *value* (V) my children eating healthfully.

THEORY AS A STRUCTURED GUIDE OR TOOL

From these early beginnings, health behavior researchers have, over the decades, added to this basic, simple "Expectations times Value" theory, other determinants of behavior that are related to each other and to behavior in a predictable way that helps us understand in greater depth why people do what they do and how they change. These coherent sets of predictive relationships are, as we noted above, *theories* about why we do what we do and how we change (DiClemente, Crosby, and Kegler 2002; Brug, Oenema, and Ferreira 2005). The dictionary defines theory as "a set of statements or principles devised to explain a group of facts or phenomena" (*American Heritage Dictionary* 2011). In short, when applied to nutrition education, theory predicts and/or explains behavior or behavior change.

These determinants or predictors of behavior change include items we have already mentioned, such as *beliefs* about outcomes of behavior, *attitudes* towards the behavior, *perceptions of risk* or disease or some other condition, *self-efficacy* or confidence in engaging in the behavior, *perceptions of barriers* to engaging in the behavior, as well as *knowledge* and *skills*. A theory describes the measurable relationships of these items with each other and with behavior. Recall that these beliefs or perceptions may be derived from nutrition science content.

Knowing about such relationships (expressed in a theory) serves as a structured guide or tool for designing nutrition education. We can then use this tool to select the appropriate nutrition education strategies to change the specific determinants that we know will help to change people's actions or behaviors.

Theory Enhances Effectiveness

Kurt Lewin said that there is nothing so practical as a good theory (Lewin 1935). Conducting nutrition education requires considerable resources in terms of time, money, and personnel, which are all usually in short supply. Thus, as nutrition educators, we want to conduct activities that make the most effective use of these resources. We can do that only if our nutrition education programs are based on evidence. Reviews of nutrition education conclude that programs are more likely to be successful when they use appropriate theory and evidence to guide their choice of activities (Contento et al. 1995; Baranowski et al. 2003; Lytle 2005; Diep et al. 2014). This is equivalent to the notion of evidence-based practice used in medicine and other areas of nutrition. If we do not use evidence-based theories, we must rely on guesswork or our own experience.

BOX 3-2 Why Theory Is a Useful Tool for Nutrition Educators: A Summary

Theory is a mental map devised, based on evidence, to predict or explain health behavior. It shows how *determinants* influence action or behavior change. Theory is important to nutrition educators for the following reasons:

- Theory provides an explanation of *why* a behavior or behavior change occurs. It is not just a list of influences on behavior or behavior change. As such, it helps nutrition educators identify the specific set of determinants of behavior change that they should use in their nutrition education intervention.

- Theory specifies the *kinds of information* that need to be gathered before designing an intervention. It helps nutrition educators separate relevant from irrelevant determinants for a given group and behavior.

- Theory also provides nutrition educators guidance on exactly *how to design* the various intervention components and educational strategies to reach people more effectively.

- Theory provides guidance on exactly what to *evaluate* to measure the impact of the intervention, and how to design accurate measuring instruments.

These may be effective, but may not be—usually there is no evidence to know.

Theory Is Generated from Evidence

The purpose of theory is to describe the nature and strength of the relationships of various hypothesized determinants to behavior change or action, such as beliefs, barriers, or self-efficacy. Theories can come from quantitative or interpretative investigations.

Experimental Studies to Generate and Test Theory

Most behavioral science theories use experimental designs to examine the extent to which determinants predict behaviors as hypothesized by theory; that is, to generate information on cause-and-effect relationships between determinants and behavior. These studies can involve quantitative research based on survey methods such as questionnaires or interviews, experiments, or randomized controlled trials, in which numerical data are analyzed quantitatively. Such methods can also be used to test theory and explore its generalizability to various populations.

Qualitative or Interpretative Studies to Generate Theory and Enhance Understanding

Qualitative studies can provide rich descriptions of food-related motivations and behaviors. In this formulation, theories are not developed for their predictive power but because they can be used to help provide a clearer understanding of people's life situations (Bisogni et al. 2012). Here, in-depth interviews and other qualitative methods are used to describe the ways people engage with food, incorporating their own meanings and understandings (Strauss and Corbin 1990). Themes that emerge are recorded, analyzed, and interpreted. Various procedures are used to ensure that findings are credible and trustworthy.

Both Experimental and Interpretive Studies Are Important

Because both the experimental and interpretative approaches attempt to more clearly understand people's motivations and actions with respect to food and nutrition and are empirical in nature, both approaches are important to use and they often converge.

None of the theories derived from research studies provides a complete explanation of food choice and dietary behavior change. Researchers can only infer the true reasons why people do what they do from what people say and what they do. Members of the public are not necessarily being untruthful about why they eat what they do; rather, people often do not know. For example, individuals, particularly adolescents, insist that they are not influenced by others in their environment, yet we all are. In addition, their reasons for what they do may change from time to time and differ by specific behavior.

Best Practices

When evidence accumulates from practice that a given technique, method, or process is more effective than others at delivering a particular outcome and can be generalized, it is referred to as "evidence-based practice" or "best practices" that can be useful to others. These practices have not been rigorously tested but can lead to "practice-based research" to test their effectiveness more formally.

MAKING THEORY EXPLICIT IS EXTREMELY USEFUL

It is helpful for us to make explicit the theory or model guiding our work, because it tells us which determinants on which to focus in our intervention. For example, theory would suggest that adding a module dealing with peer pressure (a psychosocial determinant) would likely enhance breastfeeding outcomes compared with teaching only the basic information about how to breastfeed (facilitating knowledge). Making a theory explicit also helps us to develop appropriate teaching activities. For example, we can use role-playing of peer pressure situations and ask the group for suggestions of how to respond. It also suggests what we evaluate (e.g., measurements of peer pressure as well as functional nutrition knowledge). The result is that we can draw conclusions from our work that will be helpful the next time around; for example, if focusing on social pressure worked but not self-efficacy, next time we may put more effort into activities involving social pressure.

An example illustrates this point: A small town in Minnesota with a strong tradition of producing and consuming lots of beer and butter found that its obesity and overweight rates were higher than the national average and the community's leading cause of death was heart disease (American Dietetic Association 2011). The community decided it wanted to do something about it. They wanted to use evidence-based strategies. So they looked to the experience of another community—that of Kerelia, Finland. That community had found out it had the highest heart disease rate in the world. The community was able

> **Clarifying Terms**
>
> Depending on their purpose, these terms are similar in terms of behavior change:
>
> > Influences = determinants = mediators
> > = constructs = variables
>
> **Determinants**
>
> Help us *understand* behavior
>
> **Mediators**
>
> Help us figure out what can *change* behavior
>
> **Constructs**
>
> When determinants or mediators are *systematically* used in a theory
>
> **Variables**
>
> The *operational definitions* of constructs in a specific situation

to turn the situation around and has reduced heart attacks significantly for more than 30 years. The team from Minnesota flew to Finland to learn about the **theoretical framework** that guided Karelia's work along with their effective strategies and techniques. The Minnesota town was able to apply the lessons learned by Karelia with success—fruit and vegetable consumption increased more than one serving per person per day, people lost weight, and their cholesterol levels dropped. This is an example of how making theory explicit can be helpful to others.

COMPONENTS OF THEORY: CLARIFYING TERMS

Some theories are more complex than are others, and some have been more thoroughly conceptualized and intensively studied than have others. Each theory uses unique terms to describe the factors influencing behavior or specific concepts that are important for the theory based on its origins. Often these terms are similar across theories; this is noted below where appropriate. Some of the themes generated from qualitative studies are also similar to **constructs** in standard health behavior change theories. Some clarifications are provided here.

Constructs and Variables

The influences on behavior that we have described so far as determinants of action or behavior change, such as beliefs, benefits, emotions, and attitudes, are the building blocks of theories. These building blocks have different names depending on their function, as described below.

- *Constructs:* When these determinants are systematically used in a particular theory, they are called *constructs*, or mentally constructed ideas about unobservable, intangible attributes (beliefs, attitudes) that are part of the theory. They exist in the mind as abstractions about some aspect of human experience. No one has observed "beliefs" about salt in the diet or "attitudes" toward breastfeeding. Yet, researchers can talk about them and measure them. For example, if a person believes that there are benefits to reducing salt intake because it reduces risk of hypertension, this belief can influence whether he or she adds salt to food. This belief about benefits becomes the "perceived benefits" construct in the health belief model.

- *Variables:* This term is often used synonymously with *constructs*, but variables are really the operational definitions of constructs, specifying how a construct is to be measured for a specific situation. They are "variables" because they can vary in value. Thus, the perceived benefits of taking a specific action, such as the benefit of eating fruits and vegetables to reduce cancer risk, can be measured on a 1 to 5 scale. Individuals may judge the same specific benefit differently: some individuals may judge eating fruits and vegetables to reduce cancer risk as highly beneficial, giving it a score of 5, whereas others as only moderately so, giving it a score of 2 or 3.

Names of Determinants or Constructs Serve as "Buckets"

Behavioral scientists give determinants/mediators/constructs/variables specific names, such as *attitudes, perceived risk, perceived benefits,* and so forth, depending on their psychosocial function. But these names are really for content-free categories or empty "buckets." The food and nutrition information for what is in each of these buckets must be obtained from any given audience or group through means such as in-depth interviews or quantitative surveys. For example, the *positive outcome expectations* (or perceived benefits) of eating fruits and vegetables bucket for adults may be their role in prevention of chronic disease (the nutrition content or items in bucket), but for adolescents, the perceived benefits may be clear skin and help in controlling weight.

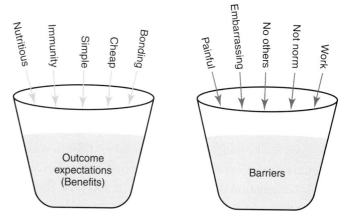

FIGURE 3-7 Determinants of breastfeeding.

In terms of breastfeeding, the *positive outcomes expectations* (bucket) or perceived benefits may be that breastmilk is nutritious for the baby, has immune substances, promotes bonding, and so forth (items in bucket). But there are also *barriers* (bucket) such as it may be painful at first; it may be embarrassing to do except in private; others, including the father, cannot be involved; and so forth (items in bucket). These are shown in **FIGURE 3-7**.

Theory, Model, and Theoretical Framework

The terms *theory, model,* and *theoretical framework* are used to describe similar ideas:

- *Theory* is usually used to describe a clearly stated set of relationships among core constructs, such as beliefs or attitudes that explain or predict behavior change or action based on evidence.

- *Model* usually just describes relationships between two or more constructs, focusing more generally on *how* they relate. Often a **model** is a composite of constructs created from several compatible theories based on evidence. Models can be used to develop a specific nutrition education program in a particular setting, where perhaps one theory alone is not sufficient. Or a model can be built with a subset of constructs from a theory.

- *Theoretical framework* refers to a description of a set of concepts in relation to each other. It is less formal than a theory or model.

These terms are overlapping and definitions are not standardized. In this book, we use the terms as given by the researchers who developed and tested them. That is, if they refer to their mental map as a theory (e.g., the "theory of planned behavior"), we use the word *theory;* if they use the term *model* (e.g., the "health belief model"), we use the word *model*. The term *theory*, when used in a general sense in this book, refers to all of the specific theories and models.

RELATIONSHIPS AMONG RESEARCH, THEORY, AND PRACTICE

Research has been defined as a "careful or diligent search; investigation or experimentation aimed at the discovery and interpretation of facts; revision of accepted theories or practical application of such new or revised theories" (Merriam-Webster 2014). Research and theory are thus interrelated. Theory is a dynamic entity. Research generates theory; at the same time, theory is guided by, and tested through, research and practice. Stated more simply, theory is not divorced from practical experience but is in fact experience that has been systematically explored and reflected upon.

Theory can be tested, refined, and modified as it is applied in interventions in practice settings and its effectiveness is evaluated (Rothman 2004). Thus theory, research, and practice all need each other.

With these definitions in hand we are now in a position to examine how theories are important to nutrition educators.

MANY THEORIES FROM THE BEHAVIORAL SCIENCES CAN BE HELPFUL

It is clear that eating behavior is complex, involving many different kinds of foods and drinks and different eating patterns, unlike, for example, smoking or alcohol use. It also involves many settings and situations, and is influenced by many personal and environmental factors that often conflict with each other. We are interested in people's health beliefs with respect to food, nutrition, and physical activity. Because food is most often eaten in social contexts and may involve negotiations with others, we are keenly interested in theories of social interactions as well. Thus we have had to draw from a variety of theories originating in the behavioral sciences, food choice research, health education, or related fields depending on our intervention or purpose. These theories were each developed to explain specific kinds of behavior that were of interest for different reasons:

- *Health behavior theories:* Psychologists interested in public health developed theories specifically to explain why people did or did not take some action that might prevent a negative health condition, such as participation in immunizations to prevent polio or screenings for HIV infection. These theories emphasize health beliefs (Hochbaum 1958).
- *Food choice theories:* Other researchers were interested in food choice. They wanted to find out what people wanted in their foods—taste, cost, convenience, texture, and so forth. Health might or might not have been an important concern. These researchers produced theories of food choice (Conner and Armitage 2002).
- *Social behaviors:* Still other theories were originally developed to explain a variety of people's day-to-day behaviors in social settings, such as purchasing various goods, voting, participating in organizations, selecting a college to attend, and so forth. These theories sought to identify and understand both intrapersonal and interpersonal influences on behavior (Ajzen 1998).

No single behavioral theory, as an abstract representation of reality, may be able to capture all the factors determining people's food- and activity-related behaviors. Different theories may be useful for different behaviors and different settings. We shall see, however, that there is a good deal of overlap among the various theories. Consequently, there has been a call for combining the determinants from different models based on current evidence (Achterberg and Miller 2004) or using more comprehensive theories (Triandis 1979; Kok et al. 1996; Institute of Medicine 2002; Baranowski et al. 2009).

WHAT SOCIAL PSYCHOLOGICAL THEORIES SHARE IN COMMON

The social psychological theories of human motivation and action have several attributes in common. This is good news for nutrition educators because we can focus on these attributes as we design our nutrition education.

The Importance of Perceptions

The theories share an emphasis on the importance of our perceptions as influences on or determinants of our behaviors. The social psychological approach proposes that although behavior certainly leads to objective consequences (such as actual impact on chronic disease or carbon footprint) the *interpretation* of these consequences by the individual has enormous influence on the person's intention to perform the behavior in the future (Lewin et al. 1944; Fishbein and Ajzen 1975, 2010).

While many social environmental and cultural forces exist in people's environment, social psychologist Triandis (1979) suggests that for any given individual, even such "external" factors as culture and social situations influence behavior because they are internalized by each individual. Thus, culture and social situations exist not only "out there" but also "in here," as subjective culture and *subjective social situations* that serve as mental maps that guide our behavior by influencing our values, norms, roles, and so forth. There is an economic world "out there," but our *perceptions* of the availability of food, cost, and time all have powerful impacts on our behaviors as well. All in all, our perception of the world appears to be a powerful influence on behavior. Indeed, often what people will or will not do is influenced as much by their *perception* of reality as by reality itself (Lewin et al. 1944; Bandura 1986; Conner and Armitage 2002; Rutter and Quine 2002).

Weighing the Pros and Cons

Individuals weigh the costs and benefits of the behavior (e.g., the inconvenience and exertion involved in exercising versus the improved muscle tone and decreased weight) to determine whether they will take action. In general, people are motivated to maximize the chances of desirable outcomes and minimize the chances of undesirable outcomes. That is, they ask the question, "What's in it for *me* (or for my family, my friends, my community, or planet Earth)?" Only when they are convinced that there is something in it for them that is personally meaningful will they be motivated to act. Goals can be short term and immediate or may be more long term and global, involving values and ethics for individuals, the community, or the planet.

Beliefs About Outcomes or Expectations of the Behavior

Some important kinds of outcomes are listed below. If individuals also value these outcomes, they are likely to take action.

- *Health outcomes:* Health outcomes are beliefs that certain actions can enhance health or reduce risk of disease.
- *Social outcomes:* Social outcomes are expectations of what others will think when an individual performs the behavior.

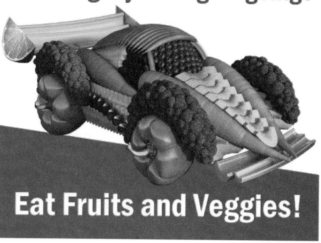

Expected outcomes that are desirable to the intended audience can be very motivating.

Reproduced from Food and Nutrition Graphics Library, United States Department of Agriculture. http://www.fns.usda.gov Accessed 1/2/2015.

BOX 3-3 What Is Motivation?

Human motivation is very complex and research has generated many descriptions and theories for it. In general, it is the internal condition that activates behavior, energizes it, and gives it direction.

Some theories focus on conditioning and rewards as motivators. Others note that motivation ranges on a continuum from extrinsic and controlled motivation to intrinsic and autonomous motivation. Extrinsic motivation comes from a desire to meet expectations from outside of the person. But motivation can come from experiencing intrinsic rewards inherent to a task or activity itself, or the satisfaction of basic human needs, such as for autonomy, competence or relatedness to others.

Motivation can also come from beliefs about the self, others, and outcomes of behavior. Social psychological theories generally emphasize that we will engage in a behavior if we believe it will bring about outcomes that we desire or value.

We want to maximize positive outcomes and minimize negative outcomes. These desired outcomes may serve immediate goals or larger intrinsic values that we possess. Health promotion generally uses social psychological theories of motivation.

■ *Self-evaluative outcomes:* Self-evaluative outcomes, such as self-esteem, self-image, or self-identity are also important for certain behaviors or situations.

Beliefs About Self-Efficacy or Confidence to Perform the Behavior

Researchers who have studied a variety of social behaviors have found that in addition to beliefs about outcomes, individuals' estimates of whether they will be able to perform the behaviors are extremely important. This construct is called self-efficacy and is central to many theories.

Influence of Culture, Life Stage, Past Experiences, and Other Factors

Other factors that are not directly changeable with a nutrition education program, such as past experiences, life stage and life trajectories, personality, socioeconomic factors, place of residence, and social and cultural context, are not specifically part of these theories. However, social psychological theories propose that although early childhood experiences with food, past life experiences, life stage, place of residence, socioeconomic situation, and one's cultural context cannot be changed, they do—if they are currently meaningful to the individual—influence behavior by influencing *current* preferences, beliefs, attitudes, values, expectations, motivations, sense of efficacy, and habits. These *current* beliefs, attitudes, and values can be captured by theory and research and targeted by nutrition education.

SOCIAL PSYCHOLOGICAL THEORY IN OUTLINE

Motivation to Take Action

In its simplest terms, then, social psychology theory suggests that for a particular action or dietary behavior change to occur, we need to possess the following convictions or beliefs about the particular behavior, referred to here as *X*. These beliefs together provide motivation for *why-to* take action. The first belief is this:

■ I want to do *X* because I expect it to lead to outcomes I value.

That is, we—as individuals or families—need to care about taking a particular action and feel that it is in our interest to do so. It is the building block of several theories and is given the name *outcome expectations*.

Example: I will breastfeed my infant because it will lead to better health for my infant and better bonding between us, both of which I value.

■ I feel confident that I can do *X*.

Once we are convinced that taking action has the desired consequences for us or our families, once we *care*, once we are motivationally ready, we need to feel confident that we can carry out the action to obtain these benefits. This too is a construct that is common to most contemporary **health behavior theories** and is referred to as *self-efficacy*. That is, we need to feel confidant that our rider will be able to script the moves.

Example: I feel confident that I will be able to breastfeed my infant.

■ I desire to do this.

These considerations lead me, or my family, to desire to do this behavior or practice. That is, the elephant in us is now on board.

■ I will do X.

If these convictions are strong, the likelihood is increased that we will decide on a given health action. This is called behavioral intention or goal intention.

Example: I will breastfeed my infant.

Facilitating Knowledge and Skills to Change Behavior

Translating intentions into actions requires information and skills for *how-to* take action:

■ I have the food and nutrition knowledge and skills to take action.

Translating intentions into actions also requires that we have the needed functional *food and nutrition knowledge and skills* to carry out the action. This is called *behavioral capability* in health psychology theory.

Example: I know how to breastfeed my infant.

■ I have the self-regulation or self-direction skills to take action.

Maintaining the behavior over the long term requires a further step: the development of the ability to think through what we want and then consciously choose our actions. This process is referred to as self-direction or *action goal-setting skills*. Here, we set small goals to achieve the outcomes we desire and monitor our actions to evaluate how well we are fulfilling our action plans or goals. We then take corrective action as necessary.

Example: I have set the action goal to breastfeed my infant exclusively for at least 3 months. I will monitor myself to see how it goes. If I have difficulties, I will know how to problem solve or where to go for help.

The Aha! Moment in Behavior Change: Chaos Theory

You have probably experienced an *aha* moment—when suddenly everything seems to come together and you can make the change you had wanted to make but could not for so long. Through nutrition education efforts, individuals may become aware of their own motivations or their behaviors, but they do not immediately take action; when they do, they may not make the decision in the orderly sequence laid out previously and as described in various models. Researchers suggest that chaos theory from physics can make sense of these phenomena (Resnicow and Page 2008).

It is known, for example, that smokers, on average, make eight attempts to quit before they successfully do so. They do so when they experience an *aha* moment. They cannot usually explain why they were successful this particular time. The determinants or theory constructs described earlier are still important and, on average, may work well. But for any given individual, the new information given about expected outcomes from taking action, the new feelings engendered, or the new skills provided may need to percolate in what may appear to be a chaotic fashion. From numerous occasions of nutrition education or individual counseling, after much rumination about the influences on their dietary or physical activity patterns and about what the individual wants out of life may come action. Because nutrition educators do not know when or why any given individual may choose to take action, we must use theory-based interventions to keep providing opportunities for individuals to contemplate and decide (Brug 2006).

Application to Different Life Stage Groups

These theories can be used in nutrition education for a variety of population and cultural groups. For different population groups, the beliefs about desired outcomes may be different, based on cultural expectations, past life experiences, life stage (e.g., mothers of young children, postmenopausal women), or role in life (e.g., mothers, husbands, businesspeople). These beliefs must be carefully explored in needs assessments or formative research using these theories to understand the behavior from the perspective of the intended audience.

Application to Different Cultural Groups

Researchers believe that when properly understood and applied, these theories can be used with many diverse cultural groups. Fishbein (2000) notes that each of the variables of the theory of planned/reasoned action approach, for example, can be found in any culture, and has been used in HIV programs in more than 50 countries in both the developing and developed worlds. In the area of diet, the relative importance of the variables may differ for different groups. For example in one study of Chinese Americans, attitudes were more important for more Western-identified individuals for performing healthy obesity-reducing behaviors, whereas perceived behavioral control, self-efficacy and perceived benefits were more important for Asian-identified individuals (Liou, Bauer, and Bai 2014). For some groups, outcome expectations based on cultural beliefs regarding food may be more important than is convenience. For others, taste preferences are more important for motivating behavior change than are health considerations. For still others, the influence of family may override all other considerations. These observations indicate that nutrition educators need to be culturally sensitive when using theory as a tool for nutrition education in different cultural groups. Working with different cultural groups is described in detail in Chapter 17.

> Theories are applied in social and cultural context when used to design nutrition education. Culture, life stage, social roles, early experiences, or socioeconomic conditions will all influence current beliefs, outcome expectations, sense of empowerment, and so forth of the audiences with whom we work. These social and cultural factors need to be sensitively and competently explored and addressed as we design and conduct nutrition education activities.

Application to Those with Diet-Related Conditions

The theories can also be used for those at high risk or who already have diet-related conditions and are attending outpatient clinics or other venues for nutritional care. The Academy of Nutrition and Dietetics in the United States has developed a model that nutrition and dietetic professionals use when working with such populations, called the Nutrition Care Process and Model (*Journal of the Academy of Nutrition and Dietetics* 2008). It asks the professional to do a careful *assessment* of the individuals' health condition and behaviors or practices as well as the various factors influencing these behaviors or practices. The process then involves an appropriate nutrition *diagnosis*, followed by *intervention* and then *monitoring* and *evaluation*. For such populations, clear direction to the rider, engaging the elephant, and shaping the path are no less important than for well populations and may indeed be more important.

Applications to Exercising Individuals and Athletes

It is often thought that athletes and others who participate in various physical activities need only accurate information about nutrition in order to eat healthfully. While accurate information is necessary, so is motivation. Indeed, motivation may be more necessary. Athletes often believe that they can eat just about anything because they will burn off the calories. They may be more interested in enhancing performance, and their choices are not necessarily healthful. So the use of theory to design motivational group and counseling sessions, posters, and hand-outs is extremely important. These can be followed by skills to put their motivations into practice.

Element of Success 4: Addressing Multiple Influences on Behavior Change with Sufficient Duration and Intensity—A Social-Ecological Approach

An important conclusion from recent research, which also supports the early conclusions of Whitehead (1973), is that nutrition education is more likely to be effective when it addresses the many levels of influences on behavior, ranging from food preferences and the sensory-affective responses to food to personal factors such as beliefs and attitudes and to the environmental and policy context.

For intentions or decisions to be translated into action and for the actions to be maintained for the long term, a supportive social and physical environment is required. At first, individuals may only adopt the behavior on a trial basis. Long-term maintenance of the behavior depends on whether they can fit it into their daily lives, whether there is social support for the behavior, and whether material conditions or social structures are in place or can be modified in some way to make it possible to carry out this new practice. Nutrition education programs thus seek to provide environmental support to individuals to enable them to act on their motivations and apply their skills.

To do this, nutrition educators work in collaboration with others—organization and community leaders, decision makers, policymakers, and legislators—to develop programs at several levels of intervention, as shown in detail in **FIGURE 3-8**.

- *Intrapersonal or individual level:* Focusing on the psychobiological core of experience with food, food preferences, and enjoyment of food, as well as beliefs, attitudes, values, functional knowledge, skills, perceived social and cultural norms, or life experience
- *Interpersonal level:* Focusing on family, friends, peers, interactions with health professionals, cultural norms and practices, social roles, and social networks
- *Environmental settings involving institutions/organizations and communities:* Focusing on availability and accessibility of healthful foods and physical activity facilities, and opportunities for taking action in workplaces or schools and other settings
- *Sectors of influence—social structure, policy, and systems:* Focusing on policies and social structures that regulate health actions

This approach is called the social-ecological model (McLeroy et al. 1988; Gregson et al. 2001; Story et al. 2008). The idea of directing interventions at various spheres of influence is now widely used in health promotion and is part of government policy in most countries (Booth et al. 2001; Green and Kreuter 2005; Story et al. 2008; U.S. Department of Agriculture and U.S. Department of Health and Human Services 2010; Hawkes 2013; McNulty 2013).

A simple diagram of nutrition education directed at several levels of intervention is shown in **FIGURE 3-9**.

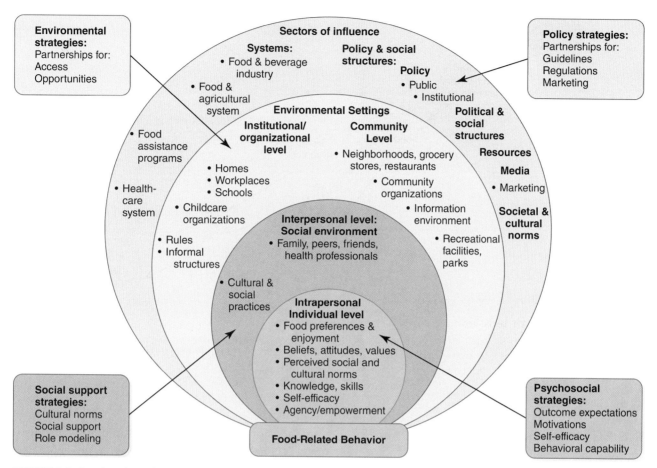

FIGURE 3-8 Social-ecological model: levels of influence for nutrition education interventions.

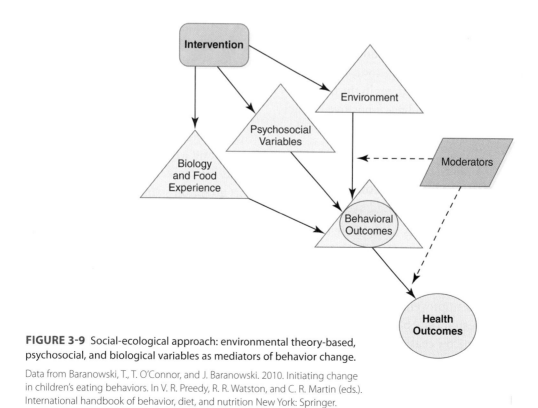

FIGURE 3-9 Social-ecological approach: environmental theory-based, psychosocial, and biological variables as mediators of behavior change.

Data from Baranowski, T., T. O'Connor, and J. Baranowski. 2010. Initiating change in children's eating behaviors. In V. R. Preedy, R. R. Watston, and C. R. Martin (eds.). International handbook of behavior, diet, and nutrition New York: Springer.

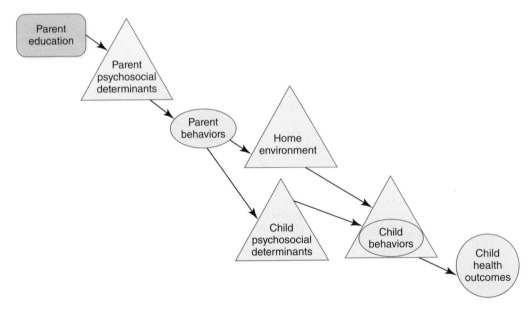

FIGURE 3-10 Social-ecological approach: Family-based programs.

Adapted from Baranowski, T., T. O'Connor, and J. Baranowski. 2010. Initiating change in children's eating behaviors. In *International handbook of behavior, diet, and nutrition,* edited by V. R. Preedy, R. R. Watston, and C. R. Martin. New York: Springer.

CHANGING BEHAVIORS THROUGH GATEKEEPERS

Many nutrition education interventions involve working with parents or families to address their children's health issues (such as child overweight) or to help their children develop healthy eating and physical activity behaviors (eating more fruits and vegetables, less screen time). In this case, the intervention works to enhance and support the parents' motivations and facilitate their food-related and parenting skills and also to make changes in the home environment of the child in order to have a positive impact on their children's behaviors (Hingle et al. 2010, 2012). This is shown in **FIGURE 3-10**.

Duration and Intensity of Intervention

Studies suggest that nutrition education that provides sufficient duration and **intensity** is more likely to be effective. A notable illustration is the "Know Your Body" program, which was designed to reduce cardiovascular risk. This program involved 30 to 50 hours per year for 3 years and achieved improvements in physiological parameters (serum cholesterol and blood pressure) as well as diet (Walter 1989; Resnicow et al. 1992). A conceptually similar intervention, CATCH, involved 15 to 20 hours per year over 3 years (third through fifth grades) and resulted

in behavior changes, though not in physiological parameters (Luepker et al. 1996). These behavioral changes were still in evidence in the eighth grade (Nader et al. 1999). Many obesity prevention studies have also found that longer duration was important for effectiveness (Khambalia et al. 2012).

A large-scale evaluation of health education programs in schools addressing a variety of behaviors found that although large effect sizes could be achieved in program-specific knowledge in about 8 hours and general knowledge in about 20, only moderate effect sizes could be achieved in attitudes and behaviors even after 35 to 50 hours (Connell, Turner, and Mason 1985).

At the same time, consumers and patients often have short attention spans, and for many practical reasons nutrition education programs are of short duration. This presents a dilemma for nutrition educators. One way to resolve this dilemma is to use a coordinated and systematic approach delivered through multiple venues to provide nutrition education using many levels of intervention and through multiple channels so that, in total, sufficient duration and intensity are delivered to individuals and the public. For example, nutrition education interventions can involve group sessions, newsletters, posters, mobile phone activities, and social marketing.

Element of Success 5: Designing Nutrition Education Using Theory- and Evidence-Based Strategies

Nutrition education is more likely to be successful when it uses behavior change strategies derived from theory to achieve its behavioral goals. For any given nutrition education intervention, we first conduct a careful assessment of the intended audience and then select the appropriate theory to use based on that assessment. The assessment should include not only objective data, but also information from the audience about their needs, assets, and desires in the context of their families, communities, and culture. We then select the strategies that go with the determinants in that theory and develop engaging and meaningful activities.

Simply put, nutrition education strategies from theory change determinants and, in turn, determinants change behaviors as shown in **FIGURE 3-11**. Each strategy can change one or more determinants, and often two or more strategies are needed to change one or more determinants. Usually several determinants are needed to change behaviors.

These determinants of behavior are shown in **FIGURE 3-12** and can be categorized into those that enhance motivation and facilitate behavior change—food-related and intra- and interpersonal determinants—and those that provide environmental supports for action. These sets of determinants influence whether individuals will make the food and nutrition-related behavior changes, which then influence nutritional status and nutritional well-being and disease risk.

Figure 3-12 acknowledges that biological factors such as age, gender, and genetics and some external physical factors such as physical activity, concurrent infections, and other issues also have impacts on health and on behaviors and that these are not modifiable by nutrition education. At the same time, people's behaviors can have effects on the environment, such as the kinds of food systems in place, through consumer demand. Hence there are arrows both ways. For example, if individuals make food choices based primarily on taste, low cost, and convenience, then that is what the food system will provide. If people make choices based on quality or concern for the viability of local farms,

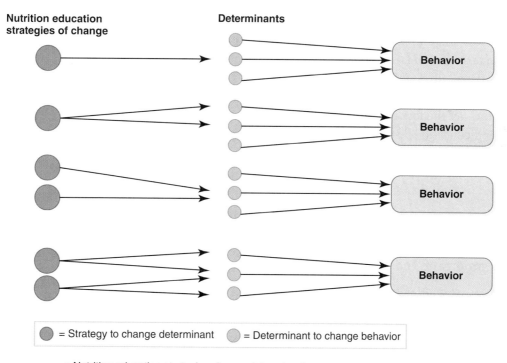

FIGURE 3-11 Using nutrition education strategies to change determinants, which then lead to behavior change.

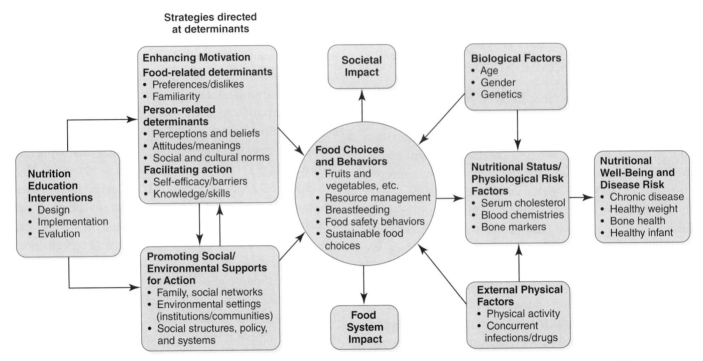

FIGURE 3-12 Strategies addressing determinants to change behaviors, and impacts on nutritional, food system, and societal well-being.

then the food system will reflect those choices. People's food-related behaviors and practices also have impacts on society, such as on farmers and farm workers and on how food-related social structures and communities are organized. The central location of behaviors in Figure 3-8 shows that behaviors are the focus of nutrition education and that developing educational strategies to change the determinants of these behaviors is the central mission of nutrition education. Strategies to address these determinants are described in great detail in Chapters 11 and 12.

BOX 3-4 *How* You Conduct Nutrition Education Is Important, Too!

Once nutrition education strategies and activities for a session or intervention have been designed, *how* they are delivered is extremely important. The activities are most effective when they are engaging, well organized, and meaningful. Educators are most effective when they are enthusiastic about what they are presenting, and seen as credible, warm, respectful, and sensitive to the cultures and social settings of their audience.

Putting It All Together: Conceptual Framework for Conducting Nutrition Education

Nutrition educators frequently assume that diet-related change is a quick, one-step process. One day individuals are eating unhealthful diets, and the next day, after "nutrition education," they are model eaters. This assumption leads us to expect that people change quickly and thus expect that a typical four- to six-session (or even one-session) program can change lifelong dietary habits. This is an unrealistic view of how we make changes in our lives, and it places unrealistic expectations on health promotion and nutrition education programs—and on ourselves.

BEHAVIOR CHANGE MAY TAKE TIME

Given so many influences on our food choices and eating patterns, it is not surprising that behavior change takes time. It may take a short time for some individuals or for some behaviors and a long time for others. Motivations have to be enhanced and skills have to be developed.

We have seen that nutrition education has three main *functions*: enhancing motivation, facilitating action through increasing factual nutrition knowledge and skills and self-direction skills, and promoting environmental supports for action. Generally the motivational function comes first as it focuses on *thinking and decision making*. This is followed by the skills development function, where the focus is on action or *doing*. An environmental support component is also important. We will refer to these as the three *components* of nutrition education. The research suggests that different processes are going on within individuals in these components and the determinants of change may be different for each (Prochaska and DiClemente 1982; Conner and Norman 1995; Schwarzer and Fuchs 1995; Norman, Abraham, and Conner 2000).

The specific behavior changes targeted by the nutrition education intervention are identified first. The conceptual framework that links the dietary change process to nutrition education practice, as shown in **FIGURE 3-13**, is explored in greater detail in the following sections.

The Motivational Component: A Focus on Enhancing Motivation (Why-to Take Action)

When individuals are in the thinking phase about dietary change, beliefs and attitudes or feelings are most important. These beliefs and attitudes can result in motivational readiness to make changes, expressed in the form of a *behavioral intention*, or choice of a specific action goal. Using the metaphor of Haidt (2006, 2012) and Heath and Heath (2010), the function of nutrition education is to engage the elephant in our audience or their emotional side, so that it is eager for the path.

- *Dietary change process within the individual:* The behavior change process going on within the individual is focused on becoming motivated to consider action and deciding whether to take action. Theory and evidence from research suggest that beliefs are important, such as whether individuals feel a sense of risk or threat regarding some issue; expectations about the outcomes of taking action, including perceived benefits and barriers; expectations of family and friends; and self-efficacy. Engaging these determinants may result in a decision-making phase in which individuals analyze the benefits versus the costs of taking action and clarify their values. When a decision is made, an intention is formed to take action.
- *Nutrition education program objective:* During this period, the objective is to increase awareness,

promote contemplation, and enhance the motivation to act.
- *Focus of nutrition education strategies:* During this time, the focus of the education program is on *why-to* take action (or motivating the elephant).

The Action Component: A Focus on How-to Take Action

When individuals decide to take action they can start making *action plans* so that intentions can be translated into action. That is, the rider now has a clear direction and can script the moves. An action plan might be "I will add to my diet a fruit for a snack 3 days this coming week."

- *Dietary change process within the individual:* At this time, the behavior change process going on within the individual is focused on initiating action and maintaining it for the long term. At first, individuals may need to learn new functional food and nutrition information and new skills, such as learning about what constitutes a serving of fruits and vegetables, how to store and prepare them, and how to read food labels, or knowing the diabetic exchange system, how to breastfeed, or how to handle family conflicts over food. These result in self-efficacy and a sense of personal agency or ability to exert influence on one's behavior as well as one's environment that can lead to development of personal food policies and to acting with others to make changes in the community through collective efficacy.
- *Nutrition education program objective:* The objective is to facilitate the individual's ability to act.
- *Focus of nutrition education strategies:* During the action phase, the focus of the education program is on *how-to* take action (or helping the rider to script the moves).

The Environmental and Policy Support Component

A supportive environment is important throughout the dietary change process. The nutrition education program objective is to educate decision-makers, policymakers, and others who have power and authority to make changes in the environment and policy about the importance of nutrition and health concerns and to work in collaboration with them to promote more supportive environments, including interpersonal social support, community activation, food and physical activity environments, and policy. The goal is to shape the path.

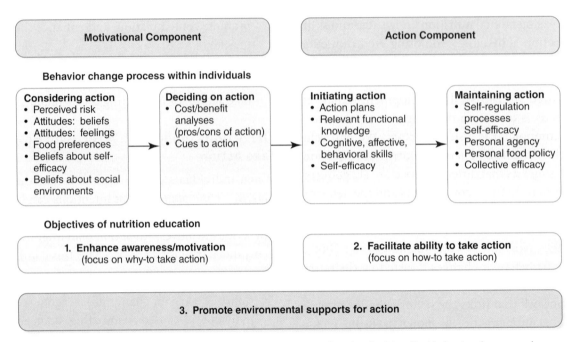

FIGURE 3-13 Conceptual framework for theory-based nutrition education for identified behavior change goals.

PUTTING IT ALL TOGETHER

In most audiences or groups, and those reached through other venues such as Web materials, newsletters, or telephone apps, people are at different phases in the change process. Thus, nutrition education in whichever venue should generally begin with motivational activities or why-to information, based on a careful assessment of and with the intended audience. This should be followed by strategies to provide skills and functional, or how-to, information to assist individuals to take action. For all audiences, but particularly those ready to take action, environmental supports are important.

The Cases of Alicia and Ray

Let us now examine the cases of Alicia and Ray again. Alicia is not very concerned about her diet. She appears to be in a pre-action mode. Yet the nutrition science literature suggests that this is the time in her life when eating a healthy diet could make a big difference in her health in the future. So, the motivational function of nutrition education would likely be most appropriate for her, with an emphasis on motivational or why-to information and activities.

Ray, on the other hand, has thought about his situation. His problem seems to be related to how to translate interest and intention into action. For Ray, strengthening his beliefs about taking action and the functional knowledge and skills to do so may be appropriate.

The next few chapters describe theory and evidence from nutrition education and health behavior research that can help you determine the kinds of strategies that might work for Alicia and Ray.

MySmileBuddy

Early childhood caries (ECC) is a serious, diet-dependent, fluoride-mediated oral disease that affects nearly one in three children before age 5. As the most common chronic disease of childhood, ECC causes tooth decay in primary teeth, often requiring extensive dental repair or even surgical extraction of teeth under general anesthesia. Children with ECC experience pain and discomfort that interferes with eating, sleeping, speaking, and behavior, resulting in diminished quality of life and self-esteem. In order to combat rising rates of ECC, a multidisciplinary team of dentists, nutrition educators, and digital media experts in New York City worked together to design a Web-based, iPad-enabled ECC risk assessment and educational tool, MySmileBudy, to help families recognize their child's risk for ECC and make positive behavior changes to reduce that risk.

Designed to be used by lay health workers (e.g., community health workers), the technology-supported MySmileBuddy tool emphasizes prevention through diet- and fluoride-related lifestyle changes and engages families through both motivational and educational activities. In addition to helping families, MySmileBuddy also presents a new way for dentists to collaborate with other health professionals (e.g., nutritionists, social workers, nurses) and lay health workers to promote nutrition-related behavior change. The program is described in **NUTRITION EDUCATION IN ACTION 3-2.**

NUTRITION EDUCATION IN ACTION 3-2 **MySmileBuddy**

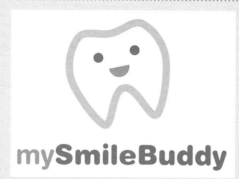

Columbia University. Developed by the MySmileBuddy research and demonstration team with support from the National Institute on Minority Health and Health Disparities, Burton Edelstein DDS MPH, PI.

MySmileBuddy includes highly visual and interactive assessment modules to calculate a child's estimated risk score for ECC, which serves to motivate families to make positive behavior changes to reduce their child's risk. Because ECC is largely a diet-dependent disease, MySmileBuddy incorporates a modified 24-hour recall in its dietary assessment module to record data on a child's reported dietary intake. It then provides clear, accurate, culturally-tailored informational videos and animations for parents on how to brush and floss their child's teeth, how to implement dietary changes to reduce ECC risk, how the ECC disease process begins and progresses, and what they can do to prevent ECC. Finally, MySmileBuddy helps families tailor personal goals to their child's specific needs. The MySmileBuddy intervention also includes educational handouts that also act as a goal-planning tool to reinforce goals and help families evaluate their progress. Through repeated use of MySmileBuddy, families are able to evaluate their progress on goals, choose new goals, and visualize how their lifestyle changes help to reduce their child's risk of ECC. Here's how theory was used to design the program:

Why-To

- Families learn that decreasing exposure to sugary foods and beverages can decrease risk of ECC by watching informational videos and talking with the health worker administering MySmileBuddy (outcome expectations).
- Families assess their child's dietary risk of ECC using the MySmileBuddy dietary assessment module, including the modified 24-hour recall (risk).

- Mothers compare their behaviors to other mothers while completing the risk assessment modules and through conversation with the health worker (social norms).
- Families express increased confidence in reducing ECC risk after using MySmileBuddy to set personalized, realistic goals (self-efficacy).

How-To

- Families learn to identify their child's current exposure to sugary foods and beverages using the MySmileBuddy dietary assessment module (self-assessment/self-regulation).
- Families choose an appropriate goal and action plan for reducing their child's exposure to sugary foods and beverages from a tailored list provided by the MySmileBuddy tool (goal-setting/self-regulation).
- Families learn to assess if they were successful at meeting their chosen goal using the goal-planning tools and by reevaluating their child's risk (self-regulation).

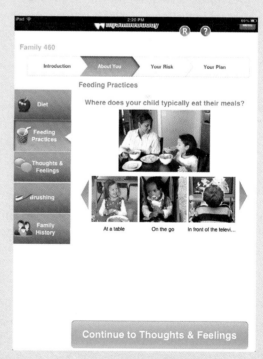

Columbia University. Developed by the MySmileBuddy research and demonstration team with support from the National Institute on Minority Health and Health Disparities, Burton Edelstein DDS MPH, PI.

(Continues)

NUTRITION EDUCATION IN ACTION 3-2 MySmileBuddy (Continued)

Evaluation

The Diet and Early Childhood Caries (DECC) study evaluated the self-reported impact of the MySmileBuddy intervention via telephone survey 1 month post-intervention. Of the parents who completed the follow-up survey:

- 68% reported that they had taken action towards their MySmileBuddy goal.
- Examples of stated actions included, ". . . buy Cheetos once per month and start buying yogurt," "Water is added to juice . . . avoid buying sweets," "Replace juice with water."

Source: Custodio-Lumsden, C., et al. 2014. The diet and early childhood caries (DECC) study: Feasibility, acceptability, and short-term impact of a novel ECC intervention. National Oral Health Conference.

NUTRITION EDUCATION IN ACTION 3-3 Cooking with Kids

Cooking with Kids is a program designed to improve children's intakes of fruits, vegetables, and whole grains (the targeted behaviors) through several kinds of activities at various levels of intervention. These are described here:

- **Individual-level intervention**: Fruit- and vegetable-tasting activities for students in the classroom; cooking fresh, affordable foods from diverse cultures; nutrition information; foods in history; food journal activities; and take-home recipes.

- **Family-level activities**: Volunteer participation; activities such as families getting together at the school during the evening and cooking and eating together, events, and incentives.

- **Institutional or environmental level**: Improvements in the meals offered at school through collaboration with others, such as farm-to-table organizations; locally grown produce included in school meals; foods cooked in the classroom adapted and served in school meals.

Evaluation

In a pilot evaluation, more than 80% of the students reported liking the foods cooked in the classroom, 75% chose the foods in the cafeteria, and 60% ate half or more of the lunch. About 50% of the parents reported that they used Cooking with Kids recipes at home, and 65% said their children now ate more fruits and vegetables at home.

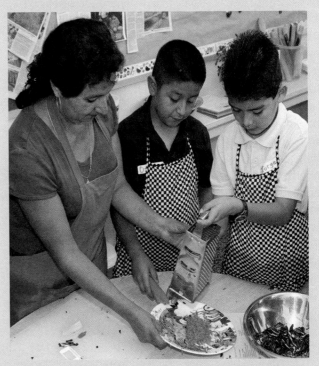

Cooking with Kids incorporates nutrition education into the classroom curriculum and involves the family.

Courtesy of Cooking with Kids.

Sources: Walters, L., J. Stacey, and L. Cunningham-Sabo. 2005. *Learning comes alive through classroom cooking: Cooking with Kids.* Presented at the annual meeting of the Society for Nutrition Education. Orlando, FL; Walters, L., and J. Stacey. Cooking with Kids. http://www.cookingwithkids.net.

Cooking with Kids

The Cooking with Kids program is based on a **social-ecological model**. The program consists of individual-level activities directed at students in the classroom, family-level activities, and institutional-level activities designed to improve foods offered at school. The program is described in **NUTRITION EDUCATION IN ACTION 3-3**.

Summary

This chapter shows that nutrition education is more likely to be successful if it includes the following key elements.

ELEMENT OF SUCCESS 1: FOCUS ON BEHAVIOR CHANGE OR ACTION

Nutrition education is most likely to be effective if it is carefully focused, usually on specific observable individual actions and behaviors or family and community practices that are of importance to individuals, communities, or the larger society. These behaviors may also serve larger goals of value to the individual or community. Critical thinking and skills are crucial.

- Check that your nutrition education sessions or intervention focuses on specific, actionable behaviors or actions.

ELEMENT OF SUCCESS 2: ADDRESS DETERMINANTS OF BEHAVIOR CHANGE OR ACTION

Nutrition education is most likely to be effective if it clearly identifies the *determinants* of the behaviors of the intended audience and makes modifying these determinants of action and behavior change the direct target of nutrition education interventions. This identification is derived from the audience participants themselves about their needs, assets and strengths, and desires, in the context of their families and communities, as well as from objective data sources. Food and nutrition content knowledge needs to be relevant to the targeted behaviors or actions: it can be used to provide motivational reasons to act (why-to knowledge) or to provide facilitating knowledge and skills to change behaviors (how-to knowledge, also called behavioral capability).

- Check that you have identified the many determinants of behavior change for your intended audience, both those determinants that are motivations for behavior change and those that are facilitators of change.

- Check that you have explored and incorporated considerations of the cultural context of your audience.

ELEMENT OF SUCCESS 3: USE THEORY AND EVIDENCE

Theory, based on evidence, provides a guide or tool that tells us which determinants of action or behavior change are more likely to result in changes in behavior by the intended audience.

- Check that you have selected an appropriate theory or created a model for your sessions or intervention.

ELEMENTS OF SUCCESS 4: ADDRESS MULTIPLE LEVELS AND DEVOTE SUFFICIENT DURATION AND INTENSITY

Nutrition education is most likely to be effective if it attends to the multiple levels of influences on food choice and eating (and physical activity) behaviors. These include influences at the individual and interpersonal levels, at the community and organizational levels, and in the physical environment, social structures, systems, and policy. A coordinated and systematic approach of sufficient intensity and duration delivered through multiple venues is essential for nutrition education to have a significant impact.

- Check if you are able to identify partners to work with you on environment and policy changes that would support the behavior change goals of your sessions or intervention.

ELEMENT OF SUCCESS 5: DESIGN APPROPRIATE STRATEGIES AND ACTIVITIES

Nutrition education is most likely to be effective if it designs strategies and activities that are based on theory and evidence to address the identified determinants of behavior change or action and their environmental contexts.

- Check that you have created engaging activities that are appropriate and meaningful for your audience in the context of their families and culture and that are based on the determinants in your theory model in order to achieve the desired behaviors of your sessions or intervention.

Use of a combination of all these key elements of success will likely enhance the effectiveness of your nutrition education intervention.

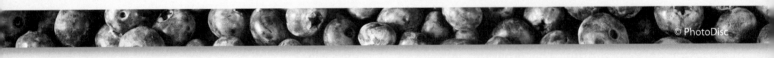

Questions and Activities

1. Describe what is meant by "behavior-focused" nutrition education. Some are concerned that this means it is about manipulating people. What would you say to them?

2. Define theory. Give three reasons why theory is considered important for effective nutrition education.

3. What does the term *theory construct* mean? How is it related to the term *determinant*?

4. Think back to a specific instance in which you gave a nutrition education session or discussed nutrition informally with a group. Do you think you used theory? If so, describe the key features of your theory. If you did not use theory, explain what guided your session.

5. Find a nutrition education program with a set of lessons that has been or is being presented to groups (these may be available online). Examine their design, content and delivery: which of the key elements of success were used? If you can find evaluation data, how effective was the program or sessions? Did the elements of success listed in this chapter contribute to their effectiveness?

6. To what extent are you personally convinced that the use of theory and evidence will help you design more effective nutrition education? Why or why not?

7. In terms of diet-related behavior change, what does motivation mean? How can nutrition educators assist individuals to become more motivated?

8. Distinguish between motivational knowledge and factual or facilitating knowledge in the area of nutrition education.

9. Nutrition education has been described as consisting of two components accompanied by environmental and policy supports. What is the primary focus of each component? How are the two components related to each other and to environment and policy?

References

Achterberg, C., and C. Miller. 2004. Is one theory better than another in nutrition education? A viewpoint: More is better. *Journal of Nutrition Education and Behavior* 36(1):40–42.

Ajzen, I. 1998. Models of human social behavior and their application to health psychology. *Psychology and Health* 13:735–739.

Ajzen, I., N. Joyce, S. Sheikh, and N. G. Cote. 2011. Knowledge and the prediction of behavior: The role of information accuracy in the theory of planned behavior. *Basic and Applied Social Psychology* 33(2):101–117.

American Dietetic Association. 2002. Knowledge, attitudes, beliefs, behaviors: Findings of American Dietetic Association's public opinion survey *Nutrition and You; Trends 2002*. Chicago: American Dietetic Association.

American Dietetic Association. 2011. Use best practices and adapt interventions from similar programs. *ADA Times* Spring:13–14.

American Heritage Dictionary of the English Language (5th ed.). 2011. Boston: Houghton Mifflin.

Ammerman, A. S., C. H. Lindquist, K. N. Lohr, and J. Hersey. 2002. The efficacy of behavioral interventions to modify dietary fat and fruit and vegetable intake: A review of the evidence. *Preventive Medicine* 35(1):25–41.

Atkinson, R. L., and S. A. Nitzke. 2001. School-based programs on obesity increase knowledge about nutrition but do not change eating habits by much. *British Medical Journal* 323:1018–1019.

Bandura, A. 1986. *Foundations of thought and action: A social cognitive theory*. Englewood Cliffs, NJ: Prentice Hall.

Baranowski, T., E. Cerin, and J. Baranowski. 2009. Steps in the design, development, and formative evaluation of obesity prevention–related behavior change. *International Journal of Behavioral Nutrition and Physical Activity* 6:6.

Baranowski, T., K. W. Cullen, T. Nicklas, D. Thompson, and J. Baranowski. 2003. Are current health behavioral change models helpful in guiding prevention of weight gain efforts? *Obesity Research* 11(Suppl):23S–43S.

Baranowski, T., L. S. Lin, D. W. Wetter, K. Resnicow, and M. D. Hearn. 1997. Theory as mediating variables: Why aren't community interventions working as desired? *Annals of Epidemiology* 7:589–595.

Bentley, M. E., D. L. Dee, and J. L. Jensen. 2003. Breastfeeding among low income, African-American women: Power, beliefs and decision making. *Journal of Nutrition* 133(1): 305S–309S.

Bisogni, C. A., M. Jastran, M. Seligman, and A. Thompson. 2012. How people interpret healthy eating: contributions of qualitative research. *Journal of Society of Nutrition Education and Behavior* 44(4):282–301.

Bonvecchio, A., G. H. Pelto, E. Escalante, E. Monterrubio, J. P. Habicht, F. Navada, et al. 2007. Maternal knowledge and use of a micronutrient supplement was improved with a programmatically feasible intervention in Mexico. *Journal of Nutrition* 137:440–446.

Booth, S. L., J. F. Sallis, C. Ritenbaugh, J. O. Hill, L. L. Birch, L. D. Frank, et al. 2001. Environmental and societal factors affect food choice and physical activity: Rationale, influences, and leverage points. *Nutrition Reviews* 59(3 Pt 2): S21–39; discussion S57–S65.

Booth-Butterfield S., and B. Reger. 2004. The message changes belief and the rest is theory: The "1% or less" milk campaign and reasoned action. *Preventive Medicine* 39: 581–588.

Brug, J. 2006. Order is needed to promote linear or quantum changes in nutrition and physical activity behaviors: A reaction to 'A chaotic view of behavior change' by Resnicow and Vaughan. *International Journal of Behavioral Nutrition and Physical Activity* 3:29.

Brug, J., A. Oenema, and I. Ferreira. 2005. Theory, evidence and intervention mapping to improve behavior nutrition and physical activity interventions. *International Journal of Behavioral Nutrition and Physical Activity* 2(1):2.

Buchanan, D. 2004. Two models for defining the relationship between theory and practice in nutrition education: Is the scientific method meeting our needs? *Journal of Nutrition Education and Behavior* 36(3):146–154.

Carbone, E. T. 2013. Measuring nutrition literacy: Problems and potential solutions. *Journal of Nutrition Disorders and Therapy* 3:1.

Carbone E. T., and J. M. Zoellner. 2012. Nutrition and health literacy: A systematic review to inform nutrition research and practice. *Journal of the Academy of Nutrition and Dietetics* 112:254–265.

Chamberlain, S. P. 2005. Recognizing and responding to cultural differences in the education of culturally and linguistically diverse learners. *Intervention in School & Clinic* 40(4):195–211.

Chesla, C. A., M. M. Skaff, R. J. Bartz, J. T. Mullan, and L. Fisher. 2000. Differences in personal models among Latinos and European Americans: Implications for clinical care. *Diabetes Care* 23(12):1780–1785.

Connell D. B., R. R. Turner, and F. F. Mason. 1985. Summary of findings of the school health education evaluation: Health promotion effectiveness, implementation, and costs. *Journal of School Health* 55(8):316–321.

Conner, M., and C. J. Armitage. 2002. *The social psychology of food.* Buckingham, UK: Open University Press.

Conner, M., and P. Norman. 1995. *Predicting health behavior.* Buckingham, UK: Open University Press.

Contento, I., G. I. Balch, Y. L. Bronner, L. A. Lytle, S. K. Maloney, C. M. Olson, S. Sharaga-Swadener. 1995. The effectiveness of nutrition education and implications for nutrition education policy, programs, and research: A review of research. *Journal of Nutrition Education* 27(6):279–418.

D'Andrade, R.G. 1984. Cultural meaning systems. In *Culture theory: Essays on mind, self, and emotion,* edited by R. A. Shweder and R. A. LeVine. Cambridge, UK: Cambridge University Press.

DiClemente, R. J., R. A. Crosby, and M. C. Kegler. 2002. *Emerging theories in health promotion research and practice.* San Francisco: Jossey-Bass.

Diep, C. S., T. A. Chen, V. F. Davies, T. Baranowski, and T. Baranowski. 2014. Influence of behavioral theory on fruit and vegetable intervention effectiveness among children: A meta-analysis. *Journal of Nutrition Education and Behavior* 46(6):506–546.

Fishbein, M. 2000. The role of theory in HIV prevention. *AIDS Care* 12(3):273–278.

Fishbein, M., and I. Ajzen. 1975. *Belief, attitude, intention and behavior: An introduction to theory and research.* Reading, MA: Addision-Wesley.

———. 2010. *Predicting and changing behavior: The reasoned action approach.* New York: Psychology Press.

Green, L. W., and M. W. Kreuter. 2005. *Health promotion planning: An educational and ecological approach.* 4th ed. New York: McGraw-Hill Humanities/Social Sciences/ Languages.

Gregson, J., S. B. Foerster, R. Orr, L. Jones, J. Benedict, B. Clarke, et al. 2001. System, environmental, and policy changes: Using the social-ecological model as a framework for evaluating nutrition education and social marketing programs with low-income audiences. *Journal of Nutrition Education* 33(Suppl 1):S4–S15.

Haidt. J. 2006. *The happiness hypothesis: Finding modern truth in ancient wisdom.* New York: Basic Books.

———. 2012. *The righteous mind: Why good people are divided by politics and religion.* New York: Vintage Books.

Hawkes, C. 2013. *Promoting healthy diets through nutrition education and changes in the food environment: An international review of actions and their effectiveness.* Rome: Nutrition Education and Consumer Awareness Group, Food and Agriculture Organization of the United Nations. http://www.fao.org/docrep/017/i3235e/i3235e.pdf Accessed 5/19/15.

Heath, C., and D. Heath (2010). *Switch: How to change when change is hard.* New York: Random House.

Hingle, M., A. Betran, T. M. O'Connor, D. Thompson, J. Baranowski, and T. Baranowski. 2012. A model of goal directed vegetable parenting practices. *Appetite* 58:444–449.

Hingle, M., T. M. O'Connor, J. M. Dave, and T. Baranowski. 2010. Parental involvement in interventions to improve child dietary intake: A systematic review. *Preventive Medicine* 51(2):103–111.

Hochbaum, G. M. 1958. *Participation in medical screening programs: A socio-psychological study.* Public Health Service Publication No. 572. Washington DC: U.S. Government Printing Office.

Institute of Medicine. 2002. *Speaking of health: Assessing health communication strategies for diverse populations.* Washington, DC: National Academies Press.

———. 2004. *Health literacy: A prescription to end confusion.* Washington, DC: National Academies Press.

Johnson, B. T., L. A. J. Scott-Sheldon, and M. P. Carey. 2010. Meta-synthesis of health behavior change meta-analyses. *American Journal of Public Health* 100:2193–2198.

Khambalia, A. Z., S. Dickinson, L. L. Hardy, T. Gill, and L. A. Baur. 2012. A synthesis of existing systematic reviews and meta-analyses of school-based behavioral interventions for controlling and preventing obesity. *Obesity Reviews* 13:214–233.

Kittler, P. G., K. P. Sucher, and M. Nelms. 2011. *Food and culture.* 6th ed. Belmont, CA: Wadsworth/Thomson Cengage Learning.

Kok, G., H. Schaalma, H. De Vries, G. Parcel, and T. Paulussen. 1996. Social psychology and health. *European Review of Social Psychology* 7:241–282.

Kreuter, M. W., S. N. Lukwago, R. D. Bucholtz, E. M. Clark, and V. Sanders-Thompson. 2003. Achieving cultural appropriateness in health promotion programs: Targeted and tailored approaches. *Health Education and Behavior* 30(2):133–146.

Kreuter, M. W., C. Sugg-Skinner, C. L. Holt, E. M. Clark, D. Haire-Joshu, Q. Fu, et al. 2005. Cultural tailoring for mammography and fruit and vegetables intake among low-income African-American women in urban public health centers. *Preventive Medicine* 41:53–62.

Lemmens, V. E., A. Oenema, K. I. Klepp, H. B. Henriksen, and J. Brug. 2008. A systematic review of the evidence regarding efficacy of obesity prevention interventions among adults. *Obesity Reviews* 9(5):446–455.

LeVine, R. A. 1984. Properties of culture: An ethnographic view. In *Culture theory: Essays on mind, self, and emotion,* edited by R. A. Shweder and R. A. LeVine. Cambridge, UK: Cambridge University Press.

Lewin, K. T. 1935. *A dynamic theory of personality.* New York: McGraw-Hill.

———. 1936. *Principles of topological psychology.* New York: McGraw-Hill.

Lewin, K. T., T. Dembo, L. Festinger, and P. S. Sears. 1944. Level of aspiration. In *Personality and the behavior disorders,* edited by J. M. Hundt. New York: Roland Press.

Liou, D., and I. R. Contento. 2001. Usefulness of psychosocial theory variables in explaining fat-related dietary behavior in Chinese Americans: Association with degree of acculturation. *Journal of Nutrition Education* 33(6):322–331.

———. 2004. Health beliefs related to heart disease prevention among Chinese Americans. *Journal of Family and Consumer Sciences* 96:21–25.

Liou, D., K. Bauer, and Y. Bai. 2014. Investigating obesity risk-reduction behaviors in Chinese Americans. *Perspectives in Public Health* 134(6):321–330.

Luepker, R. V., C. L. Perry, S. M. McKinlay, G. S. Parcel, E. J. Stone, L. S. Webber, et al. 1996. Outcomes of a field trial to improve children's dietary patterns and physical activity. The Child and Adolescent Trial for Cardiovascular Health. CATCH Collaborative Group. *Journal of the American Medical Association* 275(10):768–776.

Lytle, L. 2005. Nutrition education, behavioral theories, and the scientific method: Another viewpoint. *Journal of Nutrition Education and Behavior* 37(2):90–93.

McLeroy, K. R., D. Bibeau, A. Steckler, and K. Glanz. 1988. An ecological perspective on health promotion programs. *Health Education Quarterly* 15:351–377.

McNulty, J. 2013. Challenges and issues in nutrition education. Rome. Nutrition Education and Consumer Awareness Group. Food and Agriculture Organization of the United Nations. http://www.fao.org/docrep/017/i3234e/i3234e.pdf Accessed 5/15/15.

Merriam-Webster. 2014. *Merriam-Webster's collegiate dictionary.* 11th ed. Springfield, MA: Merriam-Webster.

Moule, J. 2012. *Cultural competence: A primer for educators.* Belmont, CA: Wadsworth/Cengage.

Nader, P. R., E. J. Stone, L. A. Lytle, C. L. Perry, S. K. Osganian, S. Kelder, et al. 1999. Three-year maintenance of improved diet and physical activity: The CATCH cohort. Child and Adolescent Trial for Cardiovascular Health. *Archives of Pediatric and Adolescent Medicine* 153(7):695–704.

Norman, P., C. Abraham, and M. Conner. 2000. *Understanding and changing health behavior: From health beliefs to self-regulation.* Amsterdam: Harwood Academic Publishers.

Ozer, E. J. 2007. The effects of school gardens on students and schools: Conceptualization and considerations for maximizing healthy development. *Health Education and Behavior* 34:846–864.

Prochaska, J. O., and C. C. DiClemente. 1982. Transtheoretical therapy: Toward a more integrative model of change. *Psychotherapy: Theory, Research, Practice* 19:276–288.

Reger, B., M. Wootan, S. Booth-Butterfield, and H. Smith. 1998. 1% or less: A community-based nutrition campaign. *Public Health Reports* 113:410–419.

Resnicow, K., L. Cohen, J. Reinhardt, D. Cross, D. Futterman, E. Kirschner, et al. 1992. A three-year evaluation of the Know Your Body program in inner-city schoolchildren. *Health Education Quarterly* 19:463–480.

Resnicow, K., and S. E. Page. 2008. Embracing chaos and complexity: A quantum change for public health. *American Journal of Public Health* 98(8):1382–1389.

Rosenstock, I. M. 1960. What research in motivation suggests for public health. *American Journal of Public Health* 50:295–301.

Rozin, P. 1982. Human food selection: The interaction of biology, culture, and individual experience. In *The psychobiology of human food selection*, edited by L. M. Barker. Westport, CT: Avi Publishing.

Rothman, A. J. 2004. "Is there nothing more practical than a good theory?" Why innovations and advances in health behavior change will arise if interventions are used to test and refine theory. *International Journal of Behavioral Nutrition and Physical Activity* 1(1):11.

Rutter, D. R., and L. Quine. 2002. *Changing health behaviour: Intervention and research with social cognition models*. Buckingham, UK: Open University Press.

Sanjur, D. 1982. *Social and cultural perspectives in nutrition*. Englewood Cliffs, NJ: Prentice Hall.

Satia-Aboud, J, R. E. Patterson, M. I. Neuhauser, and J. Elder. 2002. Dietary acculturation: applications to nutrition research and dietetics. *J Am. Dietetic Association* 102(8):1105–1118.

Satia, J. A., R. E. Patterson, A. R. Kristal, T. G. Hislop, Y. Yasui, and V. M. Taylor. 2001. Development of scales to measure dietary acculturation among Chinese-Americans and Chinese-Canadians. *Journal of the American Dietetic Association* 101(5):548–553.

Schwarzer, R., and R. Fuchs. 1995. Self-efficacy and health behaviors. In *Predicting health behavior*, edited by M. Conner and P. Norman. Buckingham, UK: Open University Press.

Silk, K. J., J Sherry, B. Winn, N. Keesecker, M. A. Horodynski, and A. Sayir. 2008. Increasing nutrition literacy: Testing the effectiveness of print, Web site, and game modalities. *Journal of Nutrition Education and Behavior* 40(1):3–10.

Silver Wallace, L. 2002. Osteoporosis prevention in college women: Application of the expanded health belief model. *American Journal of Health Behavior* 26:163–172.

Spiro, M. E. 1984. Some reflections on cultural determinism and relativism with special reference to emotion and reason. In *Culture theory: Essays on mind, self, and emotion*, edited by R. A. Shweder and R. A. LeVine. Cambridge, UK: Cambridge University Press.

Stein, K. 2009. Cultural competency: Where it is and where it is headed. *Journal of the American Dietetic Association* 109(2 Suppl):S13–S19.

———. 2010. Moving cultural competency from abstract to act. *Journal of the American Dietetic Association* 110(2):180–184, 186–187.

Story, M., K. M. Kaphingst, R. O'Brien, and K. Glanz. 2008. Creating healthy food and eating environments: Policy and environmental approaches. *Annual Review of Public Health* 29:253–272.

Strauss, A. L., and J. Corbin. 1990. *Basics of qualitative research: Grounded theory procedures and research*. Newbury Park, CA: Sage Publications.

Suarez-Balcazar, Y., J. Friesma, and V. Lukvanova. 2013. Culturally competent interventions to address obesity among African-American and Latino children and youth. *Occupational and Therapeutic Health Care* 27(2): 113–128.

Supermarket Nutrition. 2013. How grocery retailers and supermarket dietitians can impact consumer health, in-store & online. http://supermarketnutrition.com/how-grocery-retailers-and-supermarket-dietitians-can-impact-consumer-health-in-store-online/ Accessed 7/24/13.

Thompson, C. A., and J. Ravia. 2011. A systematic review of behavioral interventions to promote intake of fruit and vegetables. *Journal of the American Dietetic Association* 111(10):1523–1535.

Triandis, H. C. 1979. Values, attitudes, and interpersonal behavior. In *Nebraska symposium on motivation*, edited by H. E. How. Lincoln, NE: University of Nebraska Press.

U.S. Department of Agriculture and U.S. Department of Health and Human Services. 2010. *Dietary Guidelines for Americans*. www.health.gov/dietaryguidelines/ Accessed 8/14/13.

Ventura, A. K. and L. L. Birch. 2008. Does parenting affect children's eating and weight status? *International Journal of Behavioral Nutrition and Physical Activity*. March 17, 5:15.

Walter, H. J. 1989. Primary prevention of chronic disease among children: The school-based "Know Your Body" intervention trials. *Health Education Quarterly* 16:201–214.

Waters, E., A. de Silva-Sanigorski, B. J. Hall, T. Brown, K. J. Campbell, Y. Gao, et al. 2011. Interventions for preventing obesity in children. *Cochrane Database of Systematic Reviews* 7;12:CD001871.

Whitehead, F. 1973. Nutrition education research. *World Review of Nutrition and Dietetics* 17:91–149.

Zoellner, J., C. Connell, W. Bounds, L Crook, and K. Yadrick. 2009. Nutrition literacy status and preferred nutrition communication channels among adults in the lower Mississippi delta. *Preventing Chronic Disease* 6(4):A128.

Zoellner, J., W. You, C. Connell, R. L. Smith-Ray, K. Allen, K. L. Tucker et al. 2011. Health literacy is associated with Healthy Eating Index scores and sugar-sweetened beverage intake: Findings for the Lower Mississippi Delta. *Journal of the American Dietetic Association* 111(7):1012–1020.

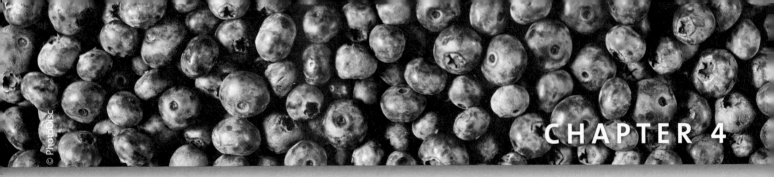

Increasing Awareness and Enhancing Motivation and Empowerment for Behavior Change and Taking Action

OVERVIEW

This chapter describes several key theories that can serve as maps or guides to help us understand motivations for behavior and dietary change. The chapter also describes how to use the theories as tools for nutrition education success through real-world examples and illustrative case studies. It focuses on the important role of beliefs, feelings, attitudes, motivations, sense of empowerment, and social and cultural perceptions in motivational nutrition education for *why to* change behavior or take action. The description of each psychosocial theory is followed by how to use the theory as a tool in nutrition education.

CHAPTER OUTLINE

- Nutrition education for enhancing motivation and empowerment: focus on why to take action
- The health belief model
- Using the health belief model in nutrition education to enhance motivation and activate audiences
- Theory of planned behavior: the reasoned action approach
- Extensions of the theory of planned behavior/reasoned action approach

- Using the theory of planned behavior in nutrition education to enhance motivation and activate audiences
- Self-determination theory
- Using self-determination theory in nutrition education to enhance motivation and activate audiences
- Summary

LEARNING OBJECTIVES

At the end of the chapter, you should be able to:

- Describe key theories that help nutrition educators understand motivation for health and nutrition behaviors, in particular the health belief model, the theory of planned behavior or reasoned action approach, and self-determination theory
- Discuss how theories and research have been used in nutrition education research and

programs to increase awareness and enhance motivation
- Describe ways to design nutrition education using these theories as tools to increase interest, enhance motivation, promote active contemplation, and facilitate formation of intentions to take action

Nutrition Education for Enhancing Motivation and Empowerment: Focus on Why to Take Action

As nutrition educators your work will most likely involve direct education by providing educational sessions for a variety of audiences, particularly those of low-income or diverse backgrounds. These educational sessions may consist of leading group discussions in communities, doing cooking demonstrations, conducting farmers' market or grocery store tours, working with school-based programs, or providing workshops for athletes and exercising individuals. Your work will also likely involve indirect activities such as developing educational materials and using mobile technology and social media. You may also participate in developing programs with a larger scope involving working with partners to embark on social marketing and a variety of activities that foster health-supportive changes in institutions, communities, and policies. Our audiences may come to us out of interest, through referral, or as a result of our efforts to seek out the underserved. They are usually busy people with many urgent matters on their minds and their diets may not be one of them.

In most developed countries, and increasingly in others, high-calorie, tasty foods are everywhere in the environment; they are usually convenient and cheap. Indeed, many of these food items are "addictive," and difficult to resist (Moss 2013). In addition, people's food choices and eating patterns develop over a lifetime and are embedded in many aspects of their lives. Many people may not be entirely satisfied with how they are eating, but their patterns generally work for them, given their life circumstances and the trade-offs they need to make. Our case example from an earlier chapter, 19-year-old Alicia, illustrates this point: she is not concerned about her diet. Yet this is the time when eating a healthy diet could make a big difference in her future health. Given the many competing desires and priorities in the lives of people such as Alicia, how do we assist them to become motivated and feel empowered to act on nutrition and health messages?

We are fortunate that we can draw on the considerable and exciting research and theory building in the fields of behavioral nutrition, health education and promotion, and nutrition education to help us answer that question.

Chapter 3 describes how, based on this foundation, we can think of nutrition education as consisting of three key components or functions: a motivational component with a focus on why-to take action, an action component where the focus is on how-to take action, and an environmental support component where the focus is on when and where to take action. This chapter focuses on the motivational component. That is, this chapter focuses on how to help individuals like Alicia with a crucial first step: becoming aware of a need to change and feeling ready and empowered to do so.

Chapter 3 also points out in a general way, that to help our audiences become motivationally ready to take action, we can emphasize several psychosocial influences or determinants of behavior, such as awareness of risk or threat of current behavior, beliefs about the benefits and costs of taking action, feelings about taking action, beliefs about self-efficacy or confidence in taking action, and beliefs about social environments. In this chapter we explore some key theories linking how these determinants influence behavior change and describe the way each theory can be applied in nutrition education to improve its effectiveness. We illustrate the theories with case studies.

These psychosocial influences or determinants of behavior come from science-based, and cultural, social, family, or personal sources. They are rooted in individuals' prior life experiences, life stage, personality, family structure and culture, and sociodemographic and historic factors that influence their behavior (Chamberlain 2005, Diaz et al. 2009). These, of course, are not modifiable by educational means. However, these background factors affect *current* beliefs, knowledge, feelings or **emotions**, **attitudes**, or

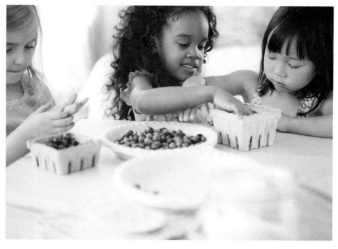

Nutrition education activities can help to motivate students.

© Jamie Grill/Getty Images.

self-identities that influence behavior, and these *current* influences can be addressed by nutrition education.

THE IMPORTANCE OF THEORIES OF MOTIVATION FOR NUTRITION EDUCATION SUCCESS

The theories of motivation that have been generated from research can help us to do two things: first, understand the motivations of our audiences from their own point of view, and second, get our audiences excited about our messages and to act on them. Some theories were developed because researchers were studying health-related behaviors specifically, whereas other theories were developed when researchers were investigating other social behaviors (such as consumer behaviors, including food choice) not necessarily related to health. The **health belief model** was developed specifically to understand and predict health behaviors. The main determinants of behavior according to this theory—perceived threat, perceived benefits, and **perceived barriers** (described in greater detail later in this chapter)—have proved to be very important and are widely used in interventions. However, the model does not help nutrition educators understand food choices and dietary behaviors that are undertaken for a variety of reasons other than health. For such understanding, other related social psychological theories prove very helpful. We describe two of them in this chapter, the **theory of planned behavior/reasoned action approach** and **self-determination theory (SDT)**. We can then use our understanding to develop nutrition education strategies that are motivational.

THE HEALTH BELIEF MODEL

> In simplest terms, the health belief model states that people's readiness to take action or make a health behavior change is influenced by their health beliefs or convictions. It was one of the earliest conceptual models to address health behavior specifically and is the most well known theory in the field of public health.

The model was developed in the 1950s by social psychologists working in the Lewin tradition who were interested in using social science to solve practical public

BOX 4-1 The Health Belief Model in Practice

The health belief model proposes that readiness to take action is based on the following beliefs or convictions:

- I am susceptible to this health risk or problem.
- The threat to my health is serious.
- I am convinced that the benefits of the recommended action outweigh the barriers or costs.
- I am confident that I can carry out the action successfully.
- Cues to action are present to remind me to take action.

health problems (Becker 1974; Rosenstock 1974). They were committed to building theories for long-term use and not merely for solving practical health problems one at a time. The model is intuitively appealing, easy for nonpsychologists to understand and apply, and inexpensive to implement. It is widely used around the world for a variety of health behaviors. Its common sense constructs or determinants (beliefs) are clearly stated, manageable in number, and easily measured in a variety of ways, from interviews to surveys (see BOX 4-1).

DETERMINANTS OF ACTION ACCORDING TO THE MODEL

The model proposes that people's likelihood of taking a specific health-related action is primarily motivated by the perceptions, beliefs, or convictions listed below. Please note that science-based information usually provides the foundation for these beliefs and convictions.

- *Perceived susceptibility*: Perceived susceptibility is the degree to which we feel personally at risk for a particular health-related condition.
- *Perceived severity*: Perceived severity is the degree to which we believe that this health-related condition is severe (such as diabetes). It may include our evaluation of the personal medical consequences (such as pain, disability, or death) or social consequences (impact on work, family life, and so forth) of the health condition, based on scientific evidence or surveillance data.

- *Perceived threat or risk*: This is the combination of perceived severity and personal susceptibility. These perceptions together result in our psychological state of readiness to take action about the risk of the condition (such as diabetes).
- *Perceived benefits*: Perceived benefits are our opinions of whether a particular action or behavior is useful or effective in reducing the risk or threat of getting the condition. The behaviors may be eating fruits and vegetables to reduce diabetes risk or safe food handling practices to reduce foodborne illness. Again these perceptions are based on scientific evidence or surveillance data.
- *Perceived barriers*: Perceived barriers are our perceptions of the difficulties of performing that action or behavior, which can be psychological as well as physical. These may include perceptions of the cost and inconvenience of eating fruits and vegetables or the perception that some fruits and vegetables may not be agreeable. The barriers or obstacles may also be environmental, such as perceptions of the lack of availability and accessibility of healthful foods or options for physical activity. We tend to weigh costs of action against the benefits of action before taking action, even if we are not always conscious of doing so.
- *Self-efficacy*: The health belief model was originally developed to explain simple health behaviors such as vaccinations or screenings, and hence did not include the role of perceived skill or ability to perform the behavior (called self-efficacy). The role of self-efficacy has now been added to the model to explain long-term behaviors such as dietary behaviors. Self-efficacy is the confidence we have that we can perform the behavior (such as selecting, storing, or preparing fruits and vegetables, or breastfeeding).
- *Cues to action*: External events, such as the illness of a friend or family member or news stories on a scientific study about the issue, or internal events, such as personal symptoms and pains, are cues that prompt us to act.

The model also states that demographic variables such as age, sex, and ethnicity indirectly influence behavior through their impact on perceived threat or perceived benefits and barriers. Likewise, sociopsychological variables such as personality, socioeconomic status, and peer and reference group pressure also influence behavior indirectly through their impact on perceived threat or perceived benefits and barriers.

PERCEIVED RISK: OVERCOMING OPTIMISTIC BIAS

Based on this model, making people aware of threat or risk is an important task of nutrition education. Indeed, studies have found that many people are falsely optimistic about their diets (Shim, Variyam, and Blaylock 2000; Discovery News 2011). For example, many think that their diets are appropriately low in fat when in fact their diets are high in fat (Glanz, Brug, and van Assema 1997). Nutrition educators can use risk appraisals and self-assessments to elucidate personal risk information. Such personalized feedback counters people's tendency to be optimistically biased and encourages them to make changes in their dietary behaviors based on their true risk. A review of studies found that knowing personal risk may indeed spur lifestyle changes (McClure 2002).

A summary of the model is shown in **FIGURE 4-1**. How the main determinants of constructs of the health belief model can be converted into practical activities for nutrition education is shown in **TABLE 4-1**.

EVIDENCE FROM RESEARCH

Because the health belief model is concerned with beliefs and concerns that can be changed through the means of communication or education, the model has been used as a framework to guide a variety of health behavior and nutrition education investigations. Here are some examples:

- In a study of individuals' likelihood to reduce their fat intake to reduce heart disease risk, perceived barriers emerged as most important, followed by self-efficacy (Liou and Contento 2001).
- In a study with older adults, the perceived threat of foodborne illness was important, but the **cues to action** from news stories or labels on food packages most strongly influenced safe food handling behaviors (Hanson and Benedict 2002).
- A study found that, for wives, the costs of or barriers to a healthy diet in terms of expense, time, unpleasantness, and confusion about recommendations had a significant effect on fat intake, whereas for their husbands, perceived threat of disease and self-efficacy had a significant effect (Shafer, Keith, and Schafer 1995).

These studies show that the relative importance of the health beliefs differed by study, most likely reflecting the specific behavior in question and the nature of

Table 4-1 Health Belief Model: Major Constructs and Use in Nutrition Education Interventions

Construct of Theory (Determinant of Behavior Change)	Definition	How to Use in Nutrition Education
Perceived susceptibility	Chances of personally experiencing a risk or getting a condition	Provide messages or activities to personalize the scientifically based risk data for a health condition by examining family history, or self-assessment tools of personal behaviors or practices.
Perceived severity	Beliefs about the seriousness of the consequences of a health condition	Provide messages through statistics, evidence, visuals, or stories about the serious personal impacts (medical and social) of conditions such as heart disease or diabetes.
Perceived threat or risk	A combination of perceived susceptibility and perceived severity	Provide clear and effective messages about the serious threat or risk posed by a condition based on scientific evidence and its possible impact on the individual and others.
Perceived benefits	Beliefs that a given action is effective in reducing risk	Provide messages based on scientific evidence on the efficacy of the behavior to reduce risk. Examine other benefits, such as taste or convenience.
Perceived barriers	Beliefs about the psychological or tangible costs or obstacles to taking the action	Identify and reduce perception of specific barriers to engaging in the action. For example, fruits and vegetables can be inexpensive if eaten in season and can be filling. Correct misconceptions.
Self-efficacy	Confidence in one's ability to carry out the action	Create activities that provide guidance on how to make the behavior or action easy to do; provide opportunities for guided practice of the targeted behavior.
Cues to action	Strategies to activate readiness to take the action	Provide reminders about the behavior: magnets for refrigerator doors, tip sheets, posters, community billboards, and media campaigns.

the particular groups of people in the different studies. The specific beliefs may also differ by cultural heritage. For example, one study found that barriers to eating healthfully among African Americans included the social and cultural symbolism of certain foods along with taste and expense (James 2004).

Using the Health Belief Model for Designing Nutrition Education

An example of how this theory was used for developing culturally appropriate weight management materials for African-American women (James et al. 2012) is described in **NUTRITION EDUCATION IN ACTION 4-1**. Focus groups were

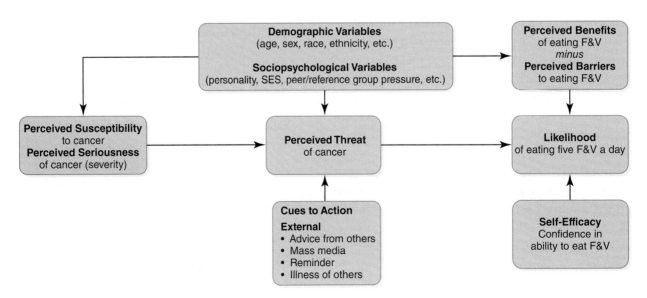

FIGURE 4-1 Health Belief Model. F&V = fruits and vegetables.

NUTRITION EDUCATION IN ACTION 4-1 Use of the Health Belief Model in the Development of Culturally Appropriate Weight-Management Materials For African-American Women

Theory Construct/Determinant of Behavior	Focus Group Results
Perceived susceptibility for obesity	Descriptions of their bodies included terms such as thick, stacked, curvy, or big boned. A healthy weight is when your jeans fit; overweight when a few pound over where you would like to be; and obese when you can't tie your shoelaces. Obesity is a dirty word, with preferred terms being really big or extremely overweight. Black women are brought up to think that big is beautiful.
Perceived severity of obesity (seriousness)	Obesity puts one at risk of heart attack or stroke and restricts what you can do.
Perceived benefits of losing weight	Healthy, look good, can wear the cute stuff; can live life more fully, with more energy, enjoy their kids.
Perceived barriers to losing weight	Lack of motivation – don't want to make the effort, difficult given so much food around, no time; don't know what works as so many different approaches are advertised, family eats junk food, so no social support.
Cues to action	Physicians noted potential health problems – diabetes, hypertension; clothes became tight.
Self-efficacy	Discouraged from prior dieting attempts – nothing works; lacking reliable information on what really works; having someone as dieting or exercise buddy.

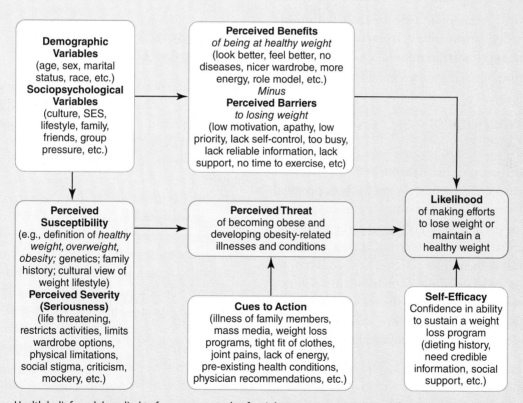

Health belief model applied to focus group study of weight management issues in African-American women

Reprinted from *Journal of the Academy of Nutrition and Dietetics* 112, James, D. C. S., J. W. Pobee, D. Oxidine et al. Using the health belief model to develop appropriate weight-management materials for African-American women, Pages 664–670, Copyright 2012, with permission from Elsevier.

held and the table shows the comments of women in terms of the health belief model constructs. The diagram shows the findings in terms of the health belief model.

TAKE-HOME MESSAGE ABOUT THE HEALTH BELIEF MODEL

When people experience a personal threat about a health condition they will likely take action, but only if the benefits of taking action outweigh the barriers, actual and psychological. Having the ability to take action also is crucial.

You will find this theory especially useful for designing nutrition education activities to enhance awareness and motivation to take action to reduce risk of a health-related condition.

Using the Health Belief Model in Nutrition Education to Enhance Motivation and Activate Audiences

How we can use the six main determinants within the health belief model as a tool to design practical educational activities to enhance motivation to take action is shown in Table 4-1. More specific examples are described below.

INCREASE AWARENESS OF RISK, CONCERN, OR NEED

To enhance motivation and activate our audiences, we start with activities to increase people's concern about personal health, community practices, the sustainability of food system practices, or another issue. People need enough knowledge of a potential concern to warrant action but not so much as to paralyze them from action. They need accurate perceptions and understandings of their own behaviors or community practices in relation to the risk or concern. Effective strategies and specific activities for this construct of determinant might involve the following:

- *Make the issues and problems relevant:* A careful needs assessment of our audiences is essential to learn what is relevant for them within the context of their families, community, and **culture**. We can then use relevant trigger films, striking national or local statistics, pictures and charts, personal stories, and other strategies to make salient issues of concern, such as the

increase in obesity rates, how much of school lunches are thrown away, the portion sizes of food products, the prevalence of bone loss or metabolic syndrome in adolescents, or the carbon footprint of various foods based on their production methods.

- *Provide self-assessment tools to compare to recommendations:* Individuals can complete short food checklists or 24-hour food intake recalls and compare intakes to a standard, such as MyPlate servings, to give themselves an accurate picture of their intake. They can also complete checklists to see how "green" their food shopping practices are (e.g., where the food comes from, degree of packaging). Such personalized feedback helps counteract optimistic bias and encourages individuals to consider changes in their dietary behaviors based on their true risk.
- *Make a community assessment of practices:* Information about community food practices could provide a true picture of the extent of risk or severity of an issue. Nutrition educators can use existing data or surveys, formal and informal.

USE THREAT OR RISK EFFECTIVELY IN COMMUNICATIONS

Using fear in communications to increase perceived risk has been the subject of some debate and discussion in health promotion. Fear and threat are conceptually distinct: fear is defined as a negative emotion accompanied by a high level of arousal, whereas threat is a cognition or thought. They are, however, intricately related, such that the higher the threat, the greater the fear experienced.

Reviews of studies have found that, overall, fear appeals can have effects on intentions and behaviors based on how people respond to the threat or risk presented (Leventhal 1973; Peters, Ruiter, and Kok 2013). For example, strong fear appeals produce high levels of perceived seriousness and susceptibility and are more persuasive than low or weak fear appeals. However, people respond to such fear appeals in two competing ways that interfere with each other: an adaptive response is to deal with the risk or danger, or a maladaptive response is denial or defensiveness. Our messages need to bring about the adaptive response as described below. It may also be that some individuals are more likely than others to respond to appeals based on threat. So we must also get to know our audience and what might work for them.

Effective Use of Threat or Risk

Fear appeals are effective only if people also feel that they can do something to protect themselves. Thus, fear appeal messages can be effective in bringing about behavior change when they do the following: (1) depict a significant and relevant threat, but only when the messages also (2) clearly specify that there are effective strategies in which people can engage to reduce the threat or fear, and that (3) these strategies appear easy to accomplish. That is, threat is effective only if self-efficacy is also increased or already high (Peters et al. 2013). Thus we need to find out whether the groups we are working with have high self-efficacy, or confidence that they are able to take the needed protective actions. To increase such self-efficacy or self-confidence, nutrition educators need to provide specific instructions on exactly when, where, and how to take action.

ADDRESS PERCEIVED BENEFITS AND BARRIERS

Explore Benefits and Barriers

In group settings, nutrition educators can help participants understand the benefits of taking action. For breastfeeding, these might include health of the baby, convenience, mother–child bonding, and so forth, depending on what is relevant for the group. Also, nutrition educators must identify barriers, such as pain of first breastfeeding, embarrassment in public situations, or wishes of others in the family. These can be identified through presentations or group discussion. These theory constructs can also be explored through the media, such as the campaign to eat five fruits and vegetables a day.

Frame Messages as Gains and Losses

How messages are framed in terms of gains and losses may be important. For example, there is some evidence that health communications about the need for people to get *checkups* (e.g., mammograms) are more persuasive if they are framed in terms of guarding against health losses (breast cancer), but to get people to adopt *preventive actions*, communications are more effective if they are framed in terms of health benefits or gains.

ENHANCE SELF-EFFICACY

Making food choices is very complex, requiring food and nutrition related facilitating knowledge and skills and the self-confidence to apply these. We can enhance individuals' self-efficacy by creating activities, tip sheets, or visuals that provide guidance for the action or behavior change. In particular it is important to provide individuals with hands-on activities and practice: we first model the behavior, then provide experiences such as worksheets on how to make changes in favorite recipes to make them more healthy, actually preparing foods, or planting a garden. Our guidance and feedback are essential in increasing individuals' self-confidence in doing these actions.

PROVIDE CUES TO ACTION

We all need reminders about doing something we say we want to do, and our audiences are no different. At the individual or group level, this may mean tip sheets to take home, magnets for refrigerator doors, calendars with reminders, and so forth. For communities, it may mean posters, community billboards, and media campaigns.

EXAMPLES OF INTERVENTIONS USING THE HEALTH BELIEF MODEL

The health belief model is especially useful for adults who are at risk for health conditions or who are beginning to think about their health. It may be less useful for children, for whom health is not a major motivator.

Below are some examples of using the health belief model in interventions and for our case example, Alicia.

Fresh Conversations with Older Adults

The Iowa Nutrition Education Network developed a program for older adults based on the health belief model. It focuses on newsletters delivered at federally funded congregate meal sites. It is described in more detail in **NUTRITION EDUCATION IN ACTION 4-2**.

Public Education or Social Marketing Campaign

A social marketing campaign based on the health belief model is described here: New York City's Pouring on the Pounds. It involved posters in subways, videos on YouTube and television commercial spots. This campaign is described in **NUTRITION EDUCATION IN ACTION 4-3**.

THE CASE OF ALICIA: USING THE HEALTH BELIEF MODEL AS A TOOL

Alicia, you recall, is a 19-year-old high school graduate who works as a receptionist in a busy dentist's office.

NUTRITION EDUCATION IN ACTION 4-2 Fresh Conversations

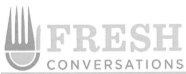

Courtesy of Iowa Department of Public Health.

The Fresh Conversations Intervention

The Iowa Nutrition Network's (INN) *Fresh Conversations* is a newsletter-centered program for adults over 60 based on the health belief model. *Fresh Conversations* consists of monthly newsletters and nutrition education sessions presented to older adults at congregate meal sites. The newsletter is the centerpiece of the intervention, but lessons composed of direct instruction, group discussion, and interactive activities and tastings based on the newsletter topics are presented when each newsletter is distributed. *Fresh Conversations* aims to increase produce and dairy consumption as well as physical activity and improve food safety practices among the target audience. State and national monitoring indicate that these behaviors are all relevant to healthy aging.

Theoretical Framework

In order to use limited resources efficiently and be able to scale the program to reach as many older Iowans as possible, the INN team recognized the importance of designing *Fresh Conversations* with a strong and consistent theoretical framework. Information gathered during focus group interviews indicated that program participants wanted their previous life experiences and prior knowledge to be valued throughout the intervention. Importantly, the participants were motivated by a drive to be self-sufficient. Program developers chose the health belief model to frame *Fresh Conversations* because it would allow them to address *real and perceived barriers* that hinder older Iowans' consumption of fruits, vegetables, and dairy; participation in physical activity; and adherence to food safety recommendations. Basing the intervention on the health belief model also focused the newsletters and lessons on the *perceived benefit* of maintaining independence as an older adult and *self-efficacy* in using their knowledge and experience to choose these healthy behaviors.

- Perceived barriers: *Fresh Conversations* addresses perceived barriers that healthy foods are more expensive.
- Perceived benefits: It also emphasizes how healthy eating can reduce the number of health issues, like diabetes, experienced by older adults.
- Self-efficacy: By including goal setting and planning exercises as well as potential challenges, *Fresh Conversations* also addresses participants' self-efficacy.

Evaluation

A 6-month pilot evaluation of *Fresh Conversations* was conducted in 2012. Participants who received the health belief model-based *Fresh Conversations* ($n = 29$) were compared to a control group ($n = 31$) who received a similar newsletter program without a theoretical basis. The two groups responded to several validated questionnaires, including the Dietary Screening Tool, the Nutrition Self-Efficacy Scale, and the U.S. Household Food Security Survey. Although self-efficacy and food security were not different between the two groups, participants who received *Fresh Conversations* had significantly increased their produce and dairy consumption and significantly lowered their nutritional risk scores.

From Iowa Fresh Newsletter:

Courtesy of Iowa Department of Public Health.

NUTRITION EDUCATION IN ACTION 4-3 **New York City's Pouring on the Pounds Campaign**

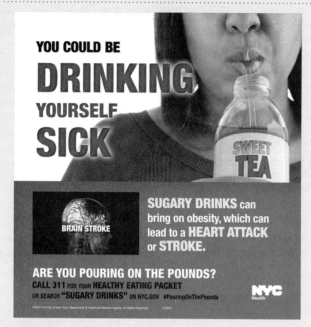

Courtesy of New York City Department of Health and Mental Hygiene.

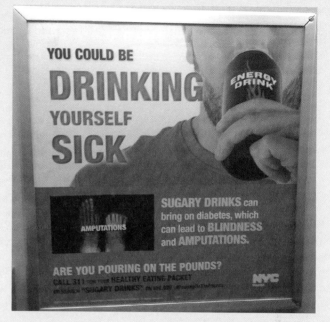

Courtesy of New York City Department of Health and Mental Hygiene.

Several variations of the New York City Department of Health's (DOH) Pouring on the Pounds campaign have run in New York City since 2009. Focus group research led DOH officials to the shocking and graphic ads that have run on subways, YouTube, and in television commercial spots. A poster is shown here. One TV spot shows a young man drinking a sweetened drink and it slowly turns into fat (see Chapter 3). Another shows the same young man having to walk through many neighborhoods and over a bridge, taking a good deal of time, to use up the calories in one large sweet drink. Other posters focus on the health consequences of drinking soda,

as shown here. The perceived threat in these materials is accompanied by a telephone number and a website for resources to help people make better choices and also by posters showing possible solutions.

The DOH reports over 313 earned media mentions since 2010 (according to Van Wye at a presentation at Yale in 2012) and that they have reached 400 community-based organizations to reduce sugary beverage consumption at their sites. Further, the percentage of adults reporting that they drank 1+ sugary drinks each day decreased from 36% to 30% from 2007–2010.

She grabs a quick lunch each day—something filling. She doesn't cook much and so tends to snack and eat fast food. Her mother recently had a heart attack and was hospitalized. Alicia was alarmed. Until now she had not thought much about her health or her diet. In her view, medical conditions were caused by biology, mostly, or luck. Now she wants to learn more about the condition and whether and how she might prevent such an attack in herself. This is a "cue to action" in the health belief model. The staff in the office told her about educational sessions offered by the nearby community clinic.

One session was called "Eat Right for Your Heart: A Focus on Fast Food and Snacks." Alicia decided to attend. Here is how the nutrition educator designed the session.

She decided that the best theory to use to address the issue of reducing risk of heart disease was the health belief model with its focus on health beliefs. She looked at research and survey data and conducted some interviews with potential audience members. She found that several behaviors were problematic, chief among them for this age group, the high consumption of snacks and fast food. She then created a theory model for her session. The diagram in CASE STUDY 4-1 shows how she operationalized the model for this session. There is a similar blank diagram at the end of this chapter that you can use to design nutrition education activities based on the heath belief model. She then developed a lesson plan from this theory model, as shown in Case Study 4-1.

CASE STUDY 4-1 The Case of Alicia: Nutrition Education Using the Health Belief Model

Audience: General adults at a community center

Behavioral Goal: Reduce consumption of fast food and snacks, and replace with fruits and vegetables

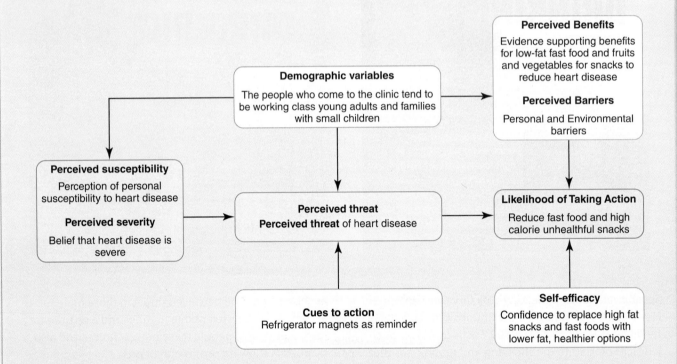

Here is the lesson plan for the session Alicia attended. Note that it focuses on specific behaviors—reducing fast foods and snacks and replacing with fruits and vegetables. The nutrition educator started with each of the determinants of change in the health belief model (shown as a heading) and then designed a specific activity to address this determinant.

"Eat Right for Your Heart: A Focus on Fast Food and Snacks"
Educational Plan for Group Session

Behavioral goal: Participants will reduce their consumption of fast food and snacks to reduce risk of heart disease.

Educational objectives to achieve behavioral goal. At the end of the session, participants will be able to:
- Evaluate the degree to which their eating patterns increase their risk of chronic disease
- Describe the impact of high-fat, high-calorie diets on their heart health
- Describe the benefits of eating more whole grains and vegetables instead of high-calorie fast food and snacks
- Identify the barriers to eating healthfully and state ways to overcome barriers
- State commitment to make changes through an action plan

Procedure:
Determinant shown in **bold**, followed by the specific activity, underlined, directed at determinant.

1. **Perceived susceptibility**
   - Self-assessment: Purpose: To help participants become aware of the high-fat foods they eat so that they can see themselves as susceptible to heart disease.

     So, as they come in, participants are asked to write down everything they ate and drank in the past 24 hours. Then, they are to circle the foods that are high in fat and discuss.

2. **Perceived severity**
   - <u>Measure fat in snack foods.</u> In order to help the participants believe that heart disease is severe, the instructor wants participants to see how much fat is in snacks and fast foods.

     The nutrition educator shows the group some examples of popular fast foods and snacks. Then, she asks a volunteer to come up and measure out, with estimates provided by the group, how many teaspoons of fat (from a container of solid cooking fat) they think is in each snack.

     Alicia and the others are shocked at the amount of fat in the food items.
   - <u>Fat clogs blood vessels.</u> To further enhance the belief that heart disease is severe, the instructor conducts a demonstration using a plastic tube to represent a blood vessel.

     She pours some "blood" through—it moves quickly through the tube. Then, she places some solid fat in the tube, and the blood now trickles through. She discusses this as illustrating the impact of a dietary pattern with large amounts of snacks and fast foods that are high in saturated fat.

     Alicia and the others are moved by the visual demonstration and their perceived risk of disease is heightened.

3. **Perceived benefits of taking action**
   - <u>Fast food options:</u> The nutrition educator provides evidence showing that choosing healthier, lower fat fast foods and snacks and eating more whole grains and fruits and vegetables can reduce risk of chronic disease.

     Alicia is now very concerned about her diet but convinced that there are things she can do to reduce her risk of heart disease.

4. **Perceived barriers**
   - <u>Identifying personal barriers:</u> The group reviews their dietary recalls and discusses their specific and personal barriers to reducing the number of fast foods and unhealthy snacks they eat.

5. **Overcoming barriers**
   - <u>Ways to overcome barriers:</u> The group brainstorms ways to reduce the number of unhealthy snacks and fast food items they eat and substitute with healthier snacks, such as fruits and vegetables or whole-grain snacks and healthier options at fast food restaurants.

6. **State likelihood of taking action**
   - <u>Set action plan:</u> The nutrition educator asks group members to write down one action they will take to reduce their consumption of unhealthy snacks and fast foods and replace them with healthier ones. This can be called an action plan.

     Alicia is pleased that there are some actions she can take to protect her heart. She decides that she will take fresh fruit or bagged baby carrots to work each day. She writes out a plan to do so. She thinks that she will also commit to a second behavior: she will select a healthier option at least once a week when she goes to fast food restaurants.

The Way We Deliver Our Sessions in Practice Is Crucial for Success!

A well-developed, theory-based educational plan is only effective with our audience if we communicate it effectively. How do we do that? By being perceived by our audience as *credible, culturally sensitive,* having some *common ground* with the audience, and having a *dynamic* personality.

- *Credibility* is based on the audience's perception of our expertise and trustworthiness. Being perceived as having *expertise* in nutrition can come from our credentials, past work, the organization or agency we represent, and being seen as organized and speaking with confidence. Perceived *trustworthiness* means the audience perceives us as not benefiting personally from what we say—financially or otherwise. We clearly believe in and are passionate about what we are presenting.

- *Cultural sensitivity* means being mindful of the cultural food-related traditions of your audience, using a participant-centered approach, facilitating an interactive process, and focusing on their capacities and strengths in order to enhance empowerment (Moule, 2012).

- *Common ground* means being seen as understanding, accepting, and respectful of the audience, and perhaps having had experiences similar to the audience in some way.

- *Dynamism* means being passionate about what you are presenting. Your enthusiasm will go a long way in helping the audience understand—and importantly, feel—the importance of what you are saying.

Theory of Planned Behavior: The Reasoned Action Approach

In its simplest terms, the theory of planned behavior or the rational action approach states that people's behavior is powerfully determined by their beliefs or convictions: beliefs about the consequences of the behavior, which leads to attitudes toward the behavior; beliefs about what others think they should do; and beliefs about whether they have control over the behavior in question. With its emphasis on convictions and attitudes the theory is especially useful for designing interventions to enhance motivation for behavior change.

The theory of planned behavior (Fishbein and Ajzen 1975), also called the rational action approach (Fishbein and Ajzen 2010), was developed to try to understand a number of social behaviors such as voting or participation in community organizations. It has been found to be a very useful tool for understanding food choice and various health and dietary behaviors. Despite its name, the theory does not imply that behaviors are necessarily rational, planned, or appropriate from an objective point of view—only that behaviors *follow reasonably or predictably, and sometimes spontaneously, from people's beliefs.* The beliefs themselves can be rational or wishful thinking, accurate or misinformed.

The theory of planned behavior helps nutrition educators in two ways: *first,* it helps us understand a given group's own reasons or convictions that motivate their current behavior. The theory does not specify what these beliefs are, only which categories of beliefs or which constructs to explore with an intended audience. As we noted before, think of these categories as empty buckets with labels on them: beliefs and attitudes about the behavior, other people's opinions, and sense of control. You have to find out what goes into each of the buckets from your investigations about the group you plan on working with, such as low-income mothers or teenagers. These sets of beliefs are not necessarily related to health. Nor does the theory imply that people consciously and systematically go through all the processes described here every time they act. Obviously, many people's health-related behaviors have become automatic or habitual, such as smoking or eating cereal at breakfast. Their underlying beliefs are automatically triggered in these instances.

The *second* way the theory can help us is when we use our understanding to help our audiences become aware of their own attitudes and beliefs that predict their behaviors and hence help them make changes if they wish to do so. This is good news. Clearly it becomes important for us to understand the nature of attitudes and beliefs, how they are formed, and how people can change them.

A summary of the theory is shown in **FIGURE 4-2**. How the main constructs of the theory (which represent the determinants of the behavior) can be applied in nutrition

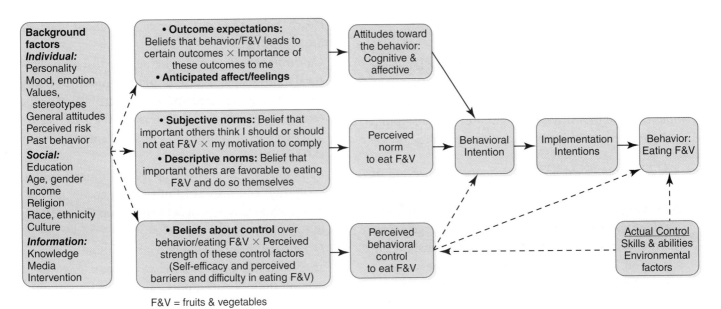

F&V = fruits & vegetables

FIGURE 4-2 Theory of planned behavior/reasoned action approach: example of behavior of eating fruits and vegetables. F&V = fruits and vegetables.

Table 4-2 Theory of Planned Behavior: Major Constructs and Use in Nutrition Education Interventions

Theory Construct (Determinant of Behavior Change)	Definition	Use in Nutrition Education
Beliefs about behavior/ outcome expectations	Individuals' beliefs that the behavior leads to certain desired or negative outcomes (in the areas of health, personal, social, etc.)	*Enhance positive expectations:* Provide messages or use strategies to enhance people's expectations about taste, health benefits, and convenience of eating F&V, including through tasting them. *Increase awareness of negative outcomes* of not taking action (i.e., not eating F&V).
Attitudes: Cognitive/instrumental	Individuals' favorable or unfavorable judgments about a given behavior	Messages and images can show healthful behavior in positive light.
Attitudes: Affective/experiential	Individuals' emotional response to the idea of performing the behavior	Provide opportunities to experience and enjoy healthful food through food tastings or food preparation and cooking experiences accompanied by eating the food prepared with others. Positive emotional messages about doing the behavior. Explore anticipated regret if action is not taken.
Perceived norms: Subjective norms (injunctive norms)	Individuals, beliefs that people who are important to the individuals either approve or disapprove of them performing a behavior	Help participants clarify expectations of friends and families for their behavior and evaluate whether they should comply or not.
Descriptive norms	Individuals' beliefs about important others' *attitudes* or *behaviors* in regard to the behavior	Give data showing that many teens do eat F&V and/or value health; correct misconceptions. Show that eating F&V is cool; use peer or valued models to encourage eating F&V.
Perceived behavioral control Self-efficacy/difficulty	Individuals' perceptions about factors that will make it easy or difficult to perform the behavior and whether there are environmental barriers to action	Provide messages that eating F&V can be easy and convenient (e.g., for bananas: "Peel, eat; how easy is that?"). Provide demonstration and guided practice on how to prepare or cook F&V; or how to select items to carry to school or work to increase self-efficacy or self-confidence.
Behavioral intentions Implementation intentions	Individuals' perceived likelihood of taking a given action	Lead group through decision-making activities to assess personal positive and negative expectations (pros and cons) of change and commitment to try the new action or behavior change. State specific plan for when and where to carry out the new action or behavior change.

Note: F&V = fruits and vegetables.

education practice is described in **TABLE 4-2**. A brief example of how the theory can be used to describe people's actions in the real world is shown in **BOX 4-2**.

BEHAVIOR

The starting point, of course, is a behavior, defined as an observable action of individuals. A behavior can be stated as a behavioral category, such as eating 5 fruits and vegetables each day, exercising 30 minutes per day, consuming fewer sugar-sweetened drinks, purchasing foods with low carbon footprints, and so forth (Conner and Norman 1995). Some studies state behaviors even more generally, reflecting practical considerations, such as "eating a MyPlate meal." Behavior can also be stated more specifically, such as eating breakfast, adding a vegetable to lunch each day,

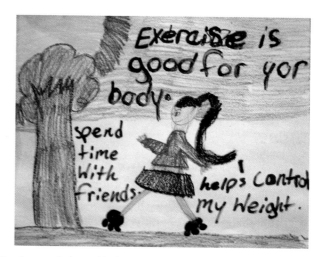

The theory of planned behavior allows us to understand what motivates people to exercise.

Courtesy of EarthFriends, Teachers College Columbia University.

BOX 4-2 The Theory of Planned Behavior/Reasoned Action Approach in Practice

The reasoned action approach proposes that individuals are likely to take a specific action if they *intend* to take that action. Intention to take action is based on the following beliefs or convictions and feelings:

- I believe that taking this action will lead to outcomes I desire.
- I believe that the positive outcomes of taking this action outweigh the negative outcomes.

- I have positive feelings about taking this action, and taking action will make me feel good about myself.
- People important to me think that I should take this action, and their opinions are important to me.
- People who are important to me have positive attitudes towards the action and do it themselves.
- I am confident that I can carry out the action, despite difficulties.

---

or eating a fruit for an afternoon snack, or drinking eight glasses of water each day. Food frequency questionnaires or behavioral checklists are often used to measure behaviors. Behaviors can also be other food-related behaviors such as breastfeeding, food safety practices, or parenting practices.

BEHAVIORAL INTENTION

We are more likely to engage in a behavior, such as eating low-fat foods or engaging in physical activity, if we intend to do so. This seems so obvious it does not need to be stated. Why the idea of intention is useful, however, is because the opposite is also true—it is unlikely we will do something if we do not intend to do so. This most immediate determinant of taking action or making a behavior change is called *behavioral intention* (BI). This state of mind can be stated simply as an *intention*, as *how likely* a person is to engage in an *expected action* (Sparks, Shepherd, and Frewer 1995) (see Table 4-2).

Research evidence has found that reported intentions are reliably and moderately correlated with a range of health actions (Armitage and Conner 2001; Fishbein and Ajzen 2010). Intention is, in turn, determined by attitudes, **social norms**, and a sense of control over the behavior.

ATTITUDES

Attitudes are our favorable or unfavorable judgments about a given behavior. We can think of attitudes as representing to some extent our motivations to take action.

Attitudes have both a cognitive/evaluative aspect (also called *instrumental attitudes*) such as how good or bad for health it would be to lose weight, and an *affective aspect* (also called *experiential attitudes)* such as how good

or bad a person would feel about him- or herself losing weight. Both components influence intentions (Ajzen 2001; Fishbein and Ajzen 2010).

Cognitive (Instrumental) Attitudes Based on Beliefs

Attitudes (or our motivations) are powerfully influenced by our *beliefs* or convictions about the outcomes or consequences of our actions and how important these consequences are to us. This is shown in Figure 4-2.

Beliefs About Expected Outcomes of Behavior as the Basis of Cognitive Attitudes

Our global, enduring and all-pervasive attitudes (or core values) influence our motivation to act. To achieve our desired ends, however, we have more immediate **cognitive** or **instrumental attitudes**, which are based on our beliefs and expectations that a behavior will lead to certain more immediate outcomes that we desire. Psychologists call these beliefs *outcome beliefs* or *outcome expectations* (OEs). Very often these beliefs are based on scientific evidence and our acceptance of the evidence. Examples are "Eating fruits and vegetables will reduce my risk of cancer/heart disease/hypertension/diabetes," or "Eating fruits and vegetables will help me to have a clear complexion."

Outcomes expectations, reasons, or convictions for a given action or behavior can be:

- *Health outcomes* that are based on scientific evidence on diet and health or diet and disease relationships, such as the relationships between eating calcium-rich foods and bone health, breastfeeding and the health of the infant, antioxidants in food and cancer, and so forth. These beliefs about the positive outcomes of the behavior can be called perceived benefits; those beliefs about negative outcomes, perceived threat or risk.

- *Personally meaningful and social outcomes* might be taste, convenience, preparation/cooking needs, cost, good value for money, contribution to personal appearance, makes a good impression on others, shows others you are a good parent, family cohesion, having more energy, and so forth. Expected outcomes can be positive (e.g., good taste) or negative (e.g., bad reaction to the food).
- *Larger, global outcomes* might include such outcomes or values as family cohesion, empowerment of communities, support of local farmers, or conservation of resources.

How important these various outcomes of a behavior are to us also needs to be considered: We may truly desire the outcome or we may not. If not, we will not take the actions no matter how beneficial they might be.

Affective (Experiential) Attitudes Based on Feelings

Attitudes (or our motivations) are also powerfully—often more powerfully—influenced by our *feelings* about the behavior (e.g., eating chocolate) (Salovey and Birnbaum 1989; Richard, van der Pligt, and de Vries 1996; Lawton, Conner, and Parker 2007; Crum et al. 2011). These feelings or emotions contribute to the **affective** component of attitudes. People's emotions and feelings, often deeply held, are often called "hot buttons" by marketers and are extensively studied. Affect or feelings are more likely to be derived from direct experience, such as physiological reactions to food (e.g., taste, smell, sight, or fillingness of food) and familiarity through frequent exposure. This is shown in Figure 4-2.

Food Preferences and Enjoyment

Our sensory-affective responses to food (taste, smell, impact on how full we feel) powerfully influence food choice and dietary behavior, as we see in Chapter 1 (Rozin and Fallon 1981; Moss 2013). Consumers consistently rate taste preferences or "liking" as a leading motivator of their dietary choices.

CONFLICTING ATTITUDES: AMBIVALENCE

We often have both positive and negative *beliefs* about the outcomes of a given behavior and this may cause us some ambivalence (Armitage and Conner 2000; Ajzen 2001). For example, we may believe that eating fruits and vegetables is desirable because doing so reduces the risk of cancer, but also believe that fruits and vegetables are expensive and inconvenient to carry around or eat.

Ambivalence may also result from a *conflict* between the cognitive aspect (chocolates are fattening) and the affective aspect of attitudes (I love the taste of chocolate) (Sparks et al. 2001). Or again, we may like the taste of meat, but may have concerns about animal welfare issues (Povey, Wellens, and Conner 2001). The relative strengths of these thoughts and feelings influence whether we will take action. Often such ambivalence immobilizes people from taking action. An important role for nutrition educators is to help people work through their ambivalences.

PERCEIVED NORMS (SOCIAL PRESSURE)

We all know about social peer pressure. Our behaviors are influenced by our perceptions of what's normal—in terms of whether others approve or disapprove of what we do, and what they themselves feel and do.

Subjective or Injunctive Norms

Our beliefs that people who are important to us either approve or disapprove of us performing a behavior are called **subjective norms** or **injunctive norms** (other people's injunctions to us) by psychologists and are experienced as social pressure (e.g., "My close friends/parents think that I should/should not eat meat"). These can be quite subtle and act almost unconsciously. For example, one study found that males who were eating with women at a fixed-price "all you can eat" restaurant ate more, perhaps to project masculinity (Sigirci, Kniffin, and Wansink 2014). How strongly we wish to comply with other people's opinions is very important to whether you will take action or not ("I do/do not think it is important to do what my friends think I should do").

Descriptive Norms, Including Perceived Cultural Norms

Our perceptions of other people's attitudes and what they do also influence our behaviors, even if they are not pressuring us as to what to do (Sheeran, Norman, and Orbell 1999; Fishbein and Ajzen, 2010). Psychologists call these **descriptive norms**. Descriptive norms include beliefs about: (a) other people's *attitudes* toward the behavior in question (group attitude), such as attitudes of our personal or social network toward drinking soda; and (b) perceptions of other people's behavior (group behavior), such as how many in our social circle drink soda. The degree to which we identify with these groups will influence how likely it is that we will follow these norms. This construct captures the strong impact of perceived cultural norms and practices.

Which Are More Important: Our Attitudes or Perceived Norms?

Individuals differ on the relative weight they place on personal attitudes and on the opinions of others. For example, subjective or injunctive norms may be more important in cultures that are more collectivist in nature, whereas attitudes may be more important in individualistic cultures (Ajzen 2001). These relative weights also differ across behaviors. Some food behaviors (such as eating low-fat foods) may be more influenced by attitudes, whereas others (such as breastfeeding) are more influenced by social norms and pressures.

PERCEIVED BEHAVIORAL CONTROL

Our perceptions of how much control we have over a behavior are an important determinant of our behaviors. Psychologists call this **perceived behavioral control (PBC)**. It also includes the notion of whether we can overcome barriers or can perform the behavior. For example, healthier foods may not be easily available in the local grocery store, or people may not know how to cook the foods. Perceived behavioral control influences both intention and behavior directly, as shown in Figure 4-2, probably because our perception of control may accurately reflect whether we, in fact, have *actual control* over being able to perform the behavior.

Perceived Behavioral Control and Self-Efficacy: Is There a Difference?

Perceived behavioral control is similar to the self-efficacy construct of social cognitive theory, which we will describe in the next chapter (Armitage and Conner 2001). Perceived behavioral control includes the notion of perceived difficulties, including personal resources and external barriers, whereas self-efficacy is generally defined in terms of **personal confidence** in being able to carry out a given behavior ("I am confident that I could successfully eat five fruits and vegetables a day if I wanted to"). Many researchers, however, consider the terms to be

interchangeable (Bandura 2000; Fishbein and Ajzen 2010; Lien, Lytle, and Komro 2002).

THE BEHAVIOR INTENTION TO BEHAVIOR LINK

We are only too aware that we do not always act on our intentions. A number of factors may be operating. These are shown in Figure 4-2. First, our *perceived behavioral control* or *self-efficacy* influences our actual behavior directly as well as our intention to take action. For many behaviors or behavior changes, we will need a degree of self-confidence or self-efficacy to carry out the actions. We need to feel that the actions are not too difficult to do.

Second, the degree to which we have *actual control* over the given behaviors is very important in translating intentions into actual behaviors. Do we have *relevant skills and abilities* to carry out the behavior, whatever our intentions? Do *environmental factors* facilitate or present a barrier to our performing the behavior? For example, are healthy foods or opportunities for physical activity available to us in our community at an affordable cost? We may have strong intentions and the needed functional knowledge and skills but still may not be able to carry out the actions because of high environmental barriers.

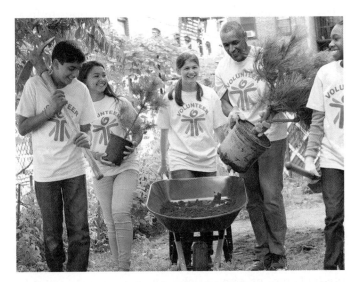

Participating in a community urban farming project improves youths' attitudes toward food and nutrition.

Extensions of the Theory of Planned Behavior/Reasoned Action Approach

EXTENSIONS OF THE THEORY OF PLANNED BEHAVIOR: A FOCUS ON ADDITIONAL BELIEFS

Research has suggested that the reasoned action approach can be expanded by incorporating additional determinants of behavior that reflect beliefs about the self, such as moral norms and self-identity. In the area of food and nutrition, these determinants have been found to make some additional independent contribution to the prediction of behavior.

FIGURE 4-3 summarizes the extended theory of planned behavior, showing the role of additional beliefs in predicting behavioral intentions and the role of implementation intentions for enacting behavior. It also includes the more complex view of attitudes and subjective norms described above.

Personal Normative Beliefs: Perceived Moral or Ethical Obligation

A number of researchers have found that people have personal norms that also influence their behaviors (Godin, Conner, and Sheeran 2005; Raats, Shepherd, and Sparks 1995; Sparks et al. 1995; Bissonette and Contento 2001; Williams-Pethota et al. 2004). Some of these are:

- *Personal normative beliefs.* An example might be, "I feel I should breastfeed my baby."
- *Moral and ethical considerations*, such as parents saying, "I feel it is my moral obligation to feed my child milk/healthful foods."

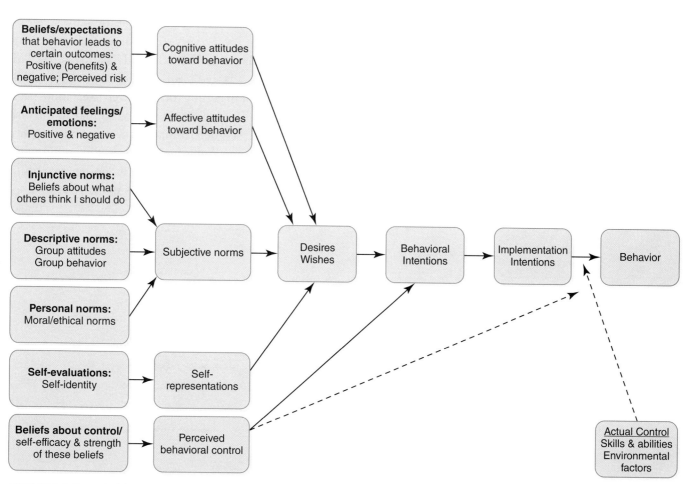

FIGURE 4-3 Extended theory of planned behavior.

Data from Abraham, C., and P. Sheeran. 2000. *Understanding and changing health behaviour: From health beliefs to self-regulation. In Understanding and changing health behaviour from health beliefs to self-regulation*, edited by P. Norman, C. Abraham, and M. Conner. Amsterdam: Hardwood Academic Publishers.

- *Personal responsibility*, such as, "I feel that I have a responsibility to buy organic foods to improve the health of the natural environment."

Self-Identity

Thoughts we have about ourselves have also been shown to contribute to the prediction of behavior (Abraham and Sheeran 2000; Sparks 2000; Bissonette and Contento 2001; Robinson and Smith 2002; Bisogni et al. 2002).

- *Self-concept* or *self-identity*. "I think of myself as a "green consumer" or "a health-conscious consumer."
- *Ideal-self versus actual-self.* We also tend to compare ourselves to some ideal. Our ideal-self versus actual-self discrepancies can lead to disappointment, sadness, or depression.
- *Ought-to-be self versus actual-self discrepancies* can result in guilt, worry, helplessness, anger, and fear: "I feel like a bad mom. I know that my kids should have better things to eat" (IFIC Foundation 1999).
- *Membership in a cultural group.* "I think of myself as [Italian] [Chinese] [Mexican] when it comes to food."

EXTENSIONS OF THE THEORY OF PLANNED BEHAVIOR: A FOCUS ON FEELINGS AND EMOTIONS

We all know that our emotions or feelings about performing the behavior are powerful motivators of dietary behaviors (Lawton et al. 2007; Lawton, Conner, and McEachan 2009;

Crum et al. 2011). Research has been very active in this area and researchers propose that although they can be considered part of outcome expectations, emotions and feelings should be made more prominent.

Desire

One model suggests that desire or wish represents the motivational state whereby our beliefs or reasons for the behavior are transformed into motivations to engage in the behavior and are the closest determinant of behavioral intentions. Consequently, "desire" should be inserted between the major TPB determinants of attitudes, social norms, perceived behavioral control and behavioral intention, and that anticipated positive and negative emotions should be more prominently shown alongside these standard determinants as contributing to desires and hence to intentions (Bagozzi, Baumgartner, and Pieters 1998; Perugini and Bagozzi 2001; Hingle et al. 2012).

Desire has been measured as "My desire to exercise in the next 4 weeks to lose weight/stay at the same weight is 'no desire at all . . . very, very strong desire'" (Perugini and Bagozzi 2001; Bagozzi, Dholokia, and Basuroy 2003). This model has been adapted for use to examine what predicts parents' behavior in getting their children to eat more fruits and vegetables. Here, desire is seen as similar to *intrinsic motivation* from self-determination theory, to be described later in this chapter, and is measured as "Encouraging my child to eat vegetables is enjoyable, frustrating, rewarding, hard" (Baranowski et al. 2013). This is shown in **FIGURE 4-4**.

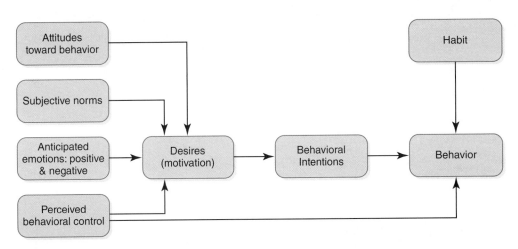

FIGURE 4-4 Model of goal directed behavior.

Data from Perugini, M., and R. P. Bagozzi. 2001. The role of desires and anticipated emotions in goal-directed behaviors: Broadening and deepening the theory of planned behavior. *British Journal of Social Psychology* 40:79–98; and Baranowksi, T., et al. 2013. Psychometric assessment scales for a model of goal directed vegetable parenting practices. *International Journal of Behavioral Nutrition and Physical Activity* 10:110.

Anticipated Positive Emotions

Our anticipated positive feelings and emotions about the consequences of involvement in a behavior are highly motivating. For example, our attitudes toward breastfeeding or eating foods with a lower carbon footprint may be motivated not only by our *belief* that it will make us healthier or will be better for the environment, respectively (the cognitive aspect of attitudes), but also by our anticipation that it will make us *feel* "delighted, satisfied, happy, proud, pleased" and generally good about ourselves (Bagozzi et al. 1998; Perugini and Bagozzi 2001; Hingle et al. 2012). This provides the motivational impetus for intentions. Thus nutrition educators can help parents increase their desire or motivation to increase fruit and vegetable consumption by their children if we can help them recognize that this will make them feel proud, satisfied, and good about themselves.

Anticipated Negative Emotions and Regret

People's anticipation that they will have a negative emotion from the behavior will influence their intention to take action, such as it will make them feel "upset, frustrated, disappointed, concerned" (Baranowski et al. 2013). People's anticipation that they might regret the consequences of acting or failing to act has also been shown to be a determinant of preventive health behavior (Sandberg and Conner 2008). For example, a study showed that anticipated regret influenced the intention of college students to eat junk foods (Richard, van der Pligt, and de Vries 1996). Our anticipated regret or worry that our diet may increase our risk of getting heart disease later may influence our food choices.

FROM "I WISH" TO "I WILL": THE IMPORTANCE OF IMPLEMENTATION INTENTIONS (ACTION PLANS)

Our personal experience suggests, and research confirms, that behavioral intentions are not sufficient for us to initiate difficult behaviors such as dietary change. Our intentions are often more like wishes. It has been found that they are more likely to be carried out if they are first translated into a practical action to-do list. These are called *implementation intentions* in this theory and they specify exactly when, where, and how we will undertake the particular behavior (Gollwitzer 1999; Armitage 2006; Garcia and Mann 2003). These are called *action plans* in other

theories. The general behavioral intention may be to eat five fruits and vegetables each day. However, to make that a reality, we need to make more specific plans, such as "I will have a midmorning snack of fruit and add one vegetable to my lunch each day this week."

Note, however, that setting an implementation intention for a healthy behavior (e.g., eating more fruit for a snack) by itself does not necessarily drive out a less healthy behavior (e.g., eating fatty snacks and sweets) (Verplanken and Faes 1999).

HABIT

Many of our behaviors appear to occur without much thought, mindless even (Wansink 2006). We develop routines or **habits** that seem to be automatic responses to situations and are often the driving force in behavior. Some of these habits may derive from cultural traditions. This is especially true of frequently performed behaviors, such as eating behavior (Triandis 1979; Brug et al. 2006; Kremers, van der Horst, and Brug 2007). These habits can be strong. This is because when we repeatedly perform a behavior in the same situation, such as breakfast, our intention (to eat cereal) becomes automatically triggered (Fishbein and Ajzen 2010). The same thing happens when we take very little time to make a decision, such as may occur in supermarket purchases (Abratt and Goodey 1990; Cohen 2008).

Habit Versus Intention

Intention and habit may be competing with each other. However, nutrition educators can help individuals recognize the behaviors that they do from habit and help them re-evaluate the habit. In addition, it has been found that targeting both intentions and perceived control over the behavior is likely to influence future behavior *despite* past behavior.

UNDERSTANDING JASON AND HIS FRIENDS

The theory of planned behavior provides us with a wonderful tool for understanding the motivations of our audiences. Let's take Jason and his friends as an example. They are 20-somethings. To determine what would motivate them to think seriously about eating more fruits and vegetables, you could use the theory to structure some interviews. **BOX 4-3** shows what they might say.

BOX 4-3 Understanding Jason and His Friends Using the Theory of Planned Behavior/Reasoned Action Approach

Jason is a 25-year-old salesperson in a clothing store. To determine the reasons, insights, or feelings that would motivate Jason and individuals like him to think seriously about why to take action now about eating more fruits and vegetables, you would have to conduct some interviews. From these, the reasons or outcome expectations, attitudes or feelings, and larger values or hot buttons in the following list might emerge. Modify and add to the following list those that you think would be powerful for Jason and his friends:

- *Attitudes:* Their attitude toward eating fruits and vegetables is positive, but weakly so.

- *Outcome expectations:* There are competing beliefs or outcome expectations about eating fruits and vegetables: these foods are known to be healthful, but they are not convenient to eat during the day, and they are expensive.

- *Anticipated emotions*: Jason and his friends say they anticipate that vegetables will not taste as good as other foods.

- *Social norms:* Jason and youth like him are busy, vibrant young people who do things together—eating fruits and vegetables is not one of them! It is just not part of their mind-set.

- *Values or hot buttons:* They feel they are now adults, able to make their own choices. Eating fruits and vegetables seems like what "good children" do. They are no longer children.

- *Self-identity:* They do not see themselves as "health-conscious eaters." They know people like that and don't want to be like them.

Nutrition education for this group needs to address all of these determinants of behavior change in order to help Jason and his friends to see "what's in it for me" to eat fruits and vegetables.

EVIDENCE FOR THE THEORY FROM RESEARCH AND INTERVENTION STUDIES

The theory of planned behavior/reasoned action approach has been studied extensively and rigorously in the social psychology field and used widely to understand health issues, including food choice and dietary and physical activity behaviors (Godin and Kok 1996; Armitage and Conner 2001).

A few specific studies are described here to indicate the range of behaviors and groups with whom the theories have been used. Here are a few examples.

Research on Food Choice and Dietary Behaviors

Studies with Adolescents

Studies with adolescents have examined a variety of diet-related behaviors:

- *Eating Healthy,* a study in children aged 8–9 years, found that attitudes, friends' and family norms, knowledge, motivation to conform to the norms, and perceived behavioral control predicted healthy eating, with sense of control being the most important (Bazillier et al. 2011).

- *For soda consumption,* the predictions by the theory were high: 64% for intention and 34% for behavior (Kassem et al. 2003). The strongest predictors were attitude and the subjects' underlying outcome beliefs (feel healthy, become hyper, gain weight, quench thirst), followed by perceived behavioral control (availability at home and school, money) and subjective norms.

- *Buying or eating local and organic foods* was best predicted by behavioral intention, beliefs about outcomes, and perceived social influences. Also significant were *perceived responsibility* for buying and eating organic foods and *self-identity* for buying and eating local food (Bissonette and Contento 2001).

Studies with Adults

Numerous studies have also been conducted with adults, both with the general population and those at risk of chronic disease:

- *Fast food consumption in adults* was most influenced by anticipated immediate outcomes—foods that are tasty, satisfying, and convenient, and not long-term health, and friends and family (injunctive norms) (Dunn et al. 2011).

- *Sweetened beverage consumption* in a rural, low-income population was most strongly influenced by behavioral intention, followed by attitudes, perceived behavioral control, and subjective norms (Zoellner et al. 2012).

- *Consumption of foods low in saturated fat* among people diagnosed with type 2 diabetes was best predicted by intentions and perceived control, while intentions were predicted by attitude and subjective norms; *planning* was an important link between intention and behavior (White et al. 2010).

- *Cultural beliefs.* Theory constructs can incorporate cultural beliefs (Blanchard et al. 2009). One study found that barriers included the *outcome beliefs* that to eat healthfully meant giving up part of their cultural heritage and trying to conform to the dominant culture. Friends and relatives (*social norms*) were also not supportive of dietary changes (James 2004).

Example from Practice

An example of how the construct of outcome expectations/perceived benefits of the theory of planned behavior is used in a nationwide Web-based campaign called Kids Cook Monday is shown in **NUTRITION EDUCATION IN ACTION 4-4**.

NUTRITION IN ACTION 4-4 Kids Cook Monday

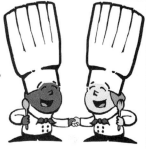

The Monday Campaigns is a nonprofit public health organization in association with Columbia University Mailman School of Public Health, Johns Hopkins Bloomberg School of Public Health and Maxwell School of Syracuse University. ©2003–2015 The Monday Campaigns Inc.

The Monday Campaigns is a nonprofit public health organization in association with Columbia University Mailman School of Public Health, Johns Hopkins Bloomberg School of Public Health and Maxwell School of Syracuse University. ©2003–2015 The Monday Campaigns Inc.

Kids Cook Monday is a nationwide, Web-based campaign that encourages families to cook and eat together. The promotional materials focus on outcome expectations, highlighting evidence that by helping to prepare food, kids are more likely to try new foods, eat more nutritious food, learn new problem-solving skills, become more confident across all aspects of their lives, and establish strong communication with their parents and caregivers. The Kids Cook Monday poster series proclaims,

"When kids help prepare dinner they help prepare themselves for life." Toolkits, family-friendly recipes, video demonstrations, and guidance about which food preparation tasks are appropriate for children of different ages are designed specifically for families and educators and emphasize self-efficacy for the adults promoting Kids Cook Monday as well as for the kids participating in the program.

Intervention Studies

Many dietary and physical activity interventions have used the key elements of the theory of planned behavior with some success.

Group-Based and Media Interventions

- *A school-based weight gain prevention* intervention for adolescents based on the theory of planned behavior and accompanied by environmental supports positively influenced several measures of body composition among both girls and boys (Singh et al. 2007).
- *A gardening program* that was effective in improving youth fruit and vegetable consumption found that perceived behavioral control was predictive of behavior in girls (Lautenschlager and Smith 2007).
- *A booklet* used with outpatients older than 65 years resulted in gains in perceived behavioral control, behavioral intention, and behaviors targeted. Those who set specific goals were much more successful in making changes than those who did not (Kelley and Abraham 2004).
- *A media campaign called "1% or Less"* encouraged people to switch from higher-fat milk to milk with 1% or less fat (Booth-Butterfield and Reger 2004). The campaign targeted behavioral beliefs and found significant effects on intention, attitudes, and behavioral beliefs; these were related to changes in self-reported milk use.

OTHER MOTIVATORS OF FOOD CHOICE AND DIETARY BEHAVIOR CHANGE

Global Values and Hot Buttons

We have seen that individuals are motivated to take action if the action will lead to outcomes or goals they value (Lewin et al. 1944). The goals about certain immediate ends, such as taste, seeming cool, losing or maintaining weight, or being liked by one's friends, are outcome expectations, as noted. Other goals or values are more global and are an important basis for action. These are often set by a person's culture or subculture and are relatively enduring. The desires to achieve these are also determinants of motivation. Notice that these values are based on people's emotions or deepest feelings about themselves or the world around them. Consequently, they are sometimes referred to as people's *hot buttons* in the mass media literature. Understanding these would likely help us design

effective nutrition education because they influence people's short-term goals.

Global Values of Rokeach

A widely used set of global goals or values is that of Rokeach (1973), which includes an exciting life, inner harmony, a sense of accomplishment, social recognition, national security, a comfortable life, pleasure, equality, happiness, mature love or sexuality, self-respect, and true friendship, to which health has been added.

Global Values of Kahle

Marketers often use Kahle's list of values (Kahle 1984; Andreasen 1995), which is somewhat similar: self-respect, sense of accomplishment, self-fulfillment, fun and enjoyment in life, security, being well respected, a warm relationship with others, and excitement. Other lists include additional values such as novelty, independence, or sense of belonging.

Other Basic Values

Other values or goals may also be important, such as family cohesion, empowerment of communities, support of local farmers, social justice, vegetarianism, feminism, or conservation of resources. For example, a study with adults found that individuals who cleaned their plates felt they did not want to waste food because it was linked to a larger value of not wasting resources (Pelican et al. 2005). Values may also differ by age group, so values for children, teens, and adults may differ.

PERSONAL MEANINGS GIVEN TO FOOD

Out of our values and specific past experiences, including cultural traditions, may emerge very personal meanings we attach to the foods we eat. Foods may be eaten because they are comfort foods—foods that remind us of positive childhood experiences—or because we want to use them to manage feelings. For example, a study with teenagers found that although they knew that eating sweets might be unhealthy, bad for their teeth, or fattening, it was also a way to deal with frustration, stress, or anger (Spruijt-Metz 1995). These meanings given to food are a form of outcome expectations. Exploring these personal meanings or desired outcomes of food and eating will help us plan more effective nutrition education programs.

TAKE-HOME MESSAGE ABOUT THEORY OF PLANNED BEHAVIOR

- People are motivated to take action if they expect the action will lead to outcomes they desire, if other people they value think it is a good idea, and if they feel they have some control over taking action. Developing specific implementation plans can help them translate intention to action.
- You will find this theory especially useful for designing nutrition education activities and mass media programs to increase awareness of issues and enhance motivation for action.
- Each of the variables of the theory has been found in relation to health behaviors in most cultures investigated, and thus the theory can be useful cross-culturally (Fishbein 2000).

Using the Theory of Planned Behavior in Nutrition Education to Motivate and Activate Audiences

The theory of planned behavior (or reasoned action approach) provides us with tools to understand that people's beliefs or convictions and affect or feelings are at the heart of their motivation to take healthful action. These tools help us design appropriate nutrition education strategies. The convictions can be about the behavior, what other people think, or whether they have control over their behavior. This is good news for nutrition educators because we now know we need to help people construct cognitive beliefs or convictions (instrumental attitudes) and affective attitudes toward behaviors that will be conducive to their health and to the community's or planet's well-being. Useful nutrition education strategies are discussed in more detail in Chapter 11.

DESIGNING MESSAGES TO ADDRESS ATTITUDES AND BELIEFS ABOUT TAKING ACTION

An exciting approach to enhancing motivation in our audiences is to design activities that focus on constructing arguments, factual and persuasive, to enhance beliefs about the potential desirable outcomes of behaviors, such as the benefits of eating healthful foods or making sustainable or "green" food choices. Such beliefs are powerful motivators

of behavior through their impact on attitudes, intentions, and formation of goals.

Identify Relevant Beliefs and Attitudes of Our Audiences

Our first step is to identify which specific *beliefs* and attitudes are relevant to the recommended nutrition- or food-related behavior in the given group through a thorough needs analysis, using surveys, focus groups, interviews, or other methods. This is a crucial step and is similar to market research in the social marketing process.

Select Potential Determinants of Change for the Group

We then select a series of key beliefs determining intentions as our intervention targets. The relative importance of different beliefs, or reasons for action, will differ depending on the behavior and the group or audience. For example, in the case of eating fruits and vegetables, being cool may be important for teenagers, improving the health of their baby may be important for pregnant women, reducing cancer risk may be important for men, and ease of preparation may be important for women. Beliefs about risk or perceived threat may also be used, but messages about risk must be accompanied by increasing the individuals' confidence that they can take action to reduce the risk.

Design Effective Messages: The Elaboration Likelihood Model (ELM)

We then convert these beliefs about valued outcomes from the recommended behavior (such as breastfeeding or eating fruits and vegetables) into messages for the mass media, group educational activities, brochures, or newsletters (Salovey Schneider, and Apanovitch 1999). These beliefs are really reasons or arguments for the benefits of valued outcomes. The elaboration likelihood model (ELM) proposes that individuals will process messages through either a central route or a peripheral route (Petty and Cacioppo 1986).

Central or mindful route for our messages. Our messages are more likely to be effective or persuasive if they are constructed in such a way as to induce our audiences to think about the messages or elaborate on them. Beliefs and attitudes changed by this route are well thought out and become integrated into individuals' belief or attitude structure, such as "It is desirable for me to eat more locally grown foods because it will support local farmers."

Note, however, that individuals are more likely to think about the message when it is personally relevant and easy to understand, people have time to think about it, and there are not many distractions.

Peripheral or mindless route for our messages. When our health message about reasons or arguments for taking action is difficult to process or does not seem relevant, individuals tend to judge the message by more superficial aspects, such as the attractiveness or credibility of the source or the associations of the food with other desirable, but not directly relevant, attributes, such as a picture of a slender, attractive woman on food packaging.

Ability and motivation to process messages. Individuals differ in their *ability* and *motivation or willingness* to process the messages through the more effective central route.

- To increase participants' *ability* to process messages, make your messages straightforward and clear, repeat or reinforce them, and present them with a minimum of distractions.
- To increase participants' *motivation* to process messages, make messages unexpected or novel, memorable, culturally appropriate, and most important, *personally relevant*, stressing positive outcomes that are important to the intended audience. In a society that increasingly only pays attention to short, pithy, graphically appealing messages, it is challenging, but essential, to make messages comprehensive and catchy at the same time!

Two examples of effective messages are shown in Nutrition Education in Action 4-4: Kids Cook Monday and **NUTRITION EDUCATION IN ACTION 4-5**: Drinking Tap Water Campaign.

ENHANCING POSITIVE ATTITUDES AND FEELINGS

One important way to increase motivation is to provide opportunities for individuals to experience and enjoy healthful food, for example, through food tastings or food preparation and cooking experiences in groups, accompanied by eating the prepared food together. Repeated experiences and familiarity are more likely to lead to positive sensory-affective responses to new foods (Grieve and Vander Weg 2003).

When appropriate, groups can explore their feelings about food, understand these feelings, and seek ways to

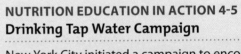

NUTRITION EDUCATION IN ACTION 4-5
Drinking Tap Water Campaign

New York City initiated a campaign to encourage people to drink water from drinking fountains.

Helped eliminate waste from

0001246

disposable plastic bottles

© ZUMA Press, Inc/Alamy

Posters above the drinking fountains say:

Can't beat the taste or the price!

I love NY water

Refills not Landfills

- Bottled water costs 1,000 times more than tap water.
- Drinking 2 liters of tap water a day costs only 50 cents per year.

When people fill their bottles, a meter senses the action and displays how many bottles have been saved from being thrown away. Each bottle filled makes the meter move up.

enjoy substituting less healthful with more healthful foods. In addition, because people's feelings and emotions are closely related to their deeply held values, emotion-based messaging has been proposed as a way to build on people's values and hot buttons, such as about being a good parent (McCarthy and Tuttelman 2005). Exploring anticipated positive feelings and anticipated regret is also important.

EXPLORING SOCIAL NORMS AND SOCIAL EXPECTATIONS

Nutrition educators can develop group activities to help participants identify what important others think that they should be doing (e.g., perceptions of the spouse's or partner's approval or disapproval of breastfeeding). In addition, educators can use materials, films, posters, and statistics to indicate how individuals similar to the group are engaging in the healthful behaviors, such as other WIC women breastfeeding, teenagers drinking water, and so forth (descriptive norms).

IDENTIFYING PERSONAL AND MORAL NORMS

Nutrition educators can help the group explore personal norms or internal standards and sense of responsibility through various activities where individuals reflect on and evaluate the importance of health in their lives and make choices about the values they wish to place on health. Moral issues can also be explored. These may derive from cultural or religious traditions.

INCREASING SELF-EFFICACY AND CONTROL: OVERCOMING BARRIERS AND DIFFICULTIES

Beliefs about self-efficacy or control over the behavior are important when individuals are in the motivational or decision-making mode about a behavior, as well as when individuals are attempting to carry it out. Self-efficacy can be seen as the mirror image of perceived barriers or difficulty in taking action. In group settings, nutrition educators can elicit perceptions of the barriers to taking action from group members and then share and discuss ways to reduce those barriers. In mass media approaches and materials, difficulties can be addressed in the messages themselves. For example, a statewide program placed a series of messages on billboards about eating fruits and vegetables, such as "Peel, eat; how easy is that!" for bananas, and "Slice, eat; how easy is that!" for tomatoes (http://www.idph.state.ia.us/INN/PickABetterSnack.aspx).

EXPLORING BELIEFS ABOUT THE SELF

Active methods of self-exploration and understanding are likely to be most effective. One strategy might be facilitated group dialogue (Norris 2003). (See Chapter 17.) This is similar to motivational interviewing for individuals (Rollnick, Miller, and Butler 2008). Films, discussions, or debates of the pros and cons of the behavior may be useful here. Self-presentations such as self-identity or social identity can be explored. Ideal-self versus actual-self discrepancies and ought-to-be self versus actual-self discrepancies

can be explored through activities that bring to awareness these discrepancies, and strategies can be provided for handling them.

RECOGNIZING HABITS, ROUTINES, AND CULTURAL TRADITIONS

Nutrition education activities can be designed to bring the less positive habits or routines (e.g., being a couch potato) to consciousness so that they can be considered and replaced by more positive habits or routines. Because these may require more effort (e.g., exercising regularly), nutrition educators can design tip sheets, checklists, or activities to assist individuals to develop these new routines. On the other hand, there may be family and cultural traditions that are supportive of healthy eating, and these can be encouraged.

MAKING DECISIONS AND RESOLVING AMBIVALENCES

Nutrition educators can help the group explore the benefits and costs of taking action as well as not taking action. This can be done verbally as a group or through an activity where individuals write out the pros and cons. In addition, educators can help group participants explore their own values by providing the group with a series of value statements to which they can respond. This is to seek to elicit their ambivalences, and then assure them that this is normal.

At the end of these activities, individuals can come to closure and write out their intention with respect to the issue or behavior that is the focus of the program and state some specific implementation plans on how exactly they will carry out their intentions.

THE CASE OF MARIA: NUTRITION EDUCATION USING THE THEORY OF PLANNED BEHAVIOR

Maria is a 23-year-old who works in a construction company office. She eats lunch each day from a mobile vendor who sells hotdogs, hamburgers, and sandwiches and drinks a soda pop or two each day for a quick pick-me-up. She has a 4-year-old daughter who goes to a Head Start program in her community. She and her husband are divorced. She knows that she and her daughter should eat more fruit each day, but they both like sweets and soda, which are cheap and convenient. These are also common practices among the other families in her community. Pamphlets at Head Start encourage families to provide healthy snacks and drinks for children at home. She wants to be a good mother and she is becoming concerned about her daughter's teeth; her daughter also is getting a little chubby. While her family and friends think children will just grow out of this phase, she wants to be sure she is doing right by her daughter. She sees that there will be a session for moms offered at the site titled "Give your child the smile of a lifetime—healthy drinks and snacking." She decides to attend. Notice that the behavior is very specific (information is not general about nutrients such as calcium). She also noticed that, like herself, the nutrition educator was Hispanic. Thus she felt comfortable attending because she believed that her cultural background would be understood.

Here is how the nutrition educator designed the session. She decided that the best theory to use to address the issue of motivating moms to help their children eat healthfully was the theory of planned behavior. She looked at research and survey data and conducted interviews and held group discussions with some Head Start mothers. She found that mothers in this low-income community had a common concern about getting their young children to eat more healthfully in the context of their culture. She then created a theory model for her session. The figure in the case study illustrates how she operationalized the model for this session. There is a similar blank form at the end of this chapter that you can use to design nutrition educations based on the theory of planned behavior. She then developed a lesson plan from this theory model, as shown in **CASE STUDY 4-2**.

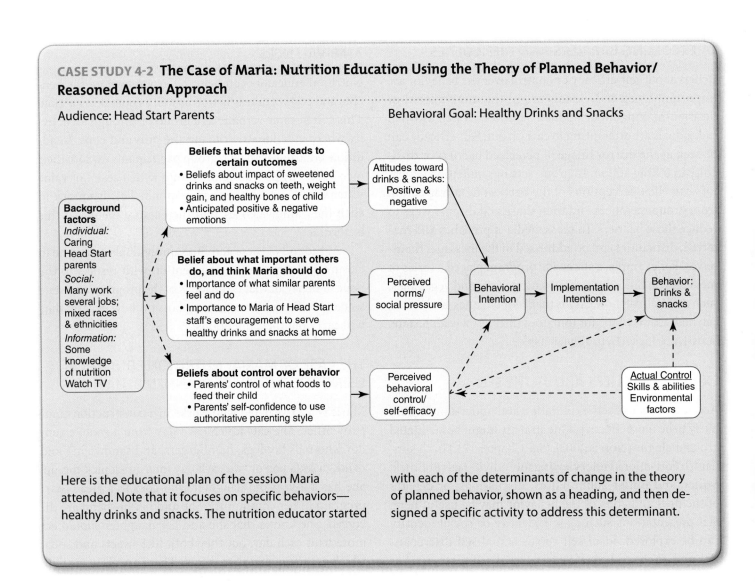

CASE STUDY 4-2 The Case of Maria: Nutrition Education Using the Theory of Planned Behavior/ Reasoned Action Approach

Audience: Head Start Parents

Behavioral Goal: Healthy Drinks and Snacks

Here is the educational plan of the session Maria attended. Note that it focuses on specific behaviors—healthy drinks and snacks. The nutrition educator started with each of the determinants of change in the theory of planned behavior, shown as a heading, and then designed a specific activity to address this determinant.

"Give Your Child the Smile of a Lifetime—Healthy Drinks and Snacking"

Education Plan for Group Session

Behavioral goal: Participating parents will offer their children healthy snacks and drinks for strong teeth and a healthy weight.

Educational objectives to reach goals: At the end of the session, participants will be able to:
- Evaluate the degree to which their child's eating patterns increase their risk of dental caries and unhealthy weight
- Describe the impact of foods and drinks high in sugar on the health of their child's teeth and weight
- Describe the benefits of water and milk for strong bones and teeth and a healthy weight
- Understand and appreciate appropriate parenting practices
- State commitment to make changes through an action plan

Procedure: (Determinant in **bold** and activity for <u>determinant</u> underlined):

Beliefs about outcomes of current behavior
- <u>Diet assessment:</u> Purpose: To help mothers become aware of the sugary drinks and snacks their child consumes. So, as they come in, participants are asked to write down everything their child ate and drank in the past 24 hours—approximate amounts only. (Head Start provides menus for foods/drinks offered there.) Then, they are to circle the drinks high in sugar and snacks high in sugar and fat.

Beliefs about outcomes of current behavior
- <u>Measure out sugar:</u> The nutrition educator brings out a variety of popular sugared drinks. Then, she asks a volunteer to come up and measure out, with estimates provided by the group, how many teaspoons of sugar (from a container of sugar) they think is in each drink. They also look at the calorie count. From the brief 24-hour recall, they calculate how many teaspoons of sugar their child gets in their drinks per day, per week, per year. They also estimate the calories and how many pounds of body weight that comes to.

  Maria and the other parents are shocked at the amount of sugar in drinks and the number of calories. She always thought that liquids had no calories.

- <u>Soda pop and teeth:</u> The instructor then shows the group a chicken bone that she has let sit in a glass of soda pop for several days. The bone is rubbery and soft compared to a bone placed in water. She points out that the same can happen to teeth, particularly when children take a sweetened drink to bed with them in a bottle.

  Maria and the other parents are again surprised that sweetened carbonated drinks could have such an effect.
- <u>Sugar in packaged snacks:</u> The nutrition educator then shows participants various packaged snacks (empty). She asks them to read the label to find out how much sugar is in each. Again, she has volunteers measure out the amount of sugar in each.
  Maria takes note of the calories in the cookies and packaged snacks she and her daughter often eat.

Importance of the outcomes
  Parents discuss that these effects on their child's health are really of concern to them. They want to take good care of their child.

Beliefs about positive outcomes of changing current behaviors
- <u>Developing strong bones and teeth:</u> The nutrition educator uses PowerPoint with relevant photos and simply written statements to provide evidence showing that drinking water and milk instead of sugared drinks and eating low-fat dairy products in the context of a healthy diet including whole grains and fruits and vegetables can help children develop strong bones and teeth and maintain a healthy weight.

Affective attitudes (experiential attitudes)
- <u>Appreciating children's smiles:</u> The nutrition educator shows pictures of strong bones and children of diverse ethnic backgrounds with beautiful teeth and smiles, and being active and full of energy.
  Maria likes the pictures she sees, and her attitude becomes more positive.

Anticipated emotions
- <u>Feelings about being a mom:</u> She will be pleased with herself making the recommended changes as a caring mom; but she is concerned that she might become frustrated and disappointed if her daughter does not want to drink less soda or eat healthier snacks.

Social norms
- <u>Mom and friends:</u> The instructor shows a film clip showing similar moms offering their children healthy snacks and talking about their experiences. The instructor also tells them that the Head Start staff truly wish the children to be healthy and will help.

Perceived control over behavior, including barriers or difficulties
- <u>Moms have dilemmas:</u> The group reviews the dietary recalls for their children. They recognize that they are the ones that choose what foods to feed their child. But they also discuss the difficulties in getting children to drink milk and water rather than sweetened drinks and to eat healthy snacks.

Actual control
- <u>Moms have actual control:</u> Head Start provides two meals a day, and these are required to be healthy. Parents agree, however, that they have a large amount of control over their children's eating: they can provide healthy options at home.

(Continues)

CASE STUDY 4-2 **The Case of Maria: Nutrition Education Using the Theory of Planned Behavior/ Reasoned Action Approach (Continued)**

Overcoming barriers (self-efficacy)
- <u>Confidence in feeding their child:</u> The nutrition educator discusses the authoritative parenting style, where the parent puts out a few healthful options such as 100% juice, milk, and water and lets the child choose, or several healthy snacks and lets the child choose which to eat. The group brainstorms different kinds of good (and tasty) substitutes for unhealthy snacks.
  Maria feels confident in what to provide her child and is eager to practice the authoritative parenting style presented.

Behavioral intention/implementation intentions
- <u>Making plans for action:</u> The nutrition educator asks group members to write down at least one action they will take during the coming week to make their child's diet healthier. She asks them to be very specific.

  Maria feels motivated to take action. She decides that she will offer a couple of healthful snacks when her daughter comes home after Head Start each day instead of the usual less healthy ones. She decides on a second action: she will not stock soda pop in the house so that she and her daughter will only drink it occasionally. Instead, she will offer milk at meals and water in between. She believes her implementation plan is feasible.

Theory as a Tool or Guide in Nutrition Education

Theory in nutrition education provides practitioners with a tool, guide, or framework, derived from evidence, to help us develop an effective program. Each theory is not the complete story, however. For example, the theories in this chapter are important for designing activities that enhance motivations for people's decisions and choices and do not address in any detail social and environmental factors.

Self-Determination Theory

In its simplest terms, self-determination theory proposes that individuals have innate psychological needs for autonomy, competence, and relatedness, which, when satisfied, enhance their autonomous motivation and well-being. The enhancement of growth and well-being requires strategies to satisfy these basic needs and supportive social conditions.

Self-determination theory (SDT) is a general theory of human motivation that begins with the assumption that people are by nature active and self-motivated, curious and interested, with innate tendencies toward psychological growth and development because growth itself is personally satisfying and rewarding. Social environments can either support or thwart these tendencies. (Deci and Ryan 1985, 2000, 2008; Ryan and Deci 2000; Ryan et al. 2008).

COMPONENTS OF THE THEORY

This natural tendency that all humans have toward growth and development requires ongoing satisfaction of basic psychological needs and supports from the social environment to function effectively.

Basic Psychological Needs

Basic psychological needs are a natural aspect of being human that apply to all people, regardless of gender, group, or culture. These are innate, universal, and essential for health and well-being. To the extent that the needs are satisfied, people will function effectively and develop in a healthy way, but to the extent that they are thwarted, people will not function optimally or in a healthy way. According to Deci and Ryan, three psychological needs motivate the self to initiate behavior, and specific "nutriments" are essential for our psychological health and well-being: the need for competence, the need for autonomy, and the need for **relatedness** to others (Deci and Ryan 2000, 2008).

- *Need for competence:* The need for competence refers to the need to experience ourselves as capable and competent in carrying out the behaviors we choose.
- *Need for autonomy (or self-determination):* The need for autonomy refers to our need to actively participate in determining our own behavior. It includes the need to experience our actions as the result of autonomous choice without external interference.

■ *Need for relatedness:* The need for relatedness refers to our need to care for and be related to others. It includes the need to experience authentic relatedness from others and to experience satisfaction in participation and involvement with the social world.

Different Types of Motivation: Controlled and Autonomous

The degree to which individuals are self-determined depends on the degree to which these needs are met and how individuals handle pressures from the environment. Different types of motivations have been described based on the degree to which motivations are controlled or autonomous.

Amotivation is when individuals have no motivation or intention to engage in a particular action or behavior. This may result from not valuing the behavior or outcome, not believing that the behavior will lead to desired outcomes, or not feeling competent to engage in the behavior.

Controlled motivation is when individuals engage in activities in response to external pressure or to achieve an external goal. These pressures and goals are extrinsic motivators, which can often undermine intrinsic motivation because they are experienced as controlling.

Autonomous motivation is when individuals initiate an activity or behavior for its own sake because it is interesting and satisfying in itself, as opposed to doing an activity to obtain an external goal. The individuals experience a full sense of choice and fully endorse the activity. Intrinsic motivation is a prototype of this experience. People engage in behaviors because of passion, pleasure, and interest. Autonomous motivation is not the same as independence, which means to function alone and not rely on others. Independent action can be undertaken autonomously and yet include engagement with and relying on others because it is satisfying. In contrast, people may be independent because they feel pressured to be independent or because they do not like being engaged with or dependent on others. In these cases, the motivation is not autonomous.

For our purposes as nutrition educators, understanding and applying these broad categories to designing nutrition education is sufficient. The difference in general is between motivations based on "having to" do something, such as eating healthfully or exercising, and "wanting to" do so. However, the theory does describe a continuum of motivations ranging from amotivation to intrinsic motivation, as shown in **FIGURE 4-5**.

Continuum of Motivations: From "Having To" to "Wanting To"

Self-determination theory states that based on the degree of autonomy and control, motivations can be aligned along a continuum ranging from being highly controlled by

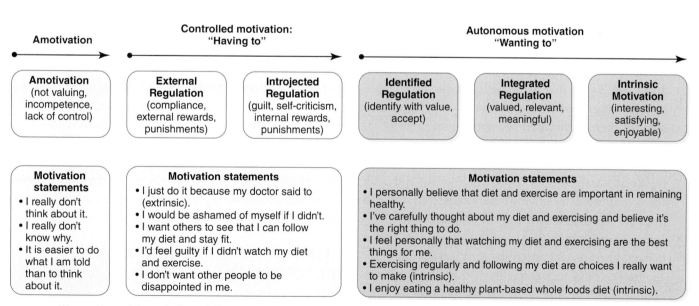

FIGURE 4-5 Self-determination theory: continuum of motivations, examples of motivation statements, and strategies for enhancing movement.

external motivators to autonomous motivation based on intrinsic motives (Ryan and Deci 2000, Deci and Ryan 2008):

- *External regulation:* On one end of the continuum is external regulation, which refers to doing something for the sole purpose of achieving a reward, avoiding a punishment, or living up to external expectations. Examples might be a child having to conform to the parental request to "clean your plate," or a heart disease patient attending an exercise program because their doctor requires it.
- *Introjected regulation:* This refers to partial internalization of extrinsic motives. Although these motivations are more internal, they are still not experienced as truly one's own, so individuals feel controlled by them. Individuals feel guilt, shame, and self-criticism when they fail and pride and self-aggrandizement after success. For example, individuals may feel guilty if they eat chocolate because they feel it is fattening or feel that they have disappointed themselves by doing so.
- *Identified regulation:* Next on the continuum, individuals accept the importance of the behavior for themselves and consciously accept it as their own. They identify with the value of the activity and willingly accept responsibility for the behavior. For example, they accept that reducing their consumption of sweet drinks is good for their health and now do so with a greater sense of autonomy and thus do not feel pressured or controlled by external factors to do the behavior.
- *Integrated regulation:* Here individuals have accepted the values and meanings of the activity or behavior to the extent that it becomes fully internalized (Deci and Ryan 2008). The behavior is personally relevant and meaningful and indeed autonomous or freely chosen. It differs from intrinsic motivation only in that the behavior is done to obtain outcomes that are not purely due to inherent enjoyment. An example is eating a plant-based diet mostly of whole grains and fresh fruits and vegetables that is freely chosen in order to improve personal health and support farmers.
- *Intrinsic motivation:* Here individuals engage in the behavior because it is interesting and satisfying. They experience positive feelings from the behavior itself. Here individuals may now eat the plant-based diet because it tastes good.

External and introjected ways of regulating behavior are clearly controlled by external motivators and are considered forms of *controlled motivation*. Identified, integrated, and intrinsic modes of behavior are forms of autonomous motivation. Examples of the kinds of statements people might make that reflect controlled and autonomous motivation are shown in Figure 4-5. Strategies for encouraging movement along the continuum are shown at the bottom of the diagram and described in detail in a later section.

Energy and Vitality

Deci and Ryan (2008) propose that satisfying our basic psychological needs leads directly or indirectly to vitality or energy available to the self. This energy allows individuals to act autonomously. Deci and Ryan point out that many theorists have posited that self-regulation or taking charge of one's life depletes energy, but SDT researchers have proposed and demonstrated that only controlled regulation depletes energy. Autonomous regulation can actually be vitalizing (e.g., Moller, Deci, and Ryan 2006).

Facilitating Individuals' Movement Toward More Internalization and Integration

Autonomous motivation is associated with more positive human experience, performance, and health consequences. Individuals move toward autonomous motivation when they feel competent (able to perform a behavior), have a sense of autonomy (where they have choice and control), and experience relatedness or connection to others.

Support for Autonomy

Studies show that self-determined behavior is enhanced by: (1) providing individuals with a meaningful rationale so that they understand why the specific behavior or activity is important, (2) acknowledging the individuals' feelings and perceptions about the behavior so that they feel understood, and (3) supporting their experience of choice and minimizing the use of pressure to do the behavior while at the same time pointing out discrepancies between individuals' behaviors and their stated desires.

RESEARCH AND INTERVENTIONS USING SELF-DETERMINATION THEORY

An increasing number of studies have been conducted with self-determination theory in the health domain (Ryan et al. 2008, Teixeira et al. 2012). Here are a few examples:

- *An intervention to promote physical activity in children* provided children with low (1 toy) or high (3 toys) choice of physically active games and mastery experiences (competence). Children played much longer when they had a choice of games (autonomy support) (Roemmich et al. 2012).

- *An obesity-prevention curriculum for middle school youth* called Choice, Control, and Change was designed to enhance autonomous motivation focused on dietary behaviors that youth had control over (such as sweet drinks and packaged snacks). The intervention provided a meaningful rationale for healthy behaviors through inquiry-based science activities, and guided goal setting where youth selected which goals to work on, promoting autonomy. Results showed that youth improved their food choices and increased their sense of competence and autonomy (Contento et al. 2010).

- *Adults with diabetes* who participated in a computer-assisted, patient-centered (autonomy-supportive) intervention increased their perception of autonomy support and competence and improvements in lipids, diabetes distress, and depressive symptoms (Williams, Lynch, and Glasgow 2007).

TAKE-HOME MESSAGE ABOUT SELF-DETERMINATION THEORY

- All people have an innate tendency toward growth and development. Maintenance of this tendency requires ongoing satisfaction of basic needs for competence, autonomy, and relatedness to others and a supportive social environment.

- Nutrition education needs to focus on supporting autonomous motivation by providing a meaningful rationale for behavior, acknowledging participants' feelings so that they feel understood, and supporting their experience of choice and hence autonomy.

Using Self-Determination Theory in Nutrition Education to Enhance Motivation and Activate Audiences

The focus of nutrition education using self-determination theory is to facilitate internalization of motivation and autonomous enactment of behaviors. Nutrition educators can do this by providing conditions that are supportive of the basic needs for competence, autonomy, and relatedness. The processes are very similar to motivational interviewing for individuals (Rollnick et al. 2008) and facilitated dialogue (Norris 2003) described in Chapter 17.

Autonomy support involves the following:

- Eliciting the understandings and feelings of the participants through reflective listening.

- Providing individuals with a meaningful rationale for taking action.

- Providing structure for explorations, ensuring that patients have relevant information about health risks and about the relations between their behaviors and the consequences likely to be associated with them.

- Helping individuals explore and resolve their ambivalences, assuring them that ambivalences are normal; expressing empathy. At the same time, pointing out discrepancies between their current behavior and what they say they would like to do.

- Respecting their frame of reference and helping them to chart a pathway of engagement in healthful eating that they can both endorse and apply.

- Minimizing control or pressure; rolling with the resistance.

- Emphasizing choice and providing a menu of effective options, including the option of not making a change.

Enhancing competence involves the following:

- Providing the food and nutrition-related knowledge and skills that they need to carry out the behaviors targeted by the intervention, which may involve specific foods and drinks such as vegetables or sweetened drinks, breastfeeding, parenting, or buying sustainably produced foods.

- Strategies to increase individual's sense of confidence or self-efficacy through mastery learning: demonstration and guided practice.

- Couching feedback for improvement in positive terms (as opposed to negative). For example, saying, "Very good, that's an excellent beginning! And I'm sure you can do even better in the future," rather than saying "Well, that's a start. Hopefully you can do a little better in the future."

- Providing opportunities for self-assessment, setting action goals, and monitoring progress towards achieving these action goals.

The overall result is that the individuals feel that they are capable of handling their situations, which could be managing their diabetes or being able to use appropriate parenting practices with their children.
Fostering a sense of relatedness involves:

- Expressing caring and concern for participants or audience
- Making the learning environment safe so participants feel secure in expressing their thoughts and feelings
- Stating personal experiences with the issue or behavior so that the audience feels a connection with you, the nutrition educator
- Encouraging interactive activities among participants that make them feel satisfaction in involvement with the others

Summary

The theories in this chapter provide us with tools to understand the motivations of our audiences in terms of dietary change. The theories also help us to design nutrition education activities to enhance motivation, promote active contemplation, and facilitate formation of intentions to take action. The theories were developed from research evidence and emphasize the importance of people's beliefs or convictions in motivating their behaviors.

THE HEALTH BELIEF MODEL

The health belief model proposes that when people experience a personal threat about a health condition they will likely take action, but only if the benefits of taking action outweigh the barriers—actual and psychological. Having the self-efficacy to take action is also crucial. Nutrition education activities make people aware of risks for health conditions, describe benefits of taking action, and provide opportunities to develop the self-confidence to take action.

THE THEORY OF PLANNED BEHAVIOR/REASONED ACTION APPROACH AND ITS EXTENSIONS

The theory of planned behavior or reasoned action approach states that people are likely to take action if they believe, expect, or are convinced the action will lead to the outcomes they desire—thus improving their attitudes if they feel the action is good, if other people they value think it is good idea, and if they feel they have some control over taking action. Their moral or personal norms as well as their self-identities are also important. Together, these create motivation to take action or change behavior. Developing specific implementation plans can help them translate intention to action.

The reasoned action approach provides us a particularly good tool for helping us develop motivational messages and activities, which are at the heart of nutrition education. Both group nutrition education and media communications are useful strategies to deliver effective messages. Media messages should be personally relevant to the intended audience, memorable, and easy to understand and process. Affect or feelings are particularly important in the case of food and eating. Thus, individuals should be provided with opportunities to taste and experience healthful foods and explore and understand their emotions with respect to food or being physically active. Nutrition educators can help individuals set specific plans to implement their intention to take action.

SELF-DETERMINATION THEORY

Self-determination theory also suggests that people's beliefs and experiences are motivators of behavior, in particular their need to believe in their competence, sense of autonomy, and relatedness to others. Activities that support these beliefs can enhance autonomous motivation. These activities include providing a good rationale for taking action, supporting people's sense of choice and control, and helping them feel understood and providing opportunities to relate to others.

OVERALL

The theories, taken together, emphasize the central role of people's beliefs or convictions for motivating people to take action as well as their affective attitudes or feelings about the action. Having some sense of control over the behavior and their ability/self-efficacy to take action is also important. Perceived social pressure can also influence people directly or indirectly. By addressing all these motivational determinants of behavior, nutrition education interventions can help to enhance motivation to change their behavior, activate decision making, and assist people to decide on intentions to act.

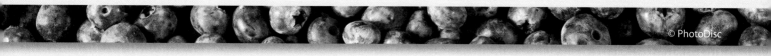

© PhotoDisc

Questions and Activities

1. A first crucial step in making diet-related behavior changes is becoming motivated. What does it mean to be motivated? What is the main educational goal of nutrition education in this first step? How can nutrition educators best achieve this goal?

2. Describe briefly what you think are the essential features of each of the following theories in terms of how they explain health motivations:
   a. The health belief model
   b. The theory of planned behavior: reasoned action approach
   c. Self-determination theory
   What do they have in common? Where do they differ? In what ways do they differ?

3. Find a friend or relative who *would like to change* an eating behavior and/or exercise more. Interview this person (take notes during the interview). Ask him or her to describe why he or she thinks the change is personally important and what is motivating the change.

   a. Decide if you think the theory of reasoned action or the health belief model better describes why your interviewee thinks the change is personally important. Briefly state why this theory is the better fit. Make a two-column table. In the first column put quotes from your interviewee. In the second column put the theory-based determinant (from your chosen theory) that fits the quote and state why this determinant fits the quote.

   b. Where do you think your interviewee is on the continuum of motivations from self-determination theory? Use what your interviewee said about *what is motivating the change* to justify his/her place on this continuum.

4. If you were asked to design media messages for a group of young people like Jason, whom you met in Box 4-3, what do you think would be one key message you would want to get across?

5. You have been asked to provide a nutrition education session with a group of young adults. Choose a behavior you will focus on. Plan the session using the health belief model by completing the diagram below:

Health belief model

If you selected the health belief model to plan a session or Intervention use this diagram to guide you. Choose ONE food-related behavior you want to focus on. In the boxes below fill in how you would operationalize each of the constructs for your target audience for your chosen behavior:

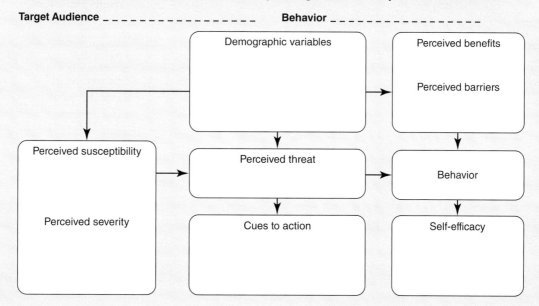

6. You have been asked to provide a nutrition education session with a group of young adults. Choose a behavior you will focus on. Plan the session using the theory of planned behavior/reasoned action approach by completing the diagram below:

Theory of Planned Behavior/Reasoned Action Approach

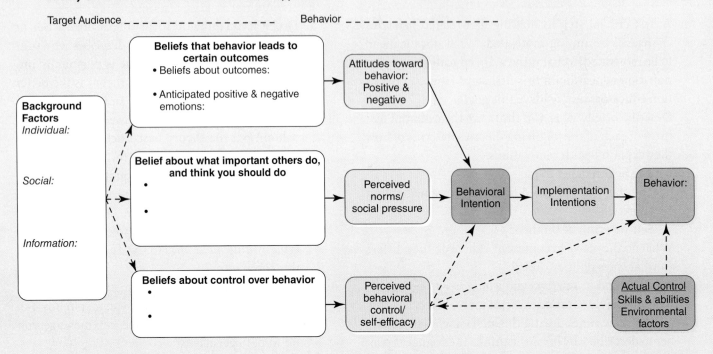

7. Describe three key strategies that nutrition educators can use to enhance movement toward autonomous motivation to eat more healthfully.

Self-Determination Theory

In order to develop an intervention for your group you are using the self-determination theory. Choose ONE of your food behaviors. In the boxes below please fill in how you move people along the motivation continuum.

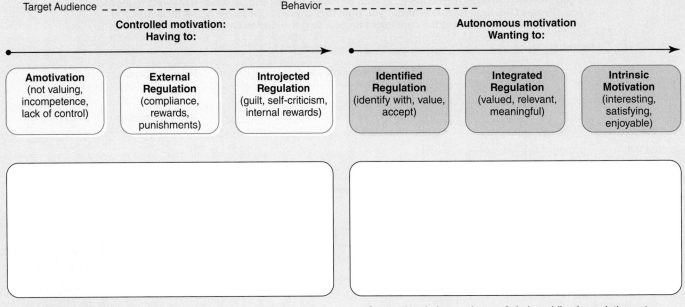

• Providing meaningful rationale for the behavior and acknowledging individuals' feelings so they feel understood

• Supporting their experience of choice while also pointing out discrepancies between current behavior and stated desires

References

Abraham, C., and P. Sheeran. 2000. Understanding and changing health behaviour: From health beliefs to self-regulation. In *Understanding and changing health behaviour from health beliefs to self-regulation*, edited by P. Norman, C. Abraham, and M. Conner. Amsterdam: Harwood Academic Publishers.

Abratt, R., and S. D. Goodey. 1990. Unplanned buying and in-store stimuli in supermarkets. *Managerial Decisions and Economics* 11:111–121.

Ajzen, I. 1998. Models of human social behaviour and their application to health psychology. *Psychology and Health* 13:735–739.

———. 2001. Nature and operation of attitudes. *Annual Review of Psychology* 52:27–58.

Andreasen, A. R. 1995. Marketing social change: Changing behavior to promote health, social development, and the environment. Washington, DC: Jossey-Bass.

Armitage, C. J. 2006. Evidence that implementation intentions promote transitions between the stages of change. *Journal of Consulting Clinical Psychology* 74(1):141–151.

Armitage, C. J., and M. Conner. 2000. Attitudinal ambivalence: A test of three key hypotheses. *Personality and Social Psychology Bulletin* 26(11):1421–1432.

———. 2001. Efficacy of the theory of planned behaviour: A meta-analytic review. *British Journal of Social Psychology* 40(Pt 4):471–499.

Bagozzi, R. P., H. Baumgartner, and R. Pieters. 1998. Goal-directed emotions. *Cognition & Emotion* 12(1):1–26.

Bagozzi, R. P., U. M. Dholokia, and S. Basuroy. 2003. How effortful decisions get enacted: The motivating role of decision processes, desires, and anticipated emotions. *Journal of Behavioral Decision Making* 16:273–295.

Bandura, A. 2000. Health promotion from the perspective of social cognitive theory. In *Understanding and changing health behavior: From health beliefs to self-regulation*, edited by P. Norman, C. Abraham, and M. Conner. Amsterdam: Harwood Academic Publishers.

Baranowski, T., A. Beltran, T. A. Chen, D. Thompson, T. O'Conner, S. Hughes, et al. 2013. Psychometric assessment of scales for a model of goal directed vegetable parenting practices. *International Journal of Behavioral Nutrition and Physical Activity* 10:110.

Bazillier, C., J. F. Verlhiac, P. Mallet, and J. Rousesse. 2011. Predictors of intention to eat healthy in 8-9-year-old children. *Journal of Cancer Education* 26(3):572–576.

Becker, M. H. 1974. The health belief model and personal health behavior. *In Health Education Monographs*. Thorofare, NJ: Charles B. Black

Bisogni, C. A., M. Connors, C. M. Devine, and J. Sobal. 2002. Who we are and how we eat: A qualitative study of identities in food choice. *Journal of Nutrition Education and Behavior* 34(3):128–139.

Bissonette, M. M., and I. R. Contento. 2001. Adolescents' perspectives and food choice behaviors in relation to the environmental impacts of food production practices. *Journal of Nutrition Education* 33:72–82.

Blanchard, C. M., J. Kupperman, P. B. Sparling, E. Nehl, R. E. Rhodes, K. S. Courneya, et al. 2009. Do ethnicity and gender matter when using the theory of planned behavior to understand fruit and vegetable consumption? *Appetite* 52(1):15–20.

Booth-Butterfield, S., and B. Reger. 2004. The message changes belief and the rest is theory: The "1% or less" milk campaign and reasoned action. *Preventive Medicine* 39(3):581–588.

Brug, J., E. de Vet, J. de Nooijer, and B. Verplanken. 2006. Predicting fruit consumption: Cognitions, intention, and habits. *Journal of Nutrition Education and Behavior* 38(2):73–81.

Chamberlain, S. P. (2005). Recognizing and responding to cultural differences in the education of culturally and linguistically diverse learners. *Intervention in School & Clinic* 40(4):195–211.

Cohen, D. A. 2008. Obesity and the built environment: Changes in environmental cues cause energy imbalances. *International Journal of Obesity* 32:S137–S142.

Conner, M., and P. Norman. 1995. Predicting health behavior. Buckingham, UK: Open University Press.

Contento I.R., P.A.Koch, H. Lee, and A. Calabrese-Barton. 2010. Adolescents demonstrate improvement in obesity risk behaviors following completion of *Choice, Control & Change*, a curriculum addressing personal agency and autonomous motivation. *Journal of the American Dietetic Association* 110:1830-1839.

Crum, A. J., W. R. Corbin, K. D. Brownell, and P. Salovey. 2011. Mind over milkshakes: Mindsets, not just nutrients, determine ghrelin response. *Health Psychology* 30(4): 424–429.

Deci, E. L., and R. M. Ryan. 1985. Intrinsic motivation and self-determination in human behavior. New York: Plenum.

———. 2000. The "what" and "why" of goal pursuits: Human needs and the self-determination of behavior. *Psychological Inquiry* 11(4):227–268.

———. 2008. Facilitating optimal motivation and psychological well-being across life's domains. *Canadian Psychology* 49:14–23.

Diaz, H., H. H. Marshak, S. Montgomery, B. Rea, and D. Backman. 2009. Acculturation and gender: Influence on healthy dietary outcomes for Latino adolescents. *Journal of Nutrition Education and Behavior* 41(5):319–326.

Discovery News. 2011. Americans falsely believe their diet is healthy. http://news.discovery.com/human/health/americans-diet-weight-110104.htm Accessed 12/5/14.

Dunn, K. I., P. B. Mohr, C. J. Wilson, and G. A. Wittert. 2008. Beliefs about fast food in Australia: A qualitative analysis. *Appetite* 51(2):331–334.

———. 2011. Determinants of fast-food consumption: An application of the Theory of Planned Behavior. *Appetite* 2011(2):349–357.

Fishbein, M. 2000. The role of theory in HIV prevention. *AIDS Care* 12(3):273–278.

Fishbein, M., and I. Ajzen. 1975. *Belief, attitude, intention and behavior: An introduction to theory and research.* Reading, MA: Addison-Wesley.

———. 2010. *Predicating and changing behavior: The reasoned action approach.* New York: Psychology Press.

Garcia, K., and T. Mann. 2003. From "I Wish" to "I Will": Social-cognitive predictors of behavioral intentions. *Journal of Health Psychology* 8(3):347–360.

Glanz, K., J. Brug, and P. van Assema. 1997. Are awareness of dietary fat intake and actual fat consumption associated?—a Dutch-American comparison. *European Journal of Clinical Nutrition* 51(8):542–547.

Godin, G., M. Conner, and P. Sheeran. 2005. Bridging the intention-behavior "gap": The role of moral norm. *British Journal of Social Psychology* 44(Pt 4):497–512.

Godin, G., and G. Kok. 1996. The theory of planned behavior: A review of its applications to health-related behaviors. *American Journal of Health Promotion* 11(2):87–98.

Gollwitzer, P. M. 1999. Implementation intentions: Strong effect of simple plans. *American Psychologist* 54(7):493–503.

Grieve, F. G., and M. W. Vander Weg. 2003. Desire to eat high-and low-fat foods following a low-fat dietary intervention. *Journal of Nutrition Education and Behavior* 35(2):98–102.

Hanson, J. A., and J. A. Benedict. 2002. Use of the Health Belief Model to examine older adults' food-handling behaviors. *Journal of Nutrition Education and Behavior* 34 (Suppl 1):S25–S30.

Hingle, M., A. Beltran, T. O'Connor, D. Thompson, J. Baranowski, and T. Baranowski. 2012. A model of goal directed vegetable parenting practices. *Appetite* 58: 444–449.

IFIC Foundation. 1999. Are you listening? What consumers tell us about dietary recommendations. *Food Insight: Current Topics in Food Safety and Nutrition.* Sept/Oct:1–6.

James, D. C. 2004. Factors influencing food choices, dietary intake, and nutrition-related attitudes among African Americans: Application of a culturally sensitive model. *Ethnicity and Health* 9(4):349–367.

James, D. C., J. W. Pobee, D. Oxidine, L. Brown, and G. Joshi. 2012. Using the health belief model to develop culturally appropriate weight-management materials for African-American women. *Journal of the Academy of Nutrition and Dietetics* 112(5):664–670.

Kahle, L. R. 1984. The values of Americans: Implications for consumer adaptation. In *Personal values and consumer psychology*, edited by R. E. Pitts Jr. and A. G. Woodside. Lexington, MA: Lexington Books.

Kassem, N. O., J. W. Lee, N. N. Modeste, and P. K. Johnston. 2003. Understanding soft drink consumption among female adolescents using the Theory of Planned Behavior. *Health Education Research* 18(3):278–291.

Kelley, K., and C. Abraham. 2004. RCT of a theory-based intervention promoting healthy eating and physical activity amongst out-patients older than 65 years. *Social Science and Medicine* 59(4):787–797.

Kremers, S. P., K. van der Horst, and J. Brug. 2007. Adolescent screen-viewing behavior is associated with consumption of sugar-sweetened beverages: The role of habit strength and perceived parental norms. *Appetite* 48(3):345–350.

Lautenschlager, L., and C. Smith. 2007. Understanding gardening and dietary habits among youth garden program participants using the Theory of Planned Behavior. *Appetite* 49(1):122–130.

Lawton, R., M. Conner, and R. McEachan. 2009. Desire or reason: Predicting health behaviors from affective and cognitive attitudes. *Health Psychology* 28(1):56–65.

Lawton, R., M. Conner, and D. Parker. 2007. Beyond cognition: Predicting health risk behaviors from instrumental and affective beliefs. *Health Psychology* 26(3):259–267.

Leventhal, H. 1973. Changing attitudes and habits to reduce risk factors in chronic disease. *American Journal of Cardiology* 31(5):571–580.

Lewin, K., T. Dembo, L. Festinger, and P. S. Sears. 1944. Level of aspiration. In *Personality and the behavior disorders*, edited by J. M. Hundt. New York: Roland Press.

Lien, N., L. A. Lytle, and K. A. Komro. 2002. Applying theory of planned behavior to fruit and vegetable consumption of young adolescents. *American Journal of Health Promotion* 16(4):189–197.

Liou, D., and I. R. Contento. 2001. Usefulness of psychosocial theory variables in explaining fat-related dietary behavior in Chinese Americans: Association with degree of acculturation. *Journal of Nutrition Education* 33(6):322–331.

McCarthy, P., and J. Tuttelman. 2005. Touching hearts to impact lives: Harnessing the power of emotion to change behaviors. *Journal of Nutrition Education and Behavior* 37 (Suppl 1):S19.

McClure, J. B. 2002. Are biomarkers useful treatment aids for promoting health behavior change? An empirical review. *American Journal of Preventive Medicine* 22(3):200–207.

Moller, A. C., E. L. Deci, and R. M. Ryan. 2006. Choice and ego-depletion: The moderating role of autonomy. *Perspectives of Social Psychology Bulletin* 32(8):1024–1036.

Moss, M. 2013. *Salt, fat, sugar.* New York: Random House.

Moule, J. 2012. *Cultural competence: A primer for educators.* Belmont, CA: Wadsworth/Cengage.

Norris, J. 2003. *From telling to teaching.* North Myrtle Beach, SC: Learning by Dialogue.

Pelican, S., F. Vanden Heede, B. Holmes, S. A. Moore, and D. Buchanan. 2005. Values, body weight, and well-being: the influence of the protestant ethic and consumerism on physical activity, eating, and body image. *International Quarterly of Community Health Education* 25(3): 239-270.

Perugini, M. and R. P. Bagozzi. 2001. The role of desires and anticipated emotions in goal-directed behaviors: Broadening and deepening the theory of planned behavior. *British Journal of Social Psychology* 40:79-98.

Peters, G-G. Y., R. A. C. Ruiter, and G. Kok. 2013. Threatening communication; A critical re-analysis and a revised meta-analytic test of fear appeal theory. *Health Psychology Review* 7(Suppl 1):S8-S31.

Petty, R. E., and T. Cacioppo. 1986. *Communication and persuasion: Central and peripheral routes to attitude change.* New York: Springer-Verlag.

Povey, R., B. Wellens, and M. Conner. 2001. Attitudes towards following meat, vegetarian and vegan diets: An examination of the role of ambivalence. *Appetite* 37(1): 15-26.

The power of others to shape our identity: Body image, physical abilities, and body weight. *Family and Consumer Sciences Research Journal* 34(1):57-80.

Raats, M. M., R. Shepherd, and P. Sparks. 1995. Including moral dimensions of choice within the structure of the theory of planned behavior. *Journal of Applied Social Psychology* 25:484-494.

Richard, R., J. van der Pligt, and N. K. de Vries. 1996. Anticipated affect and behavioral choice. *Basic and Applied Social Psychology* 18:111-129.

Robinson, R., and C. Smith. 2002. Psychosocial and demographic variables associated with consumer intention to purchase sustainably produced foods as defined by the Midwest Food Alliance. *Journal of Nutrition Education and Behavior* 34(6):316-325.

Roemmich, J. N., M. J. Lambiase, T. F. McCarthy, D. M. Feda, and K. F. Kozlowski. 2012. Autonomy supportive environments and mastery as basic factors to motivate physical activity in children: a controlled laboratory. *International Journal of Behavioral Nutrition and Physical Activity* 9:16.

Rokeach, M. 1973. *The nature of human values.* New York: Free Press.

Rollnick, S., W. R. Miller, and C. C. Butler. 2008. *Motivational interviewing in health care: Helping patients change behavior.* New York: Guilford Publications.

Rosenstock, I. M. 1974. Historical origins of the health belief model. *Health Education Monographs* 2:1-8.

Rozin, P., and A. E. Fallon. 1981. The acquisition of likes and dislikes for foods. In *Criteria of food acceptance: How man chooses what he eats*, edited by J. Solms and R. L. Hall. Zurich: Foster Lang.

Ryan, R. M., and E. L. Deci. 2000. Self-determination theory and the facilitation of intrinsic motivation, social development, and well-being. *American Psychologist* 55(1):68-78.

Ryan, R. M., H. Patrick, E. L. Deci, and G. C. Williams. 2008. Facilitating health behavior change and its maintenance: Interventions based on Self-Determination Theory. *European Health Psychologist* 10:1-4.

Salovey, P., and D. Birnbaum. 1989. Influence of mood on health-relevant cognitions. *Journal of Personality and Social Psychology* 57(3):539-551.

Salovey, P., T. R. Schneider, and A. M. Apanovitch. 1999. Persuasion for the purpose of cancer risk reduction: A discussion. *Journal of the National Cancer Institute Monographs* 25:119-122.

Sandberg, T., and M. Conner. 2008. Anticipated regret as an additional predictor in the theory of planned behavior: A meta-analysis. *British Journal of Social Psychology* 47:589-606.

Shafer, R. B., P. M. Keith, and E. Schafer. 1995. Predicting fat in diets of marital partners using the Health Belief Model. *Journal of Behavioral Medicine* 18:419-433.

Sheeran, P., P. Norman, and S. Orbell. 1999. Evidence that intentions based on attitudes better predict behaviour than intentions based on subjective norms. *European Journal of Social Psychology* 29:403-406.

Shim, Y., J. N. Variyam, and J. Blaylock. 2000. Many Americans falsely optimistic about their diets. *Food Review* 23(1):44-50.

Sigirci, O., K. M. Kniffin, and B. Wansink. 2014. Eating together: Men eat heavily in the company of women. *Journal of the Society for Nutrition Education and Behavior* 46(Suppl):S105.

Singh, A. S., A. Paw, M. J. Chin, J. Brug, and W. van Mechelen. 2007. Short-term effects of school-based weight gain prevention among adolescents. *Archives of Pediatric and Adolescent Medicine* 161(6):565-571.

Sparks, P. M. 2000. Subjective expected utility-based attitude-behavior models: The utility of self-identity. In *Attitudes, behavior, and social context: The role of norms and group membership*, edited by D. J. Terry and M. A. Hoggs. London: Lawrence Erlbaum.

Sparks, P., M. Conner, R. James, R. Shepherd, and R. Povey. 2001. Ambivalence about health-related behaviours: An exploration in the domain of food choice. *British Journal of Social Psychology* 6(Pt 1):53-68.

Sparks, P., R. Shepherd, and L. J. Frewer. 1995. Assessing and structuring attitudes toward the use of gene technology in food production: The role of perceived ethical obligation. *Basic and Applied Social Psychology* 163:267-285.

Spruijt-Metz, D. 1995. Personal incentives as determinants of adolescent health behavior: The meaning of behavior. *Health Education Research* 10(3):355-364.

Teixeira, P. J., E. V. Carraca, D. Markland, M. N. Silva, and R. M. Ryan. 2012. Exercise, physical activity, and self-determination theory: A systematic review. *International Journal of Behavioral Nutrition and Physical Activity* 9:78.

Triandis, H. C. 1979. Values, attitudes, and interpersonal behavior. In *Nebrask A symposium on motivation*, edited by H. E. How. Lincoln: University of Nebraska Press.

Verplanken, B., and S. Faes. 1999. Good intentions, bad habits, and effects of forming implementation intentions on healthy eating. *European Journal of Social Psychology* 29:591–604.

Wansink, B. 2006. *Mindless eating: Why we eat more than we think*. New York: Bantam Dell.

White, K. M., D. J. Terry, L. A. Rempel, and P. Norman. 2010. Predicting the consumption of foods low in saturated fats among people diagnosed with type 2 diabetes and cardiovascular disease. The role of planning in the theory of planned behavior. *Appetite* 55(2):348–354.

Williams, G. C., M. Lynch, and R. E. Glasgow. 2007. Computer-assisted intervention improves patient-centered diabetes care by increasing autonomy support. *Health Psychology* 26(6):728–734.

Williams-Pethota, P., A. Cox, S. N. Silvera, L. Moward, S. Garcia, N. Katulak, and P. Salovey. 2004. Casting messages in terms of responsibility for dietary change: Increasing fruit and vegetables consumption. *Journal of Nutrition Education and Behavior* 36(3):114–120.

Zoellner J., P. A. Estabrooks, B. M. Davy, Y. C. Chen, and W. You. 2012. Exploring the theory of planned behavior for sweetened beverage consumption. *Journal of Nutrition Education and Behavior* 44(2):172–177.

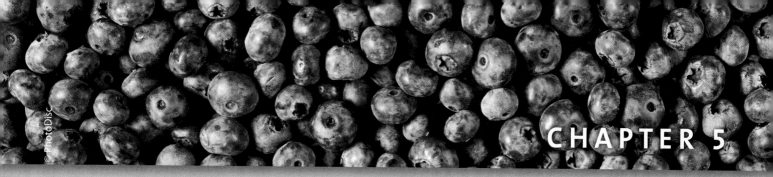

CHAPTER 5

Facilitating the Ability to Change Behavior and Take Action

OVERVIEW

This chapter describes several key theories that can serve as tools to help us facilitate the behavior change process within individuals. It also describes how each theory can be translated into successful nutrition education practice by providing real-world examples of nutrition education in action and illustrative case studies. It focuses on the key roles of food and nutrition knowledge and behavioral skills, and self-regulation or self-direction processes in building capacity in individuals and facilitating their ability to change behavior, emphasizing "how-to" take action. The description of each psychosocial theory is followed by how to use the theory as a tool in nutrition education.

CHAPTER OUTLINE

- Nutrition education to facilitate the ability to change behavior: focus on how to take action
- Understanding the determinants of action and behavior change strategies
- Social cognitive theory
- Using social cognitive theory in nutrition education to facilitate behavior change

- Self-regulation models: focus on planning and self-efficacy
- Grounded theory approach: personal food policies
- Transtheoretical model and the stages of change construct
- Using the transtheoretical model in nutrition education
- Summary

LEARNING OBJECTIVES

At the end of the chapter, you should be able to:

- Describe key theories of health behavior change, including social cognitive theory, self-regulation models such as the health action process model, and stage models such as the transtheoretical model
- State key concepts in these theories and describe their application to practice

- Demonstrate understanding of how theory and research have been used in interventions to assist people to take action and maintain change
- Describe nutrition education strategies to facilitate initiating and maintaining action or behavior change

Nutrition Education to Facilitate the Ability to Change Behavior: Focus on How to Take Action

To change a behavior or take action, individuals have to believe it is desirable, effective, and feasible; fits their values and culture; and is what they feel they want to do in the context of their life situations. Enhancing this process is the first function of nutrition education and is described in Chapter 4. However, translating desires and intentions into action is not always easy. We all know this from our own experience of making resolutions at New Year's or on our birthdays or some other landmark occasion. Following through on our resolutions is often the hard part. Our case example, Ray, knows he needs to lose some weight and watch what he eats if he is to avoid getting diabetes. He makes a resolution to do so each birthday. Within days, he has forgotten about his resolution. It is particularly difficult when we wish to help our entire family make some healthy changes.

BRIDGING THE INTENTION–ACTION GAP: NUTRITION EDUCATORS AS COACHES

How can we, as nutrition educators, help individuals and families bridge the intention–behavior gap? How do we help them move from motivation to action, from intention to reality, from thinking to doing?

Evidence suggests that one of the most effective ways for people to change their behaviors or take action on their motivations and intentions is to make specific plans to do so. These plans are often referred to as *action plans* or *action goals*. To carry out action plans or goals, individuals need specific knowledge and skills and they need environments that are supportive.

Nutrition educators can act as coaches to assist individuals and families to make action plans and carry them out by helping to build their abilities and skills, made easily accessible in useful formats. These activities are the subject of this chapter. We can also help make the environment more supportive of the change they seek. Such activities are the subject of the next chapter.

Understanding the Determinants of Action and Behavior Change Strategies

What useful tools can theory provide nutrition educators to assist individuals and groups to translate their intentions into action?

Beliefs, feelings, and motivations predominate when people are thinking about or contemplating taking action or changing their behavior. However, to move from contemplation and intention to behavior change, people need to be able to set specific action goals or plans to carry out their motivations. They also need the relevant food- and nutrition-specific knowledge and skills. The most useful tools come from **social cognitive theory (SCT)** (Bandura 1986, 1997, 2001), *models of self-regulation* (by which psychologists mean our skills in being able to think through, make conscious choices about what to do, and hence direct or "regulate" our own behavior) (Bagozzi 1992; Gollwitzer 1999, Schwarzer and Fuchs 1995; Sniehotta, Scholz, and Schwarzer 2005), and the *transtheoretical or stages of change model* (Prochaska and DiClemente 1984). These theories and models identify determinants that increase motivation for health behaviors, as do the theories described in Chapter 4. However, in addition, these theories provide us with guidance on ways to facilitate people's ability to take action and make changes in their behavior. These key theories are described here.

Social Cognitive Theory

Social cognitive theory, as proposed and developed by Bandura (1977, 1986, 1989, 1997, 2001, 2004) to analyze and understand human thought, motivation, and action in general, has become the most widely used theory for designing nutrition education and health promotion programs. In addition to providing a unified and comprehensive framework for understanding the determinants of behaviors, it describes potential procedures for behavioral change that nutrition educators can use to design activities to assist and empower people to take action.

Social cognitive theory proposes that personal, behavioral, and environmental determinants work in a dynamic and reciprocal fashion to influence health behavior. *Personal determinants* involve people's thoughts or beliefs and their feelings. *Behavioral determinants* include their food-, nutrition-, and health-related facilitating knowledge and skills, together called **behavioral capability**, and their skills in regulating, directing, and taking charge of their own behaviors, called self-regulation skills. *Environmental determinants* include those factors external to individuals, such as the physical and social environments.

In its simplest terms, social cognitive theory proposes that behavior is the result of personal, behavioral, and environmental factors that influence each other in a dynamic and reciprocal fashion. Individuals' personal beliefs and feelings influence their behaviors. Environments also shape individuals' behaviors, but at the same time, individuals have agency—the capacity to exert influence over the environment as well as over their own behaviors through their self-regulation or self-direction skills. The theory helps nutrition educators to design strategies that address people's beliefs and feelings, help empower people to make changes through knowledge and **action goal setting** skills, and increase environmental supports for action.

The relationships of these determinants to each other and to behavior are shown in **FIGURE 5-1**. The determinants on the left in the figure are the various personal determinants of behavior (described later). The many arrows that go in both directions illustrate how these personal determinants of behavior are reciprocally related to behavior, as shown in the middle of the figure, and to environment. The consequences of the behavior provide a feedback loop to influence thoughts and abilities, which will in turn influence future behavior.

Recall that determinants of behavior change are given specific names by health psychologists, such as **outcome expectations** or *behavioral capability*. These can be seen as labels placed on a series of buckets: what exactly is in the buckets—their content—comes from your interviews with your audience or information from the literature or surveys about groups that are similar.

TABLE 5-1 provides a summary of the determinants of behavior change according to social cognitive theory and how they can be used in the design of nutrition education. Recall, too, that determinants are called *theory constructs* when they are in a theory.

PERSONAL DETERMINANTS: A FOCUS ON HUMAN AGENCY AND EMPOWERMENT

According to social cognitive theory, our behavior is influenced by a host of thoughts or beliefs about ourselves. The theory gives special emphasis to our ability to think and plan ahead, to be reflective about our own abilities and actions, as well as the meaning and purposes of our life pursuits. We are thus capable of intentional or purposive action. Although future events cannot serve as determinants of current behavior, their cognitive representations in the present through our symbolic capability can have a strong motivating impact on current behavior. Among the many person-related factors, two major determinants that are important in motivating behavior are outcome expectations and **self-efficacy** (see Figure 5-1).

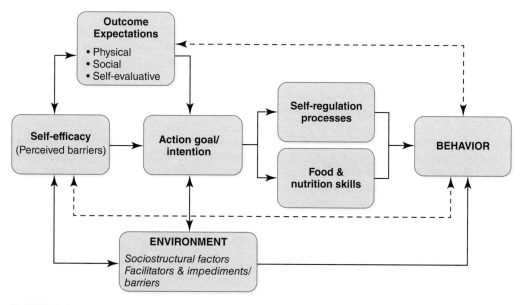

FIGURE 5-1 Social cognitive theory.

Data from Bandura, A. 2004. Health promotion by social cognitive means. *Health Education and Behavior* 31(2):143–164.

Table 5-1 Social Cognitive Theory: Major Constructs and Use in Nutrition Education Interventions

Theory Construct (Determinant of Behavior Change)	Definition	Use in Nutrition Education
Individual Factors		
Outcome expectations (physical or material), positive and negative	What individuals believe or expect will happen to them physically (e.g., health) if they make a behavior change	Provide activities to enhance awareness of negative outcomes of current behavior such as risk of disease (perceived threat); or enhance the importance of positive outcomes (perceived benefits) of taking action, for example, through messages about the positive effect of F&V on cancer risk reduction.
Outcome expectations (social)	What individuals believe or expect will happen to them socially if they make a behavior change	Design messages and activities to make eating appropriate portions and healthy eating the social norm (e.g., make eating F&V cool for teens; show breastfeeding moms similar to audience).
Outcome expectations (self-evaluative)	What individuals believe or expect they will feel about themselves if they make a behavior change	Emphasize self-satisfaction and self-worth from behavior (e.g., "When I eat local F&V, I am being good to the environment by reducing my carbon footprint").
Expectancies	The values individuals place on these physical, social, and self-evaluative outcomes	Discuss social impact and media influence on behavior to help individuals examine how much they value these outcomes.
Barriers or impediments	Include the *perceptions* of *personal* barriers or challenges to taking action (which are integral to self-efficacy assessments) and actual *environmental* barriers (which reside in socio-structural factors)	Help individuals identify their *perceived barriers* that impede their ability to take health actions, and empower them through knowledge and skills by making the actions easy to understand and do. For *environmental barriers*, assist group to develop collective efficacy to take collective action; work with policymakers and decision-makers to create supportive environments.
Self-efficacy	Individuals' confidence in their personal ability to perform the given behavior	Assist individuals to achieve success by delivering clear, targeted messages and planning changes in small steps. Create modeling and mastery experiences about food and nutrition (e.g., label reading, cooking, gardening, advocacy). Provide feedback and encouragement. Alleviate concerns about responses to the new food or behavior.
Behavioral capability/capacity	Individuals' food- and nutrition-related knowledge and cognitive, affective, and behavioral skills needed to enact the behavior	Provide necessary *knowledge and cognitive skills* for taking action through presentations, handouts, demonstrations, videos, and other channels, as well as discussions and debates to develop critical thinking skills. Also build *affective skills*, such as handling stressful situations, and *behavioral skills,* such as food purchasing and storage, cooking skills, safe food handling and preparation behaviors, and growing vegetables. Use a repeated, multimedia approach to reinforce skills.
Self-regulation/self-direction skills	The ability to direct their own actions or behaviors through conscious, intentional choices; involves skills in being able to create appropriate action plans and to follow through with them	Provide instruction and practice opportunities for individuals to develop skills in consciously choosing behaviors to act on: assessing their values and current behaviors, setting action goals or plans, monitoring self in attaining goals, self-rewards, and problem solving. Emotional coping and stress-management skills are also included as are ways to enlist social support.
Environmental Factors		
Observational learning/ modeling	Learning to perform a behavior through observing someone modeling the behavior and the consequences of that behavior	Use credible, recognizable, or relatable role models. Conduct food demonstrations relating to the target behavior, such as making a whole grain recipe. Provide opportunities for the group to practice the recipe, with guidance, to enhance mastery.
Reinforcement	Responses to individuals' behavior that increase or decrease the likelihood of its occurrence	Provide external reinforcement in the form of rewards or incentives, such as T-shirts, key chains, and raffle tickets for goal attainment. Provide opportunities to develop internal or self-reinforcement for own accomplishments.

Beliefs About Outcomes of Behavior Change (Outcome Expectations)

Social cognitive theory posits that much of our behavior is regulated or directed by our beliefs about anticipated outcomes from engaging in a specific behavior or pattern of behavior and the degree to which we value these outcomes. For example, a mother will breastfeed her baby if she believes that breastfeeding will make her baby healthy and she wants her baby to be healthy. As such, *outcome expectations* are similar to *beliefs about outcomes* of behavior in the theory of planned behavior and to **perceived benefits** of behavior in the health belief model. Outcome *expectancies* are the values people place on these outcomes (e.g., moderately valued or highly valued) and are also called incentives by Bandura (1986).

Social cognitive theory states that we will choose to perform an action that maximizes the anticipated positive outcomes and minimizes the anticipated negative outcomes. Beliefs about the outcomes of behavior or *outcome expectations* can take three forms:

- *Physical outcomes*: These are the perceived physical and health effects that accompany the behavior. According to Bandura (2004), *negative* physical outcomes include **perceived risk** of disease from not engaging in healthy behaviors, similar to the perceived threat in the health belief model. *Positive* outcomes are similar to perceived benefits in other theories.
- *Social outcomes*: These are the perceived social consequences of the behavior. Behaviors that fulfill social norms bring positive reactions, such as soda drinking for teenagers, whereas outcomes that violate social norms bring social censure, such as breastfeeding in public in cultures where this is not the norm.
- *Self-evaluative outcomes*: These are the positive and negative reactions we have to our own behaviors. We engage in behaviors that bring satisfaction and a sense of self-worth, for example, success in breastfeeding, being a good parent, or in being able to walk an hour a day. We avoid behaviors that lead to dissatisfaction, for example, because a given action "will make me feel I am not taking good care of my family." Bandura (2004) believes that self-satisfaction for personal accomplishments is a powerful motivator of behavior, often more important than tangible rewards.

Self-Efficacy

Although our beliefs about health outcomes or risks of a behavior are a precondition for change, we need a sense of self-efficacy to overcome barriers or impediments to adopting and maintaining healthy behaviors (Bandura 1989, 2004). Self-efficacy is the confidence we have that we can carry out the intended behavior successfully or overcome barriers to engaging in the behavior. Self-efficacy involves both the skills and the confidence that we can effectively and consistently use these skills. Extensive research indicates that the higher the level of perceived self-efficacy, the more effort we will expend and the longer we will persist in a newly learned behavior, especially in the face of difficulties. Indeed, self-efficacy is considered to be the major motivator of changing behavior as well as a facilitator of action. See **BOX 5-1** for strategies to enhance self-efficacy in individuals.

Self-efficacy tends to be specific for a given behavior. For example, an individual may have confidence that he or she can prepare a simple healthful meal for the family, but not run 3 miles a day. The concept of self-efficacy has been incorporated into recent versions of other theories such as the health belief model, the theory of planned behavior/reasoned action approach, and the **transtheoretical model (TMM)** as applied to the area of diet and health.

Taking Charge of Our Lives: Personal Agency and Empowerment

Social cognitive theory posits that not only can we develop self-efficacy for individual behaviors, but we can see ourselves as agents who are able to take charge of our lives. This notion of **personal agency** or *sense of empowerment* can be defined as a strong sense of our ability to consciously choose to exercise influence over our own thoughts, feelings, and behaviors and over environmental conditions that affect our lives, in order to produce effects we desire (Bandura 1989, 2001). Unless we believe that we can achieve desired outcomes through our own actions, we have little incentive to take action. Such a sense of personal agency is based on learning a set of skills, not willpower.

Bandura (1989) points out that a robust sense of personal agency and the ability to recover quickly from difficulties and setbacks help people succeed in their endeavors. For example, James Joyce's book *The Dubliners*

BOX 5-1 Methods for Enhancing Self-Efficacy

We can help to strengthen the self-efficacy of our audiences by these strategies:

1. *Personal mastery experiences*: Practice is the most effective way of creating a strong sense of personal efficacy. We can provide guided practice in order to help individuals master the behavior through setting and achieving increasingly challenging action goals.

2. *Social modeling*: We can show our audiences that others similar to themselves have succeeded in the behavior. For example, the nutrition educator can show films of similar moms successfully breastfeeding, or demonstrate the steps involved in cooking a healthy dish.

3. *Social persuasion*: Providing (realistic) encouragement can help people overcome self-doubts. We can also help people measure success against their own improvement, not against what others are doing.

4. *Modification of emotional or physical responses to the behavior*: People rely partly on information from their physiological states to judge their own abilities. This can be misleading. For example, people often have a negative physiological reaction to eating high fiber foods and give up trying. We can assure them that this is normal and that the reaction will diminish with time.

Adapted from Bandura, A. 1997. *Self-efficacy: The exercise of control.* New York: WH Freeman.

---

was rejected by 22 publishers, and a manuscript by E. E. Cummings was rejected 12 times, but each author kept sending them in for consideration. They are now both considered major literary works.

Collective Efficacy

Social cognitive theory extends the notion of self-efficacy to collective efficacy, which emphasizes the human capacity for collective action. Collective efficacy is the ability of individuals to work in a group to bring about changes in environments, including social structures and policy, to benefit the entire group (Bandura 1997). It can result in collective agency or empowerment. This construct is described in detail in Chapter 6.

Impediments or Barriers

Some barriers are personal, including our judgments of our self-efficacy—or lack thereof—to surmount obstacles (see Figure 5-1). According to Bandura (2004), assessing our barriers is part of our assessment of self-efficacy because this process allows us to judge whether we will be able to carry out a behavior even under difficult circumstances, such as cooking a healthy meal when we are tired from a day at work or have several children clamoring for something quick to eat. Some impediments are external, or reside in the environment, such as lack of availability

or accessibility of healthful foods or venues for physical activity and lack of health resources.

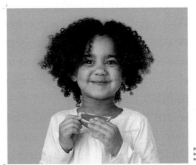
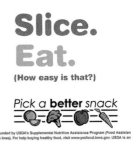

Overcoming barriers: making the action easy.
Courtesy of Iowa Department of Public Health.

Goals and Goal Intentions

Goals can refer to values that serve an orienting function for the long term, such as being healthy, living an ethical life, and so forth. These are extremely important because they represent the internal standards or values we develop from a variety of sources, against which we can judge our current behaviors. These provide context but may be too broad to guide changes in the specific behaviors or actions we wish to undertake.

Goals also can refer to immediate goals that contribute to our long-term goals but are actionable. In this

Wash. Bite.

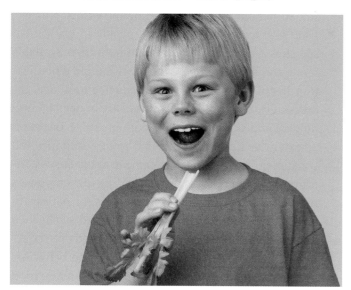

(How easy is that?)

When they come home hungry,
have fruits and veggies ready to eat.

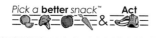

Funded by USDA's Supplemental Nutrition Assistance Program, an equal opportunity provider and employer. In addition, this institution works with the Iowa Department of Public Health. Iowa Food Assistance can help you buy healthy food. Visit www.yesfood.iowa.gov for more information.

Overcoming barriers: making the action easy.

Courtesy of Iowa Department of Public Health.

text, we call these *action goals*. They are similar to the *implementation intentions* of the theory of planned behavior. In the context of a behavior change process, action goals represent a commitment to take action. This commitment comes about when our outcome expectations are positive (perceived benefits) and self-efficacy is high.

Reinforcements

Reinforcements are the responses to a person's behavior that increase or decrease the likelihood of occurrence of that behavior. We are providing external reinforcement when we use an action or item that is known to have reinforcement value for the individual or group, such as gold stickers for children completing a task in school or T-shirts, certificates, or other rewards for completing a health program. Internal reinforcement is individuals' own perceptions that the behavior had some value for them that will encourage them to do the action again.

Relapse Prevention

Relapse prevention focuses on strategies used to maintain the new behaviors. These strategies include *cognitive restructuring*, which involves substituting alternative positive thoughts for negative, dysfunctional, or distorted thoughts about healthful eating behaviors ("I am a bad person because I ate that chocolate cake"), *controlling the environment* by removing or avoiding *cues* to less healthful eating (such as avoiding stocking the household pantry with sweets), and adding cues for more healthful eating (such as leaving washed fruit out on the counter at home).

BEHAVIOR-RELATED DETERMINANTS

Behavioral factors include *food- and nutrition-related* knowledge and skills needed to engage in the behavior, and *self-regulation/self-direction* skills—the ability to exercise influence over our own behavior through our conscious choices and actions.

Behavioral Capabilities: Food and Nutrition Knowledge to Facilitate Change

Behavioral capabilities are the food- and nutrition-related knowledge and skills that individuals need to carry out the behavioral action goals that they have selected. Here, knowledge is of the functional or *how-to* kind:

- *Factual knowledge*: **Factual knowledge** includes food and nutrition information and how to use it, such as information about nutrients and food sources, MyPlate eating patterns, or the Dietary Guidelines messages *and* relatively simple skills such as how to read food labels. The information must be specific to the behavior that has been chosen if it is to be helpful to the individuals or families attempting to carry out the behavior.
- *Nutrition literacy*: Nutrition literacy is similar to factual knowledge and is defined as the degree to which people have the capacity to obtain, process, and understand the basic health (nutrition) information and services they need to make appropriate health (nutrition) decisions (Osborne 2005; Zoellner et al. 2011; Carbone and Zoellner 2012). Nutrition literacy is particularly important for the low-literacy audiences with whom many of us work as they need the most help understanding basic food and nutrition guidance information (Silk et al. 2008; Zoellner et al. 2009). It is also very important for those with nutrition-related health

conditions who need to understand instructions in order to manage their conditions (Institute of Medicine 2004). It is consequently important for nutrition educators to use the appropriate literacy level, plain language, and graphics with low-literacy audiences to ensure understanding. Such communication issues are discussed in detail in Chapters 16 and 17.

■ *Procedural knowledge:* **Procedural knowledge** is the knowledge about *how* to do something, or decision rules for solving given cognitive tasks. Included are relatively simple skills such as how to read a recipe, or more complex tasks such as how to breast-feed. Through the acquisition of such knowledge, people develop *knowledge structures* or *schemas*—personal conceptual frameworks, if you will—for given areas of information.

■ *Critical thinking and problem-solving skills:* **Critical thinking skills** involve the integration of the higher order thinking skills of analysis, evaluation, and synthesis. It includes problem-solving skills for decision-making. Such skills are needed in many everyday situations people face such as making choices about what foods to prepare for the family, selecting the best parenting practices for their children, or managing food budgets. Food choice criteria have also become more complex, involving not only health concerns, but also, for many people, concerns about the ecological consequences of consumption (e.g., conventional, organic, local), moral/ethical concerns (to eat meat or not), social justice concerns (e.g., who produced the food, under what working conditions), and food safety concerns. Thus, people need critical thinking skills to make informed trade-offs between criteria in making food choices.

Behavioral Capabilities: Behavioral Skills Related to Food and Nutrition

■ *Behavioral skills:* Additional mechanisms are needed to get from knowledge structures to skilled action. Learning by doing (or "enactive learning") is the translating vehicle, according to Bandura (1986). People develop behavioral skills through performing the behaviors and practicing them, such as preparing healthful snacks, cooking plant-based recipes, practicing safe food handling behaviors, breastfeeding, or practicing appropriate food-related parenting skills. Nutrition educators can facilitate the acquisition of such skills

by first demonstrating the skills and then providing the opportunity for individuals to practice them. This is sometimes referred to as modeling and guided practice.

■ *Food literacy and skills:* While people in traditional societies are very knowledgeable about their available foods and how to prepare them, with rapid globalization in this fast food and convenience food age, increasingly, many people of all ages are in need of food literacy and skills (Fordyce-Voorham 2011). Based on an extensive study, international home economics and consumer science educators came to a consensus definition: "Food literacy is the scaffolding that empowers individuals, households, communities, or nations to protect diet quality through change and strengthen dietary resilience over time. It is composed of a collection of inter-related knowledge, skills, and behaviors required to plan, manage, select, prepare, and eat food to meet needs and determine intake. At its simplest, food literacy can be interpreted as the tools needed for a healthy lifelong relationship with food" (Vidgen and Gallegos 2014, p. 54). Given how important it is for the world's food systems to remain sustainable, any definition of food literacy additionally needs to include an understanding of the complex systems that produce, process, transport, and market food and how these systems impact health, ecological sustainability, social justice, the economy, and the ability to use this understanding to make informed choices that support people's health, communities, and the environment.

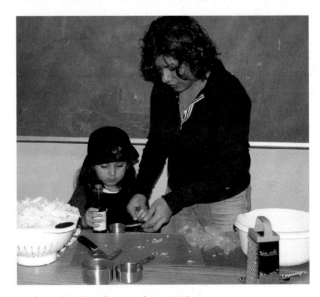

A mom helps her daughter cook at a WIC center.
Courtesy of USDA.

Self-Regulation and Action Goal Setting Skills

Self-regulation is the term that psychologists use to describe the process through which individuals develop the ability and are empowered to think through and make conscious choices about what they want to do and thus direct their own actions through their own efforts. This process is often referred to as *self-control*. However, what is meant by the term is the ability to take control or make voluntary decisions and choices about one's actions and so *self-direction* is a more accurate term.

Self-regulation is not achieved through willpower but by learning a set of skills, in particular, what are called *action goal setting skills* by health psychologists (Bandura 1986; Cullen, Baranowski, and Smith 2001; Shilts, Horowitz, and Townsend 2004a, 2004b, 2009). Action goal setting skills involve being able to create specific action plans and to follow through with them. Consequently, we call this process *action goal setting*. Individuals then learn the food and nutrition-related knowledge and skills to carry out the behaviors stated in the action plans.

Why setting action goals is important. Setting action goals (also referred to as *action plans*) increases our motivation to act because it signals that we have made a specific commitment to take action, cultivates our intrinsic interest because we are actively involved in the process, builds our perceptions of our self-efficacy and mastery, and creates self-satisfaction and a sense of fulfillment from having achieved the goals. It also reduces stress and effort because it involves planning ahead so that we will not need to make a new decision in each new situation (Gollwitzer 1999). Chapter 12 describes in detail how to set action goals that are *Specific, Measurable, Achievable, Realistic,* and *Time-bound* or SMART.

ENVIRONMENTAL FACTORS

Social cognitive theory distinguishes between situation, which is people's perception or cognitive representation of the environment, and environment, which relates to the objective factors affecting their behavior that are external to them.

Influences of the Environment on Behavior

Numerous environmental factors influence behavior, as we saw in Chapter 2. Many physical and sociostructural environments have an impact on us whether we like it or not. Examples are the physical availability of specific healthy

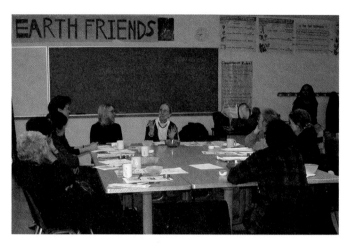

Learning to set action plans for healthy living.
Courtesy of Fredi Kronenberg.

foods at the workplace or in the local corner store, and the social environment, such as whether family or friends eat fruits and vegetables.

People's Influences on the Environment

At the same time, we can control how we *react* to environments, *act within* them, or work to *change* them. For example, we might influence what the family purchases or advocate for policies within workplaces or schools to improve nutrition at the site. We might advocate for legislators to enact policies to improve the built environment, such as more supermarkets in low-income neighborhoods or food deserts or more walkable streets. Because we are constantly interacting with our environments—choosing how to interpret and react to them, negotiating with them, or changing them—we influence our environments even as our environments influence us. Nutrition educators thus seek to work with policymakers and others to create environments that are supportive. How to do so is described in more detail in Chapter 6.

Observational Learning from the Environment

The environment is also the source for modeling of behaviors. Trial-and-error learning from experiences—that is, feedback from the consequences of our own behavior—is one source of learning. However, we also learn by observing the behavior of others and the consequences that follow from their behavior, whether or not we are conscious of it. Such **observational learning** is a very important construct in social cognitive theory. For example, children, who are trying to figure out the world, learn from

---

NUTRITION EDUCATION IN ACTION 5-1 Using Social Cognitive Theory to Promote Stair Use: Modeling

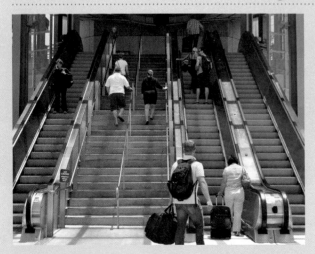

Courtesy of Marc Adams.

An Active Living Research program study examined the effect of natural models (i.e., passersby) and experimental models (i.e., research confederates) on stair use in the

San Diego airport. Researchers videotaped and coded the behavior of over 15,000 people when confronted with the choice to take the escalator or stairs when ascending or descending during busy times at the airport. Stair use was observed without manipulating the environment, with (a) research confederates acting as models, and (b) a pair of research confederates acting as models while verbalizing their choice to take the stairs. The researchers considered demographic factors, including gender; youth, adult, or senior status; and race, as well as amount of luggage, type of shoes and dress, presence of children, and presence of a social group.

Regardless of whether a model was part of the research staff, stair use increased in the presence of models. Men who observed a model on the stairs were up to 3 times more likely to use the stairs, and women who observed a model on the stairs were up to 2.5 times more likely to use the stairs.

Source: Adams, M. A., M. F. Hovell, V. Irvin, J. F. Sallis, K. J. Coleman, and S. Liles. 2006. Promoting stair use by modeling: An experimental application of the behavioral ecological model. *American Journal of Health Promotion* 21(2):110–118.

---

observing their parents. Teenagers learn from observing the food-related behaviors of their peers, valued adults, and relevant celebrities and public figures. Nutrition educators can use modeling as a strategy by pointing to positive role models for the behavior or by demonstrating food-related skills, such as in cooking.

EVIDENCE FROM RESEARCH AND INTERVENTION STUDIES

Numerous intervention studies in the domain of food and diet have been conducted using social cognitive theory, although the full model is not usually used in most studies. A few studies are described here to illustrate the theory.

Questionnaire study.

- *Questionnaire study with adolescents:* Theory can be used as the basis of questions in open-ended interviews or in questionnaires. **TABLE 5-2** gives an example of how social cognitive theory was used to construct questions to determine the influences on fruit and vegetable consumption by low-income black American adolescents (Molaison et al. 2005).

Studies with children.

- The *Coordinated Approach to Child Health (CATCH)* program is a school-wide comprehensive program consisting of curriculum for grades K–5 based on social cognitive theory and environmental supportive components involving physical education, school meals, and family engagement (Luepker et al. 1996; Hoelscher et al. 2010). Many studies have been conducted on the CATCH program over the years with recent versions of CATCH now focusing on reducing obesity risk through increasing consumption of fruits and vegetables and physical activity and decreasing consumption of sweetened beverages and sedentary behaviors (Coleman et al. 2005; Hoelscher et al. 2010). The results have been positive for some behaviors and weight.
- *Choice, Control, and Change* was an obesity prevention program for middle school students that focused on fostering personal agency by using an inquiry-based science education to address outcome expectations or why-to take action, and goal setting and self-regulation skills for how-to take

Table 5-2 Using Social Cognitive Theory to Guide Questions About Influences on Fruit and Vegetable Consumption in a Sample of Low-Income Black American Adolescents

Open-Ended Questions	Social Cognitive Theory Construct
Environment	
If you looked in the refrigerator or the kitchen cabinet of your home right now, what kinds of fruits (vegetables) would you find?	Environmental
Do you ever eat fruits (vegetables) away from home? What are some other places that you eat fruit (vegetables)?	Environmental
Behavioral skills	
Do you help prepare the meals and snacks in your home? What kinds?	Behavior
Personal beliefs	
What do you think would happen if you don't eat fruits (vegetables)?	Outcome expectancies
What would make you want to eat more fruits (vegetables)?	Outcome expectancies
If you wanted to eat more fruits or vegetables, would you be able to? Why or why not? How would you get them?	Self-efficacy
Family and friends	
Do you think your friends (family members) would help you eat more fruits and vegetables?	Social support
What would you do if no one is eating fruits (vegetables), but you would like to eat fruits (vegetables)?	Social expectations
What are some reasons you and your friends eat fruits (vegetables)?	Social expectations

Data from Molaison, E. F., C. L. Connell, J. E. Stuff, M. K. Yadrick, and M. Bogle. 2005. Influences on fruit and vegetable consumption by low-income black American adolescents. *Journal of Nutrition Education and Behavior* 37(5):246–251. Used with permission of the Society for Nutrition Education.

action. It involved a randomized controlled study of 10 schools from low-income, minority neighborhoods in New York City. An evaluation found that students in intervention schools compared to the control schools reported consumption of significantly fewer sweetened drinks and packaged snacks, smaller sizes of fast food, increased intentional walking, and decreased leisure screen time, although it found no increases in their intakes of vegetables or water. They showed significant increases in positive outcome expectations about the behaviors, self-efficacy, goal intentions, competence, and autonomy (Contento et al. 2007, 2010). See Nutrition Education in Action 12-2 in Chapter 12 for further details.

- *EatFit*, an intervention with middle school students, was directed at both dietary and physical activity behaviors (Horowitz, Shilts, and Townsend 2004). It was found that adding a guided goal setting component to the intervention improved students' dietary behavior, physical activity behavior, and physical activity self-efficacy compared with the same intervention without goal setting (Shilts et al. 2009). See **NUTRITION EDUCATION IN ACTION 5-2.**

- *A review of eight studies on increasing fruit and vegetable intake in children* found the following to be important for success: a supportive environment, building behavioral skills or capacity, helping youth evaluate social and media influences, and role modeling by peers and parents and by recognizable or relatable characters in comic books, videos, or social media (Gaines and Turner 2009).

Studies with adults.

- *ALIVE* is a randomized control study using email to reach employees with a 16-week program involving individually tailored, small-step goals; a personal homepage with tips; educational materials; and tracking and simulation tools. Results showed increases in moderate and vigorous physical activity, walking, and in fruit and vegetable intake, and decreases in saturated fat intake (Sternfeld et al. 2009).

- *A community-based diabetes education program* resulted in positive impacts on knowledge, health beliefs, and the self-reported behaviors of using herbs in place of salt, cooking with olive or canola oil, and

NUTRITION EDUCATION IN ACTION 5-2 EatFit: A Goal-Oriented Intervention that Challenges Adolescents to Improve Their Eating and Fitness Choices

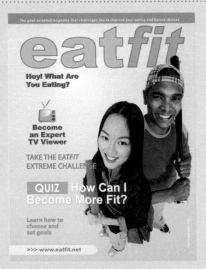

Courtesy of Marilyn S. Townsend.

Surveys show that the diets of youth do not meet those recommended by the Dietary Guidelines, and neither do youth engage in recommended amounts of physical activity. This program was designed to improve the dietary and physical activity behaviors of middle school students. It consisted of a classroom curriculum for the teacher or leader, a workbook for each student, a Web-based interactive program in which students received personalized assessment based on a 24-hour diet record that they completed, personalized dietary feedback,

goal setting, and a contract. The program was based on social cognitive theory:

Outcome expectancies. Motivators identified from focus groups were as follows: improved appearance, increased energy, and increased independence. These were used in the lessons.

Self-efficacy. Students were provided opportunity to practice skills (recipe preparation and tasting, physical activities), receive encouragement, and develop social support among the group.

Self-Regulation

- Self-monitoring of their own diets and physical activity patterns
- Setting goals
- Monitoring their progress toward the goals
- Problem-solving activities to overcome perceived barriers (e.g., how to select fast foods that support their goals)
- Rewards or positive reinforcements for attaining goals

Details of how the food choice determinants or theory constructs were operationalized in the program are shown in the following table.

Examples of Use of Social Cognitive Theory in EatFit	
Theory Construct/Strategy	**Theory-Based Activities**
Self-efficacy/skills mastery	Students increase their self-efficacy in choosing foods that meet their selected dietary goals. They learn how to read food labels and practice those skills by answering questions on dozens of foods that are specific to their goals.
Modeling	Students interview a parent or guardian about their goal setting experiences.
Barriers counseling	During the parent interview, students ask about barriers/hurdles encountered during parent's goal progress and the resolution of those hurdles.
Self-monitoring	Students complete self-assessments of current dietary and fitness practices.
Goal setting	Students set physical activity goals using results from the self-assessments.
Contracting	Students complete contracts for their dietary and fitness goals. This contract specifies the goal and the motivation for attainment and has space for signatures from student, a friend, and a parent.
Cue management	A teacher-led discussion asks, "What are some negative cues that may prevent you from reaching your fitness goal?"
Social support	To strengthen social support networks, students are placed into groups based on chosen goals.

Reinforcement	Students receive raffle tickets for goal attainment.
Cognitive restructuring	By restructuring the way students think about breakfast, options open up for their morning meal such as leftover pizza or a microwaveable burrito, thus making breakfast easier to obtain.
Relapse prevention	The student workbook includes a section devoted to helping students maintain, set, and achieve new goals after the completion of the intervention.
Environment/reciprocal determinism	Homework assignments focus on the role of the environment on behavior change. For example, students identify five locations where they could exercise after school, the hours of operation, and cost. Students find one food from an on-campus source that meets their dietary goals.

Data from Horowitz, M., M. K. Shilts, and M. S. Townsend. 2004. EatFit: A goal-oriented intervention that challenges adolescents to improve their eating and fitness choices. *Journal of Nutrition Education and Behavior* 36:43–44. Used with permission of the Society for Nutrition Education.

using artificial sweeteners in baking. Participants increased their self-efficacy in changing their diet and preparing healthful meals (Chapman-Novakofski and Karduck 2005).

- *A 10-week Web-based intervention with college students* found that goal setting had a positive effect on fruit and vegetable consumption and physical activity, although the impact was stronger for fruits and vegetables, possibly because physical activity in the students was already high at baseline (O'Donnell, Greene, and Blissmer 2014).

- *A review of studies for physical activity* involving 44 studies found that self-efficacy and goal setting were consistently associated with physical activity and that outcome expectations and sociostructural factors were less so (Young et al. 2014).

EXAMPLES FROM NEW MEDIA

Many programs from reputable online sources focus on skill building. Examples include the many how-to tip sheets, recipes, and videos provided online from government, university, cooperative extension, and nutrition professional organizations. The U.S. Department of Agriculture (USDA) provides "10 tips" for each of the behaviors targeted by the Dietary Guidelines as well as others (http://www.choosemyplate.gov/healthy-eating-tips/ten-tips.html). Other countries provide similar information. And any Internet search will generate numerous recipes for just about any kind of food or prevention tips for any nutrition-related condition. Tools for goal setting are also readily available. One

example is the USDA's SuperTracker, which is discussed in **NUTRITION EDUCATION IN ACTION 5-3**.

TAKE-HOME MESSAGE ABOUT SOCIAL COGNITIVE THEORY

- Social cognitive theory states that individuals are agents who can develop skills to become empowered to consciously choose to exercise influence over their own thoughts, feelings, and behaviors and over environmental conditions that affect their lives, in order to bring about both personal and social change. These skills are based on being convinced that performing a given behavior will be effective in leading to the outcomes they desire, and that they can carry out the behavior even in the face of difficulties and setbacks. Therefore, self-efficacy is a major determinant of change. Developing behavioral and self-regulation/self-direction skills, especially goal setting, is the major procedure for personal change. Relevant food and **nutrition knowledge** and skills are also crucial. The importance of action goal setting is summarized in **BOX 5-2**.

- Because the environment influences, but is also influenced by, people's behaviors, people can take collective action with others in their community to work with policymakers and decision-makers to create supportive environments and bring about social change.

- This theory is especially useful if your nutrition education wishes to address both motivation and skills, and both individual and families and the environment.

NUTRITION EDUCATION IN ACTION 5-3   USDA's SuperTracker

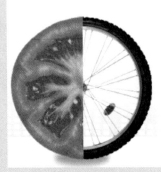

SuperTracker:
My foods. My fitness. My health.
- Get your personalized nutrition and physical activity plan.
- Track your foods and physical activities to see how they stack up.
- Get tips and support to help you make healthier choices and plan ahead.

Reproduced from Supertracker.USDA.gov. United States Department of Agriculture. http://www.supertracker.usda.gov/

The USDA's Center for Nutrition Policy and Promotion developed MyPlate, a multifaceted health communication plan, in support of the 2010 Dietary Guidelines for Americans (DGA). SuperTracker is positioned as a real-time, Web-based tool that empowers users with personalized feedback based on self-identified areas for improvement.

SuperTracker can be used to:

- Identify personalized recommendations of what and how much to eat.
- Track diet and activity.
- Compare choices to 2010 DGA and 2008 Physical Activity Guidelines for Americans.
- Search nutrition and energy balance information for foods and activities.

SuperTracker provides personalized features, including My Top 5 Goals, My Weight Manager, My Journal, and My Reports. These features allow users to:

- Choose personal goals (My Top 5 Goals).
- Sign up for tips and support from a virtual coach.
- Track weight loss progress over time.
- Compare weight history to trends in calorie intake and physical activity.
- Track factors of personal importance, such as meal location and mood.
- View reports of meal summaries and diet analyses of nutrient and food intake.

Importantly, SuperTracker aims to capitalize on social media use to help motivate SuperTracker users to change their behavior by encouraging them to share tips and successes with their personal social networks via Facebook and Twitter.

http://www.choosemyplate.gov/supertracker-tools.html

BOX 5-2 Why We Need Action Plans/Goal Setting: Bridging the Intention to Behavior Gap

Action plans (or implementation intentions) are highly effective in bridging the intention to behavior gap for many reasons:

- Stating a clear action plan means committing to an action, resulting in a sense of control, determination, and also obligation to realize the action or behavior.
- The decision is made ahead of time so that when the situation arises we do not have to think and make a new decision each time. Such *planning ahead* means

the behavior will require less mental effort each time.

- Because the action plan is made in advance, it is also on our mind.
- Developing action plans increases our intrinsic interest through active involvement in the process.
- Action plans increase motivation through anticipation that we will feel good about achieving the action goals.

Using Social Cognitive Theory in Nutrition Education to Facilitate Behavior Change

Social cognitive theory provides us with a tool for designing effective nutrition education that helps to motivate our audiences with why-to change behavior and also how-to do so. As we have seen, social cognitive theory emphasizes that taking a health-related action requires that people become aware of health risks, believe in the benefits of taking action, and set action goals to make changes. They then need relevant food- and nutrition-related knowledge and skills to accomplish the action goals as well as self-regulation skills so that they feel empowered to direct or take charge of their health-related behaviors (Bandura 1989, 2004). Self-efficacy is key. Changes in the environment to support these changes are also important; individuals and groups can advocate for these changes and develop collective efficacy. Specific strategies derived from social cognitive theory that can help improve the effectiveness of what we do are described here.

An example of how social cognitive theory is used in a farm-to-school program is shown in **TABLE 5-3**, the Vermont Food Education Every Day (VT FEED) program (Berlin et al. 2013a, 2013b). For many youth, engagement with food and the food system is more effective for dietary change than a focus on health.

In addition, it must be remembered that all of the beliefs and skills of individuals are embedded in their culture, and thus their cultural norms and expectations need to be carefully considered when designing nutrition education (more detailed discussions are presented in Chapters 3, 4, and 17).

OUTCOME EXPECTATIONS

Increasing Awareness of Risk or Benefits of Current Behaviors or Actions

We can enhance motivation in our audiences by designing activities to increase the relevance of specific issues or perceived risk of current behaviors in relation to personal health, community practices, or the sustainability of food system practices. Benefits of current practices can also be explored. Effective strategies and specific activities might involve the following:

- *Increasing the relevance of risks or concerns*: We can use trigger films, striking national or local statistics, pictures and charts, personal stories, and other strategies to make issues relevant to people, such as the increase in obesity rates, the portion sizes of food

Table 5-3 Using Social Cognitive Theory for Farm-to-School Activities: The Example of the Vermont Food Education Every Day Program	
Activity	**Social Cognitive Theory Construct**
Taste tests	Outcome expectations, positive reinforcement
Breakfast program using whole fresh foods	Outcome expectations
"Eat your colors" week	Outcome expectations
Nutrition education in the classroom	Outcome expectations, self-efficacy, functional knowledge
Teachers model by eating school lunch	Outcome expectations: social support
Farmers visit the classroom regularly	Outcome expectations
Farm-to-school bulletin board	Outcome expectations
In-class food preparation and sharing	Behavioral capability, self-efficacy, outcome expectations
Salad bar training for students	Behavioral capability, self-efficacy
Cooking club	Behavioral capability, self-efficacy
Students help design, build, and tend school gardens	Behavioral capability, self-efficacy
Students visit local farms	Reciprocal determinism, environment
Students apprentice on local farm	Behavioral capability, self-efficacy
Community celebrations featuring local foods	Outcome expectations: social support; environment: reciprocal determinism

products, or the prevalence of metabolic syndrome in adolescents.

- *Providing self-assessment compared to recommendations*: Individuals and families can complete short checklists, food frequency questionnaires, or 24-hour food intake recalls and compare intakes to a standard, such as MyPlate servings, to give themselves an accurate picture of their intake. For low-literacy audiences, these can be highly visual, using few words. The foods on the checklists need to be culturally appropriate.
- *Making a community assessment of practices*: Information about community food practices could provide a true picture of the extent of risk for a condition. We can use existing data or surveys, formal and informal. However, it is best to actively engage the potential audience or community members in this self-assessment, taking particular note of existing strengths and assets.

Increasing Awareness of Positive and Negative Effects of Changing Current Behaviors or Taking Action

- *Physical outcomes*: In group settings, nutrition educators can help participants understand the pleasurable and negative outcomes of taking action. For breastfeeding, for example, the benefits might include health

of the baby, convenience, mother–child bonding, and so forth. However, there are also costs or barriers, such as pain of first breastfeeding. These can be identified through presentations, videos, or group discussion.

- *Social outcomes*: Behavior is partly regulated by the social approval and disapproval of others. In the case of breastfeeding, this might include embarrassment in public situations or wishes of others in the family.
- *Self-evaluative outcomes*: These are the positive and negative outcomes we expect of our own behaviors. In the case of breastfeeding, we might help mothers recognize that they may gain satisfaction from feeling they are being good mothers.

BEHAVIORAL CAPABILITY: INCREASING FOOD- AND NUTRITION-RELATED KNOWLEDGE AND COGNITIVE SKILLS

Facilitating Knowledge and Nutrition Literacy

After individuals become motivated, they need specific knowledge and skills to act on their motivation. For example, individuals need to know how to select foods for optimal health from the 50,000-item supermarket; evaluate the nutrition information that bombards them from magazines, newspapers, advertising, and friends; and interpret personal medical information provided by their physicians. We can help build capacity in our audiences by providing information and opportunity to develop the cognitive skills that empower people to act on their desire to be healthy.

Now is the time to provide how-to information (factual knowledge) about foods, nutrients, dietary guidelines, label reading, or MyPlate and ways to apply this information in people's daily eating plans (procedural knowledge). If a low-fat diet is the focus of the program, important knowledge is the fact that chicken eaten with skin has 3 times the calories as chicken without skin and has 5 to 10 times the calories (because of fat) if it also is battered and deep-fried. Lectures, group discussion, activities, slides, handouts, tip sheets, newsletters, flyers, and Web-based displays of information are all suitable here, depending on the behavior or practice and the channel chosen (e.g., mass media or in person).

Decision-Making and Critical Thinking Skills

Food and nutrition issues are often complex, and research findings sometimes contradictory. Individuals

---

Reminder: The Way in Which We Deliver Our Sessions in Practice Is Crucial for Success!

A well-developed, theory-based educational plan is only effective with our audience if we communicate it effectively. How do we do that? By being:

- *Credible.* This means being perceived as having *expertise* in nutrition from our credentials and being seen as knowledgeable, organized, and not benefiting personally from what we say.
- *Passionate.* This means being personally passionate about what we are presenting,
- *Culturally sensitive.* This means respecting our audience's cultural traditions and focusing on their capacities and strengths in order to enhance empowerment.
- *Respectful of audience.* This means being seen as understanding, warm, and empathetic of the audience and the challenges they face.

need the ability to evaluate evidence and understand reasoned arguments for different options for decision making, such as whether to reduce dietary fat or sugar to lose weight and improve health, or what parenting practices are most effective to get children to eat fruits and vegetables. They need critical thinking skills to understand complex issues related to health and food policies. We can provide the opportunities to develop these skills using activities such as trigger films to stimulate discussion, debates, or written or oral critiques.

BUILDING BEHAVIORAL SKILLS IN FOODS AND NUTRITION AND ENHANCING SELF-EFFICACY

Self-efficacy is not the same thing as physical skills such as food preparation or safe food handling, although it is likely to increase with increased skills. Self-efficacy involves both skills and the confidence that individuals can consistently use them even in the face of impediments or barriers. We can help our audiences build their food- and nutrition-related behavioral skills by modeling the behavior, such as through food demonstrations accompanied by clear instructions. However, individuals learn best and their self-efficacy is enhanced if we also provide them with opportunities to practice the behavior. Our verbal encouragement can help to overcome self-doubts. This process is often called *guided mastery experience*. Social cognitive theory emphasizes that it requires actual experience to develop physical skills such as cooking, safe food preparation practices, and other food-related skills, and to increase self-efficacy. Refer to Box 5-1 for details.

USING NEW MEDIA TO EMPOWER OUR AUDIENCES

Most adults in the United States, and increasingly in the developing world, have access to new technologies such as mobile phones, smartphones and the Internet. For example, at this time in the United States 70–92% of low-income individuals have text messaging, applications "apps," and Internet capabilities (Ahlers-Schmidt et al. 2011) and about two-thirds of low-income, low-education, minority adults use social media (Lefebvre and Bornkessel 2013). These venues can be used to provide needed knowledge and skills to make healthy choices in the grocery stores or even food pantries. See Chapter 16 for more details.

SETTING ACTION GOALS

Besides skills in food and nutrition, behavior change also requires individuals to feel empowered to make the changes they wish. This comes from learning how to set goals or action plans and to follow through with them (Bandura 1986; Cullen et al. 2001; Shilts et al. 2004a). We can help individuals develop action goal setting skills by providing opportunities for them to practice the following steps, recognizing that these steps are taken in the context of family culture and needs (Shilts et al. 2004b, 2009):

- *Conducting self-assessments or observations:* The purpose is to identify ways in which individuals' current actions or behaviors contribute to the issue or problem they are concerned about. We can provide individuals with a method to conduct a self-assessment such as behavioral checklists, food frequency forms, or group 24-hour recalls.
- *Setting action goals:* Individuals set action goals to address the problems identified in the self-assessment. These action goals should be *Specific, Measurable, Achievable, Realistic,* and *Time-bound* (or SMART); for example, stating exactly when they will add fruits and vegetables to their daily diet and how much.
- *Making a commitment:* Commitment to the action goal is strengthened when individuals actually make binding pledges, often called *contracts*. Such pledges have motivational impact because there are consequences or costs to not following through on an agreement. These consequences may be personal, such as self-reproof, or social, if the commitments were made in public or involve others, where the costs may include embarrassment or social disapproval. The process works best when you provide them with a form to complete—more open-ended or more specific, depending on the age group you are working with or their literacy level. See Figures 5-2a and 5-2b for examples.
- *Acquiring relevant facilitating knowledge and skills:* Information and skills to attain the action goal are needed next. These we are good at providing!
- *Monitoring of progress toward the goal:* We can help individuals monitor how they are doing, focusing on positive accomplishments rather than failures.
- *Attaining goals:* Attaining an action goal can result in a sense of self-efficacy, self-satisfaction, and accomplishment that sustains effort or leads to the setting of increasingly more difficult behavior change goals.

- *Using problem-solving and decision-making strategies:* These strategies are mobilized if the action goal is not achieved. We can help individuals modify their action goal or set a new, more achievable goal.

Action Goal Setting Worksheets for Different Audiences

We can help our audiences to develop action plans if we provide them with some kind of form for them to complete. A blank sheet of paper generally will not be effective! The simpler the better, because it makes it easier to complete, particularly for low-literacy audiences. The use of action goal setting was specifically studied in a pilot program with low-income women (Heneman et al. 2005). Women significantly increased their fruit intake. In terms of their stages of change, they moved toward acceptance of vegetable consumption. The "Contract for Change" that was used in the study is shown in **FIGURE 5-2A**. An action planning form was developed for elementary school children for the Food Day Curriculum. It is shown in **FIGURE 5-2B**. It is also helpful to have some way for group participants to monitor how they are doing on their action plans. One format used in the USDA Supplemental Nutrition Assistance Program Education (SNAP-Ed) for older adults is shown in **FIGURE 5-2C**. A simple self-monitoring log is included as part of the action plan form.

MAINTAINING CHANGE

Nutrition education activities designed to assist individuals to maintain their chosen action should focus on teaching individuals the strategies that are shown in **BOX 5-3**.

ENVIRONMENTAL SUPPORTS FOR CHANGE

Social cognitive theory emphasizes that the physical and sociostructural environment influences people's behavior and that people's behaviors can also influence the environment in a reciprocal fashion. Nutrition educators thus seek to work in collaboration with various community stakeholders and decision-makers to make changes in the environment that are supportive of healthful dietary behaviors. How we do so is described in detail in Chapter 6.

The aim of this is to help you make and keep healthy eating habits.

1. Goals: List two ways you can eat more fruits and vegetables.

1) _____

2) _____

2. Setting a goal: Choose one goal from the above two lines and make it into something you can do.

   Action goal:

   What will you do differently? _____

   _____

   How often? _____

   How much? _____

   Where? _____

   With whom? _____

3. Make a plan: List two reasons why this change may be hard.

1) _____

2) _____

What will you do to beat these problems?

1) _____

2) _____

Let's try to make this change!

FIGURE 5-2A Example of a contract for setting goals.

Data from Heneman, K., A. Block-Joy, S. Zidenberg-Cherr, et al. 2005. A "contract for change" increases produce consumption in low-income women: A pilot study. *Journal of the American Dietetic Association* 105(11):1793–1796.

Sample:

My Action Plan:

I am going to eat _____**an apple**_____ instead of _____**a fruit roll up**_____
          whole food   overly processed food

Time of day (check one):   Days of the week (check as many as you like)

    ☐ At breakfast   ☐ Sunday
    ☐ In the morning   ☒ Monday
    ☐ At lunch   ☐ Tuesday
    ☒ In the afternoon   ☒ Wednesday
    ☐ At dinner   ☐ Thursday
    ☐ In the evening   ☒ Friday
                              ☐ Satuday

My Action Plan:

I am going to eat __**grilled chicken breast**__ instead of _____**chicken nuggets**_____
          whole food   overly processed food

Time of day (check one):   Days of the week (check as many as you like)

    ☐ At breakfast   ☐ Sunday
    ☐ In the morning   ☐ Monday
    ☐ At lunch   ☐ Tuesday
    ☐ In the afternoon   ☒ Wednesday
    ☒ At dinner   ☐ Thursday
    ☐ In the evening   ☐ Friday
                              ☒ Satuday

My Action Plan:

I am going to eat _____ instead of _____
          whole food   overly processed food

Time of day (check one):   Days of the week (check as many as you like)

    ☐ At breakfast   ☐ Sunday
    ☐ In the morning   ☐ Monday
    ☐ At lunch   ☐ Tuesday
    ☐ In the afternoon   ☐ Wednesday
    ☐ At dinner   ☐ Thursday
    ☐ In the evening   ☐ Friday
                              ☐ Satuday

FIGURE 5-2B Action planning form, food day school curriculum 2014.

Reproduced with permission from Food Day, Center for Science in the Public Interest.

Here we can mention several strategies that fit well with other activities of social cognitive theory:

- *Behavioral economics*, which emphasizes making the healthy choices the easy choices through changes in the environment to increase the convenience, attractiveness, and normative nature of healthy foods (Wansink et al. 2012; Hanks, Just, and Wansink 2013). This nudges people towards healthier choices of their own volition.
- *Farm-to-school and farm-to-cafeteria programs* where the institutions buy and feature foods from local farms and may include school, worksite, hospital gardens, or visits to local farms (USDA 2014).

THE CASE OF RAY: NUTRITION EDUCATION USING SOCIAL COGNITIVE THEORY

Ray, you recall, is in his mid-40s. His weight just crept up on him, a pound or two each year, and now he is about 40 pounds overweight. His job is as a salesman in a large appliance store, where he is mostly on the phone or standing around and he is not very active. He buys packaged snacks from the vending machine and nibbles when he is bored or anxious. He goes to a nearby fast food restaurant for lunch with a couple of coworkers most days. When he goes home he just wants to sit and watch TV and drink a few beers. His wife is interested in eating more healthfully, but he likes a hearty meal and always a dessert.

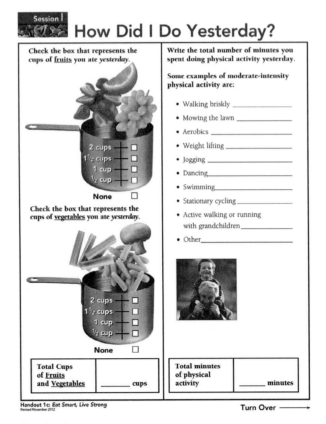

FIGURE 5-2C From Eat Smart, Live Strong activity kit, session 1.

http://snap.nal.usda.gov/snap/ESLS

His doctor tells him that he is at risk of diabetes and that his "bad" serum cholesterol is on the high side. The physician tells Ray that the clinic offers nutrition education sessions and he might benefit from attending. Ray sees one session titled "Right size it!" and decides to attend. This hypothetical session is shown here.

Here is how the nutrition educator designed the session. She looked at research and survey data and conducted some interviews with potential audience members. She found that several behaviors were problematic, chief among them for this age group, the high consumption of snacks and fast food. However, many were already concerned but just did not seem to be able to make the changes they knew they needed to make. She decided that the best theory to use to address the issue of reducing weight and risk of diabetes was social cognitive theory, with its emphasis on action goal setting and attention to the environment. She then created a theory model for her session. The diagram presented in CASE STUDY 5-1 shows how she operationalized the model for this session. There is a similar blank diagram at the end of this chapter that you can use to design nutrition education activities based on the social cognitive theory. How she and Ray addressed his work environment is discussed in Chapter 6.

Self-Regulation Models: Focus on Planning and Self-Efficacy

Our ability to think through, make conscious choices, plan ways to follow through with those choices, and generally take charge of or "regulate" our behaviors is a key process in initiating and maintaining health behavior change, according to research (Bagozzi and Dholakia 1999). Central to this process are planning and self-efficacy, which are the primary focus of some "self-regulation" models (Bagozzi 1992; Gollwitzer 1999; Gollwitzer and Sheeran 2006; Sniehotta 2009; Koring et al. 2012). These models are similar to social cognitive theory, but note that becoming motivated to initiate a behavior requires a different mind-set and different tasks from maintaining a behavior once we have started taking action. In the *motivation phase*, a deliberative—or thinking—mind-set predominates, and in the *action phase* an implementation—or doing—mind-set predominates (Abraham, Sheeran, and Johnson 1998; Gollwitzer 1999; Wiedemann et al. 2009). Self-efficacy is considered key in both phases, with motivational self-efficacy important in the first phase, coping self-efficacy in the second phase, and planning self-efficacy linking the two.

CASE STUDY 5-1 The Case of Ray: Nutrition Education Using the Social Cognitive Theory

Target Audience: Adults at Risk for Chronic Disease

Behavioral Goal: Consume Appropriate Sizes of High-Energy Foods and Drinks

Social cognitive

Target Audience **Health Clinic Clients**　　　　　　　　　　　Behavior **Small Size SSB, PPS, FF**

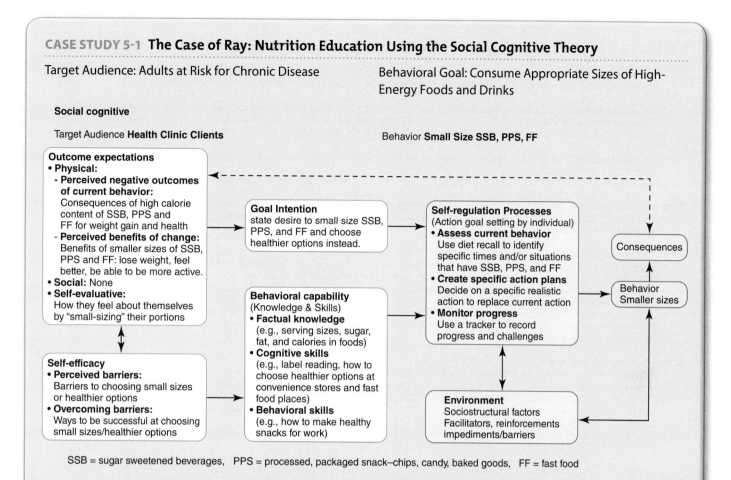

SSB = sugar sweetened beverages,　PPS = processed, packaged snack–chips, candy, baked goods,　FF = fast food

Here is the educational plan of the session Ray attended, along with many other people around his age. Note that it focuses on specific behaviors—consuming smaller sizes of sweetened beverages, fewer packaged processed snacks, and less fast food. The nutrition educator started with each of the determinants of change in social cognitive theory (shown as a heading in the educational plan) and then designed a specific activity to address this determinant.

"Small Size It!"

Education Plan for Group Session

Behavioral goal: Participants will consume smaller sizes of sweetened beverages, packaged processed snacks, and fast food.

Educational objectives to reach goals. At the end of the session, participants will be able to:
- Evaluate the degree to which their eating patterns increase their risk of chronic disease and unhealthy weight
- Describe the impact of large sizes of foods and drinks high in sugar and fat on their health and weight
- Describe the benefits of smaller sizes and healthier options on disease risk and a healthy weight
- State commitment to make behavior changes through an action plan

Procedure: (Determinant in **bold** and activity for determinant <u>underlined</u>):

Perceived physical outcomes of current behavior (self-assessment of risk)
- <u>Diet self-assessment:</u> The participants are asked to write down everything they ate and drank in the past 24 hours. Then, they are to circle the sweetened beverages, snacks, and fast food they consumed.

Perceived physical outcomes of current behavior (health risk)
- <u>Scientific evidence for health risk:</u> The instructor uses a slide presentation to tell the participants about the scientific evidence about the impact of excess weight on health, in particular diabetes.
- <u>Measure out sugar:</u> Instructor shows the group containers (empty) of different sizes of a popular drink. Then, she asks a volunteer to come up and measure out, with estimates provided by the group, how many teaspoons of sugar (from a container of sugar) they think is in each size of container of drink. She provides them with a worksheet where they check which size of beverage they usually drink and

(Continues)

---

how often. They then calculate how many calories a year that would be for each bottle size. She also explained that whenever people consume about 3,500 calories in the diet beyond need, their bodies deposit the extra calories as a pound of fat.

Ray and the others are surprised at the number of calories in drinks. He did not think liquids had calories. He asks if beer also has calories and learns that it does indeed. At about 300 calories a day in beverages he is consuming, that would be about 10,000 calories a year. That would translate to nearly 3 pounds a year. He now understood how his extra weight crept up.

- Calories in fast food: The instructor then shows participants a slide presentation that depicts the number of calories in some key fast food items. For example, a medium cheeseburger had 650 calories, a large French fries had 500 calories, and a medium milkshake had 500 calories. *Ray and the others are shocked by the presentation, and they are now truly concerned about their health risks.*

Beliefs about positive outcomes of taking action to change current behaviors
- Benefits of smaller sizes: The instructor provides the evidence using slides that choosing healthier options and smaller sizes can help them reach or maintain a healthy weight.

Perceived barriers or impediments to taking action
- Review of self-assessment: Group members review their dietary recalls and circle the sweet drinks, packaged snacks, and fast food. They discuss what keeps them from choosing smaller sizes or healthier options.

Self-efficacy/overcoming barriers
- Brainstorm ways to overcome barriers: The group brainstorms ways to select healthier options, and comes up with the kinds of fruits and vegetables that could serve as snacks to bring to work, whole grain crackers when they wanted something crunchy, and nonfat yogurt with fruit as dessert.

Action goal-setting/action plans
- Assess current behaviors: The instructor asks group members to use their diet recall from the beginning of the session to determine a specific time of day and/or situation that they have a large size of sweetened beverages, packaged processed snacks or fast food.
- Create specific action plans: The instructor asks group members to decide on a specific action they will take in the coming week to reduce the size of their portions (e.g., instead of choosing a 24-oz bottle of iced tea get the 12-oz can). She helps all participants have a realistic, concrete plan.
- Monitor progress: The instructor gives participants a tracker to record when they follow their plan and when they do not, with space for notes about what made it easy to make the change and what challenges they had.

Ray is now very concerned about his diet and energized/motivated to do something about it. He chooses two actions he will take: he will switch from a cheeseburger to a grilled chicken sandwich for lunch, and he will have only one beer at home and make that a near beer with very few calories. (All he really wants is the bubbly bitter taste.) He intends to come back to a session next week to learn about reading food labels and he plans on setting additional goals for actions he could take such as making his own sandwiches to take for lunch.

BOX 5-3 **Meeting the Challenge of Maintaining Healthful Behaviors**

Maintaining chosen behaviors over the long term requires "self-regulatory skills" by which individuals develop the ability to influence their own actions through their own efforts by making conscious choices, setting action goals, and following through. Some of the strategies that are helpful are listed here.

Maintaining Goals

- *Prioritizing competing goals*: All individuals have competing goals at any one time. To maintain their chosen behavioral goal, they need to protect it from being interrupted or given up prematurely as a result of competing goals. They can also seek ways of satisfying both their health goal and other goals at the same time.

- *Mindful eating: protecting action goals from distractions:* Individuals can become busy and distracted by the presence of friends or colleagues or of non-healthful foods, and without thinking, they may fail to follow their action plan. Sticking with their plan is not about being rigid or about denial. It is about being mindful about their eating and thinking about whether this is what they really want to be doing. In the current environment, eating healthfully and being physically active require conscious attention.

- *Focusing on the big picture*: Individuals can remember that if they eat foods they had not planned to on one occasion, they can always compensate for it on another occasion so that overall they achieve their goal.

- *Linking action goals to their self-identity*: Sometimes it can help for individuals to remember that they now have a new identity—for example, as individuals who want to take care of themselves or as active people.

- *Correctly attributing their successes and failures*: This allows individuals to claim successes and feel good about them and recognize that failures may be caused by circumstances beyond their control.

Developing Routines and Habits

- Sticking with action plans can make the chosen behavior become more routine; new habits are developed.

Substituting with Helpful Thoughts

- Individuals can substitute alternative, more helpful thoughts about making changes for less helpful ones.

Coping Self-Efficacy

- Strong beliefs about their ability to deal with barriers—the conviction that they can carry out their intentions even under difficult circumstances—can be very helpful at this stage.

Creating Personal Environments to Achieve Action Goals

- *Controlling stimuli*: Individuals can restructure their personal environment to make it more supportive by removing cues to less healthful eating and adding cues for more healthful eating.

- *Seeking social support*: Individuals can seek the help of those around them.

Enjoying Healthful Food: Coming to Like What One Eats

- Eating healthfully becomes enjoyable as healthful foods become familiar and when individuals learn the skills to make them tasty.

Developing Personal Policies: Expressing Agency and Empowerment

- Individuals can create their own personal food policies or systems to manage, over the long term, the numerous and conflicting values they hold about their food choices. For example, they may have a policy that they will always have breakfast before leaving the house, even if it is modest.

RELATED CONSTRUCTS: SELF-REGULATION, EFFORTFUL CONTROL, AND EXECUTIVE FUNCTION

As we have seen, self-regulation involves making consciously chosen voluntary choices, goal setting, monitoring our behavior, and managing the environment. There are a few related constructs to keep in mind. *Effortful control* can act in service of self-regulation because it involves the ability to control the impulse to respond to a stimulus and supports the ability to focus on important stimuli while disregarding distractions (Gardner, Dishion, and Connell 2007). Being able to ignore or inhibit a dominant response, such as the taste of a highly palatable food item, to respond to the less dominant one, such as the choice of fruit, can clearly serve our desire to focus on our chosen health goals. There may be individual differences in this ability to control emotional and attentional responses that are related to termperament (Rothbart, Ellis, and Posner 2013). *Executive function* is the neurological mechanism by which the

brain assigns attention to stimuli (Kuhn 2008). So we can see that these constructs are related to each other.

HEALTH ACTION PROCESS APPROACH MODEL

The health action process approach model is a simple self-efficacy model that also includes a time dimension (Schwarzer and Fuchs 1995; Schwarzer and Renner 2000; Sniehotta et al. 2005; Ziegelmann and Lippke 2007). It is shown in **FIGURE 5-3**. The model proposes two phases—a pre-action phase and an action phase—and focuses on the important role of self-efficacy at various points in the dietary change process, as shown in the figure. Planning is also central.

Motivational Phase

The focus in the motivational phase is on beliefs and affect or feelings, and a deliberative mind-set prevails. Individuals' intention to adopt a valued health behavior

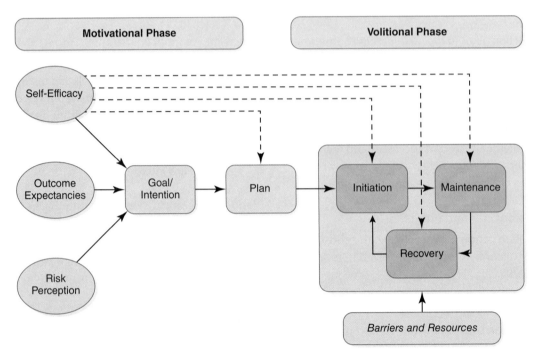

FIGURE 5-3 The Health Action Process Approach.

Reproduced from R. Schwarzer, Freie Universitat Berlin, Germany. Used with permission.

(such as eating a low-fat, high-fiber diet) depends on three sets of beliefs as shown in Figure 5-3:

- *Risk perceptions:* The belief that we are at risk for disease (e.g., diabetes)
- *Outcome expectancies:* The belief that a change in behavior would reduce the health risk (e.g., "If I eat healthful foods, I will reduce my risk for diabetes")
- *Self-efficacy:* The belief that we are sufficiently capable of exercising control over a difficult behavior (e.g., "I am capable of controlling my diet to make it healthful in spite of temptations to eat sweets")

Planning

Strategic planning has been found to greatly enhance the translation of intentions into action (Ziegelmann and Lippke 2007; Scholz et al. 2008). Here we begin to make plans to carry out the behavior, and developing confidence or self-efficacy in being able to make plans becomes important.

Action or Volitional Phase

In the action phase, the mind-set is one of implementation (or doing), and the focus is on conscious choices, making plans based on those choices, and following through (Gollwitzer 1999). Coping self-efficacy is important in this phase.

Initiating Action: Planning Ahead

In this subphase we convert intentions (e.g., eating four and a half cups of fruits and vegetables each day) into *action plans* or *implementation intentions, specifying when, where, and how we will take action* ("I will add orange juice at breakfast each day next week; I will have a fruit for a snack 3 days this coming week"). Making very specific action plans has been shown to be effective in assisting individuals to initiate action (Gollwitzer 1999; Armitage 2004; de Nooijer et al. 2006). See Box 5-2 for more details about why planning ahead helps people translate intentions into action.

Maintaining Action: Skills for Agency and Empowerment

In this subphase individuals become empowered to take charge of their own actions through their own efforts and maintain their chosen behavior change using their food and nutrition and behavioral skills (Taylor, Bagozzi, and Gaither 2005). See Box 5-3 for details on these self-regulation skills. A major challenge for us at this stage—indeed, an ongoing challenge in maintaining healthful practices—is setting priorities between conflicting goals or desires. We may want to eat more healthfully, but we also have work-related aspirations that do not leave much mental and physical time for planning and eating healthfully. At this time, the chosen behavioral goal, such as to eat healthful lunches at work, needs to be protected from being interrupted or given up prematurely because of competing intentions, such as the desire to be a productive worker and work through lunch. We need to keep the overarching long-term goals in mind and ignore the more immediate distracting action imperatives.

Self-Regulation: The Synergistic Effect of Planning and Self-Efficacy

When individuals consider their risk from the current condition, their desired outcomes, and their self-efficacy they will normally become motivated to state an intention to make the desired change. To actually initiate change, however, they will need to do some planning. Self-efficacy is crucial here. Self-efficacy is important at many stages: initiating action, planning, maintaining the behavior, and recovery after we have not been able to follow our action plans.

Planning and Initiation Self-Efficacy

Studies have found that when individuals feel self-efficacious, planning is more likely to be translated into action (Koring et al. 2012). Put another way, planning will not be translated into action if people harbor self-doubts. Self-efficacy comes from building confidence in food and nutrition skills through mastery experiences, role modeling, and verbal assurances. Self-efficacy is important here because many desirable food- and nutrition-related practices require effort, for example, learning to cook in order to gain control over what ingredients are in the food eaten. Nutrition educators should note that implementing a new, more healthful behavior, such as adding fruit to the diet, does not automatically reduce less healthful habits such as eating high-fat, high-sugar snacks (Verplanken and Faes 1999).

Coping Self-Efficacy: Mindfulness

Self-efficacy and empowerment to maintain desired behaviors rely on conscious control and attention; in short, being mindful. Maintaining desired behaviors also relies on strategies for coping with our emotions, such as the ability to ignore feelings of worry or of disappointment in not meeting the set goals.

Optimistic beliefs about our ability to deal with difficulties, although a major hindrance in getting us motivated, may be helpful here because a new behavior may turn out to be much more difficult to adhere to than we

had anticipated. These beliefs are sometimes referred to as coping self-efficacy. An example is "I can stick with a healthful diet even if I have to try several times until it works" or "even if I need a long time to develop the necessary routines" (Schwarzer and Renner 2000). The aim here is for the new behavior to become habitual and routine.

Just as initiation of a behavior is based on our *anticipation* of the satisfaction we can obtain from a behavior, so maintenance of the new behavior is based on our *experience* of the satisfaction of the *actual outcomes* we obtain from the new behavior (Bandura 1997).

Recovery Self-Efficacy

Individuals may not be able to maintain their goal behaviors at all times. Recovery self-efficacy—the conviction that they will be able to get back on track after being derailed from the goal or after they experience setbacks—now becomes important. High recovery self-efficacy enables individuals to get back on track.

Evidence for Self-Regulation Models from Research Studies

Several studies have examined the importance of these variables in relation to diet and physical activity (Taylor et al. 2005; Ziegelmann, Lippke, and Schwarzer 2006; Lippke et al. 2009):

- *A study of four health behaviors*, including dietary behavior and physical activity, found that self-efficacy and planning were the immediate predictors of behavior, while **risk perception** was an early phase factor (Schwarzer et al. 2007).
- *For physical activity behavior*, planning and self-efficacy had a synergistic effect (Koring et al. 2012).
- *In a study of fruit and vegetable intake*, outcome expectations predicted progression from pre-intention to intention, whereas social support predicted progression to the action phase. Low levels of planning were associated with relapse to the pre-action phase. Self-efficacy emerged as a universal predictor of phase transitions (Wiedemann et al. 2009).
- *Dietary interventions* based on these findings were used successfully to increase fruit and vegetable consumption (Kreausukon et al. 2012; Lange et al. 2013), decrease unhealthy snacking (Tam, Bagozzi, and Spaniol 2010) and cope with hypertension (Taylor et al. 2005). A comparison of information-only and self-regulation

strategies with a group of adult women found that both groups initially increased their intake of vegetables, but only those who had learned self-regulation skills maintained this increased intake 2 years later (Stadler, Oettingen, and Gollwitzer 2010).

Grounded Theory Approach: Personal Food Policies

Some studies using a grounded theory approach or interpretative approach for studying dietary behavior have found that individuals develop **personal food policies** or systems to manage, over the long term, the numerous and conflicting values they hold about their food choices (Furst et al. 1996; Bisogni et al. 2012; Contento et al. 2006). We can see that many of the strategies people use in their food choices and in making changes are similar to variables in the theories described.

For example, some people balance criteria for food choice:

- Some studies found that individuals can choose one value and use it predominantly, such as choosing the least expensive option, the one that tastes the best, or the healthiest, regardless of other criteria (Connors et al. 2001). (These are outcome expectations.) But they can modify these depending on the situation (Jastran et al. 2009).
- A study with adolescents obtained similar kinds of personal policies: they balanced "unhealthy foods" with "healthy foods" within a meal, between meals (less-healthy lunches with peers and healthful dinners at home), and between weekdays and weekends to serve various purposes (Contento et al. 2006). (These are outcome expectations.)

Others develop personal policies for managing healthy eating over the long term:

- Managing healthy eating for some adults meant joining community supported agriculture (CSA). One study found that after joining a CSA, families hit a "learning curve," in which they must learn to adapt to the structure of getting a weekly bounty of fresh vegetables. The steepness and duration of the learning curve depends on families' skills in the kitchen and on their ability to consume large quantities of sometimes-unfamiliar

vegetables. Once families traverse the learning curve, CSAs become part of who they are (Iwaki et al. 2014). (These represent self-efficacy.)

- For those experiencing food insecurity, personal food policies were chosen to cope with the lack of sufficient quantity of wholesome, nutritious food. Here the personal food policies included substituting less expensive foods for more expensive (e.g., dried beans instead of canned beans or canned fruits instead of fresh), reducing or omitting unaffordable ingredients, looking for foods from atypical sources such as food pantries, and putting children's food needs first (Hoisington, Shultz, and Butkus 2002). (These are outcome expectations.)

- People who are diagnosed with type 2 diabetes as adults need long-term maintenance of behavior change. They are required to adopt and maintain a number of dietary patterns and self-care behaviors to achieve and sustain control of their blood sugar. They use many of the strategies described previously: making action plans and protecting their action plans from competing goals, being mindful about their eating so that they are not distracted by alternative intentions, and making personal food policies. (These are self-regulation skills.) A study that examined diabetics' beliefs and perceptions about their diets and how to manage them is described in **NUTRITION EDUCATION IN ACTION 5-4**.

Transtheoretical Model and the Stages of Change Construct

> In its simplest terms, the transtheoretical model (TTM) proposes that self-change in behavior is a process that occurs through five stages and that individuals use a variety of psychological and behavioral processes in making changes.

The transtheoretical model has become one of the most widely used models in the study of health behavior change (Prochaska and DiClemente 1984; Prochaska and Velicer 1997; Prochaska 2007; Wright, Velicer, and Prochaska 2009). It originated from an analysis of 18 systems of psychotherapy that identified common processes that individuals use to make changes in their own behavior (Prochaska and DiClemente 1984), hence the name *transtheoretical*.

NUTRITION EDUCATION IN ACTION 5-4 Food Selection and Eating Patterns Among People with Type 2 Diabetes

People with type 2 diabetes are required to adopt and maintain for the long term many dietary and self-care behaviors in order to achieve and sustain control of their blood sugar. This study used semi-structured, in-depth interviews to explore the beliefs and perspectives of those with type 2 diabetes about dietary requirements, food selection and eating patterns, as well as attitudes about self-management practices. These interviews were analyzed for themes, which are captured in the accompanying diagram.

Prior history with food selection and weight control efforts are linked to current challenges involving avoiding favorite foods and choosing more healthful alternatives, managing weight, dining out, and exercising restraint in terms of portions. Their prior knowledge was helpful in using strategies to manage their diets.

The determinants that facilitated or impeded their food selection behaviors and eating patterns were as follows:

- Level of social support, particularly support of spouse.

- Degree of self-efficacy or confidence that they would be able to stay with their eating plans even in difficult situations, such as when eating with coworkers who were eating fast foods they liked or resisting rich baked goods at family gatherings.

- Time management, which was a problem because they always had to plan ahead of time what they were going to eat and stick with a schedule. They had to time their insulin or oral medication to food intake.

In general, they developed specific practices, routines, or personal policies to support their self-management efforts.

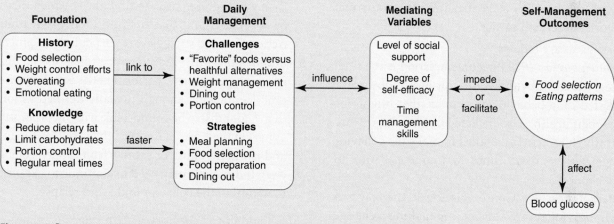

Elements Influencing Food Selection and Eating Patterns Among People with Type 2 Diabetes

Reproduced from Savoca, M., and C. Miller. 2001. Food selection and eating patterns: Themes found among people with type 2 diabetes mellitus. *Journal of Nutrition Education* 33:224–233. Figure used with permission of the Society for Nutrition Education.

During this analysis, Prochaska and DiClemente found that behavior change seemed to occur through a series of stages. The model has now been applied to a range of health behaviors, including smoking, safer sex practices, mammography screening, weight control, and diet and physical activity behaviors.

The transtheoretical model proposes that self-change in behavior is a process that occurs through five stages. It also proposes that there are two determinants of change

(decisional balance based on pros and cons of change, and self-efficacy) and 10 processes of change. The transtheoretical model is a model of behavior change, not a model predicting behavior. It is shown in **FIGURE 5-4**.

THE STAGES OF CHANGE CONSTRUCT

The transtheoretical model proposes that health behavior change is a gradual, continuous, and dynamic process that

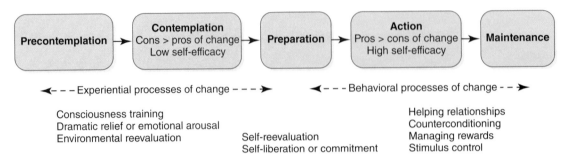

FIGURE 5-4 Transtheoretical Model

can be seen as occurring through a series of stages based on people's readiness to change. Knowledge of the stage or readiness of individuals and groups can be used to inform intervention design. Many studies use the **stages of change construct** without using the transtheoretical model's "processes of change," making the underlying theory a stages of change model. In some studies, the stages are collapsed into pre-action and action/maintenance stages, resulting in a stage structure similar to some of the theories described earlier.

The stages as are follows:

1. *Precontemplation (PC):* Precontemplation is the time during which individuals are not aware of, or not interested in, a behavior or practice that might enhance their health. Also included in this category are those who have tried and failed to make the behavior change, perhaps many times, and no longer want to think about it.

2. *Contemplation (C):* Contemplation is the stage in which individuals are considering making a change sometime in the near future, usually defined as within the next 6 months. They are more aware of the pros of changing but are especially aware of the costs of changing. They struggle between thinking about the positive outcomes of the behavior and the amount of time, energy, and other resources that will be needed to change. This can cause enormous ambivalence, resulting in "chronic contemplation" or procrastination (Prochaska, DiClemente, and Norcross 1992). Individuals at this stage need motivational activities rather than action-oriented, behavioral change strategies.

3. *Preparation (P):* Preparation is the stage in which individuals intend to make a change in the immediate future, usually defined as 1 month, and may have already taken some steps in that direction. Individuals

in this stage are ready for action-oriented strategies that will help them initiate action.

4. *Action (A):* Action is the stage in which individuals have started to engage in the new behavior or practice (often defined as within the previous 6 months). They may adopt the practice (e.g., eat more whole grains) on a small scale at first or try out alternative practices, such as eating whole grain breakfast cereals rather than whole grain pasta, to find one at which they can be successful and that fits into their usual routine. Action-oriented strategies are particularly helpful here.

5. *Maintenance (M):* Maintenance refers to the period in which people have performed the new behavior or practice for long enough (usually defined as longer than 6 months) to be comfortable with incorporating it as part of their way of life (e.g., they now routinely buy and use nonfat milk or eat five fruits and vegetables a day). Individuals may need to continue to exert effort to maintain the behavior and avoid relapse.

For addictive behaviors, a sixth stage, termination, is included, during which individuals no longer succumb to any temptation and feel total self-efficacy. For dietary behaviors, this stage may not be practical or applicable because everyone has to eat; hence, a more realistic goal is a lifetime of maintenance.

Different Stages for Different Behaviors

Nutrition educators should note that individuals can be, and usually are, at different stages of change for different diet-related behaviors. For example, individuals wanting to "eat more healthfully" may be at the action stage in terms of adding fruits and vegetables to their diets but still contemplating cutting down on high-fat, high-sugar food products; or people may have started making changes in diet but not physical activity (Boudreaux et al. 2003).

Nutrition Education for Different Stages

A major contribution of the stages of change construct is a reminder that most nutrition education programs are "action centered," assuming a certain degree of readiness to take action on the part of program participants. They thus fail to address the needs of those who are not yet emotionally prepared to act.

Changes in stage are not always linear. The transtheoretical model acknowledges that change is more like a spiral than a straight line, with a great deal of back and forth movement and recycling between the stages (Kristal et al. 2000; De Nooijer et al. 2006).

Research studies have found that in the area of diet, the stages are often not clearly delineated.

DETERMINANTS OF CHANGE

The theory proposes two determinants of change: the pros and cons of change and self-efficacy.

Decisional Balance: The Pros and Cons of Change

Decisional balance, or the weighing of the pros and cons of change, is an important construct in the transtheoretical model. Pros are people's beliefs about the anticipated benefits of changing, and cons are the costs of changing. Decisional balance is based on a model of decision making that proposes that behavior change emerges when the pros, or anticipated benefits, outweigh the cons, or costs, of the change. The pros and cons of change are similar to the perceived benefits and barriers constructs of the health belief model and the outcome expectations construct of the theory of planned behavior and social cognitive theory.

Examples of pros of change are "Eating healthy food is helpful in preventing cancer" and "Eating healthful food will improve the way I look." Examples of cons of change include "I would find it hard to give up some of my favorite foods to follow a healthier diet" and "It is too expensive to eat organic foods."

In a review of 27 diet-related studies, the average increase of pros was almost two times greater than the decrease in cons from precontemplation to action stages (Di Noia and Prochaska 2010a). The crossover point in the diet and physical activity areas is generally between the contemplation and the preparation and action stages. Thus, it can be concluded that only when perceived benefits outweigh perceived barriers will contemplators move into preparation and action. This suggests that nutrition education may need to place considerable emphasis on raising the benefits of change to overcome the barriers to change (Prochaska and Velicer 1997).

Self-Efficacy

The self-efficacy construct was integrated into the transtheoretical model from social cognitive theory. It is the confidence that people have that they can carry out the behavior across different challenging situations and not relapse to their previous, less healthy behavior. Self-efficacy tends to decrease between the precontemplation stage and contemplation stage, probably because during the precontemplation stage individuals have an optimistic bias about what they can do, and it is during the contemplation stage that they first realize how difficult the new behavior may be. Self-efficacy then steadily increases through the action and maintenance stages (Sporny and Contento 1995; Campbell et al. 1998; Ma et al. 2002).

THE PROCESSES OF CHANGE

The processes of change are overt and covert strategies that individuals use to move themselves through the stages of change. Each of the change processes is a category of similar activities and experiences that facilitate individuals' progress through the stages. Ten processes have been proposed. These include experiential or cognitive processes that focus on thoughts, feelings, and experiences, and behavioral processes that focus on behaviors and reinforcement. The transtheoretical model proposes that behavior change is facilitated if interventions focus on change processes that are matched to the stage of change of individuals.

The processes associated with change are as follows:

Experiential processes.

- *Consciousness-raising* occurs when we increase our awareness about the causes, consequences, and cures for a health issue and seek new information about healthy behaviors. For example, "I seek out magazine articles to learn more about how eating fruits and vegetables can affect health."
- *Dramatic relief or emotional arousal* occurs when we experience and express the negative emotions or feelings (fear, anxiety, worry, sense of threat) about our problems, followed by reduced emotion if appropriate action is seen as possible. For example, "Warnings

about how diet can contribute to the risk of developing heart disease make me anxious."

- *Self-reevaluation* is when we reassess our beliefs, knowledge, feelings, or self-image about a particular unhealthy food-related behavior or practice in relation to ourselves (e.g., an image of self as a junk food eater) For example, "I think about how I would be a healthier person if I ate more fruits and vegetables."

- *Environmental reevaluation* happens when we examine our positive and negative beliefs and feelings about the impact of our personal diet-related behaviors on others. This could also include evaluation of ourselves as a role model to others, positive or negative. For example, "I realize that I may be able to keep local farmers in business if I join a community-supported agriculture farm" or "I realize that I would be a role model to my children if I ate more fruits and vegetables daily."

- *Self-liberation or commitment* occurs when we believe that we can change and make a conscious choice and firm commitment to make the change. For example, "I am committed to eating more fruits and vegetables each day."

Behavioral processes.

- *Helping relationships* are those in which we enlist the trust, caring, and acceptance in our relationships with others to help us change (such as making pacts with coworkers not to eat donuts for snacks).

- *Counterconditioning* occurs when we learn to replace less healthful behaviors with more healthful ones, such as eating fruit instead of high-fat, high-sugar desserts.

- *Managing rewards* is when we reevaluate the way in which we use food as a reward or punishment. Evidence suggests that self-changers use rewards more than punishment to manage their behaviors.

- *Stimulus or environmental control* occurs when we remove cues or triggers for undesirable behavior (e.g., avoiding walking past a bakery that makes our favorite pastries) and add cues or prompts for more healthful alternatives, such as putting a reminder on the office calendar to walk during lunch hour.

- *Social liberation* happens when we become aware of environmental factors that influence our dietary patterns and use the external environment to help us get started or to stay with a change. For example, if individuals are trying to eat more vegetables, they

will choose a restaurant that offers salads and vegetable entrees for lunch. This process also involves the notion of advocacy, for example, to increase the availability of more healthful foods in schools and communities.

PROCESSES OF CHANGE AT DIFFERENT STAGES

Studies have provided evidence that individuals use these processes in self-change to different extents as they move through the stages (Prochaska and Velicer 1997). In the area of diet, it has been found that experiential and behavioral processes often increase together through the stages (Greene et al. 1999; Rosen 2000).

Precontemplation

The transtheoretical model proposes, and research evidence confirms, that when people are in the precontemplation stage, they use all of these processes significantly less than in all the other stages.

Contemplation

In the contemplation stage, people become open to consciousness-raising strategies, such as observations, self-assessments, and other strategies to raise awareness about their behavior. For example, they may conduct self-assessments of their fruit and vegetable intakes per day and look for information about the benefits of fruits and vegetables for health or disease risk.

During contemplation, people are also open to emotionally arousing experiences, such as stories about the impact of diabetes on given individuals, which can lead to dramatic relief as they make changes (e.g., based on information about the efficacy of fruits and vegetables for reducing disease risk). As individuals become more conscious of themselves and the nature of their food-related issues, they are more likely to reevaluate themselves, their values, and their problems both cognitively and affectively. They also evaluate the effects of their behaviors on those around them and on the physical environment. Movement through the contemplation stage involves increased use of the cognitive, affective, and evaluative processes of change.

Action

People begin to take action when they believe that they have the autonomy to make changes through a self-liberation process, and then make a firm commitment to change. As they take action, they call on skills in counterconditioning (substituting more healthful foods for those that are less healthful) as well as environmental or stimulus control such as making sure not to keep large supplies of energy-dense foods in the house to help them maintain their weight.

Maintenance

Successful maintenance of change involves the use of behavioral processes to prevent relapse to less healthy patterns of behavior. Here nutrition education can assist individuals to acquire and practice these skills. Social support can be important, as well as rewards given by others or by individuals themselves. Most important to maintenance is the sense people have that they are becoming who they want to be.

RESEARCH AND INTERVENTION EXAMPLES

A number of studies show support for the stages of change construct in the area of diet (Di Noia and Prochaska 2010a). For example, those individuals in the action and maintenance stages have lower intakes of fat and higher intakes of fiber and of fruits and vegetables compared with those in the pre-action stages (Sporny and Contento 1995; Glanz et al. 1998). In studies, the stage of change is useful in several ways: as a predictor of health behavior change, as a way to stratify people in order to match interventions to individuals on the basis of their readiness to change, and as an intermediate outcome measure to indicate progress toward health behavior change.

Determinants of Change and Stages

The motivating forces for movement through the stages (or determinants of change), according to the transtheoretical model, are the balance of pros and cons of change (perceived benefits and barriers) and self-efficacy.

Numerous cross-sectional studies have examined the relationship between these variables and stages of change in the area of diet and physical activity. Psychosocial constructs from the other theories are often also included (Sporny and Contento 1995; Brug, Glanz, and Kok 1997; Campbell et al. 1998; Kavookjian et al. 2005; Henry et al. 2006; Buchanan and Coulson 2007; Wright et al. 2009). Taken together, these and other studies suggest that although there is considerable moving back and forth among stages, perceived benefits or

pros are especially important in the early stages, where they serve a motivational role, and must become greater than cons if change is to take place (Di Noia and Prochaska 2010a). Self-efficacy has been found to influence movement through the stages (O'Hea et al. 2004; Henry et al. 2006).

Stage-Matched Interventions Tailored to Individuals

One of the main implications of the stages of change model is that nutrition educators should use different kinds of nutrition education activities with individuals at different stages of psychological readiness to change (Velicer and Prochaska 1999). Here the stages of change construct is used to design interventions that are specifically tailored to individuals at different stages of change (Prochaska et al. 1993). Tailoring differs from targeting in that targeted interventions are directed at groups or populations with similar characteristics, whereas tailored interventions are directed at individuals within target populations. Here individuals complete a questionnaire by phone, on paper, or online to assess their pros and cons, self-efficacy, and stages of change and are then provided with individualized feedback reports based on their responses. They are next provided with information (e.g., through newsletters, email, or the Internet) on the processes of change that they can use, appropriate to their stage.

In the area of diet, tailored interventions have been conducted with individuals in a variety of group settings, such as primary care settings (Salmela et al. 2009), health departments (Jacobs et al. 2004), worksites (Campbell et al. 2002; De Bourdeaudhuij et al. 2007), after-school programs with youth (Di Noia, Contento, and Prochaska 2008), and families (De Bourdeaudhuij et al. 2002). Other channels have also been used, such as the Web (Oenema, Tan, and Brug 2005; Park et al. 2008) and multimedia programs (tailored soap opera and interactive infomercials) (Campbell et al. 1999). These studies suggest that tailoring the intervention to a given individual's stage of psychological readiness to take action can enhance the effectiveness of nutrition education (Horwath et al. 2013). Two studies are summarized here, and a study with seniors is shown in detail in **NUTRITION EDUCATION IN ACTION 5-5**.

- *Clinic-based program:* In one study, the transtheoretical model processes of change were used in a clinic-based

NUTRITION EDUCATION IN ACTION 5-5 The SENIOR Project Intervention

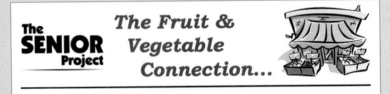

Courtesy of Senior Project.

The Study of Exercise and Nutrition in Older Rhode Islanders (SENIOR project) promoted fruit and vegetable consumption and exercise among community-dwelling adults over the age of 60. The yearlong study included 1,277 older adults.

Theoretical Framework

The SENIOR project was designed using the transtheoretical model of behavior change because of previous success using TTM among young adults, and the ease with which TTM can be used for individual tailoring and technological applications.

Intervention Components

- Manual: Each participant was provided with a binder that explained the processes and strategies for behavior change associated with each stage of change. The manuals included interactive activities and acted as a reference guide for participants. The manual also included community-specific resources.

- *Tailored reports*: These reports, given to each participant at months 4, 8, and 12, were based on data collected from participants in phone interviews. The tailored information provided to each participant included: their *stage of change*; their reported *pros and cons* for changing their behavior (*decisional balance*); the *processes of change* they used and how these compare to their previous assessment and the processes others have used to successfully change; their *self-efficacy*

in tempting situations; and the strategies that are most likely to help them take small steps toward the next stage.

- *Monthly newsletters*: These tailored mailings provided engaging educational information appropriate for the recipient's *stage of change*.

- *Coaching calls*: Participants also received phone calls from "personal behavior change coaches" who used brief motivational interviewing techniques matched to the participant's *stage of change* to help the participant enhance their *motivation* for change.

Evaluation

The SENIOR project was evaluated using validated dietary assessment measures from the National Cancer Institute as well as measures of stage of change, decisional balance, situational self-efficacy, and processes of change. Participants who received the SENIOR Project's fruit and vegetable intervention increased their fruit and vegetable intake by 0.5–1 serving more than the control group (who received a fall prevention intervention). In support of the transtheoretical model, the researchers found that TTM variables differed between participants who reached the maintenance stage or progressed in their stage of change and those who relapsed or failed to progress. Analyses further demonstrated that stimulus control and self-reevaluation had the strongest effect on increasing fruit and vegetable consumption, highlighting the importance of experiential processes in maintaining dietary change.

Data from Clark, P., C. Nigg, G. Greene, D. Riebe, S. Saunders, and SENIOR project team. 2002. The Study of Exercise and Nutrition in Older Rhode Islanders (SENIOR): translating theory into research. *Health Education Research* 17(5), 552–561.; Greene, G., N. Fey-Yensan, C. Padula, et al. 2008. Change in fruit and vegetable intake over 24 months in older adults: Results of the SENIOR project intervention. *Gerontologist* 48(3), 378–387.

program that focused on a healthy lifestyle approach to weight management that also included exercise. It was successful in promoting changes in exercise and dietary behaviors, weight loss, increased cardiorespiratory fitness, and improved lipid profiles (Riebe et al. 2003).

- *Study with adolescents*: A computer-based program for urban youth in after-school community programs tailored the intervention to the stages of change of the youth and vignettes, stories, and activities on the processes of change. It resulted in improved intakes of fruits and vegetables (Di Noia, Contento, and Prochaska 2008; Di Noia and Prochaska 2010b; DiNoia and Thompson 2012).

Stage-Matched Interventions with Groups

In a group or population-wide setting, nutrition educators cannot provide interventions that are specific to each individual's stage of readiness to change. However, assuming that there will be people at all stages of change in a group, educators can sequence activities in a stepwise fashion, as shown in the two examples here.

- *Study with college students*: One study with college students was delivered in a group setting (Finckenor and Byrd-Bredbenner 2000). The first half of the sessions focused on the processes of consciousness raising and emotional arousal. The later sessions focused on self-evaluation and social liberation, which included some skill building.
- *Worksite study to increase fruit and vegetable intake and reduce fat intake*: Activities were sequenced as follows:
  - Promotional activities to promote awareness and enhance motivation, targeting those in the pre-action stages
  - Action and skills training, targeting those in the action stage
  - Social support and maintenance of behavior
  - Environmental supports

Results showed that those in pre-action stages at baseline were much more likely to move into action and maintenance stages than were controls. Changes in stage were associated with decreases in fat intake and increases in fiber, fruit, and vegetable intake, for example (Glanz et al. 1998; Kristal et al. 2000).

TAKE-HOME MESSAGE ABOUT THE TRANSTHEORETICAL MODEL

- The transtheoretical model emphasizes that individuals are at different stages in terms of their readiness to engage in a health- or food-related behavior and that, consequently, nutrition education interventions must be designed to meet the needs of individuals at each stage of change. The majority of people are not ready for action in terms of healthy behaviors and will not be well served by traditional action-oriented programs.
- To enhance effectiveness, nutrition education interventions can address the determinants of change—pros and cons of change and self-efficacy—and base activities on the 10 processes of change, matched to the individual's or group's stage of change.

Using the Transtheoretical Model in Nutrition Education

The construct of stages of change, along with the determinants of pros and cons of change and self-efficacy, can be used to tailor nutrition education to individuals through a variety of media as described earlier (Prochaska, 2007, Di Noia and Prochaska 2010b). The 10 processes of change are also useful in nutrition education. **TABLE 5-4** describes in detail how transtheoretical model constructs are translated into educational strategies.

Summary

NUTRITION EDUCATION AS COACHING

Once convinced of the desirability, effectiveness, and feasibility of an action, individuals may state an intention to take action. However, to help individuals convert their intentions to action, nutrition educators can help individuals build on their abilities and skills to act on their motivations through coaching. This chapter focuses on facilitating the ability to take action. Several theories are useful here.

SOCIAL COGNITIVE THEORY

Social cognitive theory states that in addition to being convinced that performing a given behavior will be effective in leading to the outcome individuals desire, they must also

Table 5-4 Transtheoretical Model: Use in Nutrition Education Interventions

Stage of Readiness to Change	Important Processes for Moving to Next Stage	Nutrition Education Intervention Strategies
Precontemplation	Increased awareness, sense of risk, understanding, and recognition of emotional adjustments needed for change	Provide personalized information on own eating pattern for consciousness-raising (e.g., fruit and vegetable intake) through self-assessment and feedback (e.g., group 24-hour recall), personalize risk (e.g., through personal testimonials about losing a friend/loved one to heart attack), and help individuals understand and express emotions about the need for change (dramatic relief). Media: trigger films, personal testimonies, and media campaigns to address feelings and personalized risks.
Contemplation	Recognition of ambivalence but increased appreciation for benefits of behavior, and confidence in one's ability to enact the recommended behavior	Guided self-evaluation imagery to understand consequences of not adopting target behavior, strategies in groups to enhance people's pros/benefits of change (e.g., taste, health benefits, convenience), discuss barriers to change, assist individuals to recognize their own ambivalence, and provide positive feedback about individuals' current abilities and assets.
Preparation	Making a commitment to change; resolving ambivalence	Have individuals state goal intention (e.g., to eat more fruits and vegetables), develop specific action plans, and start taking small steps toward goal; reinforce attempts to change (self-liberation).
Action	Building skills and seeking social support	Teach food- and nutrition-specific knowledge and skills needed for behavior change, goal setting, and self-monitoring; provide encouragement and support; and encourage seeking of social support network (helping relationships).
Maintenance	Self-management and relapse prevention skills creating social and environmental support	Teach new ways of thinking about behavior (counterconditioning), restructuring environment, and rewarding themselves; anticipate and plan for potential difficult situations; create buddy systems; problem-solve if they lapse; and strengthen skills to advocate for environments that support healthful food practices.

believe that they can carry out the behavior even in the face of difficulties and setbacks. The environment both influences and is influenced by people's behaviors. Therefore, self-efficacy and skills are the major facilitators of change. Individuals need skills in self-regulation, which consist of setting action goals for themselves, also called action plans, and monitoring their progress toward their goals. They need food and nutrition knowledge and cognitive, affective, and behavioral skills that will enable them to achieve their goals. Nutrition education focuses on assisting audiences in *how-to* take action, using modeling, guided mastery, and interactive and generally hands-on activities. These skills help contribute to a sense of personal agency and empowerment so they can make active choices about their lives. Individuals also need a supportive environment and collective efficacy to work to change the environment.

SELF-REGULATION MODELS

Self-regulation models such as the health action process model emphasize that moving from intention to action requires moving from a thinking mind-set to a doing mind-set and that planning and self-efficacy are both central and synergistic in this process—self-efficacy to initiate action and coping self-efficacy to maintain action. Nutrition education can thus focus on helping individuals set realistic action goals and develop strategies to cope with distractions so as to maintain the behavior change. Mindfulness and planning are also important here.

TRANSTHEORETICAL MODEL

The transtheoretical model emphasizes that individuals are at different stages in terms of their readiness to engage in a health- or food-related behavior and that consequently, nutrition education interventions must be designed to meet the needs of individuals at each stage of change. The determinants of change are the pros and cons of change and self-efficacy. To enhance effectiveness, nutrition education interventions can base activities on the 10 processes of change, matched to the individual's or group's stage of change.

OVERALL FOCUS FOR NUTRITION EDUCATION TO FACILITATE BEHAVIOR CHANGE AND ACTION

Nutrition educators' main focus in this component of nutrition education is to assist individuals to develop relevant food and nutrition-related skills, skills in choosing and directing their own behaviors, including goal setting and planning, and developing personal food policies to cope with their life situations and to maintain the changes they have sought. The desired result of this process is empowered individuals, able to act on their own desired behavior changes.

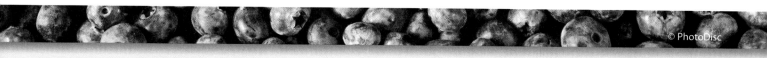

© PhotoDisc

Questions and Activities

1. Social cognitive theory is widely used in nutrition education and health promotion. Why do you think this is so—what specific features of the theory make it so useful?

2. Find a friend or relative who has recently been *successful at making a change* to an eating behavior and/or has started exercising more. Interview this person (take notes during the interview). Ask him or her to describe *specifically what he or she did to be successful at making the change*. Ask the person to share any thoughts on how he or she *plans to maintain this change in the future*.

   a. Write about *what made this person successful* using the language of social cognitive theory and the transtheoretical model. Discuss some of the following: the knowledge and skills the person learned in order to increase chances of success, how the person's self-efficacy increased, the self-regulation

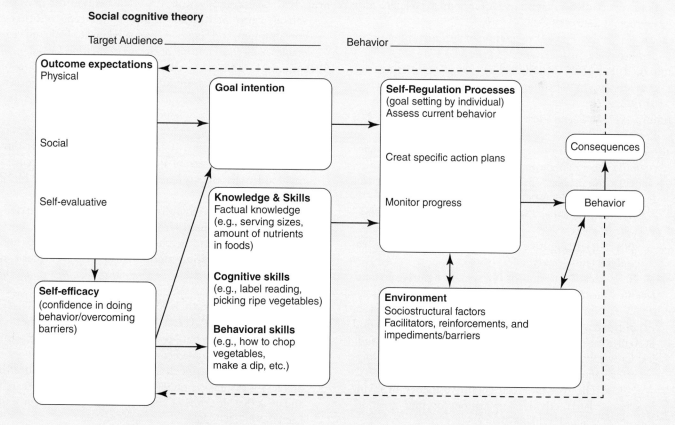

techniques the person used, the "processes of change" that were important, and anything else that helped increase success.

   b. Look at Box 5-3 and discuss if your interviewee is using any of these strategies to *maintain the change*. Any other strategies? If you want, share some of these strategies with your interviewee and write about if the person thought these strategies would be helpful.

3. What strategies can be used to increase self-efficacy in individuals?

4. Why is action goal setting (or stating action plans) so important? What does it accomplish? What are some key steps?

5. Describe an instance where you used SMART action goals to make a dietary or physical activity change yourself. What were your reactions? How effective was the procedure for you?

6. You have been asked to provide a nutrition education session with a group of young adults. Choose a behavior you will focus on. Plan the session using social cognitive theory by completing the diagram on the previous page.

References

Abraham, C., P. Sheeran, and M. Johnson. 1998. From health beliefs to self-regulation: Theoretical advances in the psychology of action control. *Psychology and Health* 13:569–591.

Ahlers-Schmidt C. R., T. Hart, A. Chesser, A. Paschal, T. Nguyen, R. R. Wittler. 2011. Content of text messaging immunization reminders: What low-income parents want to know. *Patient Education and Counseling* 5(1):119–121.

Armitage, C. J. 2004. Evidence that implementation intentions reduce dietary fat intake: A randomized trial. *Health Psychology* 23(3):319–323.

Bagozzi, R. P. 1992. The self-regulation of attitudes, intentions, and behavior. *Social Science Quarterly* 55:178–204.

Bagozzi, R. P. and U. M. Dholakia. 1999. Goal setting and goal striving in consumer behavior. *Journal of Marketing* 63:19-32.

Bandura, A. 1977. *Social learning theory*. Englewood Cliffs, NJ: Prentice Hall.

———. 1986. *Foundations of thought and action: A social cognitive theory*. Englewood Cliffs, NJ: Prentice Hall.

———. 1989. Human agency in social cognitive theory. *American Psychologist* 44:1175–1184.

———. 1997. *Self efficacy: The exercise of control*. New York: WH Freeman.

———. 2001. Social cognitive theory: An agentic perspective. *Annual Review of Psychology* 51:1–26.

———. 2004. Health promotion by social cognitive means. *Health Education and Behavior* 31(2):143–164.

Berlin L., K. Norris, J. Kolodinsky, and A. Nelson. 2013a. Farm-to-school: Implications for child nutrition. Food System Research Collaborative, Center for Rural Studies, University of Vermont. *Opportunities for Agriculture Working Paper Series* 1:1.

———. 2013b. The role of social cognitive theory in farm-to-school-related activities: implications for child nutrition. *Journal of School Health* 83:589–595.

Bisogni, C. A., M. Jastran, M. Seligson, and A. Thompson. 2012. How people interpret healthy eating: Contributions of qualitative research. *Journal of Nutrition Education and Behavior* 44(4):282–301.

Boudreaux, E. D., K. B. Wood, D. Mehan, I. Scarinci, C. L. Taylor, and P. J. Brantley. 2003. Congruence of readiness to change, self-efficacy, and decisional balance for physical activity and dietary fat reduction. *American Journal of Health Promotion* 17(5):329–336.

Brug, J., K. Glanz, and G. Kok. 1997. The relationship between self-efficacy, attitudes, intake compared to others, consumption, and stages of change related to fruit and vegetables. *American Journal of Health Promotion* 12(1):25–30.

Buchanan, H., and N. S. Coulson. 2007. Consumption of carbonated drinks in adolescents: A transtheoretical analysis. *Child Care and Health Development* 33(4):441–447.

Campbell, M. K., L. Honess-Morreale, D. Farrell, E. Carbone, and M. Brasure. 1999. A tailored multimedia nutrition education pilot program for low-income women receiving food assistance. *Health Education Research* 14(2):257–267.

Campbell, M. K., M. Symons, W. Demark-Wahnefried, B. Polhamus, J. M. Bernhardt, J. W. McClelland, et al. 1998. Stages of change and psychosocial correlates of fruit and vegetable consumption among rural African-American church members. *American Journal of Health Promotion* 12(3):185–191.

Campbell, M. K., I. Tessaro, B. DeVellis, S. Benedict, K. Kelsey, L. Belton, et al. 2002. Effects of a tailored health promotion program for female blue-collar workers: Health Works for Women. *Preventive Medicine* 34(3):313–323.

Carbone E. T., and J. M. Zoellner. 2012. Nutrition and health literacy: A systematic review to inform nutrition research and practice. *Journal of the Academy of Nutrition and Dietetics* 112:254–265.

Chapman-Novakofski, K., and J. Karduck. 2005. Improvement in knowledge, social cognitive theory variables, and movement through stages of change after a community-based diabetes education program. *Journal of the American Dietetic Association* 105(10):1613–1616.

Coleman K. J., C. L. Tiller, J. Sanchez, E. M. Heath, O. Sy, G. Milliken, et al. 2005. Prevention of the epidemic increase in child risk of overweight in low-income schools: The El Paso coordinated approach to child health. *Archives of Pediatric and Adolescent Medicine* 159(3):217–224.

Connors, M., C. A. J. Sobal, and C. M. Devine. 2001. Managing values in personal food systems. *Appetite* 36(3):189–200.

Contento, I. R., P. A. Koch, A. Calabrese-Barton, H. Lee, and W. Sauberli. 2007. Enhancing personal agency and competence in eating and moving: Formative evaluation of a middle school curriculum—Choice, Control, and Change. *Journal of Nutrition Education and Behavior* 39:S179–S186.

Contento I. R., P. A. Koch, H. Lee, and A. Calabrese-Barton. 2010. Adolescents demonstrate improvement in obesity risk behaviors after completion of Choice, Control and Change, a curriculum addressing personal agency and autonomous motivation. *Journal of the American Dietetic Association* 110(12):1830–1839.

Contento, I. R., S. S. Williams, J. L. Michela, and A. B. Franklin. 2006. Understanding the food choice process of adolescents in the context of family and friends. *Journal of Adolescent Health* 38(5):575–582.

Cullen, K. W., T. Baranowski, and S. P. Smith. 2001. Using goal setting as a strategy for dietary behavior change. *Journal of the American Dietetic Association* 101(5):562–566.

De Bourdeaudhuij, I., J. Brug, C. Vandelanotte, and P. Van Oost. 2002. Differences in impact between a family- versus an individual-based tailored intervention to reduce fat intake. *Health Education Research* 17(4):435–449.

De Bourdeaudhuij, I., V. Stevens, C. Vandelanotte, and J. Brug. 2007. Evaluation of an interactive computer-tailored nutrition intervention in a real-life setting. *Annals of Behavorial Medicine* 33(1):39–48.

De Nooijer, J., E. de Vet, J. Brug, and N. K. de Vries. 2006. Do implementation intentions help to turn good intentions into higher fruit intakes? *Journal of Nutrition Education and Behavior* 38(1):25–29.

Di Noia, J., I. R. Contento, and J. O. Prochaska. 2008. Intervention tailored on Transtheoretical Model stages and processes of change increases fruit and vegetable consumption among economically disadvantaged African American adolescents. *American Journal of Health Promotion* 22: 336–341.

Di Noia, J., and J. O. Prochaska. 2010a. Dietary change and decisional balance: A meta-analytic review. *American Journal of Health Behavior* 34(5):618–632.

———. 2010b. Mediating variables in a transtheoretical model dietary change intervention program. *Health Education and Behavior* 37(5):753–762.

Di Noia, J., and D. Thompson. 2012. Processes of change for increasing fruit and vegetable consumption among economically disadvantaged African American adolescents. *Eating Behavior* 13(1):58–61.

Finckenor, M., and C. Byrd-Bredbenner. 2000. Nutrition intervention group program based on preaction-stage-oriented change processes of the Transtheoretical Model promotes long-term reduction in dietary fat intake. *Journal of the American Dietetic Association* 100(3):335–342.

Fordyce-Voorham, S. 2011. Identification of essential food skills for skill-based healthful eating programs in secondary schools. *Journal of Nutrition Education and Behavior* 43(2):116–122.

Furst T., M. Connors, C. A. Bisogni, J. Sobal, and L. W. Falk. 1996. Food choice: a conceptual model of the process. *Appetite* 26:247–266.

Gaines, A., L. W. Turner. 2009. Improving fruit and vegetable intake among children: A review of interventions utilizing the social cognitive theory. *California Journal of Health Promotion* 7(1):52–66.

Gardner, T.W., T. J. Dishion, A. M. Connell. 2007. Adolescent self-regulation as resilience: Resistance to antisocial behavior within the deviant peer context. *Journal of Abnormal Child Psychology* 36:273–284.

Glanz, K., A. R. Kristal, B. C. Tilley, and K. Hirst. 1998. Psychosocial correlates of healthful diets among male auto workers. *Cancer Epidemiology, Biomarkers, and Prevention* 7(2):119–126.

Gollwitzer, P. M. 1999. Implementation intentions—strong effects of simple plans. *American Psychologist* 54:493–503.

Gollwitzer, P. M., and P. Sheeran. 2006. Implementation intentions and goal achievement: A meta-analysis of effects and processes. *Advances in Experimental Social Psychology* 38:69–119.

Greene, G. W., S. R. Rossi, J. S. Rossi, W. F. Velicer, J. L. Fava, and J. O. Prochaska. 1999. Dietary applications of the stages of change model. *Journal of the American Dietetic Association* 99(6):673–678.

Hanks, A. S., D. R. Just, and B. Wansink. 2013. Smarter lunchrooms can address new school lunchroom guidelines and childhood obesity. *Journal of Pediatrics* 162:867–869.

Heneman, K., A. Block-Joy, S. Zidenberg-Cherr, et al. 2005. A "contract for change" increases produce consumption in low-income women: A pilot study. *Journal of the American Dietetic Association* 105(11):1793–1796.

Henry, H., K. Reimer, C. Smith, and M. Reicks. 2006. Associations of decisional balance, processes of change, and self-efficacy with stages of change for increased fruit and vegetable intake among low-income, African-American mothers. *Journal of the American Dietetic Association* 106(6):841–849.

Hoelscher D. M., A. E. Springer, N. Ranjit, C. L. Perry, A. E. Evans, M. Stigler, et al. 2010. Reductions in child obesity among disadvantaged school children with community involvement: The Travis County CATCH trial. *Obesity* 18(1 Suppl):S36–S44.

Hoisington, A., J. A. Shultz, and S. Butkus. 2002. Coping strategies and nutrition education needs among food pantry users. *Journal of Nutrition Education and Behavior* 34(6):226–233.

Horowitz, M., M. K. Shilts, and M. S. Townsend. 2004. EatFit: A goal-oriented intervention that challenges adolescents to improve their eating and fitness choices. *Journal of Nutrition Education and Behavior* 36(1):43–44.

Horwath, C. C., S. M. Schembre, R. W. Motl, R. K. Dishman, and C. R. Nigg. 2013. Does the Transtheoretical Model of behavior change provide a useful basis for interventions to promote fruit and vegetable consumption? *American Journal of Health Promotion* 27(6):351–357.

Institute of Medicine. 2004. *Health literacy: A prescription to end confusion*. Washington, DC: National Academies Press.

Iwaki, T. J., J. D. Gussow, I. R. Contento, I. S. Goodell. 2014. Gateway to Green: The family experience of community supported agriculture. *Journal of Nutrition Education and Behavior* 46(4 Suppl):P202.

Jacobs, A. D., A. S. Ammerman, S. T. Ennett, M. K. Campbell, K. W. Tawney, S. A. Aytur, et al. 2004. Effects of a tailored follow-up intervention on health behaviors, beliefs, and attitudes. *Journal of Women's Health* 13(5):557–568.

Jastran, M. M., C. A. Bisogni, J. Sobal, C. Blake, and C. M. Devine. 2009. Eating routines. Embedded, value based, modifiable, and reflective. *Appetite* 52(1):127–136.

Kavookjian, J., B. A. Berger, D. M. Grimley, W. A. Villaume, H. M. Anderson, and K. N. Barker. 2005. Patient decision making: Strategies for diabetes diet adherence intervention. *Research in Social and Administrative Pharmacy* 1(3):389–407.

Koring, M., J. Richert, S. Lippke, L. Parschau, T. Reuter, and R. Schwarzer. 2012. Synergistic effects of planning and self-efficacy on physical activity. *Health Education & Behavior* 39:152–158.

Kreausukon, P., P. Gellert, S. Lippke, and R. Schwarzer. 2012. Planning and self-efficacy can increase fruit and vegetable consumption: A randomized controlled trial. *Journal of Behavioral Medicine* 35:443–451.

Kristal, A. R., K. Glanz, B. C. Tilley, and S. Li. 2000. Mediating factors in dietary change: Understanding the impact of a worksite nutrition intervention. *Health Education and Behavior* 27(1):112–125.

Kuhn, D. (2008). Adolescent thinking. In *Handbook of Adolescent Psychology*, 3rd ed., edited by R. M. Lerner and L. Steinberg. Hoboken, NJ: John Wiley and Sons, pp. 152–186.

Lange, D., J. Richert, M. Koring, N. Knoll, R. Schwarzer, and S. Lippke. 2013. Self-regulation prompts can increase fruit consumption: A one-hour randomized controlled online trial. *Psychology & Health* 28(5):533–545.

Lefebvre, R. C., and A. S. Bornkessel. 2013. Digital social networks and health. *Circulation* 127(17):1829–1836.

Lippke, S., J. P. Ziegelmann, R. Schwarzer, and W. F. Velicer. 2009. Validity of stage assessment in the adoption and maintenance of physical activity and fruit and vegetable consumption. *Health Psychology* 28(2):183–193.

Luepker, R. V., C. L. Perry, S. M. McKinlay, et al. 1996. Outcomes of a field trial to improve children's dietary patterns and physical activity. The Child and Adolescent Trial for Cardiovascular Health. CATCH Collaborative Group. *Journal of the American Medical Association* 275(10):768–776.

Ma, J., N. M. Betts, T. Horacek, C. Georgiou, A. White, and S. Nitzke. 2002. The importance of decisional balance and self-efficacy in relation to stages of change for fruit and vegetable intakes by young adults. *American Journal of Health Promotion* 16(3):157–166.

Molaison, E. F., C. L. Connell, J. E. Stuff, M. K. Yadrick, and M. Bogle. 2005. Influences on fruit and vegetable consumption by low-income black American adolescents. *Journal of Nutrition Education and Behavior* 37(5):246–251.

O'Donnell, S., G. W. Greene, and B. Blissmer. 2014. The effect of goal setting on fruit and vegetable consumption and physical activity level in a web-based intervention. *Journal of Nutrition Education and Behavior* 46(6):570–575.

Oenema, A., F. Tan, and J. Brug. 2005. Short-term efficacy of a Web-based computer-tailored nutrition intervention: Main effects and mediators. *Annals of Behavioral Medicine* 29(1):54–63.

O'Hea, E. L., E. D. Boudreaux, S. K. Jeffries, C. L. Carmack Taylor, I. C. Scarinci, and P. J. Brantley. 2004. Stage of change movement across three health behaviors: The role of self-efficacy. *American Journal of Health Promotion* 19(2):94–102.

Osborne, H. 2005. *Health literacy from A to Z: Practical ways to communicate your health message*. Sudbury, MA: Jones and Bartlett.

Park, A., S. Nitzke, K. Kritsch, K. Kattelmann, A. White, L. Boecknr, et al. 2008. Internet-based interventions have potential to affect short-term mediators and indicators of dietary behavior of young adults. *Journal of Nutrition Education and Behavior* 40(5):288–297.

Prochaska, J. M. 2007. The transtheoretical model applied to the community and the workplace. *Journal of Health Psychology* 12(1):198–200.

Prochaska, J. O., and C. C. DiClemente. 1984. *The transtheoretical approach: Crossing the traditional boundaries of therapy*. Homewood, IL: Dow Jones-Irwin.

Prochaska, J. O., C. C. DiClemente, and J. C. Norcross. 1992. In search of how people change. Applications to addictive behaviors. *American Psychologist* 47(9):1102–1114.

Prochaska, J. O., C. C. DiClemente, W. F. Velicer, and J. S. Rossi. 1993. Standardized, individualized, interactive, and personalized self-help programs for smoking cessation. *Health Psychology* 12(5):399–405.

Prochaska, J. O., and W. F. Velicer. 1997. The transtheoretical model of health behavior change. *American Journal of Health Promotion* 12(1):38–48.

Renwick, K. 2013. Food literacy as a form of critical pedagogy: implications for curriculum development and pedagogical engagement for Australia's diverse student population. *Home Economics Victoria Journal* 52(20):6–17.

Riebe, D., G. W. Greene, L. Ruggiero, K. M. Stillwell, and C. R. Nigg. 2003. Evaluation of a healthy-lifestyle approach to weight management. *Preventive Medicine* 36(1):45–54.

Rosen, C. S. 2000. Is the sequencing of change processes by stage consistent across health problems? A meta-analysis. *Health Psychology* 19:593–604.

Rothbart, M. K., L. K. Ellis, and M. I. Posner. 2013. Temperament and self-regulation. In *Handbook of self-regulation: Research, theory and applications*, edited by K. D. Vohs and R. F. Baumeister. New York, NY: The Guilford Press, pp. 441–460.

Salmela, S., M. Poskiparta, K. Kasila, K. Vahasarja, and M. Vanhala. 2009. Transtheoretical model-based dietary interventions in primary care: A review of the evidence in diabetes. *Health Education Research* 24(2):237–252.

Scholz, U., B. Schuz, J. P. Ziegelmann, S. Lippke, and R. Schwarzer. 2008. Beyond behavioural intentions: Planning mediates between intentions and physical activity. *British Journal of Health Psychology* 13(Pt 3):479–494.

Schwarzer, R., and R. Fuchs. 1995. Self-efficacy and health behaviors. In *Predicting health behavior*, edited by M. Conner and P. Norman. Buckingham, UK: Open University Press.

Schwarzer, R., and B. Renner. 2000. Social-cognitive predictors of health behavior: Action self-efficacy and coping self-efficacy. *Health Psychology* 19(5):487–495.

Schwarzer, R., B. Schuz, J. P. Ziegelmann, S. Lippke, A. Luszczynska, and U. Scholz. 2007. Adoption and maintenance of four health behaviors: Theory-guided longitudinal studies on dental flossing, seat belt use, dietary behavior, and physical activity. *Annals of Behavioral Medicine* 33(2):156–166.

Shilts, M. K., M. Horowitz, and M. S. Townsend. 2004a. Goal setting as a strategy for dietary and physical activity behavior change: A review of the literature. *American Journal of Health Promotion* 19(2):81–93.

———. 2004b. An innovative approach to goal setting for adolescents: Guided goal setting. *Journal of Nutrition Education and Behavior* 36(3):155.

———. 2009. Guided goal setting: Effectiveness in a dietary and physical activity intervention with low-income adolescents. *International Journal of Adolescent Medicine and Health* 21(1):111–122.

Silk, K. J., J. Sherry, B. Winn, N. Keesecker, M. A. Horodynski, and A. Sayir. 2008. Increasing nutrition literacy: Testing the effectiveness of print, Web site, and game modalities. *Journal of Nutrition Education and Behavior* 40(1):3–10.

Sniehotta, F. F. 2009. Towards a theory of intentional behavior change: Plans, planning, and self-regulation. *British Journal of Health Psychology* 14:261–273.

Sniehotta, F. F., U. R. Scholz, and R. Schwarzer. 2005. Bridging the intention–behaviour gap: Planning, self-efficacy, and action control in the adoption and maintenance of physical exercise. *Psychology and Health* 20:143–160.

Sporny, L. A., and I. R. Contento. 1995. Stages of change in dietary fat reduction: Social psychological correlates. *Journal of Nutrition Education* 27:191–199.

Stadler, G., G. Oettingen, and P. M. Gollwitzer. 2010. Intervention effects of information and self-regulation on eating fruits and vegetables. *Health Psychology* 29(3):274–283.

Sternfeld, B., C. Block, C. P. Quesenberry Jr., G. Husson, J. C. Norris, M. Nelson, et al. 2009. Improving diet and physical activity with ALIVE: A worksite randomized trial. *American Journal of Preventive Medicine* 36(6):475–483.

Tam, L., R. P. Bagozzi, and J. Spaniol. 2010. When planning is not enough: The self-regulatory effect of implementation intentions on changing snacking. *Health Psychology* 29(3):284–292.

Taylor, S. D., R. P. Bagozzi, and C. A. Gaither. 2005. Decision making and effort in the self-regulation of hypertension: Testing two competing theories. *British Journal of Health Psychology* 10(Pt 4):505–530.

U.S. Department of Agriculture. 2014. Farm to institution initiatives. http://www.usda.gov/documents/6-Farmtoinstitution.pdf Accessed 1/14/15.

Velicer, W. F., and J. O. Prochaska. 1999. An expert system intervention for smoking cessation. *Patient Education and Counseling* 36(2):119–129.

Verplanken, B., and S. Faes. 1999. Good intentions, bad habits, and effects of forming implementation intentions on healthy eating. *European Journal of Social Psychology* 29:591–604.

Vidgen, H. A. and D. Gallegos. 2014. Food literacy and its components. *Appetite* 76:50–59.

Wansink B., D. R. Just, C. R. Payne, and M. Z. Klinger. 2012. Attractive names sustain increased vegetable intake in schools. *Preventive Medicine* 55(4):330–332.

Wiedemann, A. U., S. Lippke, T. Reuter, B. Schuz, J. P. Ziegelmann, and R. Schwarzer. 2009. Prediction of stage transitions in fruit and vegetable intake. *Health Education Research* 24(4):596–607.

Wiedemann, A. U., B. Schuz, F. Sniehotta, U. Scholz, and R. Schwarzer. 2009. Disentangling the relation between intentions, planning, and behavior: A moderated mediation analysis. *Psychology and Health* 24(1):67–79.

Wright, J. A., W. F. Velicer, and J. O. Prochaska. 2009. Testing the predictive power of the transtheoretical model of behavior change applied to dietary fat intake. *Health Education Research* 24(2):224–236.

Young, M. D., R. C. Plotnikoff, C. E. Collins, R. Callister, and P. J. Morgan. 2014. Social cognitive theory and physical activity: A systematic review and meta-analysis. *Obesity Reviews* 15(12):983–995.

Ziegelmann, J. P., and S. Lippke. 2007. Planning and strategy use in health behavior change: A life span view. *International Journal of Behavioral Medicine* 14(1):30–39.

Ziegelmann, J. P., S. Lippke, and R. Schwarzer. 2006. Adoption and maintenance of physical activity: Planning interventions in young, middle-aged, and older adults. *Psychology and Health* 21:145–163.

Zoellner, J., C. Connell, W. Bounds, L. Crook, K. Yadrick. 2009. Nutrition literacy status and preferred nutrition communication channels among adults in the lower Mississippi delta. *Preventing Chronic Disease* 6(4):A128.

Zoellner, J., W. You, C. Connell, R. L Smith-Ray, K. Allen, K. L. Tucker et al. 2011. Health literacy is associated with Healthy Eating Index scores and sugar-sweetened beverage intake: Findings for the Lower Mississippi Delta. *Journal of the American Dietetic Association* 111(7):1012–1020.

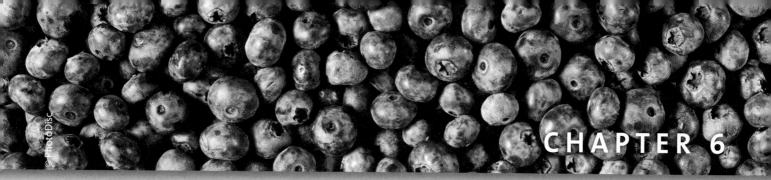

CHAPTER 6

Promoting Environmental Supports for Behavior Change

OVERVIEW

The focus of this chapter is on strategies for promoting environmental supports for individuals' motivation and ability to make healthful behavior changes based on a social ecological model. A logic model is introduced as a framework for planning strategies at the interpersonal, institutional, community, and public policy levels of influence and may involve policy, social systems, and environmental change activities.

CHAPTER OUTLINE

- Environmental support to make healthful choices easier
- A social ecological approach
- Interpersonal-level social environment change: family, peers, and social networks
- Environmental settings: strategies for organizational-level change
- Environmental settings: community-level activities for change
- Sectors of influence: policy and systems change activities
- A logic model approach for planning nutrition education
- Summary

LEARNING OBJECTIVES

At the end of the chapter, you should be able to:

- Describe key features of a social ecological model for promoting healthful diets and active living, within environmental settings and involving several levels of influence
- Appreciate the important role nutrition educators can serve as environmental and policy change agents by working in collaboration with others
- Describe effective strategies that nutrition educators can use, by collaborating with others, to address interpersonal, organizational, community, and policy and systems determinants of behavior to support people's

motivation and ability to change their behaviors and take action
- Define the concepts of social support, collaboration, and community capacity building and show how they have been used for promoting environmental and policy supports for behavior change or action
- Describe ways to evaluate environmental and policy activities that are designed to support behavior change goals
- Evaluate the relationship between education and policy for fostering behavior change or action

Environmental Support to Make Healthful Choices Easier

Our nutrition education efforts may enhance the motivation of our audiences as to *why-to* take action and help them bridge the intention to action gap by empowering them with needed nutrition-related and goal setting skills for *how-to* take action, but the environments in which they live and work may present considerable challenges to carry out their desired actions.

High-calorie foods are everywhere, convenient, and cheap; escalators and elevators are ubiquitous; and attractive and safe parks are not readily available. The desired foods may not be available at a price people can afford or accessible when they need them, and their actions may be constrained by what other members of their families do, by the norms and practices in their communities, by policies at their schools or places of work, and by the structure of their communities. All of this makes it difficult to eat healthfully and be physically active even when people have the intention to do so.

This leads us to the importance of the third function of nutrition education in our framework: promoting environmental and policy supports for behavior change and action. We need to seek ways to make the healthful actions the easy ones. For our case examples discussed previously—Maria, Alicia, and Ray—environmental supports and policy changes were very helpful as they tried to carry out their chosen food and activity action plans: Maria joined a support group and loved it; Alicia found that calorie counts on the menu boards of fast food restaurants were helpful; and Ray found that changes in his workplace made it easier to eat healthfully. We explore their experiences in greater detail later.

Many nations are concerned about the high rates of obesity and chronic disease—in some countries occurring alongside malnutrition—and have increasingly recognized that the environment has a hand in this situation. From government policymakers to public health officials to food companies, all say that they are interested in being part of the solution rather than part of the problem.

There is growing awareness within the food and nutrition profession that changes in environments can help to make food and activity choices easier. Expanding community nutrition education to include such changes is increasingly being embraced as part of the role of nutrition educators (Hill, Dickin, and Dollahite 2012;

Chipman 2013). This role of nutrition educator as change agent in the community and beyond presents exciting possibilities and also new challenges because it requires new approaches and different skills from those associated with traditional nutrition education interventions (Lu, Dickin, and Dollahite 2012). Studies have shown that these new approaches and skills can be incorporated into the roles of nutrition educators (Dickin and Dollahite 2012) but may require additional training and new job descriptions.

In this chapter we describe ways in which nutrition educators can help foster policies, social systems, and environments that are supportive of the behavioral goals established for a program. We first examine social and physical environmental and policy determinants that facilitate behavior change. We then examine recent studies that suggest strategies for promoting environments that are supportive of the targeted behavioral goals.

DEFINING TERMS

First, we need to define some terms. The terms *environment* and *ecology* can have different meanings in different contexts.

Environment

The field of health promotion uses the term *environment* to refer to factors that are external to the individual. It refers not only to the physical environment, but also the social environment. For example, our *social networks* of important others are external to us and are therefore considered environmental determinants of behavior change. On the other hand, a *social norm* is a perception that influences behavior but is not classified as an environmental determinant of behavior because it is our perception of the environment and is not external to us. Culturally based community practices and social structures such as family meals or community holiday practices are also considered part of the environment.

Environmental interventions are those that involve strategies for changing the social environment, physical surroundings, information environment, organizational systems, or policy to provide support for healthy eating and active living.

Ecology and Social Ecology

The term *ecology* is derived from the biology literature, where it refers to the relationship between organisms and their natural environments. Within the field of food and nutrition, it usually also refers to issues related to food and the natural environment, such as the impact of agricultural practices on the amount of carbon dioxide in the atmosphere, or carbon footprint.

In the health promotion field, the contexts in which people live are called *social ecologies*. Thus, social ecological models refer to approaches that address several social ecologies or levels of influence on behavior change or action at once. These levels are often labeled intrapersonal factors, interpersonal processes and primary groups, institutional factors, community factors, and social structures and public policy (McLeroy et al. 1988; Green and Kreuter 2004; Story et al. 2008). In the social ecological model, activities and initiatives are designed to change institutions, communities, policies, and legislation in order to foster individual, family, and community health. Such social ecological approaches to intervention thus address environmental determinants in addition to personal determinants of behaviors and behavior change.

Policy

Policy activities are part of environmental influences on action. *Policy* usually refers to a deliberate plan of action to guide decisions and achieve rational outcomes. Policies can be seen as the arrangement of political, management, and financial mechanisms to reach specified goals—a set of rules and understandings that govern behavior and practice. Institutions, organizations, and corporations all have such *institutional policies*. *Public policy* usually refers to a course of action taken by governmental entities with respect to a particular issue or set of issues—a set of agreements about how government will make decisions about societal needs and spend public funds.

How Might the Environment Influence Individuals?

The physical availability and accessibility of healthful foods and the means to be physically active are, of course, paramount for healthful living. That is the *direct* way environments affect people's food choices. The fact that healthful foods are present, though, does not mean that people will eat them. The environment also affects individuals' actions or behaviors in *indirect* ways through conscious and unconscious processes (Kremers et al. 2006).

- *Conscious processes.* Here the environment impacts behavior through impacts on conscious beliefs and attitudes. For example, the lack of healthful foods in a neighborhood may reduce people's sense of *self-efficacy* or perceived control, and high prices for such foods may result in a negative *attitude* toward healthful foods.

- *Unconscious processes.* These processes operate through an automatic or "mindless" route in which behaviors are automatically elicited by the environment through environment–behavior links (Wansink 2006). This route exists because our cognitive capacity is limited and automatic processes free our conscious capacity from having to consider, make choices, and deal with every aspect of our lives all the time. We automatically and unconsciously engage in many actions in response to environmental cues. For example, whenever there is an advertising break in a television program, many people head for the refrigerator for a snack. In addition, marketing practices and environmental cues are often arranged in order to unconsciously influence our choices. Many purchases in supermarkets are unplanned and, of those, about two-thirds are influenced by visual displays and other marketing devices (Abratt and Goodey 1990). The exact same dinner tastes better if we like the person with whom we are dining. Restaurant ambiance and how the food is described on the menu also can influence the amount people spend on food and drink (Wansink 2006; Cohen 2008). Many cultural expectations about foods to eat as well as when and where are habitual and unconscious. Thus, even with motivation, knowledge, and skills, people often still face difficulties in changing their behaviors or taking action because of automatic, unconscious responses to the environment. Consequently, the environment must be addressed if nutrition education is to be effective.

A Social Ecological Approach

Dietary behaviors are complex and the influences on them are many, as we saw in Chapter 2. Nutrition education is more likely to be successful if it focuses on specific behaviors or actions related to an issue of concern, identifies the determinants of these behaviors or actions, uses theory to design strategies to address them, and attends to the multiple levels of influences on these behaviors.

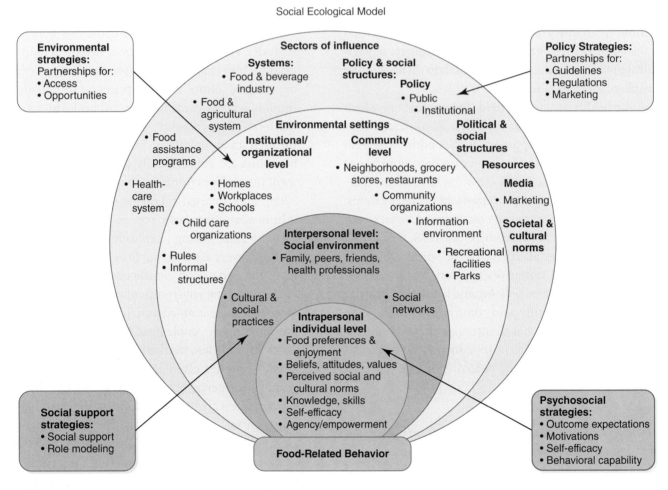

FIGURE 6-1 Social ecological model: Strategies at different levels of intervention.

Data from Dietary Guidelines for Americans. 2010. http://www.dietaryguidelines.gov; Story, M., K. M. Kaphingst, R. O'Brien, and K. Glanz. 2008. Creating healthy food and eating environments: Policy and environmental approaches. *Annual Review of Public Health* 29:253–272.

Different theories and strategies are relevant for the different levels of intervention directed at specifically identified behaviors or practices, as shown in **FIGURE 6-1**.

Individual-Level Determinants of Behavior Change

Many psychosocial influences are determinants of individuals' behaviors. As shown in Figure 6-1, nutrition education at this level focuses on enhancing motivations based on beliefs about benefits (or outcome expectations) and affective attitudes for why-to change behavior or take action; food- and nutrition-related skills for how-to change behavior (called behavioral capability); self-efficacy or confidence in being able to change behavior; and self-regulation or self-direction skills for how-to make conscious choices and direct our own behaviors, with a focus on goal setting

or action planning. The nutrition education strategies appropriate for intervention at this level, along with their theory base, are described in great detail in chapters 4 and 5, and hence will not be described here.

Interpersonal-Level Influences and Social Support

Approaches at this level use our understandings about people's families, friends, and other social networks to help to provide social support for the goal behaviors of the program. Strategies might include creating support groups for the program participants, conducting facilitated group dialogues where members support each other, working with **peer educators**, role modeling, shaping social norms, or developing family components to support school- and worksite-based programs.

Environmental Settings: Organizational and Community Level

Our role as nutrition educators in these settings is first to educate decision-makers and leaders in organizations and communities about the importance of issues that are the focus of our programs and then to develop collaborations with them to bring about change. This will involve the active engagement of nutrition educators in coalitions or partnerships with organizations and agencies to bring about access, availability, and opportunities in our program participants' food and activity environments.

Sectors of Influence: Policies, Systems, and Social Structures

Creating supportive policies and changes in social structures and systems usually requires that nutrition educators educate new audiences about the importance of actions or issues of concern and work in collaborations and partnerships with them so as to bring about supportive action. These new audiences may include those who have decision-making power and authority in other fields that affect the lives of program participants, such as school and workplace administrators, community leaders, policymakers, legislators, and regulators. The policy actions include developing guidelines, regulations, legislation, and changes in the media environment.

This chapter explores each of these levels of influence in greater detail. Studies show that activities directed at the individual, the physical, and the social and policy environments are important for behavior change because the barriers to healthful eating are both personal and environmental. In addition, this chapter discusses nutrition education and other strategies that can be used to address these levels of influence.

USING A SOCIAL ECOLOGICAL MODEL TO ASSESS AND DESIGN INTERVENTION: THE INTERNATIONAL PRO CHILDREN PROJECT

An example of how the social ecological model can be used to design an intervention to provide multilevel support for behavior change is the Pro Children Project. Its purpose was to design, implement, and evaluate an intervention program, applicable across nine European countries, for promoting consumption of fruits and vegetables among schoolchildren and their parents (Klepp et al. 2005). In order to design the intervention, the researchers first conducted a careful and comprehensive assessment using the social ecological model shown in **FIGURE 6-2**. They

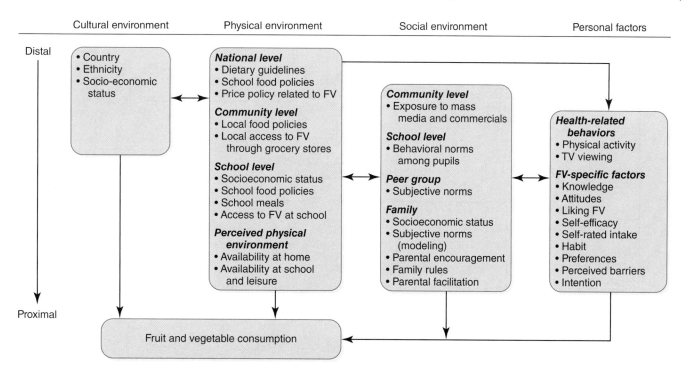

FIGURE 6-2 Social ecological framework applied to the Pro Children project for increasing fruit and vegetable consumption in children.

Reproduced from Klepp, K-I., C. Perez-Rodrigo, I. De Boureauhuij, et al. 2005. Promoting fruit and vegetable consumption among European schoolchildren: Rationale, conceptualization and design of the Pro Children project. *Annals of Nutrition and Metabolism* 49:212–221.

collected information on children's fruit and vegetable intakes as well as personal, social, and environmental determinants of these intakes. A theory-based intervention was then created using these determinants and implemented in these countries (Sandvik et al. 2007). Program activities included provision of fruits and vegetables in schools, guided classroom activities, computer-tailored feedback and advice for children, and activities completed at home with the family. Additionally, optional intervention components for community reinforcement included incorporation of mass media, school health services, or grocery stores. School project committees were supported (Perez-Rodrigo et al. 2005). The intervention led to positive results in some countries, particularly for fruit (Te Velde et al. 2008).

We can see that a specific behavior was chosen and that some of the determinants of the behavior of eating fruits and vegetables are more closely related—*proximal* to the behavior, while others are more far removed—*distal*.

The core activities addressed the more proximal determinants, but more distal determinants were also addressed.

USING THEORY WITHIN A SOCIAL ECOLOGICAL MODEL TO DESIGN INTERVENTION: JUST FOR YOU PROGRAM FOR POST PARTUM LOW-INCOME WOMEN

The social ecological model can also be used for a very small-scale intervention, in this case the Just For You program from the Expanded Food and Nutrition Education Program (EFNEP) for low-income women during the first year after childbirth (Ebbeling et al. 2007). Focus group participants indicated they preferred a mom-centered program, because "everybody forgets about you" and moms felt they needed "a little attention." The literature and assessments suggested the key messages of eating more fruits and vegetables, less red meat, and performing more physical activity. The program focused on the *intrapersonal-level*

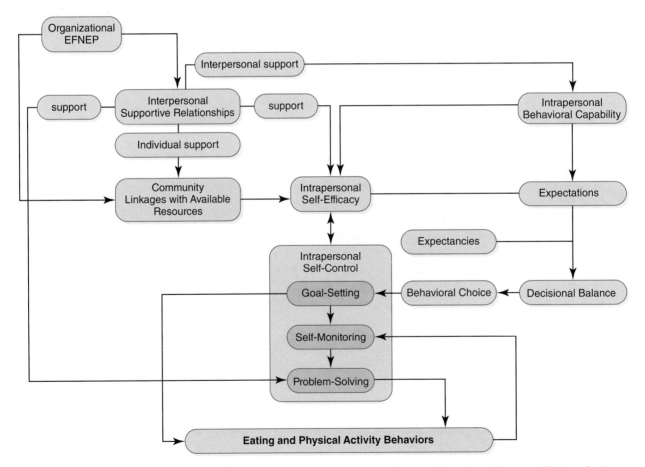

FIGURE 6-3 Conceptual model for interactions among theoretical constructs within a social ecological framework for Just for You program.

Reprinted from *Health Promotion Practice* 8(1), Ebbeling, Pearson, Sorensen, et al., Conceptualization and development of a theory-based healthful eating and physical activity intervention for postpartum women who are low income, Pages 50–59, Copyright 2007, with permission from SAGE Publications.

factors of outcome expectations (perceived benefits), behavioral capability (knowledge and skills), self-efficacy, and self-regulation skills; *the interpersonal-level* factors of supportive relationships; the *organizational-level* factor of EFNEP; and the *community-level* factor of linking the moms to available community resources. The intervention used a participant-centered approach based on principles of nonformal adult education. (See Chapter 17 for more details.) The intervention was delivered in the home by peer educators from EFNEP who were referred to as "health mentors." The conceptual framework that links the various theory constructs for the individual sessions to the social ecological environment is shown in **FIGURE 6-3.**

Interpersonal-Level Social Environment Change: Family, Peers, and Social Networks

We all live within a network of social relationships. These networks involve family, friends, neighbors, peers, coworkers, and those in various organizations to which individuals belong. These social relationships greatly influence individuals' food choices and dietary behaviors. The United States, and many other parts of the world, are becoming increasingly multicultural. People's social networks and relationships are thus often embedded in cultural traditions. Strategies to promote supportive environments need to address these relationships in the social environment.

FAMILIES

Many nutrition educators work with families, therefore, understanding families and their cultural identities and how to work with them is important. Americans eat about two-thirds of their calories from foods prepared in the home. Among the factors associated with healthful dietary behaviors, the most important are foods present in the home (household food availability), whether foods are easily accessible to family members, the frequency of family meals, and parents' own intakes and parenting practices when it comes to their children (Cullen et al. 2003; Patrick and Nicklas 2005; Fulkerson et al. 2008; Burgess-Champoux et al. 2009; O'Connor et al. 2009; Blissett 2011). Helpful parenting practices include modeling eating healthful foods and encouragement to try them,

and moderate restriction of less healthy foods, all in an atmosphere of emotional warmth (O'Connor et al. 2009; Blissett 2011), as well as involving children in decisions and providing positive feedback (Dickin and Seim 2013). Mealtime structure is also an important factor related to children's eating patterns (Berge et al. 2013). Chapter 2 describes these influences in greater detail.

The resemblances of food choice behaviors within the family are significantly greater than between family members and their friends, based on shared experience, shared foods, or cultural traditions. On the other hand, family members and others who live together may not all like or want to eat the same foods. Thus, there is a need to negotiate with the family or others about what to buy or eat (Furst et al. 1996; Feuenekes et al. 1998; Contento et al. 2006). Increasing the quality of foods in the home and at family meals and making specific changes in the food environment at home have been associated with positive dietary changes in children (Fulkerson et al. 2010; Hendrie et al. 2013). An important role for nutrition educators working with both adults and children, therefore, is to understand these family forces and develop strategies to encourage support for healthy eating in the home.

Nutrition Education Strategies for Family Support

Enhancing Family Support for Children in the Home

The most common strategy used in working with parents is the use of workshops that help parents provide healthy food for the family. These workshops are widely offered in many settings in most countries. In the United States, EFNEP has for decades been successfully offering workshops for families (Dollahite, Kenkel, and Thompson 2008).

Strategies you can use to increase family support for the behavioral goals of your program are shown here:

- *Workshops for parents or family members.* Active research documenting a link between parenting styles and practices and healthful eating and child weight status suggests that, as nutrition educators, we should design parent workshops that help parents hone their parenting skills as well as provide the food and nutrition knowledge parents need to support healthy eating for the family. One example is a series of workshops that is designed to address both behavior change

NUTRITION EDUCATION IN ACTION 6-1 Healthy Children, Healthy Families: Parents Making a Difference

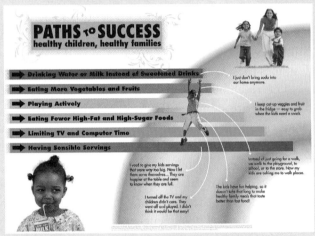

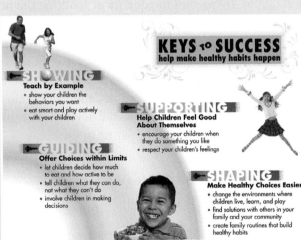

Cornell University, Center for Technology Licensing.

Healthy Children, Healthy Families (HCHF) is a workshop series developed by Cooperative Extension that integrates key nutrition and physical behavioral objectives with parenting practices to help prevent childhood obesity and improve children's health. It is designed for low-income parents and caregivers with children aged 3 to 11 years.

Theoretical Framework

The workshop series is based on social cognitive theory that emphasizes the importance of self-efficacy and behavioral skills as well as nutrition- and food-related knowledge and skills. It also uses research evidence on helpful parenting styles and practices.

The Curriculum

The curriculum consists of 8 weekly workshops of 1.5 hours each. It focuses on six key nutrition and physical activity behavioral objectives called *Paths to Success*: drinking water or milk instead of sweetened drinks, eating more vegetables and fruits, limiting high-fat and high-sugar foods, playing actively, limiting TV and recreational computer time, and having sensible servings (i.e., starting with moderately sized, age-appropriate amounts and paying attention to hunger cues and satiety). In terms of parenting practices, the HCHF curriculum promotes an authoritative or "firm and responsive" approach. These practices are called *Keys to Success*, focusing on *Showing*—teaching by example or role modeling, *Supporting*—helping children feel good about themselves, *Guiding*—offering choices within limits, and *Shaping*—structuring home environments to make healthy choices easier.

Intervention Strategies

HCHF uses a learner-centered facilitated dialogue approach (described in more detail in Chapter 15) to engage participants in discussions, hands-on activities, and role-plays to apply the behavioral and parenting skills. Each workshop includes tasting a simple, healthful recipe and an "active play break" where parents participate in an active game they can play at home with their children. Each week, participants set action goals for a new behavior to try, called "take a healthy step," which helps make progress on one of the *Paths to Success*.

Evaluation

An evaluation was conducted with 210 low-income mothers who completed the HCHF workshops. Mean scores improved significantly for most behaviors of adult and child, such as fruits and vegetables, sweet drinks, physical activity, and screen time, and in particular, fast food.

Source: Lent, M., R. F. Hill, J. S. Dollahite, W. S. Wolfe, and K. L. Dickin. 2012. Healthy Children, Healthy Families: Parents Making a Difference. A curriculum integrating key nutrition, physical activity, and parenting practices to help prevent childhood obesity. *Journal of Nutrition Education and Behavior* 44:90–92.; Dickin, K. L., T. F. Hill, and J. Dollahite. 2014. Practice-based evidence of effectiveness in an integrated nutrition and parenting education intervention for low-income parents. *Journal of the Academy of Nutrition and Dietetics* 114(6):945–950.

objectives and parenting practices called Healthy Children, Healthy Families (Lent et al. 2012; Dickin, Hill, and Dollahite 2014). It is described in greater detail in **NUTRITION EDUCATION IN ACTION 6-1.**

- *Materials, resources, and interactive tools from online sources.* Given that parents are very busy and often do not have time to attend workshops, new technologies are being explored. The majority of individuals, including low-income, low-education, and minority individuals in the United States, now have access to mobile phones with Internet capabilities (Lefebvre and Bornkessel 2013) and even computers. Governments, universities, and extension services (including, in the United States, eXtension Communities of Practice) provide interesting tools, activities, recipes, and so forth for families.

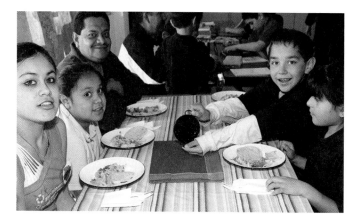

Parents and their children enjoy a meal together at their school's "Family Night."

Courtesy of Cooking with Kids.

Engaging Family Support for School-Based Nutrition Education

Many interventions in schools have focused on involving the family as a way to enhance home support for the dietary behavioral goals of school curricula. Direct methods to engage parents, such as workshops or family activities at the school, are more likely to report positive results than indirect methods such as newsletters. However, indirect methods that require children to engage their parents in some planned activity can make these indirect methods more effective (Hingle et al. 2010). Useful strategies include the following:

- *Student–parent activities conducted together at home.* Send home packets containing games and activities that require parental or adult involvement to complete along with the child (Hingle et al. 2010).
- *Family fun nights at school.* Design Family Fun Nights, in which families actually come together over a meal for a food-and-game experience (Harrington et al. 2005). In one study, each of seven sessions offered a game, new recipe choices, intervention messages to parents, a children's fun page that reinforced program themes, optional conversation topics, and menu suggestions. Such activities with families need to be solidly based on understanding the cultural context of the families.
- *Innovative technology and social media.* In today's world of cell phones and other mobile devices, use of these to convey messages to parents, for example

through text-messaging or social media, is a promising avenue to pursue, perhaps in conjunction with the other strategies. Parents report that they want tailored, themed, and simple information through multiple mediums, with a voice of authority and with appropriate duration and frequency (Bhana et al. 2014).

Family Support in Adults

Nutrition educators can develop programs to involve the family of adult participants; for example, in programs with employees and other settings. A study with employees showed that total fruit and vegetable intake increased by 19% in the worksite-plus-family group, 7% in the worksite intervention–only group, and 0% in the control group (Sorensen et al. 1999). The family component included a learn-at-home program, family newsletter, family festival, and materials mailed home at regular intervals.

Likewise, programs can involve families of those who are attending outpatient clinics or cardiac rehabilitation centers who need help with their diets. This can be done through workshops at the sites, newsletters, online programs, or learn-at-home materials.

THEORY BASE FOR NUTRITION EDUCATION AT THE FAMILY LEVEL: THE EXAMPLE OF MARIA

Please note that in parent workshops and activities, parents or family members become a secondary audience for nutrition education. Designing sessions for them is the same as designing sessions for any other group. Thus you need to select the behaviors or family practices that need to be targeted and identify the psychosocial determinants of these behaviors that you will address in your sessions. In our case example in Chapter 4, Maria was concerned about the amount of soda and sweet snacks her young daughter was consuming and their effect on her teeth and her weight. The nutrition education session she attended was stated as being about the snacking behavior of the child, but the behavioral focus of the session was on the *behaviors of the parents or caregivers*. Thus it needed to be directed at the psychosocial determinants of behavior change of the parent. The session was based on the theory of planned behavior (or the reasoned action approach), you will recall. The nutrition educator focused on helping parents understand the impact of sugary drinks and snacks on children's health, and provided tips for ways to overcome the barriers parents experience in trying to offer water and healthy snacks instead. Maria found the evidence on health impacts convincing, and she realized she needed to make some changes in her parenting behaviors. She chose *two behaviors that she could do as a parent* that would be supportive of developing healthy dietary habits in her daughter: she will not stock her house with soda pop and she will offer her daughter more healthful snacks when she comes home after Head Start. In similar fashion, for the sessions and activities that you design to enhance family support, you can select the specific supportive parenting practices that you wish to promote.

SOCIAL NETWORKS AND SOCIAL SUPPORT

It has been shown that social relationships influence health status, probably through both direct effects and their ability to buffer the negative effects of life stressors on health (Berkman and Glass 2000; Heany and Israel 2008). In particular, emotional support is related to good health and to reduced all-cause mortality.

Social Networks

Social networks refer to the web of social relationships that surround individuals. In the area of diet, food choices and eating patterns are directly influenced by social networks. Relationships with peers and those with whom people work also have an impact on individuals' day-to-day choices. Social networks can have the following characteristics (Heaney and Israel 2008):

- *Density*: The extent to which members know and interact with each other

- *Proximity*: The degree to which individuals in the network are located in close proximity, which today could include Internet connectedness through social media
- *Interaction*: The frequency of contact, the variety of functions that the network serves (complexity), and how close members are emotionally (intensity)
- *Reciprocity*: The extent to which individuals help each other with resources and support

Some individuals have very extensive social networks of family and friends who are in frequent contact with each other, whereas others have few friends and family with whom they interact.

Social Support

Social support refers to the support that individuals in social networks provide each other in various areas:

- *Emotional support*: Involves empathy, trust, caring, and esteem. This may be found in expressions such as "he listens to me when I talk to him about things," "some people look down on you: well, she doesn't," and "she is someone I trust and I know she will keep what I tell her confidential."
- *Instrumental support*: Involves money or other tangible resources and help, such as with babysitting or shopping. This is reflected in "she helped me by talking with the owners and convincing them to wait a while for the rent money."
- *Informational support*: Involves advice and information useful in solving problems. This might include "he offered suggestions about what I could do."
- *Appraisal support*: Involves constructive feedback and self-evaluation. This is reflected in statements such as "he seems to have faith in me."

Again, individuals differ in the degree to which they receive social support for their eating and physical activity patterns.

Examples of Social Network Theory in Action

Social support is incorporated into many health interventions and indeed has been identified as one of the elements that contributes to effectiveness (Ammerman et al. 2002). Weight loss interventions (e.g., Weight Watchers) routinely incorporate social support groups. Interventions in schools and workplaces have also incorporated social support in various forms, as have community-based nutrition education. Community-based group nutrition education, usually with low-income audiences, has taken advantage of the often strong relationships that can develop among groups facing similar challenges. A few illustrations are provided here for nutrition education.

Social Support in Workplaces

In worksite interventions, social support is operationalized as peer support at the worksite and involvement of family. Some interventions have attempted to make these existing social networks more supportive of health. Interactive strategies such as group education classes and contests were more effective in terms of nutritional outcomes (e.g., eating more fruits and vegetables) than were one-time activities such as kickoffs or more passive efforts such as use of printed materials (Patterson et al. 1997) and thus should be used.

Workplace, Family, and Peer Support

More specifically, nutrition educators can develop activities to involve peers at work and engage family support. Coworker support for healthful eating in one study was measured by asking questions such as how often coworkers "encourage you to eat vegetables," "compliment your attempts to eat a healthy diet," or "bring fruit to work for you to try" (Sorensen et al. 2002). Coworker support increased significantly as a result of nutrition education. Taken together, these studies suggest that we can incorporate social support into nutrition education interventions to make them more successful.

Community-Based Group Nutrition Education

Community-based group nutrition education, usually with low-income audiences, has taken advantage of the often strong relationships that develop among group members facing similar challenges. In the United States, the Women, Infants, and Children (WIC) program uses a collaborative process of developing client-centered nutrition education, which allows members to learn from one another, thus ensuring commitment from all levels of staff (Isbell et al. 2015).

USEFUL STRATEGIES FOR ADDRESSING THE INTERPERSONAL SOCIAL ENVIRONMENT

As nutrition educators, we can have an important role in enhancing social support for our audiences by strengthening their existing networks or providing structured social support groups.

Enhancing Existing Social Networks

To enhance social support for the key food- and nutrition-related behavioral change goals of a program (e.g., increasing breastfeeding rates, increasing the consumption of fruits and vegetables), we can call upon and expand existing social networks. For example, we can work with parent associations in schools, employee associations at workplaces, and groups that meet regularly in communities, cultural associations, and organizations to increase their interest in being supportive of the targeted behaviors or practices.

Developing New Social Network Linkages Through Support Groups

We can initiate social support groups through which new social network linkages are built. For example, we can develop a support group for those in a workplace who are interested in weight control or weight acceptance. We can initiate support groups at a health center for those with HIV/AIDS, or provide cooking classes and behavioral change sessions for those attending outpatient clinics.

Many of the facilitated discussion groups in the Women, Infants and Children (WIC) program and other similar programs serve this function. See Chapter 17 for a detailed discussion of how to conduct such groups. Weight management groups that meet over a long period can also provide support to members. The social support approach is especially useful for those who have been diagnosed with type 2 diabetes. Controlling blood sugar and preventing complications are unending challenges and require changes in diet for a lifetime. Consequently, the impact of receiving a diagnosis can be devastating. Social network intervention and social support have been found to be effective for helping people manage their condition (Shaya et al. 2014).

In all these situations, as nutrition educators, we can provide group members an opportunity to process their feelings with others like them through a series of structured activities. We can also help individuals develop action plans, and group members can meet to share challenges and successes. Such groups can provide emotional support, involving empathy and caring; informational support in the form of advice and information useful in solving problems; and appraisal support in terms of accurate feedback. They do not usually provide instrumental support. In addition to groups that meet physically, the groups could "meet" through social media of various kinds.

Providing Social Support Through New Technologies and Social Media

New technologies are increasingly being used to provide social support, in particular for disease management. Text-messaging holds promise (Cole-Lewis and Kershaw 2010). Nutrition educators can investigate these and other channels for social support, such as social media. These are described in detail in Chapter 16.

SOCIAL SUPPORT IN THE CASE EXAMPLES OF MARIA AND ALICIA

At the end of the workshop Maria attended at her daughter's Head Start program, the nutrition educator offered to continue to meet monthly with the moms, along with moms from other centers. Maria decided to join the group. She absolutely loved it! The group decided on the nutrition or parenting behavior they wished to work on each month. The nutrition educator facilitated the sessions, encouraging the moms to share their challenges and triumphs. They supported each other. The nutrition educator added evidence-based tips on handling the given behavior, where appropriate. The sessions closed with each person setting some kind of action goal for the next month.

Alicia is the 19-year-old who attended a session on "Eat Right for Your Heart" because her mother had a heart attack and she was now aware and concerned about her own heart health. She was also interested in social support. However, she felt she was too busy to attend any more sessions and chose text-messaging instead. The nutrition educator would text her about once per week to ask how she was doing and to encourage her in sticking with her goal to choose healthier options when she went to fast food restaurants.

Environmental Settings: Strategies for Organizational-Level Change

As nutrition educators we can contribute to making the environment in organizations more supportive of healthful eating and being active, by: (1) first educating the decision-makers and leaders by communicating food- and nutrition-related information on the importance of these actions, and (2) working in partnership or collaboration with the organization to make healthful foods more available and accessible in the given setting, such as in schools, workplaces, child care, health care, and other settings.

To educate the decision-makers and leaders, the *diffusion of innovations theory* (Rogers 2003) can serve as a helpful tool, with our nutrition education message or a proposed nutrition education program being defined as the innovation. This theory says that our message or a proposed program will be more likely to be adopted if it is seen as better than what was there before (relative advantage), fits with the organization (compatibility), is easy to use or implement (complexity), can be tried before making a final decision to adopt (trialability), and its results will be visible and easy to measure (observability). We will thus want to address these issues as we seek to educate decision-makers and develop partnerships with them. For example, if we want a program to be adopted by a school or institution, we can seek to demonstrate its *relative advantage* by presenting evidence of its effectiveness. We can show its *compatibility* by showing policy-makers that it fits with educational standards (schools) or the mission of the institution (worksites). We can reduce its *complexity* by providing simple, graphically attractive and user-friendly materials. We can help schools pilot the program first or place the program on a website for the organization or community to try out. We can also use demonstrations to show its effects in order to create *observability*. See **BOX 6-1**.

Senior-level decision-makers, such as school principals, worksite managers, and child care or healthcare organization directors, are likely to be more important at the stage of deciding on and initiating the program while midlevel individuals such as teachers and child care or healthcare staff are more important at the implementation stage. Our skills in presentation and collaboration will stand us in good stead here.

STRATEGIES FOR SCHOOL SETTINGS

In the United States, the National School Lunch Program (NSLP) provides healthy meals in schools, with reduced price and free meals available to those who qualify. Many students throw away much of the lunch, particularly

---

BOX 6-1 **Diffusion of Innovations**

An innovation is something thought to be new or novel by an individual, organization, or community, whether it is a new idea, practice, device, or program. The diffusion of innovations theory can serve as a very useful tool or framework for the work of nutrition educators in institutions and communities if we consider our messages or programs as the innovation. A number of factors determine how quickly, and to what extent, an innovation will be adopted and diffused.

The Innovation

An innovation (e.g., our behavioral messages or program) is more likely to be adopted if:

- *Relative advantage*. It is seen as better than what was there before.

- *Compatibility*. It is seen as having an appropriate fit with the existing values and needs of our audiences, cultures, or organizational and community environment.

- *Complexity*. This factor has to do with how easy it is to understand and implement the innovation.

- *Trialability*. It is advantageous if people or organizations can first try out the behavior or program on an experimental basis before making a major commitment in terms of time, effort, or money.

- *Observability*. This factor reflects the degree to which the results will be visible and easy to measure.

Communication Channels

The innovation can be diffused through various channels, from interpersonal to social and mass media and include both formal and informal channels.

Time

The process of adoption and diffusion of the innovation may take time; people, organizations, and communities can be *innovators*, *early adopters*, *early majority*, *late majority*, or *laggards* in terms of adopting messages and programs.

Source: Rogers, E. M. 2003. *Diffusion of innovations*, 5th ed. New York: Simon and Shuster.

---

the vegetables, saying it is unappetizing. Participation declines with age, with about two-thirds of elementary school children participating, down to about one-half in middle school and one-third in high school. Foods available in other venues tend to be higher in fat and sugar and less nutritious. With collaborations between nutrition educators and decision-makers such as school principals and food service providers, some school environment changes have been found to be useful. These may also work for those in countries where food is sold in schools without subsidies.

Fruit and Vegetable Access Interventions

Numerous interventions have focused on increasing fruit and vegetable intake. One intervention introduced a number of changes in the school environment: it improved the variety and attractiveness of the fruits and vegetables served at lunch, it made an extra fruit item available as a choice at lunch when a dessert was served,

and placed point-of-purchase signs in the cafeteria (Perry et al. 1998; Reynolds et al. 2000). Results showed that the interventions increased the combined intake of fruits and vegetables.

Fresh Fruit and Vegetable Programs

In the United States, eligible schools can obtain funding to receive baskets of fresh fruits and vegetables each day for each classroom. In one study, surveys at the end of the academic year showed that high school students in intervention schools compared to those in schools not receiving the program were more likely to report eating more fruit and to be drinking 100% fruit juice although there was no change in vegetable intake (Davis et al. 2009). Nutrition educators can work with schools to apply for this program and choose the best ways to implement it.

A program in Canada found that providing free fruits and vegetables in schools, with and without nutrition education, led to improved intakes (He et al. 2009).

Behavioral Economics Approach: Smarter Lunchrooms Initiative

A different approach involves behavioral economics, which examines the effect of social, cognitive, and emotional factors on the economic decisions of individuals and institutions and the consequences for market prices, returns, and the resource allocation. In applying it to the food and nutrition field, it means making changes in the environment that make the healthy choices the easy choices. In the Smarter Lunchrooms Initiative, small changes are made that increase the convenience, attractiveness, and normative nature of healthy foods in the lunchroom but do not restrict choices, with the objective being that this would encourage students to make healthier choices of their own volition (Hanks, Just, and Wansink 2013). Such an approach has been found not to increase the cost of meals. *Convenience* involves placing fresh fruit next to the cash register or fruit juice boxes in the freezer next to the ice cream, *attractiveness* involves lunch menus with attractive color photos of the fruits and vegetables served or fresh fruit displayed attractively in bowls or baskets, and making eating fruits and vegetables *seem normal* can be achieved by the persons serving the lunch saying, "Would you like to try . . . ?" Such an approach of making minor changes in how food is offered increased fruit and vegetable consumption. Likewise, giving attractive names to vegetables such as "X-Ray Vision Carrots" increased and sustained their consumption (Wansink et al. 2012). Nutrition educators can work with school service directors to make these small changes.

Farm-to-School Programs

Farm-to-school programs connect schools with local farms (National Farm to School Network, 2014; Feenstra and Ohmart 2012; U.S. Department of Agriculture [USDA] 2014a). Schools buy and feature foods such as fruits, vegetables, eggs, honey, meat, and beans on their menus or offer farm-fresh salad bars as part of the NSLP. These programs also provide students with experiential learning opportunities through farm visits, classroom visits by farmers, cooking demonstrations, school gardens, and recycling and composting programs. Through these programs, farmers have access to a new market and participate in a program designed to educate children about local food and agriculture. Such programs require the participation of a wide variety of people and organizations, and nutrition educators can have a key role.

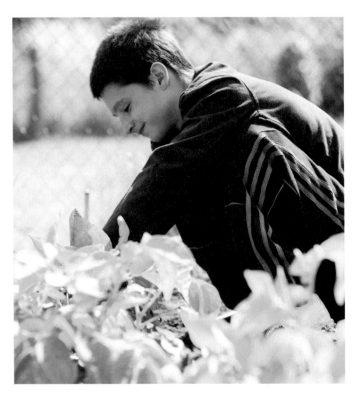

Community gardens, where youths can grow fresh produce, support healthy behaviors.

© Adrian Britton/ShutterStock, Inc.

School Policy, Environment, and System Changes in Mexico City

The rate of overweight and obesity is growing rapidly in Mexico, as in many other parts of the world, particularly among children. The school is a good place to intervene due to the feasibility of combining environmental and behavioral strategies within a common setting. The Nutridinámicos program focused on environmental policy and social structures to make healthy choices easier (Safdie et al. 2013b). It is described in greater detail in **NUTRITION EDUCATION IN ACTION 6-2**.

STRATEGIES FOR WORKPLACES

A majority of adults are employed in workplaces of some sort. Hence, what is available in and around such places can have an impact on food choices. The U.S. Centers for Disease Control and Prevention (CDC) has developed a Worksite Health ScoreCard, which employers can use to assess the status of their health promotion strategies (programs, policies, and environmental supports) (http://www.cdc.gov/dhdsp/pubs/docs/HSC_Manual.pdf).

NUTRITION EDUCATION IN ACTION 6-2 A School Environment Intervention in Mexico: Nutridinámicos

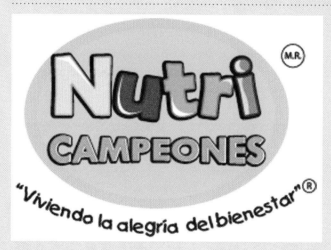

The rate of overweight and obesity is growing in Mexico, particularly among children, as it is in many countries around the world. Schools where children eat foods brought from home or buy from vendors and where there is a lack of active physical education are obesigenic. The Nutridinámicos program was directed at policy and environmental change to foster change in children's eating and physical activity behaviors and, consequently, weight status. The primary audience was fourth to sixth graders in low-income areas of Mexico City.

Theoretical Framework

The program used a social ecological model as an over-arching framework and involved many intervention components and partners. The intervention itself was based on social cognitive theory with elements from the theory of planned behavior and health belief model.

Intervention

The intervention focused on existing school infrastructure and policy with no additional investment, so that it would be sustainable. The targeted behaviors, based on a detailed assessment, were: eating more fruits and vegetables, drinking plain water, being more physically active, and bringing a healthy lunch. The intervention consisted of:

- Student workshops, twice per year for 2 years, focusing on motivation and skills

- Teacher workshops, twice per year for physical education teachers, to make classes more active

- Health screening of teachers and administrators so they would be more committed to the health of their students

- School-wide communication: posters and interactive bulletin boards; pamphlets for parents, teachers, and vendors

- School environment and policies: reduce eating opportunities to recess only (and not in class), ensure water was available in containers in each classroom, improved school premises and more sports equipment so that children can play

- Family workshops, once per year and newsletters, four times per year, focusing on skills to promote better eating and more physical activity at home and preparing healthy lunches for their children

- Vendor workshops to help vendors modify their cooking skills to make foods served at recess healthier, for example, baking instead of frying of traditional foods. The goal was to migrate to foods with fewer fat and sugar calories.

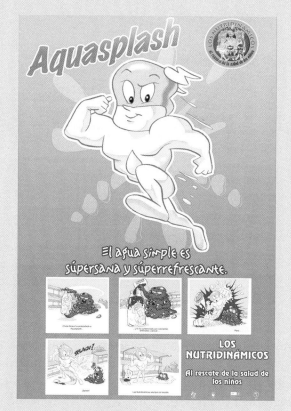

Courtesy of Nutri Campeones.

(Continues)

NUTRITION EDUCATION IN ACTION 6-2 **A School Environment Intervention in Mexico: Nutridinámicos (Continued)**

Evaluation

In a randomized controlled trial, the availability of healthy foods increased with a concomitant decrease in unhealthy food availability in the intervention schools.

Food intake showed the same trend. There were no changes in physical activity in class or weight status, however, suggesting that more prolonged and intense programs may be needed.

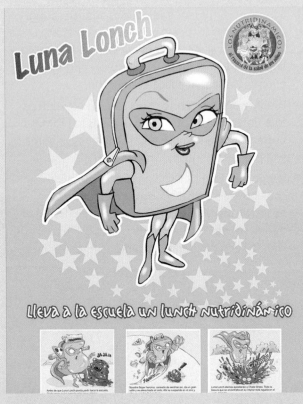

Courtesy of Nutri Campeones.

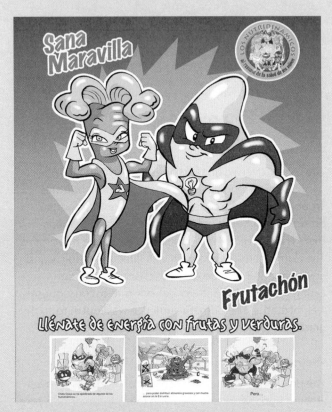

Courtesy of Nutri Campeones.

Source: Safdie, M., L. Levesque, I. Gonzalez-Casanova, et al. 2013b. Promoting healthful diet and physical activity in the Mexican school system for the prevention of obesity in children. *Salud Publica Mexico* 55(Suppl 3):S357–S373.; Safdie, M., N. Jennings-Aburto, L. Levesque, et al. 2013a. Impact of a school-based intervention program on obesity risk factors in Mexican children. *Salud Publica Mexico* 55(Suppl 3):S374–S387; Bonvecchio A, Théodore FL, Safdie M, Duque T, Villanueva MA, Torres C, and J Rivera. 2014. Contribution of formative research to design an environmental program for obesity prevention in schools in Mexico City. *Salud Publica Mexicana* 56(suppl 2):S139-S147. Bonvecchio A, Theodore F, Hernández-Cordero S, Campirano-Núñez F, Islas A, Safdie M y Rivera-Dommarco JA 2010. La escuela como alternativa en la prevención de la obesidad: la experiencia en el sistema escolar mexicano [The school as an alternative for the prevention of childhood obesity: Experience from the Mexican school system]. *Rev Esp Nutrition Comunitaria* 16(1):13–16.

A number of health promotion interventions in workplaces have attempted to make changes in the food environment by increasing the number of healthful low-fat and high-fiber foods, fruits, and vegetables available in the employee cafeteria and other sources of food at work, such as vending machines (e.g., Sorensen et al. 1990; Sorensen et al. 1996). Rewards and incentives for "good health behaviors" have also been used with some success (Merrill et al. 2011). These behaviors included periodic physical examinations, attending educational lunchtime programs, exercise classes, and screenings.

Nutrition educators and health professionals work with worksite decision-makers to develop a variety of activities for the worksite. Using educational, promotional, organizational, and policy activities, these interventions have had a positive impact on eating patterns (Sorensen et al. 1999; Engbers et al. 2005; Geany et al. 2013). Here are a few examples.

Use of Technology Channels

Several worksites have used interactive software programs, sending emails and text-messaging and creating personalized websites for health promotion. In the ALIVE (A Lifestyle Intervention Via E-mail) 16-week program, employees could choose among several behaviors: fruits and vegetables, saturated fat, trans fats and added sugars, and physical activity (Sternfeld et al. 2009). Messages were individually tailored, focusing on small-step changes, and sent via email. Results were positive. In the Health First Program, participants received three coaching sessions from a nutrition educator and were then assigned to teams to provide social support. Teams logged points on a Web program for attending sessions, weight loss, and so forth, and competed with each other over a 12-week period (Daubert et al. 2012). They could attend sessions in person or via PowerPoint online. The behaviors were those of the DASH diet or Mediterranean diet, and some positive outcomes were achieved.

Treatwell Program

An example of a worksite program to increase fruit and vegetable consumption that addressed multiple levels of influence is summarized in **NUTRITION EDUCATION IN ACTION 6-3**. The Treatwell program randomly assigned 22 worksites into three groups: minimal intervention controls, worksite intervention, and worksite-plus-family (Sorensen et al. 1998; Sorensen et al. 1999). The worksites were community health centers with racially and ethnically diverse employees, providing services to low-income community residents. The behavioral goal of the program and hence the expected outcome of the intervention was that the employees in these worksites would increase their consumption of fruits and vegetables. Nutrition Education in Action 6-3 lists the theoretical models that were used. The study also tested whether the intervention had an impact on the potential determinants of behavior change. These are shown in the table, along with how the changes were measured. (The results were described earlier in this chapter in the section titled "Social Support in Workplaces.")

Local Foods at Workplaces

Increasing the purchase of locally grown produce through worksite sales was the objective of another intervention (Ross et al. 2000). Workers were given the opportunity to order local produce that was delivered to the worksite. This environmental change was accompanied by promotional materials about the farms that grew the produce and an opportunity to sample the produce. The delivery was very public so that friends' ordering and satisfaction could be observed to provide a social normative influence. Results showed that workers who ordered local foods at the worksite were motivated to purchase locally grown produce outside the worksite as well.

The Case of Ray

You will recall that Ray, who had put on some weight over the years and is at risk of diabetes, attended several sessions offered by a nutrition educator at his physician's clinic. He is energized to make some behavioral changes in his eating patterns at work and to drink less beer at home. However, he notices that the vending machine at work has only sweetened beverages and high-calorie snacks, and he buys several of these a day. He talks with the nutrition educator about what he should do. The nutrition educator meets him at his place of work and they go to meet the manager.

The nutrition educator uses key features from the *diffusion of innovations* theory to make her case for replacing some of the sweetened drinks and snacks with healthier options: the change would be better than what was there before (relative advantage) as it would satisfy some employee needs; it would fit with the organization (compatibility) as no new space or resources would be needed; it would be easy to implement (complexity); and it could be tried before making a final decision to adopt (trialability). The educator had done her homework by contacting the vending machine company, who said they would be willing to try out the changes for a 6-month period. The manager agreed to conduct a survey to find out what the other employees thought of the idea and to take action if there was agreement to do so. Ray agreed to make a pitch to his colleagues about the issue. Most colleagues agreed to the change and it was made. The results would be visible and easy to measure (observability) by viewing sales figures and satisfaction ratings of employees.

NUTRITION EDUCATION IN ACTION 6-3 Theories Used and Potential Determinants of Behavior Change in the Treatwell 5-a-Day Worksite Program

Level of Influence	Intervention Audience	Theoretical Models	Hypotheses About Determinants of Behavior Change	Measures
Intrapersonal	• Worker	• Social cognitive theory	• Higher self-efficacy about dietary change is associated with increased fruit and vegetable consumption. • Knowledge of the diet–cancer link (outcome expectations: perceived risk) is associated with increased fruit and vegetable consumption.	• Self-efficacy • Outcome expectations
Intrapersonal	• Family • Coworkers	• Social support • Social networks and ties • Social cognitive theory	• High family and coworker support for dietary change is associated with increased fruit and vegetable consumption. • High family support for dietary change is associated with increased availability of fruits and vegetables in the home. • The type of family ties will influence the strength of the relationships between family support and changing eating habits.	• Family support • Coworker support • Social norms • Availability of fruits and vegetables in the home • Type of family ties
Organizational	• Worksite	• Organizational change and development • Diffusion of innovations • Policy	• Worksite mean increases in fruit and vegetable consumption will be greatest where fruits and vegetables are most available and a catering policy supports the purchase of healthy foods. • Program implementation and participation will be highest where effective communication channels exist and policies permit employee change agents to participate. • Coworker support for dietary changes will be highest in worksites with high coworker cohesion and positive labor–management relations.	• Worksite characteristics
Community	• Media (national campaign) • Grocery store	• Social marketing	• Workers reporting awareness of the national campaign are more likely to increase consumption of fruits and vegetables. • Workers reporting participation in grocery store programs are more likely to report increased consumption of fruits and vegetables.	• Awareness of grocery store campaign • Participation in grocery store campaign

Source: Sorensen, G., M. K. Hunt, N. Cohen, et al. 1998. Worksite and family education for dietary change: The Treatwell 5-a-Day program. *Health Education Research* 13:577–591. Used with permission.

Environmental Settings: Community-Level Activities for Change

Nutrition educators are being increasingly called upon to expand their roles to include promoting health-supportive environments for the groups and communities they serve (Hill, Dickin, and Dollahite 2012; Dickin and Dollahite 2012). This can be accomplished in most cases only by developing partnerships and participating in collaborations with other groups who have similar goals to bring about community environment changes that are supportive of the behavioral goals of the nutrition education program. We have two key tasks here: first, to seek out and develop such community partnerships and collaboration, and second, to work together to develop strategies and build community capacity to bring about change. Most often we start by gaining awareness of the issues by identifying potential partners in the short term and then a commitment to change in the medium term, before reaching desired environmental change goals.

BUILDING PARTNERSHIPS AND COLLABORATIONS

Our first task is to build community partnerships and collaborations. A *community* refers to both a physical locality where a group of people live and a group of people who share common interests. Collaborations include a range of structural relationships, and different terms are often used to describe these, such as partnerships and coalitions (Rosenthal 1998).

Clarifying Terms

Collaboration has been described as "a fluid process through which a group of diverse, autonomous actors (organizations or individuals) undertakes a joint initiative, addresses shared concerns, or otherwise achieves common goals. It is characterized by mutual benefit, interdependence, reciprocity, concerted action, and joint production" (Rosenthal 1998, p. 246). In degree of involvement, collaboration ranges from loose networks through cooperation and coordination of effort to full collaboration. *Partnerships* are formed for reasons of organizational self-interest and pragmatism and can be for the long or short term. Partners have distinct resources and expertise that, if pooled, can expand possibilities for everyone: the whole becomes greater than the sum of its parts. Partners share responsibility and ownership of the effort or product.

Coalitions or *consortia* are another arrangement in which organizations, institutions, and sectors unite to develop a comprehensive approach. The focus is on social change, **empowerment**, and community building, and the activities include planning, community organizing, advocacy, and program development.

We use the general terms *collaboration* and *partnership* to describe the variety of arrangements, formal or informal, in which nutrition education is involved.

Successful Partnerships or Collaborations

Collaborations can mobilize material resources and people's knowledge, skills, and enthusiasms to achieve desired goals in a way that is not possible for small groups alone.

Factors that are likely to enhance successful collaboration include the following: a shared vision and mission, reached by consensus through open dialogue and negotiation; a unique purpose that is meaningful to members; tasks that are clear and empowering; a sense of productivity and efficiency; open and frequent communication; all parties feeling that they benefit from participating; relationships that are based on trust, openness, and respect; and power sharing.

> "Collaborating is ultimately about relationships, and relationships do not thrive based on a rational calculus of costs and benefits but rather because of genuine caring and mutual vulnerability.
>
> Building the capacity to collaborate is hard work and demands the best of people, particularly when it involves people from different organizations with different goals and with little history of working together—maybe even with histories of distrust and antagonism.
>
> In particular, we have found that building this capacity rests on three capabilities: convening, listening and nurturing shared commitment."
>
> —Senge et al. 2010 p. 233.

Skills in Building Collaborations

To build and participate in collaborations or partnerships, it is important to become knowledgeable about the various food- and nutrition-related agencies and organizations in the community and how your program might complement their mission. Honing your networking interests and skills is also very important. Most communities have a number of existing collaborations and task forces in which you can participate, such as food systems networks, food forums, coalitions for healthy school food, or health coalitions, which often hold open network meetings, breakfasts, brownbag lunches, and so forth. It is helpful for you to participate, where relevant, in order to build up a network of colleagues to call upon when you need support for your programs. Once your partnerships are set up, it still requires spending time with them to nurture the relationships and work on projects. Your genuine interest in, and commitment to, this expanded role for nutrition educators is important because it is a change in job description to allow you to include these activities (Dickin and Dollahite 2012).

Community Collaborations and Partnerships: Examples

Building Breastfeeding-Friendly Communities

An example in the United States of a collaboration regarding a very specific behavior is a program wherein WIC nutritionists worked with other food assistance programs and a variety of community partners to build breastfeeding-friendly communities (Singleton et al. 2005). The aim was to increase public awareness, acceptance, and community support for breastfeeding. The program in one state included a public forum with 145 key community stakeholders to develop a blueprint for action to assist communities, families, schools and child care centers, healthcare systems, policymakers, and worksites in their efforts to make breastfeeding the norm for infant feeding. The partnership also initiated a public awareness campaign and activities to advocate for changes in healthcare systems, the insurance industry, the business community, and educational systems to encourage breastfeeding, and advocacy for changes in the availability of resources for community organizations and families.

Collaboration for Health, Activity, and Nutrition in Children's Environments

Collaboration for Health, Activity, and Nutrition in Children's Environments (CHANCE) is an initiative within EFNEP in New York State. It uses a social ecological approach to support families with children aged 3–11 years through education on nutrition, physical activity, and parenting skills using a curriculum called Healthy Children, Healthy Families: Parents Making a Difference (Lent et al. 2012) and through actions to support healthy environments for children by CHANCE educators collaborating on the following activities (Cornell University Division of Nutritional Sciences, n.d.):

- Developing a diverse coalition of agencies, including social service providers, healthcare providers, municipalities, and educational institutions, to work together on childhood obesity prevention efforts

- Providing training for agency staff who serve children, including day care and Head Start staff, to encourage offering healthy snacks, reducing TV time, increasing active play, and modeling healthy behaviors
- Serving on task forces that coordinate efforts such as increasing access to bike lanes and low-cost fruit and vegetable carts in low-income communities
- Leading support groups for parents who want to continue to learn and support one another after participating in the Healthy Children, Healthy Families workshops
- Providing funding to community agencies that serve children for small projects to increase access to healthy food and active play on site
- "Adopting a bodega" to encourage and support a corner store owner in stocking healthy choices and displaying them attractively

Nutrition Education Networks

Nutrition education networks have also come into existence in many states in the United States, with funding from the USDA's Supplemental Nutrition Assistance Program (SNAP) and other sources. Nutrition educators play a key role in these networks. The networks work with health departments, school districts, and community-based organizations to promote healthful diets and physical activity habits in low-income school-aged children and their families. Examples are the Network for a Healthy California, which sponsors a wide range of nutrition education activities through multiple venues in this large state (http://www.cdph.ca.gov/programs/cpns/Pages/AboutUs.aspx), and the Iowa Nutrition Network (http://www.idph.state.ia.us/INN/Default.aspx), where the program has been shown to result in increased consumption of fruits and vegetables and nonfat or low-fat milk in place of regular milk, and increased willingness to try a new kind of vegetable (Long et al. 2013; USDA 2013)

COMMUNITY CAPACITY BUILDING

Our second key task is to participate in building community capacity to work toward change. *Community capacity* may be described as the characteristics of communities that affect their ability to identify, mobilize, and address social and public health problems (Goodman et al. 1999). Once collaborations are in place, nutrition educators can work with them to increase the community's capacity to take action through various strategies, in particular through enhancing collective efficacy and through increasing sense of empowerment.

Enhancing Collective Efficacy

Collective efficacy is the belief of groups and community members that they have the capacity to take collective action to create change in their environment. Bandura (2001) notes that because human functioning is rooted in social systems, personal agency operates within a broad network of social structures that individuals, in turn, also help to create. Thus, personal agency and social structures operate interdependently. According to Bandura (2001), personal agency is not about self-centered individualism; rather, studies show that a high sense of efficacy tends to promote a prosocial orientation, involving cooperativeness and an interest in each other's welfare.

Collective efficacy can be enhanced by "equipping people with a firm belief that they can produce valued effects by their collective action and providing them with the means to do so" (Bandura 1997). The process for building collective efficacy is rather like a group goal setting process: group members identify the issue of concern, set small goals to address the concern, and, when these produce tangible results, come to believe that they have the capability to change the social and political environments in which they live. This leads them to believe that they can overcome even more difficult problems and hence to set more ambitious goals. There is evidence that skills in advocacy and community building raise both personal and collective efficacy, which can result in collective actions that may, in turn, change community practices and policies.

Strengthening Empowerment

Empowerment, a term that is used loosely and has many definitions, is similar to the process of collective efficacy of social cognitive theory. While it includes a personal process in which individuals develop and use needed knowledge, competence, or confidence for making their own decisions (somewhat like self-efficacy), empowerment can be seen as broader than that. It involves an enabling process through which individuals or communities take control over their lives and environments (Wallerstein 1992). It involves some sense of gaining political and social power as well as personal power (Israel et al. 1994).

Empowerment strategies generally involve some sort of process whereby group participants are asked to draw on their own knowledge and experiences to try to understand their lives in relation to a given problem. Group members, through dialogue, come to a collective understanding of the root causes of the problem and begin to see how they can make changes in their situation (Travers 1997a; Minkler 2004). They then set goals for actions that they will take to transform their reality through making changes in the social or political condition of their lives. In these settings, the role of the nutrition educator may be to facilitate the process at the beginning, if needed, until the group has developed its own agendas and procedures and no longer needs the nutrition educator. Another possibility is that a group has already initiated community action and needs the nutrition educator as a resource person or to provide technical assistance. Such approaches have been useful in the food and nutrition domain (Kent 1988; Rody 1988; Travers 1997b).

Project Focusing on Empowerment: Parent Center

An example of empowerment through nutrition education involved low-income women who used to meet informally every week over coffee at a parent center (Travers 1997b). The issue of common concern to them was feeding their families on a low income. The nutrition educator posed questions that led to group dialogue and discussion, out of which emerged the group's perception that foods cost more in low-income neighborhoods. This led them to make a structured comparison study of prices for foods in their local stores and prices in stores of the same chain in middle-income neighborhoods.

- *Role of the nutrition educator.* The nutrition educator provided technical assistance on this task. When their findings showed that prices in inner-city stores were consistently higher than in middle-income neighborhoods, the women came to realize that the difficulty they had in getting adequate nutrition was partly the result of social inequities. They came to the decision to write to the stores to express their concern about inequities in pricing and quality. This resulted in the chain store lowering the prices within the low-income neighborhoods. The nutrition educator facilitated the process by obtaining a word processor and writing the letter with them. This success led to a sense of empowerment. The activity also led them to recognize that

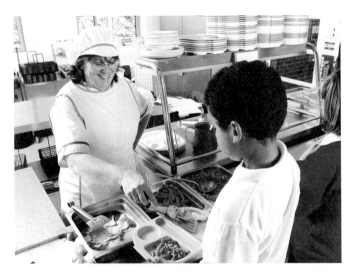

Schools can provide opportunities for children to eat healthy foods.
© Andrew Olney/Getty Images.

their welfare allowances were not adequate to meet their needs. The impact of this information on them personally was a relief from self-blame as they realized that their inability to purchase enough food for their families was not because of their personal inadequacies but because of government policy.

- *Parent action.* This discovery led them to decide to take action toward change. They wrote letters to political leaders and worked with other community groups, resulting in some increase in the welfare allowances. Finally, some time later, when there was an attempt to close the parent center because of budget cuts, the women organized a march on city hall and got media attention, which prevented closure.

COMMUNITY-LEVEL INTERVENTIONS

Community interventions can be very small scale, such as a community garden, or large scale such as Shape Up Somerville (Economos and Tovar 2012; Matson-Koffman et al. 2005; DeMattia and Denney 2008). Nutrition educators are often key players. Here are a few examples.

Shape Up Somerville (SUS): Eat Smart, Play Hard

SUS is a community-based participatory research project that illustrates the social ecological approach. It addresses concerns about childhood obesity by addressing children's before-school, during-school, after-school, home, and community environments. The intervention resulted in significant decreases in obesity in the children that were

maintained over a 2-year period (Economos et al. 2013). It is described in **NUTRITION EDUCATION IN ACTION 6-4**.

Farmers' Markets

Many communities have initiated farmers' markets, where local growers can bring their produce and other farm products into cities at markets set up by the community. In the United States, low-income individuals participating in SNAP use Electronic Benefit Transfer (EBT) cards to access their benefits at grocery stores. These cards are often accepted at farmers' markets, making fresh local foods available to low-income residents in communities. New York City initiated a direct point-of-purchase incentive called Health Bucks, which provides SNAP recipients with a $2 coupon for every $5 spent using SNAP benefits at participating farmers' markets. A study found that use of Health Bucks resulted in increased sales using the SNAP EBT cards at participating farmers' markets, thus increasing purchase of fresh produce (Baronberg et al. 2013). Nutrition educators have been in the forefront of participating in this program.

Community Gardens

Community gardens have, of course, been active since there were communities. Often, members of a community band together to use an unused city lot and start planting. They can produce enough to feed their families. There are now community garden coalitions and movements with nutrition educators as active members in most countries and states within the United States. GreenThumb in New York City, the largest urban gardening program in the United States, has 600 gardens and 20,000 garden members. (http://www.nycgovparks.org/about/history/community-gardens/movement). Additionally, community gardens are often a key feature in many healthy city and community programs around the world. These involve local leadership and resources, volunteers and community partners, and skills-building opportunities for participants (Twiss et al. 2003).

THE BUILT ENVIRONMENT: NEIGHBORHOOD SUPERMARKETS AND WALKABILITY

There is evidence that neighborhoods have an impact on obesity and health (Harrington and Eliot 2009; Dengel et al. 2009). Within neighborhoods are many retail food stores such as supermarkets and grocery stores, as well as

NUTRITION EDUCATION IN ACTION 6-4 Shape Up Somerville (SUS)—Eat Smart, Play Hard: A Social Ecological Approach

Environmental factors at the community level may contribute to the development and maintenance of obesity. Children, in particular, have very little control over their food choices and options for physical activity. School-based programs have been developed, but school time accounts for less than 50% of children's waking hours. Shape Up Somerville was developed to change the environment to prevent obesity in elementary school children.

Program

This 3-year program was directed at children in grades 1 through 3 and was designed to bring about energy balance by increasing physical activity options and availability of healthful foods within children's before-, during-, and after-school, home, and community environments. It used a multifaceted collaborative community-based participatory research (CBPR) approach. The community was involved in all phases: designing, implementing, and evaluating the intervention, and identifying how the data would be used to improve the health of the community. The intervention involved not only children, parents, and teachers, but also food service providers, city departments, policymakers, healthcare providers, restaurants, and the media.

Evaluation

Three matched, culturally diverse communities were assigned to intervention and control conditions. About 1,200 children in public schools in the intervention community participated in the classroom curriculum and pre- and post-evaluations.

Results

- *Students*: The intervention resulted in a significant decrease in the BMI z-scores in children ($P = 0.001$) at the end of 1 year that was maintained a year later.

- *School environment*: More fruits, vegetables, whole grains, and low-fat milk products were available; menus and à la carte items were brought into closer compliance with guidelines; attitudes of students, parents and guardians, school faculty, and food service staff improved; and policies related to food in schools were adopted.

- *Restaurants*: About one-third of the restaurants that were actively recruited became SUS-approved restaurants, agreeing to serve smaller portions and offer healthier options. SUS approval was marketed to the community.

Components of the SUS Program	
Before school	*Home*
■ Breakfast program ■ Walk to school campaign	■ Parent outreach and education ■ Family events ■ Child's "Health Report Card"
During school	*Community*
■ School health office ■ School food service ■ SUS classroom curriculum 　■ 30-minute nutrition and physical activity lesson each week 　■ 10-minute daily "Cool Moves" ■ Enhanced recess ■ School wellness policy development	■ SUS community advisory council ■ Ethnic-minority group collaborations ■ City employee wellness campaign ■ Farmers' market initiative ■ SUS "approved" restaurants ■ Annual 5K family fitness fair ■ Media—columns and ads ■ City ordinances on walkability/bikeability
After School	
■ SUS after-school curriculum ■ Walk from school campaign	

Sources: Economos, C. D., R. R. Hyatt, J. P. Goldberg, et al. 2007. A community intervention reduces BMI z-score in children: Shape Up Somerville first year results. *Obesity* 15:1325–1336; Economos, C. D., S. C. Folta, J. P. Goldberg, et al. 2009. A community-based restaurant initiative to increase availability of healthy menu options in Somerville, Massachusetts: Shape Up Somerville. *Prevention of Chronic Disease* 6(3). http://www.cdd.gov/pcd/issues/2009/jul/o8_0165.htm; Goldberg, J. P., J. J. Collins, S. C. Folta, et al. 2009. Retooling food service for early elementary school in Somerville, Massachusetts: The Shape Up Somerville experience. *Prevention of Chronic Disease* 6(3):A103; and Economos, C. D., R. R. Hyatt, A. Must, et al. 2013. Shape Up Somerville two-year results: a community-based environmental change intervention sustains weight reduction in children. *Preventive Medicine* 57(4):322–327.

restaurants and fast food outlets. There is an association between access to supermarkets and healthier food intakes, such as increased fruit and vegetable intakes, mostly because supermarkets tend to offer a greater variety of foods at a lower cost. Nutrition educators have worked in collaborations with others to provide interventions within grocery stores using point-of-choice information, increased availability, increased variety, pricing, advertising, and promotional strategies , which have resulted in moderate improvements in healthy eating behavior such as fruit and vegetable consumption (Glanz 2007; Escaron et al. 2013).

The term *food deserts* has come to describe areas within urban centers as well as in rural areas where low-income people do not have ready access to fruits, vegetables, and other wholesome, healthful foods at affordable costs (USDA 2014b). Researchers are using geographic information systems (GISs) to map locations of supermarkets in geographic areas to identify such deserts. Nutrition educators have worked in coalition with others to change city zoning and related policies in order to encourage supermarkets to locate in these deserts.

The built environment and walkability of neighborhoods have also been shown to be associated with health conditions. Walkability includes the notion of safe streets, attractive sidewalks with places of interest, and connections to places people need to go. Higher neighborhood walkability, for example, is associated with more walking, lower BMI, and lower blood pressure (Rohere, Pierce, and Dennison 2004; Rundle et al. 2009; Li et al. 2009). Again, in coalition with others, nutrition educators have worked to increase availability of safe and attractive places for people to walk and bicycle.

Sectors of Influence: Policy and Systems Change Activities

Policy activities are extremely important to help make the healthful choices the easy ones. Policy usually refers to a deliberate plan of action to guide decisions and achieve outcomes. Policy is enacted in all sectors of influence on behavior: organizational, community and national. Policies enable changes in systems and social structures to make healthful food and physical activity behaviors easier to do. Policy complements education and environmental change (Rothschild 1999).

RELATIONSHIP AMONG EDUCATION, ENVIRONMENTAL CHANGE, POLICY, AND SYSTEMS

Education, as we have seen, involves a combination of theory-based strategies to increase awareness, enhance motivation, and facilitate the voluntary adoption or maintenance of behaviors that are conducive to health. Some researchers note that education does not provide, on its own, direct or immediate reward or punishment for the behaviors (Rothschild 1999). Sometimes, the anticipated outcomes nutrition educators bring to the public's attention are far into the future, such as "If you drink milk now, you are less likely to develop osteoporosis when you are old."

Environmental change attempts to make the environment favorable for the new behavior. Changing the environment can help individuals make voluntary changes in behavior by offering them the benefits they want and reducing the barriers they are concerned about, for example, by increasing the availability of fruits and vegetables in grocery stores in the audience's community and making them more accessible through pricing incentives. In social marketing this is accompanied by effective communications or persuasion to enhance motivation.

Policy complements these approaches and can also have an important and positive role here. Policies, guidelines and regulations can make it easier for people to perform a desirable behavior when it would be difficult to carry out because of social pressure to do something different. For example, food policies or nutrition standards for all foods available in school could make it easier for students to eat more fruits and vegetables or drink fewer sweetened beverages, even though less healthy options might be more appealing to students and financially desirable to schools. Nutrition educators need to participate in relevant food policy decisions. This may require them to serve as advocates for healthy policies to policymakers and even lawmakers at the local or national level.

Systems changes, often linked to policy change, can be made to be more supportive of healthful action. A system is a group of independent but interrelated and interacting elements—individuals, institutions, and infrastructure—that form a unified whole. Examples include the healthcare system, school system, or parks and recreation system. Thus, the individuals, institutions, and infrastructure that make up the food system are involved in the interconnected activities of producing, processing, distributing, retailing, preparing, and consuming food. Systems are not static but constantly changing and evolving. Public policy, organizational policy, and other actions can bring about changes in systems. System change complements other venues for making the healthful action easier.

POLICY INTERVENTIONS: WHAT WORKS?

While policy interventions to promote healthy eating can take many forms, some policy analysts see them as consisting of two broad categories: interventions related to information, such as regulations about food advertising, nutritional labeling, or conducting public information campaigns, or those directed at the market environment, such as guidelines, regulations about food and diet standards, and fiscal measures (Brambile-Macias et al. 2011). A review of interventions found that those directed at the information environment have been successful in raising awareness, but not always in changing behavior. Policy interventions related to changing the market environment (e.g., incentives, regulations) are more intense or intrusive but more likely to be effective.

ORGANIZATIONAL-LEVEL POLICY AND SYSTEM CHANGE ACTIVITIES

Organizational policies regarding school, worksite, and community food environments influence people's food choices and eating patterns. Thus, an important venue for nutrition education is to work with policymakers to develop or modify existing policies to make them more supportive of healthy eating and active living.

School Food Policies and Systems Change Activities

Many food-related environmental issues that influence what youth eat in schools need to be addressed by institutional policy action rather than, or in addition to, classroom education because the school food environment is challenging in the United States:

- *Food used in school fundraising.* Short of funds, many schools sell food products to raise money; these products are usually high-fat or high-sugar items such as candy, chips, or sweetened beverages.

- *Food is often used in the classroom as a reward or incentive.* Again, most often such foods tend to be high-fat and high-sugar, largely because these are liked by students.

- *Food advertising.* In schools, advertising of food occurs directly on vending machines, book covers, wall boards, hallway decorations, and sports scoreboards, in student publications and yearbooks, and indirectly through coupons to fast food outlets given for academic achievement.

Over the years, nutrition educators have advocated that schools form school nutrition advisory councils or health councils made up of teachers, administrators, parents, students, and intervention staff to assess the overall school food environment, consider and discuss issues, and advance school-level policy that promotes a healthful food environment in order to make the healthful choice the easy choice (Kubik, Lytle, and Story 2001). In the United States, such an approach is now in place. Each local educational agency or school district participating in the NSLP is required to establish a local school **wellness policy**, which at a minimum has to include the following (Child Nutrition and WIC Reauthorization Act 2004; USDA 2005):

- Goals for nutrition education, physical activity, and other school-based activities that are designed to promote student wellness

- Nutrition guidelines selected by the local school for all foods available on campus during the school day, with the objectives of promoting student health and reducing childhood obesity

- Involvement of parents, students, and representatives of the school food authority, school board, administrators, and public in development of the policy

- A plan for measuring implementation of the policy

A nutrition educator is not specifically required to be part of the team, but can offer his or her services as a member of the public or as a parent.

Although all schools or school districts have such policies in place, the comprehensiveness of the policies differ and the degree to which they are implemented in schools also differ. Much still needs to be done for full implementation and nutrition educators can help with the process in collaboration with the schools.

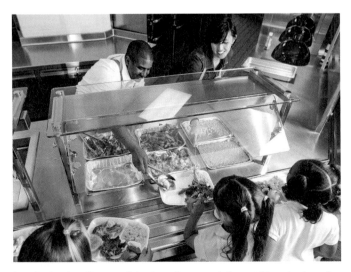

Local school wellness policies have improved the nutritional value of school lunches.

© Steve Debenport/iStock

Health Promoting Schools

The Health Promoting Schools approach, initiated by the World Health Organization (WHO) in the 1900s and widely used throughout the world, integrates multilevel and comprehensive interventions addressing school environment, curriculum, policy-making, and relevant social and cultural factors such as school ethos, cultural group membership, communication across all participants in the setting, and community involvement to promote the health of children (WHO 1996, 2013). Many schools using such an approach are effective in fostering a healthy school climate (Gugglberger and Dur 2011; Lee and Stewart 2013). Nutrition educators can play an important role in helping schools implement this approach and provide assistance in the nutrition education component of the approach.

Workplace Policy and Systems Change Activities

Many interventions in the worksite have tested a comprehensive, multilevel approach to creating an environment supportive of healthy eating by addressing organizational policy as well as the physical and social environments (Sorensen et al. 1998; Beresford et al. 2001). Nutrition educators are very important for educating decision-makers and management about the importance of food and health issues and convincing them to take action. They also can initiate programs and provide services and technical support. However, they need to work in collaboration with both employees and management to develop policies and

procedures in order to implement and institutionalize programs.

A review of such studies finds that a number of organizational factors are related to program effectiveness (Sorensen et al. 2002):

- Management commitment and supervisory support are essential. Policies need to be modified, and this requires management support.
- Worker involvement in planning and implementation is just as important. This can be done through such mechanisms as an "employee advisory board" at each site and through delivery of the intervention by peers. The employee advisory board chooses the intervention components to be implemented in the individual worksite setting, disseminates program messages and information throughout the worksite, and encourages long-term incorporation of the program into the worksite (Sorensen et al. 1990; Sorensen et al. 1992; Cousineau et al. 2008).

The more that employees are involved, the greater the number of activities implemented (Hunt et al. 2000). Worksite management must put in place policies to permit and encourage employees to take work time to participate in these health promotion activities (Williams et al. 2007).

COMMUNITY- AND CITY-LEVEL POLICY AND SYSTEM CHANGE ACTIVITIES

Many community organizations focus on food policy. For example, state and local food policy councils are composed of stakeholders from various segments of a state or local food system. Councils can be officially sanctioned through a government action such as an executive order, or they may be grassroots efforts. The primary goal of many food policy councils is to examine the operation of a local food system and provide ideas or recommendations for how it can be improved. Nutrition educators are often members of such councils to broaden the scope of the councils, in which members may be more concerned with emergency food assistance or agriculture policy (see http://www.state-foodpolicy.org).

Various community food security coalitions and farm and food projects also work to analyze and develop policy initiatives to link local farmers and communities. Important roles for nutrition educators have been proposed in terms of education about food and gardening, participation in community food recovery projects, advocacy in terms of public policy, and research (Hamm and Bellows 2003).

Cities have also become involved in food and physical fitness policy. Some cities, such as New York City, have initiated regulations that require chain fast food restaurants to post calorie counts of food items on the menu board itself. City government officials around the world have proposed and often enacted food policies, such as the comprehensive Healthy and Sustainable Food Policy in San Francisco (http://sfgov.org/sffood/).

Public Information Media Interventions

Information provided in public forums can serve as a nutrition education tool in several ways. It can provide motivational (why-to) or instrumental (how-to) information on an important issue. However, the information can also help to establish social and community norms that are supportive of dietary change. For example, numerous posters about breastfeeding or eating fruits and vegetables can encourage people to see these behaviors as the social norm. They can also serve as cues to action. In addition to posters in schools, at work, or in community centers, billboards in the community can help establish norms and serve as cues to action. Studies have shown that posters could increase stair use in blue- and white-collar worksites, shopping centers, and other locations (Kerr, Evans, and Carroll 2000, 2001; Kwak et al. 2007).

The New York City Department of Health provides posters for use in multiple settings. Two are shown in **FIGURE 6-4** and **FIGURE 6-5**. One poster is for use in small neighborhood grocery stores. As you can see, the graphic

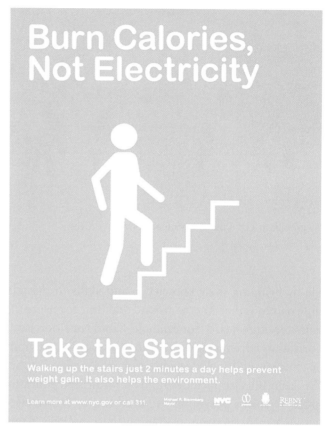

FIGURE 6-5 New York City Department of Health and Mental Hygiene: Exercise.

Courtesy of the New York City Department of Health and Mental Hygiene.

provides why-to, or motivational, information: "Move to 1% Milk. Your Heart and Your Waistline Will Thank You," and how-to, or instrumental, information: "1% Milk Available Here." The second poster is about taking the stairs rather than taking the elevator and can be used in any building. It links a "green" message with a health message: "Burn Calories, Not Electricity. Take the Stairs."

Information on the number of calories on menu items in fast food restaurant chains has become required in many communities around the world. This can signal to people that this is an important feature to consider and may have some impact on food choices (Bassett et al. 2008; Harnack et al. 2008).

PUBLIC POLICY

The main vehicle for national public policy in relation to food is through advocacy action in relation to proposed or existing legislation. In the United States, several laws related to food and nutrition come up for reauthorization every few years. Nutrition educators can play an important

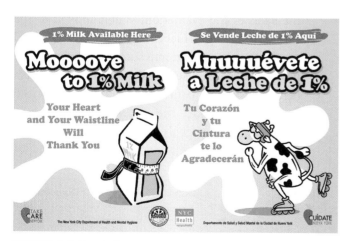

FIGURE 6-4 New York City Department of Health and Mental Hygiene: Diet.

Courtesy of the New York City Department of Health and Mental Hygiene.

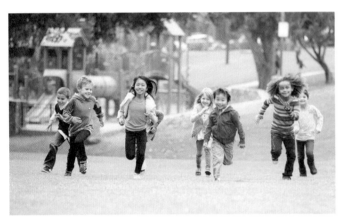

Playgrounds in a community encourage physical activity.

© Mark Bowden/iStock.

role by bringing their knowledge and skills to the relevant coalitions that emerge around that time to ensure that their voices are heard. For example, Child Nutrition Reauthorization covers many of the food assistance programs for children and includes education and wellness policy. The Farm Bill also includes funds for nutrition education through various programs. We need to stay informed so that we can participate in shaping these policies. These activities are described in greater detail in Chapter 18.

A Logic Model Approach for Planning Nutrition Education

How should we address all these different levels of influence as they impact the behavioral goals of a given program? How should we convert our understanding of these many determinants into an intervention plan? A tool that is being used in many fields and that has been applied to nutrition education programs is helpful here: the *logic model*, which is a simplified but very logical model for how to plan a nutrition education program (Medeiros et al. 2005). It shows that in planning, nutrition educators need to think about the following:

- The resources that will go into a program (the *inputs*)
- The activities the program will undertake (the *outputs*)
- The changes or benefits that result (the *outcomes*)

In its simplest form, it consists of the components shown in **FIGURE 6-6**.

As nutrition educators we can use a logic model for community nutrition education as follows.

- First, we determine the *priority behavior changes or actions* that will be the focus of our program, based on the situation and issues of concern arising from nutrition science evidence, health policy, assessment of the intended audience, and other considerations. The priority behaviors in the USDA Community Nutrition Education (CNE) Model are related to diet quality and physical activity, food security, food safety practices, and resource management. However the model can be applied to other behaviors such as dietary practices supportive of sustainable food systems. With the behavioral focus clearly delineated, we are ready to consider:
- *The inputs.* These are resources such as the staff and volunteers of the program, time, materials, money, space, partners, and collaborators.
- *The focus.* We can use the logic model to design direct or indirect nutrition education with individuals and families, or interventions directed at several levels of the social ecological model.
- *The outputs are what nutrition educators do.* Outputs consist of the strategies and activities that we design: conducting classes, facilitating groups, and developing printed and visual materials, products, Internet activities, and other resources; working with families, community partners, and public policymakers; and working with media. These activities need to be directed at the potential determinants of change identified by theory and research evidence.
- *The outcomes are the results nutrition educators obtain from the theory-based strategies that they designed and implemented.* These outcomes become the basis of the evaluation. When applied to the several levels of influence of the social ecological model, the ultimate desired outcomes are improved health, decreased disease risk, and other long-term benefits, such as community actions or revised policies to support the intervention's targeted behavioral change goals.

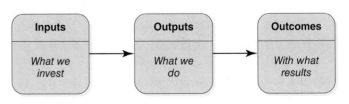

FIGURE 6-6 Components of the logic model.

Promoting policies, systems, and environments that facilitate individuals' ability to make changes in the behaviors targeted by the intervention does not come easily, as we have seen in in this chapter. In the short term, it may mean we focus on increasing the awareness of key decision-makers and policymakers regarding the importance of the issues that the program is seeking to address. In the medium term, it may mean obtaining their commitment to change. Finally, in the long term, it means working in collaboration with others to achieve the behavioral goals of the program.

FIGURE 6-7 shows a community nutrition education logic model that addresses multiple levels and sectors of influence on core behaviors that are the targets of U.S. government programs: diet quality and physical activity, food security, food safety, and food resource management. This figure is complex, combining the activities in all the settings and sectors of influence on all these behaviors in the same logic model.

We start in the left column with a statement of the *situation or issues of concern* along with the *priority behaviors* that will address the concerns, and the *inputs needed* (financial, materials, and people as well as a comprehensive needs assessment process). The *focus or level of intervention* is shown in the next column, followed by the *outputs or activities* conducted by an intervention and the participants at these levels:

- *Individuals and families*: Provide direct nutrition education involving active learning with an educator. The educational activities at both the individual and interpersonal levels address personal determinants of behavior change or action, such as beliefs, attitudes, affect, and skills, with outcomes for individuals that can be achieved within a short-, medium-, and long-term time frame.
- *Environmental settings (organizations and communities)*: Activities involve providing support for intervention behavioral goals by developing local partnerships and with them identifying challenges and opportunities to supporting intervention goals in the short term, developing plans of action in the medium term, and actually putting in place environmental changes that improve targeted behaviors in the long term.
- *Sectors of influence (policy and social systems)*: Activities involve influencing, creating, or revising social systems and policies related to intervention behavioral goals.

Finally, the desired *outcomes* at these different levels of activity are shown. On the right of the outcomes are several columns showing examples of indicators or methods to measure the outcomes in several areas targeted by U.S. government programs: diet quality and physical activity, food security, food safety, and food resources management.

Although environmental settings, policy, and systems are conceptually distinct, in most settings changes in environment require changes in policy, and changes in policy very often result in changes in the environment.

Clearly, strong networking and coalition-building skills will serve nutrition educators well as they take on the role of environmental change agents at these varying levels and sectors of influence, in addition to providing nutrition education to groups and through various media.

Summary

The social ecological model suggests that to motivate and facilitate people's move to healthy eating and active living requires that we not only conduct individual-level nutrition education activities, but also create supportive actions in the interpersonal social environment, in environmental settings such as organizations and communities, and in policies, systems, and social structures in order to ensure that the healthy actions are the easy ones.

NUTRITION EDUCATION STRATEGIES DIRECTED AT THE INTERPERSONAL-LEVEL SOCIAL ENVIRONMENT

Activities at the interpersonal level involve helping to make family context and social networks more supportive.

Enhancing Family Support

Nutrition education strategies for increasing family support usually involve workshops with parents or caregivers that are designed to integrate education about nutrition, physical activity and parenting practices; engage family support for school-based nutrition education by creating student–family activities conducted at home or at family fun nights at school; and use newer technologies such as text-messaging and social media. You can also conduct workshops or other activities for families of employees,

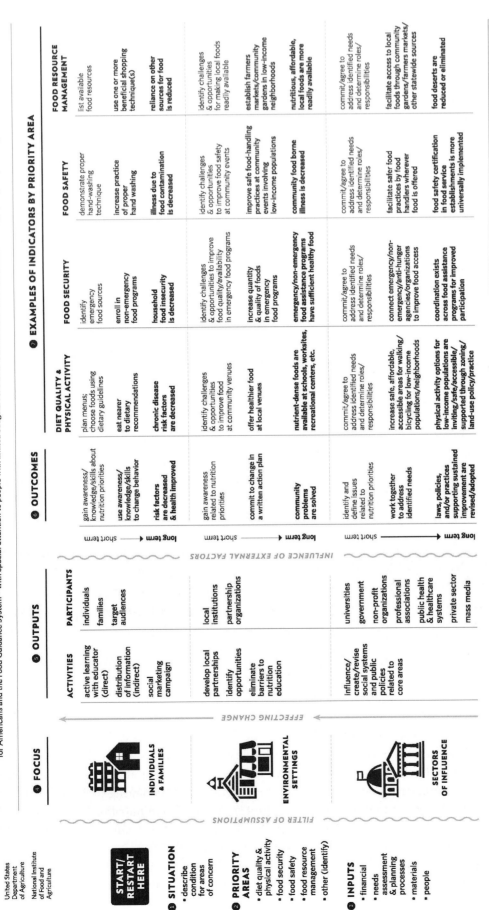

FIGURE 6-7 Community nutrition education logic model framework addressing multiple levels of intervention.

Revision 3 of the CNE Logic Model. (February 2014). Aligns with Dietary Guidelines for Americans, 2010. Contact Helen Chipman, National Program Leader, Food and Nutrition Education, NIFA/USDA. Used with permission. http://www.nifa.usda.gov/nea/food/fsne/logicmodeloverview.pdf

those attending outpatient clinics, or cardiac rehabilitation centers to help them be supportive.

Enhancing Existing Social Networks or Creating New Networks

Nutrition education programs can work with existing networks, such as parent associations in schools, employee associations at workplaces, or community groups, to make them more supportive of the targeted behaviors or practices. Nutrition educators can also initiate a social support group through which new social network linkages are built. For example, a group can be developed for those in a workplace who are interested in weight control or weight acceptance. Support groups can be developed at a health center for those with HIV/AIDS, or cooking classes and behavioral change sessions can be created for participants in a program. Social media provide an ideal way for participants to support each other.

NUTRITION EDUCATION STRATEGIES DIRECTED AT POLICY AND SYSTEM CHANGES IN ENVIRONMENTAL SETTINGS

Environmental interventions and policy and system change activities seek to enhance access and opportunities for people to engage in healthful food and activity behaviors. Addressing environmental determinants of people's health-related action takes many different approaches and involves a variety of venues. They involve collaboration and partnerships. Nutrition educators can be more effective if they hone their collaboration and networking skills.

Organizational Environmental Change

Nutrition educators can assist organizations to develop appropriate policies with respect to foods offered on site. Thus, in schools, they can work with local wellness councils or nutrition committees made up of teachers, school food service staff, administrators, community members, and students. They can provide technical assistance to these councils to review and help evaluate the effectiveness of policies to encourage healthful food environments such as food used in school fundraising or in the classroom as a reward or incentive, food advertising in schools, and beverage sales in schools. Within workplaces and other settings, vendors are usually for-profit entities. However, even here, food policies can be developed so that healthful foods are more available and accessible.

Community Environmental Change

Working toward environmental change in communities requires that nutrition educators work in collaboration or partnership with various sectors within the community, perhaps community centers, health centers, clinics, food banks, churches, community gardens, schools, restaurants, and so forth. The role of the nutrition educator can vary considerably, from being a member of the team and only providing technical expertise in the food, nutrition, and activity areas, to providing more of a coordinating or organizing role. This means that the role of nutrition educator is expanded to include being an agent of environmental change. This may require new skills in developing and nurturing collaborations and in building community capacity. This also means that the nutrition educator must have a deep understanding of the community and respect for a diversity of backgrounds.

Community and National Policy

Many community organizations and national organizations focus on food policy. Nutrition educators can work within them to advocate for, create, or revise policies that are supportive of the behaviors or issues that are important for nutritional health. Here, nutrition educators can provide technical assistance as well as influence. Nutrition educators also can bring their knowledge and skills to food assistance programs and public health agencies. Nutrition educators need to stay informed about policies and issues as they come up and participate, where possible and appropriate, to have a voice in how these policies will be developed and implemented. Some of these national policy activities are described in Chapter 18 of this book.

MAKING THE HEALTHFUL CHOICE THE EASY CHOICE

In all settings and through all sectors of influence, the goal of our activities with our partners and collaborators is to support healthful diets and active living by making the healthful choice easier. Adopting these comprehensive approaches enhances the likelihood of improving the effectiveness of nutrition education interventions for individual and environmental change.

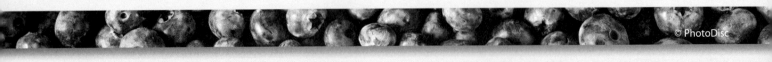

© PhotoDisc

Questions and Activities

1. Think about one or two dietary changes you have tried to make. What factors in the environment have been helpful in supporting your change, and what factors have not been helpful? List five of each. Based on this chapter, what do you think that nutrition educators could have done to be helpful to you?

2. What would the ideal healthful food and activity environment look like to you—at work or school or in the community? What role do you think nutrition educators should play in promoting an environment that is supportive of healthful eating?

3. What is the social ecological approach to nutrition education? Describe the levels of influence in this approach and the role of nutrition educators in each.

4. Define the following terms and describe how they relate to nutrition education. Give examples:
   a. Social networks
   b. Collaboration
   c. Policy

5. What is community capacity? How can it be strengthened? What is the role of nutrition educators in the process?

6. If you were asked to name three things that schools could do to support healthy eating and active living, what would they be? What is the evidence for your recommendations?

7. If you were asked to name three things that worksites could do to support healthy eating and active living, what would they be? What is the evidence for your recommendations?

8. What do we mean by policy in relation to diet and physical activity? How are education, environmental change, and policy related? What is the role of nutrition educators in policy making?

9. What skills do you think nutrition educators should have to be able to work with others to bring about environments and policy that are supportive of health? What role would you like to see yourself play in these activities? What skills do you already possess to do this work and what new skills would you like to develop? How might you obtain these skills?

10. Here are a couple of scenarios for you to work on in teams of two or three:
    - The administrative support staff in the financial aid department of the local university is looking for advice to implement a worksite health promotion program. The staff members spend a lot of time at their desks because they have a lot of calls and meetings with students who have questions about their financial aid. Sometimes it's just easier to sit at their desk and work through lunch. Also, it always seems as if every week is another birthday or holiday and there is cake in the breakroom. What barriers are unique to this population? What strategies could the worksite program use to improve the health of these employees? How will you evaluate effectiveness?
    - The warden of the state correctional facility is concerned about the health of his employees. The correctional officers pack their meals, and knowing that they might have to stay after their shift if the prison is put into lockdown, they tend to pack a large cooler with days' worth of food. Oftentimes, they will be standing guard with this cooler by their side and eat the entire contents in a single shift. Many of the employees state it is a high stress job and this contributes to their overeating. What barriers are unique to this population? What strategies would the worksite program use to improve the health of these employees? How will you evaluate effectiveness?

References

Abratt, R., and S. D. Goodey. 1990. Unplanned buying and in-store stimuli in supermarkets. *Managerial Decisions and Economics* 11:111–121.

Ammerman, A. S., C. H. Lindquist, K. N. Lohr, and J. Hersey. 2002. The efficacy of behavioral interventions to modify dietary fat and fruit and vegetable intake: A review of the evidence. *Preventive Medicine* 35(1):25–41.

Bandura, A. 1997. *Self efficacy: The exercise of control*. New York: WH Freeman.

———. 2001. Social cognitive theory: An agentic perspective. *Annual Review of Psychology* 51:1–26.

Baronberg, S., L. Dunn, C. Nonas, R. Dannefer, and R. Sacks. 2013. The impact of New York City's Health Bucks program on Electronic Benefit Transfer spending at farmers' markets, 2006–2009. *Preventing Chronic Disease* 10.

Bassett, M. T., T. Dumanovsky, C. Huang, L. D. Silver, C. Young, C. Nonas, et al. 2008. Purchasing behavior and calorie information at fast-food chains in New York City, 2007. *American Journal of Public Health* 98(8):1457–1459.

Beresford, S. A., B. Thompson, Z. Feng, A. Christianson, D. McLerran, and D. L. Patrick. 2001. Seattle 5 a Day worksite program to increase fruit and vegetable consumption. *Preventive Medicine* 32(3):230–238.

Berge, J. M., S. W. Jin, P. Hannan, and D. Neumark-Sztainer. 2013. Structural and interpersonal characteristics of family meals: Associations with adolescent body mass index and dietary patterns. *Journal of the Academy of Nutrition and Dietetics* 113(6):816–822.

Berkman, L. F., and T. Glass. 2000. Social integration, social networks, social support, and health. In *Social Epidemiology*, edited by L. F. Berkman and I. Kawachi. New York: Oxford Press.

Bhana, H., A. Islas, R. Paul, A. Rickards, I. R. Contento, H. Lee et al. 2014. Food, Health and Choices: Using focus group data to determine effective family supports. *Journal of Nutrition Education and Behavior* 46(4S):S134.

Blissett, J. 2011. Relationships between parenting style, feeding style and feeding practices and fruit and vegetable consumption in early childhood. *Appetite* 57(3):826–831.

Brambile-Macias, J., B. Shankar, S. Capacci, M. Mazzocchi, F. J. Perez-Cueto, F. J. Verbeke, and W. B. Traill. 2011. Policy interventions to promote healthy eating: A review of what works, what does not, and what is promising. *Food and Nutrition Bulletin* 32(4):365–375.

Burgess-Champoux, T. L., N. Larson, D. Neumark-Sztainer, P. J. Hannan, and M. Story. 2009. Are family meal patterns associated with overall diet quality during the transition from early to middle adolescence? *Journal of Nutrition Education and Behavior* 41(2):79–86.

Cornell University Division of Nutritional Sciences. n.d. Collaboration for Health, Activity, and Nutrition in Children's Environments. https://fnec.cornell.edu/Our_Initiatives/CHANCE.cfm

Child Nutrition and WIC Reauthorization Act. 2004, June 30. Local wellness policy. Section 204 of Public Law 108–265. Enacted by the 108th Congress of the United States of America.

Chipman, H. 2014. Community Nutrition Education (CNE) Logic Model Overview, Version 3. http://www.nifa.usda.gov/nea/food/fsne/logicmodeloverview.pdf Accessed 6/15/14.

Cohen, D. A. 2008. Obesity and the built environment: Changes in environmental cues cause energy imbalances. *International Journal of Obesity* 32:S137–S142.

Cole-Lewis, H., and T. Kershaw. 2010. Text-messaging as a tool for behavior change in disease prevention and management. *Epidemiological Reviews* 32:56–69.

Contento, I. R., S. S. Williams, J. L. Michela, and A. B. Franklin. 2006. Understanding the food choice process of adolescents in the context of family and friends. *Journal of Adolescent Health* 38(5):575–582.

Cousineau, T., B. Houle, J. Bromberg, K. C. Fernandez, and W. C. Kling. 2008. A pilot study of an online workplace nutrition program. *Journal of Nutrition Education and Behavior* 40:160–167.

Cullen, K. W., T. Baranowski, E. Owens, T. Marsh, L. Rittenberry, and C. de Moor. 2003. Availability, accessibility, and preferences for fruit, 100% fruit juice, and vegetables influence children's dietary behavior. *Health Education and Behavior* 30(5):615–626.

Daubert, H., D. Ferko-Adams, D. Rheinheimer, and C. Brecht. 2012. Metabolic risk factor reduction through a worksite health campaign: A case study design. *Online Journal of Public Health Infomatics* 4(2):e3.

Davis, E. M., K. W. Cullen, K. B. Watson, M. Konarik, and J. Radcliffe. 2009. A Fresh Fruit and Vegetable Program improves high school students' consumption of fresh produce. *Journal of the American Dietetic Association* 109(7):1227–1231.

DeMattia, L., and S. L. Denney. 2008. Childhood obesity prevention: Successful community-based efforts. *Annals of the American Academy of Political and Social Science* 615:83–99.

Dengel, D. R., M. O. Hearst, J. H. Harmon, A. Forsythe, and L. A. Lytle. 2009. Does the built environment relate to the metabolic syndrome in adolescents? *Health Place* 15(4):946–951.

Dickin, K. L., and J. Dollahite. 2012. The socio-ecological approach to healthy lifestyles: What do nutrition practitioners need to become environmental change agents? International Society for Behavioral Nutrition and Physical Activity Annual Meeting, Portugal:P041.

Dickin, K. L., T. F. Hill, and J. Dollahite. 2014. Practice-based evidence of effectiveness in an integrated nutrition and parenting education intervention for low-income parents. *Journal of the Academy of Nutrition and Dietetics* 114(6):945–950.

Dickin, K. L., and G. Seim. 2013, Sept. 13. Adapting the Trials of Improved Practices (TIPs) approach to explore the acceptability and feasibility of nutrition and parenting recommendations what works for low-income families? *Maternal and Child Health*. Epub ahead of print.

Dollahite, J., D. Kenkel, and C. S. Thompson. 2008. An economic evaluation of the Expanded Food and Nutrition Education Program. *Journal of Nutrition Education and Behavior* 40(3):134–143.

Ebbeling, C. B., M. N. Pearson, G. Sorensen, et al. 2007. Conceptualization and development of a theory-based healthful eating and physical activity intervention for postpartum women who are low income. *Health Promotion Practice* 8(1):50–59.

Economos, C. D., R. R. Hyatt, A. Must, J. P. Goldberg, J. Kuder, E. N. Naumova et al. 2013. Shape Up Somerville two-year results: A community-based environmental change intervention sustains weight reduction in children. *Preventive Medicine* 57(4):322–327.

Economos, C. D., and A. Tovar. 2012. Promoting health at the community level: Thinking globally, acting locally. *Childhood Obesity* 8:19–22.

Engbers, L. H., M. N. van Poppel, A. Paw, M. J. Chin, and W. van Mechelen. 2005. Worksite health promotion programs with environmental changes: A systematic review. *American Journal of Preventive Medicine* 29(1):61–70.

Escaron A. L., A. M. Meinen, S. A. Nitzke, and A. P. Martinez-Donate. 2013. Supermarket and grocery-store interventions to promote healthful food choices and eating practices: A systematic review. *Preventing Chronic Disease* 10:120–156.

Feenstra G., and J. Ohmart. 2012. The evolution of the school food and farm to school movement in the United States: Connecting childhood health, farms, and communities. *Child Obesity* 8(4):280–289.

Feuenekes, G. I. J., C. De Graff, S. Meyboom, and W. A. Van Staveren. 1998. Food choice and fat intake of adolescents and adults: Association of intakes within social networks. *Preventive Medicine* 26:645–656.

Fulkerson, J. A., D. Neumark-Sztainer, P. J. Hannan, and M. Story. 2008. Family meal frequency and weight status among adolescents: Cross-sectional and 5-year longitudinal associations. *Obesity* (Silver Spring) 16(11):2529–2534.

Fulkerson, J. A., S. Rydel, M. Y. Kubic, L. Lylte, K. Boutelle, M. Story et al. 2010. Healthy Home Offerings via the Mealtime Environment (HOME): Feasibility, acceptability, and outcomes of a pilot study. *Obesity* (Silver Spring) 18(Suppl 1):S69–SS74.

Furst, T., M. Connors, C. A. Bisogni, J. Sobal, and L. W. Falk. 1996. Food choice: A conceptual model of the process. *Appetite* 26(3):247–265.

Geaney, F., C. Kelly, B. A. Greiner, J. M. Harrington, I. J. Perry, and P. Beirne. 2013. The effectiveness of workplace dietary modification interventions: A systematic review. *Preventive Medicine* 57:438–447.

Glanz, K. 2007. Nutrition Environment Measures Survey in Stores (NEMS-S): Development and evaluation. *American Journal of Preventive Medicine* 32(4):282–289.

Goodman, R. M., et al. 1999. Identifying and defining the dimensions of community capacity to provide a basis for measurement. *Health Education and Behavior* 25:258–278.

Green, L. W., and M. W. Kreuter. 2004. *Health promotion planning: An educational and ecological approach.* 4th ed. New York: McGraw-Hill Humanities/Social Sciences/Languages.

Gugglberger, L., and W. Dur. 2011. Capacity building in and for health promoting schools: Results from a qualitative study. *Health Policy* 101(1):37–43.

Hamm, M. W., and A. C. Bellows. 2003. Community food security and nutrition educators. *Journal of Nutrition and Behavior* 35(1):37–43.

Hanks, A. S., D. R. Just, and B. Wansink. 2013. Smarter lunchrooms can address new school lunchroom guidelines and childhood obesity. *Journal of Pediatrics* 162:867–869.

Harnack, L. J., S. A. French, J. M. Oakes, M. T. Story, R. W. Jeffery, and S. A. Rydell. 2008. Effects of calorie labeling and value size pricing on fast food meal choices: Results from an experimental trial. *International Journal of Behavioral Nutrition and Physical Activity* 5:63.

Harrington, D. W., and S. J. Eliot. 2009. Weighing the importance of neighborhood: A multilevel exploration of the determinants of overweight and obesity. *Social Science and Medicine* 68(4):593–600.

Harrington, K. F., F. A. Franklin, S. L. Davies, R. M. Shewchuk, and M. B. Binns. 2005. Implementation of a family intervention to increase fruit and vegetable intake: The Hi5+ experience. *Health Promotion Practice* 6(2):180–189.

He, M., M. Sangster Bouck, R. St. Onge, S. Stewart et al. 2009. Impact of the Northern Fruit and Vegetable Pilot Programme—a cluster-randomized trial. *Public Health Nutrition* 12(11):199–208.

Heany, C. A., and B. A. Israel. 2008. Social networks and social support. In *Health behavior and health education: Theory, research, and practice.* 4th ed., edited by K. Glanz, B. K. Rimer, and K. Viswanath. San Francisco: Jossey-Bass, pp. 189–210.

Hearn, D. M., T. Baranowski, J. Baranowski, et al. 1998. Environmental influences on dietary behavior among children: Availability and accessibility of fruits and vegetables enable consumption. *Journal of Health Education* 29:26–32.

Hendrie G., G. Sohonpal, K. Lange, and R. Golley. 2013. Change in the family food environment is associated with positive dietary change in children. *International Journal of Behavioral Nutrition and Physical Activity* 10:4.

Hill, T., K. Dickin, and J. S. Dollahite. 2012. Nutrition educators expand their roles to build capacity and community partnerships promoting healthy foods and active play in low-income children's environments. *Journal of Nutrition Education and Behavior* 44(Suppl 1):S16–S17.

Hingle, M. D., T. M. O'Connor, J. M. Dave, and T. Baranowski. 2010. Parental involvement in interventions to improve child dietary intakes: a systematic review. *Preventive Medicine* 52(2):103–111.

Hunt, M. K., R. Lederman, S. Potter, A. Stoddard, and G. Sorensen. 2000. Results of employee involvement in planning and implementing the Treatwell 5-a-Day worksite study. *Health Education and Behavior* 27(2):223–231.

Isbell, M. G., J. G. Seth, R. D. Atwood, and T. C. Ray. 2015. Development and implementation of client-centered nutrition education programs in a 4-stage framework. *American Journal of Public Health* 105(4):e65–70.

Israel, B., B. Checkoway, A. Schulz, and M. Zimmerman. 1994. Health education and community empowerment: Conceptualizing and measuring perceptions of individual, organizational, and community control. *Health Education Quarterly* 21(2):149–170.

Kent, G. 1988. Nutrition education as an instrument of empowerment. *Journal of Nutrition Education* 20:193–195.

Kerr, J., F. Evans, and D. Carroll. 2000. Posters can prompt less active individuals to use the stairs. *Journal of Epidemiology and Community Health* 54:942–943.

Kerr, J., F. Evans, and D. Carroll. 2001. Six-month observational study of promoted stair climbing. *Preventive Medicine* 33:422–427.

Klepp, K-I., C. Pérez-Rodrigo, I. De Bourdeaudhuij, P. Due, I. Elmadfa, J. Haraldottir, et al. 2005. Promoting fruit and vegetable consumption among European schoolchildren: Rationale, conceptualization and design of the Pro Children project. *Annals of Nutrition and Metabolism* 49:212–221.

Kremers, S. P. J., G-J. de Bruijn, T. L. S. Visscher, W. van Mechelen, N. K. de Vries, and J. Brug. 2006. Environmental influences on energy-balance-related behaviors: A dual-process view. *International Journal of Behavioral Nutrition and Physical Activity* 3:9.

Kubik, M. Y., L. A. Lytle, and M. Story. 2001. A practical, theory-based approach to establishing school nutrition advisory councils. *Journal of the American Dietetic Association* 101(2):223–228.

Kwak, L., S. P. J. Kremers, M. A. van Baak, and J. Brug. 2007. A poster-based intervention to promote stair use in blue- and white-collar worksites. *Preventive Medicine* 45(2–3):177–181.

Lefebvre, R. C. and A. S. Bornkessel. 2013. Digital social networks and health. *Circulation* 127(17):1829–1836.

Lee, P. C., and D. E. Stewart. 2013. Does a socio-ecological school model promote resilience in primary schools? *Journal of School Health* 83:795–804.

Lent, M., R. F. Hill, J. S. Dollahite, W. S. Wolfe, and K. L. Dickin. 2012. Healthy Children, Healthy Families: Parents Making a Difference. A curriculum integrating key nutrition, physical activity, and parenting practices to help prevent childhood obesity. *Journal of Nutrition Education and Behavior* 44:90–92.

Li, F., P. Harmer, B. J. Cardinal, and N. Vongjaturapat. 2009. Built environment and changes in blood pressure in middle aged and older adults. *Preventive Medicine* 48(3):237–241.

Long, V., S. Cates, J. Blitstein, K. Deehy, P. Williams, R. Morgan, et al. 2013. *Supplemental Nutrition Assistance Program Education and Evaluation Study (Wave II)*. Prepared by Altarum Institute for the U.S. Department of Agriculture, Food and Nutrition Service.

Lu, A., K. L. Dickin, and J. S. Dollahite. 2012. The socio-ecological approach to healthy lifestyles: What do nutrition practitioners need to become environmental change agents? International Society for Behavior Nutrition and Physical Activity annual meeting, Texas.

Matson-Koffman, D. M., J. N. Brownstein, J. A. Neiner, and M. L. Greaney. 2005. A site-specific literature review of policy and environmental interventions that promote physical activity and nutrition for cardiovascular health: What works? *American Journal of Health Promotion* 19(3):167–193.

McLeroy, K. R., D. Bibeau, A. Steckler, and K. Glanz. 1988. An ecological perspective on health promotion programs. *Health Education Quarterly* 15:351–377.

Medeiros, L. C., S. N. Butkus, H. Chipman, R. H. Cox, L. Jones, and D. Little. 2005. A logic model framework for community nutrition education. *Journal of Nutrition Education and Behavior* 37(4):197–202.

Merrill, R. M., S. G. Aldana, J. Garret, and C. Ross. 2011. Effectiveness of a workplace wellness program for maintaining health and promoting healthy behaviors. *Journal of Occupational and Environmental Medicine* 53(7):782–787.

Minkler, M. 2004. *Community organizing and community building for health*. 2nd edition. New Brunswick, NJ: Rutgers.

National Farm to School Network. 2014. www.farmtoschool.org Accessed 4/10/14.

O'Connor T. M., S. O. Hughes, K. B. Watson, T. Baranowski, T. A. Nicklas, J. O. Fisher et al. 2009. Parenting practices are associated with fruit and vegetable consumption in preschool children. *Public Health Nutrition* 13(1):91–101.

Patrick, H., and T. A. Nicklas. 2005. A review of family and social determinants of children's eating patterns and diet quality. *Journal of the American College of Nutrition* 24(2):83–92.

Patterson, R. E., A. R. Kristal, K. Glanz, D. F. McLerran, J. R. Hebert, J. Heimendinger, et al. 1997. Components of the Working Well trial intervention associated with adoption of healthful diets. *American Journal of Preventive Medicine* 13(4):271–276.

Perez-Rodrigo, C., M. Wind, C. Hildonen, M. Bjelland, K. I. Klepp, and J. Brug. 2005. The Pro Children intervention: Applying the intervention mapping protocol to develop a school-based fruit and vegetable promotion program. *Annals of Nutrition and Metabolism* 49(4):267–277.

Perry, C. L., D. B. Bishop, G. Taylor, D. M. Murray, R. W. Mays, B. S. Dudoviz, et al. 1998. Changing fruit and vegetable consumption among children: The 5-a-Day Power Plus program in St. Paul, Minnesota. *American Journal of Public Health* 88(4):603–609.

Reynolds, K. D., F. A. Franklin, D. Binkley, J. M. Raczynski, K. F. Harrington, K. A. Kirk, et al. 2000. Increasing the fruit and vegetable consumption of fourth-graders: Results from the High 5 project. *Preventive Medicine* 30(4): 309–319.

Rody, N. 1988. Empowerment as organizational policy in nutrition intervention programs: A case study from the Pacific Islands. *Journal of Nutrition Education* 20:133–141.

Rogers, E. M. 2003. *Diffusion of innovations.* 5th ed. New York: Simon and Schuster.

Rohere, J., J. R. Pierce Jr., and A. Dennison. 2004. Walkability and self-rated health in primary care patients. *BMC Family Practice* 5:29.

Rosenthal, B. B. 1998. Collaboration for the nutrition field: Synthesis of selected literature. *Journal of Nutrition Education* 30(5):246–267.

Ross, N. J., M. D. Anderson, J. P. Goldberg, and B. L. Rogers. 2000. Increasing purchases of locally grown produce through worksite sales: An ecological model. *Journal of Nutrition Education* 32(6):304–313.

Rothschild, M. L. 1999. Carrots, sticks, and promises: A conceptual framework for the management of public health and social issues behaviors. *Journal of Marketing* 63: 24–37.

Rundle, A., K. M. Neckerman, L. Freeman, G. S. Lovasi, M. Purciel, J. Quinn, et al. 2009. Neighborhood food environment and walkability predict body mass index in New York City. *Environmental Health Perspectives* 117(3): 442–447.

Safdie, M., N. Jennigs-Aburto, L. Levesque, I. Janssen, F. Campirano-Nunez, N. Lopez-Olmedo et al. 2013a. Impact of a school-based intervention program on obesity risk factors in Mexican children. *Salud Publica Mexico* 55(Suppl 3):S374–S387.

Safdie, M., L. Levesque, I. Gonzalez-Casanova, D. Salvo, A. Islas, S. Hernandez-Cordero, A Bonvecchio, and J. A. Privera. 2013b. Promoting healthful diet and physical activity in the Mexican school system for the prevention of obesity in children. *Salud Publica Mexico* 55(Suppl 3):S357–S373.

Sandvik, C., R. Giestad, J. Brug, M. Rasmussen, M. Wind, A. Wolf et al. 2007. The application of a social cognition model in explaining fruit intake in Austrian, Norwegian, and Spanish school children using structural equation modeling. *International Journal of Behavioral Nutrition and Physical Activity* 14:57.

Senge, P., B. Smith, N. Kruschwitz, J. Laur, and S. Schley. 2010. *The necessary revolution: How individuals and organizations are working together to create a sustainable world.* New York: Broadway Books, Random House.

Shaya, F. T., V. V. Cirikov, D. Howard, C. Foster, J. Costas, S. Snitker, et al. 2014. Effect of social networks intervention in type 2 diabetes: A partial randomization study. *Journal of Epidemiology and Community Health* 68(4):326–332.

Singleton, U., A. Williams, C. Harris, and G. G. Mason. 2005. *Building breastfeeding friendly communities with community partners.* Washington, DC: U.S. Department of Agriculture, Food and Nutrition Service.

Sorensen, G., J. Hsieh, M. K. Hunt, D. H. Morris, D. R. Harris, and G. Fitzgerald. 1992. Employee advisory boards as a vehicle for organizing worksite health promotion programs. *American Journal of Health Promotion* 6(6):443–450, 464.

Sorensen, G., M. K. Hunt, N. Cohen, A. Stoddard, E. Stein, J. Phillips, et al. 1998. Worksite and family education for dietary change: The Treatwell 5-a-Day program. *Health Education Research* 13(4):577–591.

Sorensen, G., M. K. Hunt, D. Morris, G. Donnelly, L. Freeman, B. J. Ratcliffe, et al. 1990. Promoting healthy eating patterns in the worksite: The Treatwell intervention model. *Health Education and Research* 5(4):505–515.

Sorensen, G., A. M. Stoddard, A. D. LaMontagne, K. Emmons, M. K. Hunt, R. Youngstrom, et al. 2002. A comprehensive worksite cancer prevention intervention: Behavior change results from a randomized controlled trial (United States). *Cancer Causes and Control* 13(6):493–502.

Sorensen, G., A. Stoddard, K. Peterson, N. Cohen, M. K. Hunt, R. Palombo, et al. 1999. Increasing fruit and vegetable consumption through worksites and families in the Treatwell 5-a-Day study. *American Journal of Public Health* 89(1):54–60.

Sorensen, G., B. Thompson, K. Glanz, Z. Feng, S. Kinne, C. DiClemente, et al. 1996. Work site-based cancer prevention: Primary results from the Working Well Trial. *American Journal of Public Health* 86(7):939–947.

Sternfeld, B., C. Block, C. P. Queensberry, T. J. Block, G. Husson, J. C. Norris, et al. 2009. Improving diet and physical activity with ALIVE: A randomized trial. *American Journal of Preventive Medicine* 36(6):475–483.

Story, M., K. M. Kaphingst, R. Robinson-O'Brien, and K. Glanz. 2008. Creating healthy food and eating environments: Policy and environmental approaches. *Annual Review of Public Health* 29:253–272.

Te Velde, S. J., J. Brug, M. Wind, C. Holdoned, M. Bielland, C. Perez-Rodrigo, and K. I. Klepp. 2008. Effects of a comprehensive fruit- and vegetable-promoting school-based intervention in three European countries: the Pro Children Study. *British Journal of Nutrition* 99(4):893–903.

Travers, K. D. 1997a. Nutrition education for social change: Critical perspective. *Journal of Nutrition Education* 29(2):57–62.

———. 1997b. Reducing inequities through participatory research and community empowerment. *Health Education and Behavior* 24(3):344–356.

Twiss, J., J. Dickerson, S. Duma, T. Kleinman, H. Paulsen, and L. Riveria. 2003. Community gardens: lessons learned from

California Healthy Cities and Communities. *American Journal of Public Health* 93(9):1435–1438.

U.S. Department of Agriculture. 2005. Healthy Schools: Local wellness policy requirements. http://www.fns.usda.gov/tn/healthy/wellness_policyrequirements.html Accessed 8/12/14.

U.S. Department of Agriculture. 2013. Supplemental Nutrition Assistance Program Education and Evaluation Study (Wave II). Nutrition Assistance Program Report. Food and Nutrition Service, Office of Policy Support, USDA. http://www.fns.usda.gov/sites/default/files/SNAPEdWaveII.pdf Accessed 6/17/15.

U.S. Department of Agriculture. 2014a. Farm to institution. www.usda.gov/documents/6-Farmtoinstitution.pdf Accessed 12/15/14.

U.S. Department of Agriculture. 2014b. Food deserts. http://apps.ams.usda.gov/fooddeserts/foodDeserts.aspx Accessed 11/30/14.

Wallerstein, N. 1992. Powerlessness, empowerment, and health: Implications for health promotion programs. *American Journal of Health Promotion* 6(3):197–205.

Wansink, B. 2006. *Mindless eating.* New York: Bantam Books.

Wansink B., D. R. Just, C. R. Payne, and M. Z. Klinger. 2012. Attractive names sustain increased vegetable intake in schools. *Preventive Medicine* 55(4):330–332.

Williams, A. E., T. M. Vogt, V. J. Stevens, C. A. Albright, C. R. Nigg, R. T. Meenan, et al. 2007. Work, Weight, and Wellness: The 3W Program: A worksite obesity prevention and intervention trial. *Obesity* (Silver Spring) 15(Suppl 1): 16S–26S.

World Health Organization (WHO). 1996. *Local action: Creating health promoting schools* (WHO/NMH/HPS/00.3). Geneva, Switzerland: Author.

World Health Organization (WHO). 2013. What is a health promoting school? http://www.who.int/school_youth_health/gshi/hps/en/ Accessed 12/1/14.

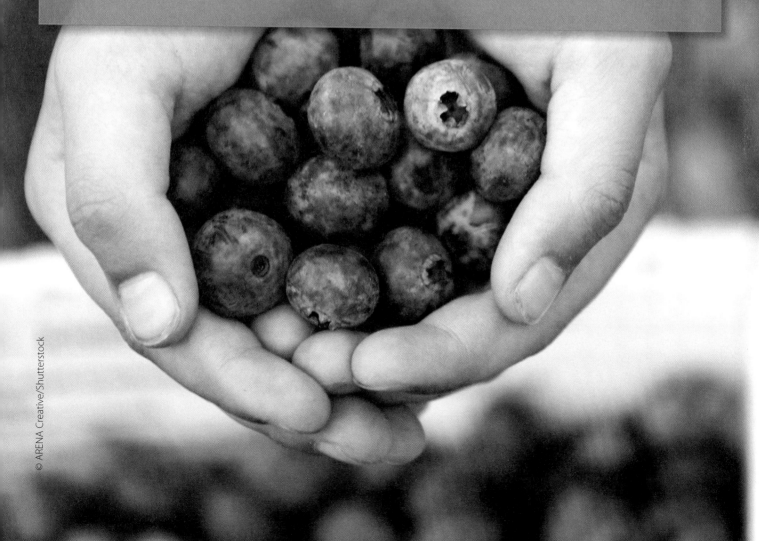

PART II

Using Research and Theory in Practice: A Stepwise Procedure for Designing Theory-Based Nutrition Education

Step 1: Deciding Behavior Change Goals of the Intervention Based on Assessing Issues and Behaviors of Audience

OVERVIEW

Nutrition education is more likely to be effective when it is carefully planned. This chapter begins a new section of the book where the ultimate goal is to develop nutrition education sessions and related activities that are engaging, evidence-based, and effective in promoting healthful eating. It provides an overview of the Nutrition Education DESIGN

Procedure, which is a simple and systematic way to link behavioral theory as a tool to guide practice with your creativity as a nutrition educator. It also describes Step 1: how to decide on the behavior change goals of your intervention based on an assessment of issues and behaviors of concern for identified audiences. A case study illustrates the procedure.

CHAPTER OUTLINE

- The importance of a systematic process for designing effective nutrition education
- Overview of the Nutrition Education DESIGN Procedure for planning theory-based nutrition education
- Using the Nutrition Education DESIGN Procedure for planning educational activities and environmental supports
- Step 1: Deciding the behavior change goals for a given audience by assessing issues and behaviors of concern

- Who is your audience?
- What can you learn about the issues and behaviors of your audience from available general sources?
- What can you learn about the issues and behaviors of your specific audience?
- Decide the behavior change goals of the program for your audience
- Case study: the DESIGN Procedure in action
- Your turn to design nutrition education: completing the Step 1 Decide Behavior Change Worksheet

LEARNING OBJECTIVES

At the end of the chapter, you should be able to:
- State why it is important to use a systematic process to identify the focus and targets for nutrition education
- Describe the six-step Nutrition Education DESIGN Procedure for planning theory-based, behavior-focused nutrition education

- Conduct assessments of the high-priority issues of concern for the intended audience and the behaviors or practices that contribute to these issues
- Identify appropriate information sources for these assessments
- Prioritize and decide on the behavior change goals for session(s) or program

The Importance of a Systematic Process for Designing Effective Nutrition Education

This chapter begins a new section of the book. So far, you have read about the foundations for effective nutrition education. It is clear that while all nutrition education involves information in some way, how this information is communicated is crucial to whether it will be effective in helping people make changes in their eating patterns. You have learned how theory from the behavioral sciences based on evidence helps us to understand why individuals take the health actions they do and how they change. You have examined how we can use such theory as a tool to communicate nutrition education in such a way as to increase the likelihood of success for our interventions. Indeed, one international term for nutrition education is *social and behavior change communication*. How exactly do nutrition educators in typical practice settings translate

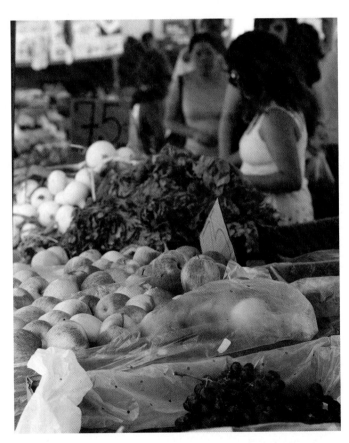

In many communities, buying produce at a farmers' market is common practice.

© Stieglitz/iStock.

these theories into a format that is usable for conducting nutrition education in the real world with real audiences? This is the central task of this book: how to use theory and evidence as a guide to design and deliver nutrition education that will be effective in practice. This is why most nutrition educators entered the field—to make a difference in people's lives.

For example, let's say a group of low-income mothers whose children attend Head Start tells the director they would like to improve their own diets to prevent diabetes, which is common in their community, and the director contacts you. How would you go about designing the nutrition education sessions? Or, the coach of a college athletic team comes to you and says that she is concerned about the eating habits of the student athletes and would like you to do some nutrition education sessions to "help them eat better for health and performance." How would you know what to talk about? What activities would you develop and why? The chapters in this section of the book are designed to help you proceed.

THE NUTRITION EDUCATION DESIGN PROCEDURE FOR EFFECTIVE NUTRITION EDUCATION

Designing nutrition education is both an art and a science. Using a systematic procedure based on research and evidence improves our chances of developing nutrition education that is effective. This is the science. Because a systematic procedure provides a broad framework for how to proceed, it frees us to be creative in developing exciting activities appropriate to our audiences. This is the art.

In this book, the systematic procedure is called the Nutrition Education **DESIGN Procedure**. It involves six steps for how to translate theory and evidence into strategies or techniques for delivery in the settings in which most nutrition educators work. This chapter describes an overview of the entire DESIGN Procedure and starts you on Step 1.

THE NUTRITION EDUCATION DESIGN PROCEDURE AS COACHING

The best way to view the Nutrition Education DESIGN Procedure is to see it as guidance from research and evidence (the science) on refining the practice of nutrition education (the art) to enhance its effectiveness. An analogy may be useful here. A young girl is a good baseball player and seems to have natural talent as a pitcher. The coach carefully analyzes her moves as she pitches, giving her specific guidance on making her moves more precise and effective. He gives her specific moves to practice, which do not come naturally at first, but she practices these moves until they become second nature, making her a formidable pitcher.

In the same way that a pitcher can have natural talent, you already have skills in nutrition education. This book offers coaching based on research evidence. Designing effective nutrition education sessions takes work and requires a systematic process. Try it out and use it a few times. With practice, this systematic process will become second nature and you will adapt it to your own style to design group sessions with ease and to plan appropriate environmental supports.

Overview of the Nutrition Education DESIGN Procedure for Planning Theory-Based Nutrition Education

An outline of the key features of the DESIGN Procedure is shown in the form of a flowchart in **FIGURE 7-1**. The steps are summarized here:

- **Step 1. *Decide* on program behavior change goals for an audience by assessing issues and behaviors of concern**. Deciding on a specific behavioral focus is extremely important for designing an effective program. To do this, we start with some questions:
  - ***Who is your audience?*** It is important to be clear who your audience is and to conduct a careful assessment of this audience.
  - ***What can you learn about the issues and behaviors of your audience from general sources?*** You can start the assessment process by collecting general

information about the issues and behaviors that are a concern for audiences similar to yours.
  - *In terms of issues of concern*: You can learn about the issues facing audiences similar to yours, such as health issues; those related to the food system; social and societal issues related to food; or other issues through sources such as research literature reviews, health surveys, national mortality and morbidity data, and government and expert panel reports. This provides the rationale for your sessions or program.
  - *In terms of behaviors of concern*: You can learn about behaviors of similar audiences that contribute to these issues of concern though research literature, consumer surveys by supermarket chains or restaurant associations, government food consumption surveys, government dietary recommendations, and so forth.
- ***What can you learn about the issues and behaviors of your specific audience?***
  - *In terms of both issues and behaviors of concern*: You can obtain information about your specific audience through group discussions, in-depth interviews of key individuals, focus groups, or surveys. You can also identify current behaviors that are already assets or strengths that can be encouraged to promote health and well-being and ask about their interests and desires for the program.
- ***Decide on the behavior change goals of the program for your audience.*** Based on your assessments, and in active collaboration with your audience to the extent possible, choose one or a few major behaviors, actions, or practices to target in your program. These become the *behavior change goals* of your direct education session(s) or indirect activities, and

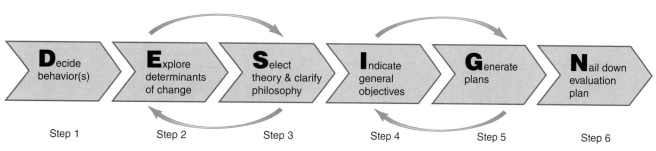

FIGURE 7-1 Nutrition Education DESIGN Procedure overview.

your environmental and policy support activities. Examples are increased breastfeeding, safe food handling behaviors, eating more fruits and vegetables, or eating local foods produced sustainably. These behaviors or practices are stated in terms of *changes* or *actions* the program or session(s) seek(s) to facilitate for the audience to achieve.

- **Step 2.** *Explore* **determinants of change for targeted behavior(s).** In this step you try to understand as fully as possible the motivations and abilities of your audience in the context of their community and culture. In particular, you use theory and research evidence to identify the personal psychosocial determinants or precursors (such as perceived benefits or perceived social and cultural norms) that are relevant and of high priority for the selected actions or behavior change goals, in your given group and setting. Because these identified determinants are those that can be modified by education, advocacy, or policy and can thus *mediate* or bring about changes in the target behaviors or practices, they are often called potential mediators of behavior change in the context of nutrition education. (See Chapter 3 for a discussion of *determinant*s and *mediators.*) Here, you also explore the degree of environmental and policy support available to help the members of your audience achieve the targeted behavior goals of the program.

- **Step 3.** *Select* **the theory you will use or create a theory model** and clarify the educational philosophy that will guide the session or intervention. These provide a framework for your intervention.

- **Step 4.** *Indicate* **appropriate general objectives for the key determinants of change.** In this step you state educational and support objectives that are directed at the key determinants of change in your theory model.

- **Step 5.** *Generate* **educational plan(s), and also environmental support plans if chosen.** Here you select behavior change strategies and practical learning experiences matched to the determinants of change in your theory model. You generate plans for environmental and policy activities to support the behavior change goals.

- **Step 6.** *Nail down* **the evaluation plan.** Finally, you will want to know whether the educational sessions, indirect education activities, and supportive activities you created are effective in achieving the general

objectives and the behavior change goal(s) that you set out. Constructing the evaluation plan at the same time that you are developing the lessons ensures that your evaluation links directly to what is in your educational plans.

Note that the DESIGN Procedure places heavy emphasis on addressing determinants of the behaviors, actions, or practices targeted by the program. The centrality of determinants, precursors, or predictors in behavior change intervention trials has been emphasized by researchers and practitioners alike (Baranowski et al. 1997; Baranowski, Cerin, and Baranowski 2009; Baker et al. 2014). Identifying and addressing determinants—the motivators and facilitators of behavior change—are thus core activities in the design process.

The end products of the procedure are educational plans for your sessions, and environmental and support plans for your program if you include this component. These end products are shown in **FIGURE 7-2**. *You want always to keep this end in sight!*

BOX 7-1   Beginning with the End in Sight— Your Products at the End of the Procedure

What you will have at the end of the design process are ready-to-use educational plans, one for each session you intend to conduct, accompanied by clearly specified supportive policy, systems, or environmental actions where appropriate and selected. You will also have a carefully designed plan to evaluate the session(s) or entire program.

Use the simple and easy-to-follow DESIGN Procedure described here and shown later in Figure 7-4 to develop a plan for nutrition education, whether it consists of only several educational sessions or includes several different kinds of activities. After you have used this process a few times, you will become comfortable with it and will go through the process relatively quickly. If you are already an experienced facilitator of theory-based, behavior-focused nutrition education groups, you can use the DESIGN Workbook short form, Figure 7-3. It is still important, however, to conduct *all* steps in the process systematically, in order to clearly link theory, research, and practice at each step.

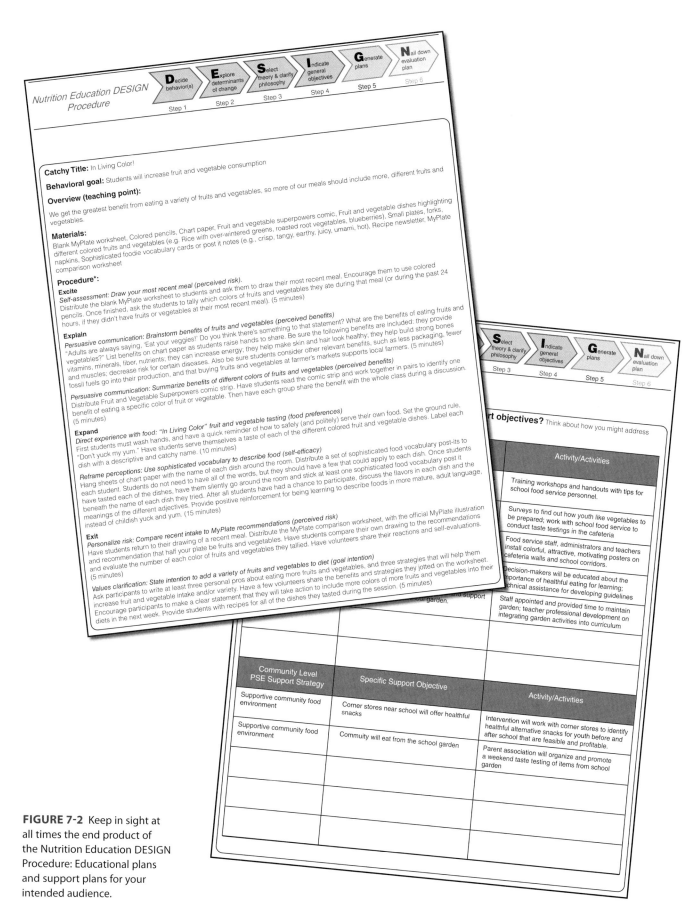

Nutrition Education DESIGN Procedure

Decide behavior(s) — Step 1
Explore determinants of change — Step 2
Select theory & clarify philosophy — Step 3
Indicate general objectives — Step 4
Generate plans — Step 5
Nail down evaluation plan — Step 6

Catchy Title: In Living Color!

Behavioral goal: Students will increase fruit and vegetable consumption

Overview (teaching point):

We get the greatest benefit from eating a variety of fruits and vegetables, so more of our meals should include more, different fruits and vegetables.

Materials:

Blank MyPlate worksheet, Colored pencils, Chart paper, Fruit and vegetable superpowers comic, Fruit and vegetable dishes highlighting different colored fruits and vegetables (e.g. Rice with over-wintered greens, roasted root vegetables, blueberries), Small plates, forks, napkins, Sophisticated foodie vocabulary cards or post it notes (e.g.. crisp, tangy, earthy, juicy, umami, hot), Recipe newsletter, MyPlate comparison worksheet

Procedure*:

Excite
Self-assessment: Draw your most recent meal (perceived risk).
Distribute the blank MyPlate worksheet to students and ask them to draw their most recent meal. Encourage them to use colored pencils. Once finished, ask the students to tally which colors of fruits and vegetables they ate during that meal (or during the past 24 hours, if they didn't have fruits or vegetables at their most recent meal). (5 minutes)

Explain
Persuasive communication: Brainstorm benefits of fruits and vegetables (perceived benefits)
"Adults are always saying, 'Eat your veggies!' Do you think there's something to that statement? What are the benefits of eating fruits and vegetables?" List benefits on chart paper as students raise hands to share. Be sure the following benefits are included: they provide vitamins, minerals, fiber, nutrients; they can increase energy; they help make skin and hair look healthy; they help build strong bones and muscles; decrease risk for certain diseases. Also be sure students consider other relevant benefits, such as less packaging, fewer fossil fuels go into their production, and that buying fruits and vegetables at farmer's markets supports local farmers. (5 minutes)

Persuasive communication: Summarize benefits of different colors of fruits and vegetables (perceived benefits)
Distribute Fruit and Vegetable Superpowers comic strip. Have students read the comic strip and work together in pairs to identify one benefit of eating a specific color of fruit or vegetable. Then have each group share the benefit with the whole class during a discussion. (5 minutes)

Expand
Direct experience with food: "In Living Color" fruit and vegetable tasting (food preferences)
First students must wash hands, and have a quick reminder of how to safely (and politely) serve their own food. Set the ground rule, "Don't yuck my yum." Have students serve themselves a taste of each of the different colored fruit and vegetable dishes. Label each dish with a descriptive and catchy name. (10 minutes)

Reframe perceptions: Use sophisticated vocabulary to describe food (self-efficacy)
Hang sheets of chart paper with the name of each dish around the room. Distribute a set of sophisticated food vocabulary post-its to each student. Students do not need to have all of the words, but they should have a few that could apply to each dish. Once students have tasted each of the dishes, have them silently go around the room and stick at least one sophisticated food vocabulary post it beneath the name of each dish they tried. After all students have had a chance to participate, discuss the flavors in each dish and the meanings of the different adjectives. Provide positive reinforcement for being learning to describe foods in more mature, adult language, instead of childish yuck and yum. (15 minutes)

Exit
Personalize risk: Compare recent intake to MyPlate recommendations (perceived risk)
Have students return to their drawing of a recent meal. Distribute the MyPlate comparison worksheet, with the official MyPlate illustration and recommendation that half your plate be fruits and vegetables. Have students compare their own drawing to the recommendations and evaluate the number of each color of fruits and vegetables they tallied. Have volunteers share their reactions and self-evaluations. (5 minutes)

Values clarification: State intention to add a variety of fruits and vegetables to diet (goal intention)
Ask participants to write at least three personal pros about eating more fruits and vegetables, and three strategies they jotted on the worksheet. Have a few volunteers share the benefits and strategies that will help them increase fruit and vegetable intake and/or variety. Have a few volunteers share how colors of more fruits and vegetables into their diets in the next week. Provide students with recipes for all of the dishes they tasted during the session. (5 minutes) Encourage participants to make a clear statement that they will take action to include more colors of more fruits and vegetables into their diets in the next week.

Select theory & clarify philosophy — Step 3
Indicate general objectives — Step 4
Generate plans — Step 5
Nail down evaluation plan — Step 6

...rt objectives? Think about how you might address

	Activity/Activities
	Training workshops and handouts with tips for school food service personnel.
	Surveys to find out how youth like vegetables to be prepared; work with school food service to conduct taste testings in the cafeteria
	Food service staff, administrators and teachers install colorful, attractive, motivating posters on cafeteria walls and school corridors.
	Decision-makers will be educated about the importance of healthful eating for learning; technical assistance for developing guidelines
	Staff appointed and provided time to maintain garden; teacher professional development on integrating garden activities into curriculum

Community Level PSE Support Strategy	Specific Support Objective	Activity/Activities
Supportive community food environment	Corner stores near school will offer healthful snacks	Intervention will work with corner stores to identify healthful alternative snacks for youth before and after school that are feasible and profitable.
Supportive community food environment	Commuity will eat from the school garden	Parent association will organize and promote a weekend taste testing of items from school garden

FIGURE 7-2 Keep in sight at all times the end product of the Nutrition Education DESIGN Procedure: Educational plans and support plans for your intended audience.

NUTRITION CARE PROCESS AND MODEL

The process described here may be new to you or similar to a process you have used before. Key features are similar to the Nutrition Care Process and Model of the Academy of Nutrition and Dietetics (American Dietetic Association 2008), which uses the following four steps in the clinical setting for individuals:

- Nutrition assessment and reassessment
- Nutrition diagnosis
- Nutrition intervention
- Nutrition monitoring and evaluation

DEFINING TERMS

The terms *behaviors*, *actions*, and *practices* are used here interchangeably, although *practices* has a connotation of long-standing behaviors or commonly practiced behaviors in the community, such as safe food handling practices, breastfeeding, or buying produce at a farmers' market. Evidence is strong that nutrition education is more likely to be effective when it is focused on clearly defined behaviors, actions, or practices.

While we are most often interested in broad food and nutrition goals, for the purposes of designing the nutrition education intervention, effectiveness is enhanced when more focused behaviors or practices are selected. For example, a school garden may be instituted for the stated goal of "improving children's eating habits" (very broad). However, it is sometimes helpful to focus on a narrower goal, such as increasing children's fruit and vegetable intakes (a behavior). Such specific actions contribute to the larger goal of "healthy eating habits." The school may also want to develop a school garden to serve non-nutrition–related goals, such as providing a venue for hands-on experiential learning, increasing the attractiveness of the campus, instilling a feeling that the school cares, and engendering a greater commitment to coming to school and hence better academic performance (Ozer 2007). These broader goals are important, and nutrition education goals may be embedded in these broader goals. However, for nutrition education activities to be effective and thus contribute to the larger goals (and for its effectiveness to be measureable), the focus needs to be clear and specific.

The term *intended audience* is used rather than target population to refer to the individuals or specific subgroup of the population with whom you will be working, to convey the sense that the group members are not a "target" of educator activities so much as partners with whom you work so that together you can address needs and issues of importance to them.

The term nutrition education *intervention* is used here to denote any set of systematically planned educational activities or learning experiences that is provided to a group in a variety of settings (along with relevant environmental supports, where appropriate). This term is problematic to some educators because it can seem to imply that nutrition educators are intervening in people's lives, possibly against their will. It is not used in that sense here; rather, it is a convenient way to describe a range of planned activities of varying scope, based on the desires and needs of the group, designed to enhance motivation, facilitate the ability to take action, and provide supports for action. Thus, the term *intervention* encompasses nutrition education of one or several sessions delivered by one person and also programs involving many components and perhaps several media and delivered by many nutrition educators and other collaborators over a long time span.

Using the Nutrition Education DESIGN Procedure for Planning Educational Activities and Environmental Supports

This part of the book aims to be very practical so that you will be able to apply the six-step process to both educational interventions directed at individuals and supportive environmental activities that include policy, systems, and environmental change.

Educational interventions can consist of *direct education activities* such as education sessions and activities delivered to groups, or *indirect education activities* such as educational materials, Internet nutrition education, communication campaigns, health fairs, or other channels. These activities focus on enhancing motivation and building skills for behavior change and action (that is, for *why-to* and *how-to* take action). All of these direct and indirect educational activities can take place within a variety of settings such as communities, outpatient clinics, schools, workplaces, fitness centers, college athletics, or private nonprofit organizations with a variety of audiences.

The intervention you design can include *environmental support activities* in addition to direct and indirect individual-level educational activities. These can consist of several components directed at policy, systems, and environments with a focus on providing supports for behavior change and action. Examples are parent and school environment components to be supportive to classroom nutrition education or institutional and community environment and policy changes to support community group education and related activities. These activities are usually conducted in collaboration with others, as we described in Chapter 6.

DESIGNING DIRECT AND INDIRECT EDUCATIONAL ACTIVITIES

Based on the mission of your program or intervention and the practical constraints and resource considerations that you know about now, think about whether your intervention will consist of only direct and indirect educational activities directed at individuals and families, or will it be possible for you to work in collaboration with others to promote environmental and policy supports for behavior change and action. That is, will the program be able to address both person-related and environmental determinants of behavior change?

Direct education activities. Direct education activities consist primarily of sessions delivered to a variety of groups (from low-income families to schoolchildren to sports teams to outpatient clinic groups). To design such sessions, follow the DESIGN Procedure steps outlined in Chapters 7–13, one of the six steps in each chapter. In order to effectively deliver what you have designed to your chosen audience(s), you will find the information in Chapters 15 and 17 helpful for honing your skills in working with groups. For these sessions, you will also develop handouts, worksheets, and so forth that you will use with your audience.

Indirect education activities. To design stand-alone indirect activities directed at individuals and families you will also use the DESIGN Procedure steps outlined in Chapters 7–13. These activities include:

- *Printed materials, visual media, Internet-based materials and activities, or health fairs.* You will use the same six steps for these venues. For example, the purpose of these activities needs to be clear as well as their theory base. You will find helpful information for making these materials attractive and useable in Chapter 16.

- *Health communication campaigns and social marketing.* These activities can be quite simple or elaborate involving many channels with a wide audience. Although these two approaches are often considered synonymous, health communication campaigns are directed at raising awareness and motivation while social marketing includes attempts to provide incentives and opportunities as well. These modalities are also described in Chapter 16.

DESIGNING ENVIRONMENTAL SUPPORT ACTIVITIES

If you also will be able to work with others to design activities or components that will provide environmental and policy supports for the behavior change goals of your program, then you will want to follow the steps outlined in Chapter 14. Chapter 14 applies all the 6 steps of the DESIGN Procedure in one chapter to activities to increase environmental supports for action. By environmental supports we mean policy, systems, and environmental activities supportive of the behavior change goals of the program.

DESIGNING EDUCATIONAL AND ENVIRONMENTAL SUPPORT INTERVENTIONS

- To design direct and indirect nutrition education interventions, use the six-step DESIGN Procedure described in Chapters 7–13.

- To design environmental activities that are intended to support the program, use the six-step DESIGN Procedure described in Chapter 14.

WORKSHEETS AND WORKBOOK

Simple *worksheets* are provided for you to use for each of the six steps in designing your nutrition education program. If you are planning group sessions, each of Chapters 7–13 describes how to complete the worksheet for that step (Steps 1 through 6), but the worksheets themselves for all six steps are placed in a *workbook* at the end of Chapter 13. Go to the end of Chapter 13 to complete each of the worksheets as you move along the planning process. If you are planning policy, systems, and environment support activities, the worksheets for all six steps are placed in a *workbook* at the end of Chapter 14. However, Step 1, deciding the behavior change goals for the intervention, is in common for both the educational and environmental support components because both kinds of interventions are directed at the exact same behavior change goals. Thus the information you gather for Step 1 in this chapter will also be used for Step 1 in Chapter 14.

A CASE STUDY: HOW THE DESIGN PROCEDURE LINKS THEORY AND RESEARCH TO PRACTICE AT EVERY STEP

This chapter introduces a case study that you will follow throughout the six steps, one step per chapter, as an example of how to complete the DESIGN Procedure worksheets. The basic steps are quite simple and easy to follow. The case study consists of both educational group sessions and environmental support activities. In Chapters 7–13, we describe the six steps as applied to the educational sessions only. A completed worksheet for each step of the DESIGN Procedure for the case study educational sessions is placed at the end of each of Chapters 7–13 to illustrate that step. In Chapter 14, we place the worksheets for all six steps of the procedure for the environmental support components of the case study.

The activities for each step of the case study are briefly described below. The case study is described in more detail at the end of this chapter. Also at the end of the chapter is the completed regular Step 1 Decide Behavior Change Worksheet for the case study.

We have also created a Nutrition Education DESIGN Procedure Workbook short form that you can use. This short form takes you through all six steps in two pages. **FIGURE 7-3** shows the completed short form for all six steps for the educational component of the case study. This "At a Glance" version gives you an overview of what goes into each step of the DESIGN Procedure.

Case study background. The organization initiating the program is a university-affiliated nonprofit organization that provides health services to youth and families in a mid-sized, racially diverse town with only one middle school. It wishes to provide nutrition education to students in this middle school. It hired a nutrition educator, who used the following steps to design the intervention.

Step 1. Decide on program behavior change goals for an audience by assessing issues and behaviors of concern. The nutrition educator investigated the major issues and behaviors of concern facing these teenagers and then decided on several behaviors to focus on.

- *Who is your audience?* In this case example, the audience is middle school students.
- *What can you learn about your audience from general sources?* In terms of *issues of concern* or rationale of the sessions, general information from research literature and national monitoring documents showed that middle school youth were at risk of obesity, along with diabetes, based on prevalence and severity of the condition. *In terms of behaviors*, government consumption monitoring data and consumer surveys on the Internet suggested that middle school youth did not eat enough fruits and vegetables; drank too many sweetened drinks; ate too many high-fat, high-sugar, highly processed snacks; ate at fast food restaurants; and were not active enough. Some of these behaviors contributed to another issue of concern: the high carbon footprint of the processing and packaging of their drinks and snacks.
- *What can you learn about your specific audience?* In terms of risk, the educator was able to review the records of the health services that the university offered to the school. The records confirmed the general information from national sources. In particular, the youth had high rates of overweight and obesity and were at risk of diabetes. In terms of behaviors, the nutrition educator gave out a survey to two of the middle school classes about their eating patterns. She found that they were eating too few fruits and vegetables; drinking too many sweetened drinks; eating too many high-fat, high-sugar, highly processed snacks; eating out frequently at fast food restaurants; and were sedentary. Some of these behaviors contributed to another issue of concern: the high carbon footprint of the processing and packaging of the snacks they ate.
- *Decide on the behavior change goals for the program.* The nutrition educator and her colleagues reviewed the data and prioritized the behaviors. They decided on addressing four of the behaviors listed above as behavior change goals: increasing intake of fruits and vegetables and physical activity and decreasing intake of highly processed, energy-dense snacks and sugar-sweetened beverages. The intervention would be delivered in health education classes over 10 sessions, with two sessions on each of the behaviors, plus an introductory session and conclusion session. Because the determinants of each of the behaviors may be different, for space reasons we will focus on only one behavior: increasing intake of fruits and vegetables.

The Nutrition Education **DESIGN** Procedure

Audience   Middle School Students (1 session)

ASSESSMENT

1: **D**ecide behavior(s)

Assess issues[a] and behaviors[b] of concern for audience from general sources.	Assess issues[a] and behaviors[b] of concern for your specific audience.
• Overweight & obesity are a priority issue for youth, especially minority youth • Adolescents consume too much added sugar & fat and not enough vegetables • They are a big market	• Higher obesity rate than national average • On average, students consume 2 sugary drinks daily, 1 serving of fruit, no vegetables • Fast food many times/week; lots of TV and not much exercise

Behavior Change Goal[c]

Increase fruit and vegetable* consumption.

* F&V

2: **E**xplore determinants of change

Motivational theory-based determinants for behavior change

What audience said and/or what you learned	Determinant
• No knowledge of health risks for a diet without F&V	• Perceived risk
• F&V are not tasty, are expensive, and are a nuisance to eat	• Perceived barriers
• Eating F&V is something you do because your parents say so	• Perceived behavioral control
• Peers set the trends; they don't eat F&V	• Social norms
• My diet is not that bad, really!	• Perceived risk (low)
• What are the benefits, really?! I feel fine with what I eat.	• Perceived benefits

Behavioral knowledge & skills theory-based determinants for behavior change

What audience said and/or what you learned	Determinant
• How much F&V should I eat each day?	• Cognitive skills
• Where do I get F&V easily?	• Behavioral capabilities (shopping)
• How do I prepare F&V so they taste good?	• Behavioral capabilities (food prep)
• I know about goal setting and tracking from my English and math classes, but never thought about doing that with what I eat.	• Goal setting self-regulation skills

INTERVENTION

3: **S**elect theory & clarify philosophy

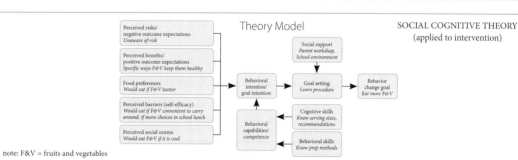

note: F&V = fruits and vegetables

Educational philosophy	Perspectives on food and nutrition
We believe that youth are responsible for their health and can make healthful food and activity choices, but that they need motivation and skills to take charge in a difficult environment. The school is responsible to provide a supportive environment. Teens need self-efficacy and a sense of agency.	We believe that youth should acquire the knowledge and skills to eat foods that are minimally processed, naturally nutrient dense, and local and fresh if possible and feasible. The issue of weight will not be addressed directly; instead, healthful eating and activity patterns will be emphasized.

FIGURE 7-3 DESIGN workbook short form for case study to illustrate steps in the procedure.

The Nutrition Education **DESIGN** Procedure (Continued)

Audience   Middle School Students (1 session)

INTERVENTION

4: Indicate general objectives & 5: Generate plans

Objectives for each determinant in your theory model	Activities to address each objective
Objectives for motivational determinants *Participants will be able to:*	
• [PERCEIVED RISK] Recognize they are not eating F&V	• Draw most recent meal, compare to MyPlate
• [PERCEIVED BENEFITS] Describe the importance of eating a variety of F&V	• Handouts with colorful photos of F&V of different colors, descriptions of nutrients in the different colors and role in body
• [FOOD PREFERENCES] Appreciate the taste of various F&V of different colors	• F&V superpower comic and discussion
• [PERCEIVED BARRIERS] Identify strategies to overcome perceived barriers to eating F&V	• Tasting F&V of different colors; discussion of flavors using sophisticated vocabulary
• [SELF-EFFICACY] Demonstrate increased confidence in their ability to eat more and/or a greater variety of F&V	• Discussion of barriers and ways to overcome them
• [SOCIAL NORMS] Recognize the influence of peers in their snacking choices	• Discussion of peer influences; identification of positive role models
Objectives for knowledge and behavioral skills determinants *Participants will be able to:*	
• [BEHAVIORAL CAPABILITIES] State the number of servings of F&V they should eat	• MyPlate handout to show amount of F&V to eat, and handouts indicating serving sizes
• [BEHAVIORAL CAPABILITIES AND SELF-EFFICACY] Demonstrate increased confidence in their ability to prepare and eat more and/or a greater variety of F&V	• Class discussion of tips for adding more F&V to their diets: how to prepare, store, and eat them at home; and selecting the vegetables at school lunch
• [BEHAVIORAL CAPABILITIES AND SELF-EFFICACY] Demonstrate ability to prepare F&V snacks	• Snack prep and tasting: cut up various F&V and make simple appropriate dips for them
• [SELF-REGULATION] Demonstrate ability to set and monitor action goals to eat more or a greater variety of F&V	• Complete an F&V action goal setting sheet
• [SOCIAL SUPPORT] Describe how they will work with their friends to help each other eat more F&V	• Sharing their F&V action goals with each other and discussing how they will help each other to stick to their goals

EVALUATION

6: Nail down evaluation plan

Outcomes you will measure	Tools to measure outcomes
• Perceived benefits	• Worksheets from sessions
• Perceived risk	• Log of discussions in class
• Perceived barriers	• Log of discussions in class
• Cognitive skills	• Pre- and post-test
• Goal setting skills	• Completed action goal setting sheet
• Increased F&V consumption	• An F&V checklist given pre and post session(s)

Process evaluation tools to measure how your session(s) went
• Observational checklist: How much was completed and what was left out?
• Observational checklist: How engaged were the students?
• Survey: How did the audience like the session? What would they improve?

---

a Issues of concern can be health (obesity, risk of type 2 diabetes), ecological (high carbon footprint of processing food) or social (farm worker rights). Your audience may or may not be told about these issues, for example you may work with children and the issue may be childhood obesity prevention, but the children just know you are doing fun classes cooking and tasting vegetables.

b These are behaviors or practices that will make the issues worse (e.g., not enough fruits and vegetables, too many sweetened beverages, too many highly processed foods).

c This is what you want your audience to do as a result of your session(s). If a behavior that contributes to issues is "not enough fruits and vegetables," your behavior change or action could be to "eat an extra vegetable at lunch and dinner" or "follow MyPlate at meals."

d Words in parentheses are the determinants of behavior change from your theory mode.

FIGURE 7-3 DESIGN workbook short form for case study to illustrate steps in the procedure (Continued).

Step 2. Explore determinants of change for targeted behavior by using theory and evidence. The nutrition educator conducted in-depth interviews of 10 middle school students and administered a survey in one class per grade (6, 7, and 8) that asked about thoughts and feelings students had about what would motivate them to eat fruits and vegetables and what would facilitate this action. These are summarized in Figure 7-3.

- *Determinants motivating action or behavior change.* The constructs from theory were used as a guide for the interviews and survey: the nutrition educator asked about students' personal sense of concern about the health issue (it was not high) and the benefits and barriers to eating fruits and vegetables (students did verbalize these). They expressed their attitudes and preferences (negative), their sense of peer pressure (peers did not eat them), and their lack of self-efficacy or self-confidence in making changes.
- *Determinants facilitating action or behavior change.* The nutrition educator then asked students about their knowledge and skills in terms of selecting and preparing fruits and vegetables and ability to set goals and follow through with their goals. The students said they did not know how to prepare fruits and vegetables and were not big on planning ahead but had learned about goal setting for other subjects in school.

Step 3. Select theory or create model to guide program and clarify philosophy. Based on the determinants that were most relevant in this assessment of the teens, the theory that was most appropriate for the intervention was social cognitive theory. The theory model as applied to this intervention is shown in the completed DESIGN Workbook short form (Figure 7-3). The program's philosophy was that it believed that while the youth were responsible for their health, it was the responsibility of the health agency to help in enhancing motivations and providing the tools to enable youth to make thoughtful and healthful choices and take charge in today's difficult food environment.

Step 4. Indicate general educational objectives for key determinants of behavior change or action. The general educational objectives are listed in the DESIGN Workbook short form as an example and are directed at motivational determinants and facilitating determinants (knowledge and skills).

Step 5. Generate educational plan(s). Select behavior change strategies and create practical activities to address determinants, through writing specific objectives. Educational objectives and activities are shown in outline form in Figure 7-3. The objectives and activities are then sequenced appropriately into an educational plan. You need one educational (lesson) plan for each session. The actual lesson plans are not shown in the short form. They are shown at the end of Chapters 11 and 12.

Step 6. Nail down the evaluation plan for the session(s). The evaluation plan for their session(s) is shown in outline in Figure 7-3.

THE DESIGN PROCEDURE IN MORE DETAIL

We can lay out the DESIGN Procedure in the form of a logic model for planning purposes. This is shown in **FIGURE 7-4**. The tasks to be accomplished and products generated for each step are also shown in this figure. You can see that Step 1 and 2 activities provide the inputs to the program and involve collecting assessment data. Steps 3, 4, and 5 are the outputs of the program and involve designing your nutrition education sessions or intervention. Step 6 addresses the outcomes of the program by nailing down a plan to evaluate the outcomes of the intervention. See Chapter 6 for a more detailed discussion of logic models.

These procedural steps for designing nutrition education activities are laid out sequentially, but in reality they are closely interrelated, so you must go back and forth between steps when designing nutrition education.

Step 1: Deciding the Behavior Change Goals for a Given Audience by Assessing Issues and Behaviors of Concern

A nutrition education activity is initiated when some individual, community, organization, or government agency expresses a concern about some issue related to diet and health, the current food system, the social impact of current practices, and so forth. The concerns may also be expressed in the form of some research finding, report, or policy document. Many food assistance programs mandate some form of nutrition education for the vulnerable populations they serve.

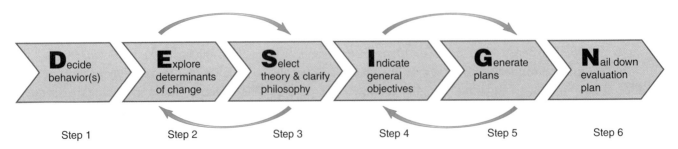

Inputs: **Collecting the Assessment Data**		**Outputs:** **Designing the Theory-Based Intervention**			**Outcomes:** **Evaluation Plan**

Tasks: • **Decide** behavior change goal(s) of the intervention, based on: • Analyzing issues and behaviors of concern for audience	*Tasks:* • **Explore** determinants of behavior change based on a variety of data sources	*Tasks:* • **Select** theory and draw intervention-specific theory model • Clarify educational philosophy • Articulate perspectives on content	*Tasks:* • **Indicate** general objectives for each determinant in your theory model	*Tasks:* • **Generate** educational plans: • Educational activities to address all determinants in theory model • Sequence for implementation using the 4 Es	*Tasks:* • **Nail down** evaluation plan • Select methods and questions to evaluate outcomes • Plan process evaluation • Create questions to measure how implementation went
Products: Statement of intervention behavior change goal(s)	*Products:* List of determinants to address in the intervention	*Products:* Theory model for intervention Statement of educational philosophy Statement of content perspectives	*Products:* A general objective for each determinant in the theory model	*Products:* Educational plans that link determinants and educational activities to achieve behavior change or action goal(s)	*Products:* List of evaluation methods and questions Procedures and measures for process evaluation

FIGURE 7-4 Nutrition Education DESIGN Procedure tasks and products.

The concern may also be expressed informally by individuals or organizations. For example, the leader of an after-school program for middle school students may be concerned about the high rates of diabetes in the community and think that the diets of the students are placing them at risk. She invites you to come and provide a couple of sessions. These concerns provide the rationale for selecting the particular behavior change goals for a nutrition education program.

"TOPICS" VERSUS A "BEHAVIORAL FOCUS" AS THE BASIS OF NUTRITION EDUCATION

When nutrition educators are asked to plan a program or some educational sessions, what comes most naturally is to think immediately about some topic or some set of knowledge and skills they think is important to convey to the audience and exciting ways to do so. We are familiar with topics because that is how we learned nutrition science.

Topics may be useful for professional development presentations when we want to know the latest on diabetes or vitamin D. For nutrition education with the public, topics tend to be broad and general, focused on disseminating some universe of information. We have seen that the evidence suggests this approach is unlikely to be effective for the purpose of behavior change, whereas a focus on behaviors that are specific to an audience and which they care about is more likely to be effective. Some nutrition educators are concerned that a behavioral focus can be too narrow. This suggests that there is some confusion regarding what focusing on a behavior means: it does not mean that nutrition content is not covered.

Remember that all nutrition education involves information in some form: it is how the information is used or conveyed that makes the difference. It means thinking about the end purpose of the information or communication. For example, the topic may be the "American food system." If all you intend to provide is a description of the food system and nothing more, then you will be presenting a topic. However, if the ultimate purpose of the educational session is for the audience to become knowledgeable about the food system in such a way that they will want to choose their foods differently, then the ultimate goal is a change in audience behaviors. Thus the session is really behaviorally focused.

Or again, the topic may be diabetes. And again, if the ultimate purpose of the session is for the audience to eat in ways that reduce their risk of diabetes, then the session is really behaviorally focused. Many nutrition education sessions are, in fact, behaviorally focused without the nutrition educator being clearly conscious of it. However, making conscious that behaviorally based end purpose is crucial, because it permits us to use the appropriate tools to identify the determinants of the behaviors and to shape our sessions accordingly. Such an approach has been shown to make nutrition education more effective.

WHY CONDUCTING ASSESSMENTS OF YOUR AUDIENCE IS CRUCIAL

Although informal judgments about your audience can sometimes suffice, a more systematic assessment has the following advantages:

- Helps you better understand your audience and the context of their lives—crucial for effective nutrition education
- Takes much of the guesswork out of nutrition education design—avoids a mismatch between what you plan and what the audience needs and wants
- Provides a basis for selecting behaviors and practices that you will focus on and developing appropriate program educational objectives to address them
- Makes clear the rationale for choosing particular priorities
- Makes it easier to use scarce resources appropriately
- Documents the need for funding or justifies expenditure of resources
- Provides a basis for measuring results

Such an assessment ensures that your food and nutrition education sessions or programs are directed at issues, needs, or interests that have been identified as important national or local priorities or that are perceived to be of concern or interest by stakeholders in the community or by the intended audience.

INVOLVING PROGRAM PARTICIPANTS ENHANCES MOTIVATION, EMPOWERMENT, AND EFFECTIVENESS

In many situations, you as the nutrition educator are the person conducting the assessments. For example, you may have been asked to conduct short-term nutrition education with a group such as an older adults' lunch program, individuals with HIV, or low-income mothers of young children. With few resources, the responsibility rests with one person: you. In other situations, a department, community group, or an agency is charged with providing nutrition education services, and several staff members may be involved. Examples might be a community program, longer-term projects such as a school curriculum, or nutrition education activities and programs sponsored or funded by Cooperative Extension or another government agency. To the extent possible and appropriate, involving people in the assessment process who have a stake in the program, such as community members, citizen groups, students, nutrition education staff, teachers, agency heads, or school principals, ensures that the program reflects their needs and desires, enhances the relevance of the sessions or program, and increases motivation to participate (Whitehead 1973; Rogers 2003; Green and Kreuter 2005).

This systematic assessment process is called by different names in different arenas. Program planners talk about "needs assessments." Social marketers talk about "market research," "formative research," or "front-end assessment" and consider this activity to be of crucial importance to the social marketing process. Also included here is identification of the assets or strengths of the group or community. Regardless of what we call it, you will seek answers to the following questions:

- Who is your audience?
- What can you learn about your audience from general sources?
- What can you learn about your specific audience?
- What will be the behavior change goals of your sessions or program, based on these assessments?

Who Is Your Audience?

The first decision you have to make is who you want to reach and about what. Your audience can be teens, mothers, older adults, Head Start teachers, low-income families, employees at a worksite, community groups, those with diabetes in an outpatient clinic, athletes, members of a fitness club, or seniors at a congregate meal site. In other words, just about anyone!

In many cases, the intended audience has been determined for you, such as by the mission of the agency or organization in which the nutrition education will be conducted or by a funding source. For example, the audience is already determined if the setting is an adolescent health clinic, a school, a Women, Infants, and Children (WIC) clinic, or a senior center. Otherwise, the choice of audience is usually based on greatest need in terms of the size of the population for whom there is an issue of concern (e.g., childhood obesity), the severity of the condition (e.g., diabetes), a population at special risk (e.g., bone health in teens), or the extent of health disparities (e.g., low-income neighborhood). It could also be based on degree of interest: people may sign up for your workshops through notices in clinics or community centers, newsletters or advertising on the Web.

What Can You Learn About the Issues and Behaviors of Your Audience from Available General Sources?

Understanding your audience in depth is crucial! Such an understanding ensures that you have a good rationale for your food and nutrition education sessions or programs based on issues or needs that have been identified as important national or local priorities or that are perceived to be of concern or interest by the community or intended audience. It also ensures that your program takes into account the current and desired behaviors and practices of the audience.

Before you have an opportunity to meet with your audience, you can learn some general information from various sources about audiences similar to yours that will be useful as you plan your nutrition education sessions or program. The information can relate to issues of concern that provide a rationale for your sessions or to behaviors and practices that make these issues worse or are assets or strengths that can be encouraged to promote health and well-being.

WHAT CAN YOU LEARN ABOUT *ISSUES* OF CONCERN FOR AN AUDIENCE FROM AVAILABLE GENERAL SOURCES?

Most often the rationale for a program is based on *health issues* facing individuals within your intended audience, such as increased risk of developing type 2 diabetes, concern about bone health, or appropriate weight gain in youth. Issues of concern can also refer to those related to the *food system*, such as those related to the carbon footprint of foods resulting from greenhouse gas emissions from excessive transportation, processing, or packaging of food and from the pollution and waste generated. In addition, issues can refer to those related to *social and societal issues related to food* such as family dynamics and cohesion, the cultural practices of communities, the impact of food marketing on the fabric of rural communities, or the working conditions of those who work in the food system, from farmers to food preparers and food servers. These are described in more detail below.

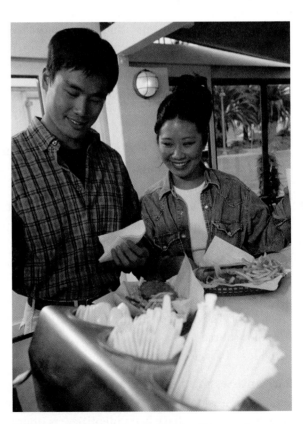

Helping teenagers learn to substitute healthier snack alternatives for french fries and chips is just one example of a nutrition education activity.

© Photodisc/Getty Images.

Health Issues from Generally Available Sources of Information

Diet-related health issues or nutritional problems can include rates of chronic diseases, malnutrition in infants, food insecurity, nutrient-deficiency diseases, breast-feeding, childhood obesity, or bone health. These are of major concern in most countries and for many different populations. Find out from the sources below to what extent these are prevalent in your population.

Sources of Information on Health Issues

Research and survey literature. You can use literature reviews, health surveys, national mortality and morbidity data, reports from scientific research, expert panels, indicators of health, or rates of disease to identify possible health concerns for audiences similar to yours.

National policy documents. Each country has developed nutrition, health, and food policy documents to guide government programs and provide information to the public. You can use these policy initiatives as the basis of your nutrition education intervention. In the United States, nutrition recommendations are spelled out in various government documents such as the Dietary Guidelines for Americans, MyPlate, Physical Activity Guidelines for Americans, and so forth. Private voluntary health organizations, such as cancer societies or heart associations, also publish guidelines for the public that you can use as a basis for choice of high-priority issues for your intervention.

Organization or funding source. You may work for an agency or organization, or the nutrition education sessions you have been asked to design will be conducted in or for an agency or organization that has its own priorities. Examples might be an after-school program, extension service program, public health department, or senior center. You might consider the expectations of the organization or funding source for the nutrition education sessions.

Food System–Related Issues of Concern from Generally Available Sources of Information

Issues of concern may not all be related directly to personal health. They can relate to other areas such as the long-term sustainability of the current industrial farming system, the impact of pollution and waste from the current farming system, the fate of local or small farms, or concern about the carbon footprint of a group's current dietary patterns. In particular, recently international organizations and national dietary guidelines are considering environmental issues as part of the rationale for dietary recommendations. The Food and Agricultural Organization outlined basic recommendations for dietary patterns that are "not only healthier but more favorable to the environment and sustainable development" (World Health Organization 2003). The Australian dietary guidelines note that "health should be considered within sustainable food systems, where the nutritional requirements of the population can be met without placing pressure on natural resources," and the Netherlands has considered dietary guidelines that can provide a win-win situation: dietary recommendations that are healthy and eco-friendly as well, in terms of land use, greenhouse gas emissions, and biodiversity (Health Council of the Netherlands 2011; Australian National Health and Medical Research Council 2013).

This same point was made in 1986 by Gussow and Clancy, who showed that following most of the dietary guidelines for health also contributed to a more ecologically sound food system (Gussow and Clancy 1986). Thus, several issues of concern can often be addressed by the same behavior. For example, reducing the number of sweetened beverages adolescents drink may reduce risks of obesity and diabetes, be good for dental health, and reduce the number of plastic bottles that make their way to garbage cans (or rubbish bins) and landfills and is thus good for the environment.

Sources of Information on Food System–Related Issues

Research and survey literature. The information you need might come from research data on the energy used for different food packaging and transportation practices, the nature of the local food supply, or food safety. Research is increasing at a rapid rate and is available through journals, websites, or publications of organizations that focus on these issues. Survey data from government and other sources may provide information on the prevalence of farmers' markets, small and medium-sized farms, and community-supported agriculture farms in the local area.

National policy documents. Concerns about the food system remaining sustainable, the carbon footprint of the food processing system, or the waste produced by the food system are described in various government documents, policy documents of food system research institutes and organizations, and publications of world health and agricultural organizations. You can consult these and other documents as you design your nutrition education sessions or program.

Organization or funding source. If your sessions are requested by an organization or are funded by a particular funding source, it is important to find out what they expect from these sessions in relation to these concerns.

Societal Concerns Related to Food from Generally Available Sources of Information

For some nutrition education programs, a choice of focus might be based on a concern about the impact of food system practices on social systems and local communities, or whether food production labor and trade practices are fair in terms of impacts on farm workers, farmers, and local communities.

Sources of Information on Societal Concerns Related to Food

Research and survey literature. Assessment data might include information about the availability to the public of foods produced through fair trade practices or institutional policies with respect to purchasing and serving such foods. It is increasingly easy for you to find such information through agriculture and food systems research journals, publications of organizations dedicated to these issues, and websites of organizations that certify and promote fair labor and trade practices. Many food system networks provide such information. Numerous books have also been published with relevant data.

National policy documents. Increasingly, governments are also incorporating concerns about societal and social justice issues related to food into their policy documents. You can consult these.

Organization or funding source. The organization or funding source for your sessions or program may have some special reason for asking you to focus on food system–related issues. It is important to find out what these may be.

WHAT CAN YOU LEARN ABOUT *BEHAVIORS* OF CONCERN FOR AN AUDIENCE FROM AVAILABLE GENERAL SOURCES?

In addition to wanting to know about the issues of concern, you will also want to understand the diet-related behaviors and practices that contribute to making these issues into those of concern; changing these behaviors

becomes the focus of nutrition education. This is a crucial step. Evidence strongly suggests that nutrition education is more likely to be effective if it focuses on specific behaviors or community practices. These behaviors or community practices may be those that are currently problematic, or they may be health-promoting behaviors and practices that could be increased or enhanced. For example, a given population or group may be consuming too many energy-dense, nutrient-poor snacks, which may constitute a problematic behavior. However, a group might already be consuming 1 cup of fruits and vegetables, which is better than none, but the group would be healthier if they ate the recommended 4 ½ cups or more. Eating more fruits and vegetables can thus be seen as a health promoting behavior to be encouraged. Note that a focus on behaviors has been shown to be important even, or especially, where resources are low and there is threat of food insecurity (Hawkes 2013), and even in interventions designed to reduce malnutrition (Bonvecchio et al. 2007; Thomson and Amoroso 2010).

The extensiveness of the information you want and the degree of accuracy you need depend very much on the nature and duration of your intervention. Even if you are providing only one or a few sessions with a given audience, it is still crucial to collect behavioral information. The Step 1 Decide Behavior Change Worksheet at the end of Chapter 13 can help you with this process. Sources of information for learning about the behaviors of the audience are presented here.

Review of the Relevant Nutrition Research Literature

Nutrition research literature is a good place to start looking for information regarding the food-related behaviors, actions, or practices that have been shown to have impacts on the specific health or food issues you identified for your intended audience. The availability of information may vary for each issue and population. It is helpful to have specific information if it is available. For example, there may be research information about the eating patterns of families in your particular cultural group, the eating practices of teenagers, or the diets of athletes of the category of interest (e.g., basketball players).

Review of Monitoring Data or Consumer Surveys

Reviewing monitoring data or consumer surveys can also provide valuable information. For example, if adolescents are the intended audience, and overweight prevention is the key health issue identified, then you will want to review existing consumer surveys, national or local monitoring data, or surveys of food purchasing practices of adolescents for information on behaviors that might contribute to the issue of overweight. Check out relevant websites for information.

Even if it is not possible to obtain information directly from the group, knowledge about the food practices and habits of people similar to the intended group is extremely helpful. This information search may yield the finding, for example, that frequent consumption of high-fat fast foods and sweetened drinks and low intakes of fruits and vegetables are contributing behaviors to overweight in similar adolescents.

Dietary Recommendations of Governmental, International, and Other Organizations

Most governments provide food-based dietary guidelines for their people (Food and Agricultural Organization 2013). In the United States it is the Dietary Guidelines for Americans (U.S. Department of Health and Human Services [HHS] 2010) and Physical Activity Guidelines for Americans (HHS 2008).

Identifying issues of concern provides a rationale for your sessions or program. However, you may or may not need to inform your audience about the underlying rationale or issue. For example, your audience may be children and the issue may be childhood obesity prevention, but you will not state that. Instead, the children just know they are doing fun classes cooking and tasting vegetables.

Behaviors of concern are behaviors or practices that make the issue worse (e.g., not enough vegetables, too many sweetened beverages, sedentary behavior, not feeding children the right foods).

Behavior change goals are what you aim for your audience to do as a result of your sessions or program. For example, if a behavior that contributes to making the issue worse is "not enough fruits and vegetables," your behavior change goal could be to "eat more fruits and vegetables" or "eat 4 ½ cups of fruits and vegetables each day."

What Can You Learn About the Issues and Behaviors of Your Specific Audience?

WHAT CAN YOU LEARN ABOUT YOUR SPECIFIC AUDIENCE IN TERMS OF *ISSUES* OF CONCERN?

The issues or needs of your specific audience may or may not be exactly the same as those that emerge from the objective data about the population in general. You can find out about the concerns of your specific audience through various methods such as those listed here.

Health Concerns

You may be able obtain specific, objective health-related data about your audience if you are working with certain groups such as an outpatient audience, athletes, or youth with diabetes. Just as important as these identified, actual, objective health and nutrition issues are the health issues and needs as perceived by the intended audience. Individuals are the experts on their own lives, so it is important to understand what they perceive as issues and dilemmas. What diet-related issues are they concerned about? What other health needs or competing, non-health–related concerns do they have? If at all possible, you should obtain information directly from, and in partnership with, the intended audience through focus group discussions, in-depth interviews of key informants, or surveys.

Food System–Related Concerns

As for health-related issues, it is important to obtain information directly from the intended audience through focus group discussions, surveys, or in-depth interviews of key informants, such as leaders within the intended audience or their communities regarding what concerns they have about the system that brings them their food, whether they are interested in farmers' markets, and so forth. Take a walk around the neighborhood to see for yourself what their food environment looks like.

Societal Concerns Related to Food

Here, too, it is important to obtain information directly from the intended audience through focus group discussions, individual interviews, or surveys.

PRIORITIZE ISSUES OF CONCERN

Whether your assessment has been comprehensive or brief, you will probably have gathered information on more issues than you have the time or resources to address. Thus, you must prioritize and focus. In addition, the information from all the various sources should be balanced. Consider the following (as suggested by Green and Kreuter 2004):

- Which issues, if appropriately addressed, are likely to have the greatest impact on the outcomes desired?
- Which issues are most amenable to intervention by educational means?
- Which issues are considered by the intended audience to be most important?
- Which issues are considered by the sponsoring agency or funding source, if any, to be most important?

WHAT CAN YOU LEARN ABOUT THE *BEHAVIORS* OF CONCERN OF YOUR SPECIFIC AUDIENCE?

Interviews or Discussion with Group

It is very important to talk to the intended audience about their behaviors and practices, if it is at all possible. Behavioral data can be obtained through individual interviews, focus groups, or intercept interviews as people leave a food store or community center. Pay special attention to culture-specific foods and practices and family patterns.

For example, which food practices contribute to the high incidence of overweight in this particular group of school-aged children? Too many sweetened beverages? Too little physical activity? Or both? Which behaviors of the audience in the context of the family or social environment lead to the intended audience's high serum cholesterol levels? Do people eat high-fat foods too often or do the food preparation methods add fat to foods (e.g., frying foods), or both? Which behaviors contribute to the low vitamin C status? Are people eating too few vegetables and fruits in their diets or are they cooking vegetables in ways that destroy the vitamin C, or both?

It is also important to ask: which healthful behaviors and practices are already being practiced by the group (i.e., what are the group's assets or strengths)? Perhaps they already practice a number of behaviors that are healthful, such as a high consumption of beans and whole grains, and can be encouraged to do more. As Heath and Heath (2010) put it: Follow the bright spots—investigate what's working and build on it!

Observations

Formal observations are difficult to do but can be very informative. Informal observations are extremely valuable and may be sufficient for most of our purposes, such as observing what children eat in school, what teenagers purchase in the school neighborhood after school, or the kinds of food stores in the neighborhood.

Surveys

If it is appropriate or possible to survey the primary audience, you should do so because questionnaires that ask about specific dietary practices provide you with specific information that is extremely useful. Informal surveys using short checklists to find out about the behaviors and practices of your audience may be sufficient for your purposes. If you need to be more systematic, you may need to use more formal instruments. Some of the kinds of data you can collect are listed here, along with methods for assessing them. An example of an instrument for low-resources audiences is given in **TABLE 7-1**.

- *Food purchasing behaviors or practices.* Specific shopping practices, such as using a shopping list, doing comparison shopping, or using coupons, can be obtained from surveys and interviews (Hersey et al. 2001).
- *Intake of specific foods or food items.* Food frequency questionnaires can be comprehensive (Willett et al. 1987; Block et al. 1992) or can be short and targeted to the behaviors of interest, in which case they often are called checklists or screeners (such as screeners for fruits and vegetables, high-fat foods, or local foods) (Block et al. 2000; Yaroch, Resnicow, and Khan 2000; Townsend et al. 2003; Hunsberger et al. 2012; McClelland et al. 2001). For nutrition education in most practice settings, short food intake checklists are sufficient.
- *Specific observable behaviors.* Examples include using skim milk instead of whole milk, taking the skin off when eating chicken, or eating whole grain bread instead of white bread. These behaviors can be assessed using questionnaires such as the Kristal food habits questionnaire (Shannon et al. 1997). Food safety behaviors belong in this category and can also be assessed; examples include cooking foods adequately, practicing personal hygiene, and keeping foods at a safe temperature (Medeiros et al. 2001).

- *Eating patterns.* Examples include whether the audience eats breakfast, eats fruit as a snack, or eats three meals a day. You can devise an instrument to fit your purposes.
- *Quality of diet.* Sometimes a single question can be used, such as "How would you describe the quality of your diet?" A simple 24-hour dietary recall can be done as a group activity and scored by the participants themselves to provide them a rough idea about their diets. They can compare what they ate with government recommendations, such as Choose MyPlate servings (U.S. Department of Agriculture [USDA] n.d.).

PRIORITIZING THE BEHAVIORS OR PRACTICES: THE CRITERIA

Given the concerns and assets you identified, you have likely gathered information on more problem behaviors or practices than you have the time or resources to address, so you have to prioritize and focus. For example,

the behaviors could be as follows: low intake of fruits and vegetables, high intake of high-calorie processed foods and snacks, sedentary behaviors, high consumption of sweetened drinks, and low consumption of milk and dairy products. These are probably more behaviors than you can address if you wish to have a meaningful impact on behavior, depending on the number of sessions or other activities planned. Certainly that is too many for one or two sessions! Rate the behaviors or practices on the basis of the criteria described below (Rogers 2003; Green and Kreuter 2004) and use the Step 1 Decide Behavior Change Worksheet at the end of Chapter 13 to record your ratings.

1. How Important Is It to Change This Behavior or Engage in This Specific Action?

You can rate the importance of each of the behaviors or practices you have identified by asking: Does this specific *behavior* clearly and significantly contribute to the *issues*

Table 7-1 Food Behavior Checklist for Limited-Resources Audiences

Scores of 1 to 5 = Never, Sometimes, Often, Usually, Always, shown as ___ in the table. Scores for those items with yes or no responses are shown in parentheses.

Fruit and vegetable items	
Do you eat more than one kind of fruit daily?	___
During the past week, did you have citrus fruit (such as orange or grapefruit) or citrus juice? (yes = 2; no = 1)	___
Do you eat more than one kind of vegetable daily?	___
How many servings of vegetables do you eat each day?	___
Do you eat two or more servings of vegetables at your main meal?	___
Do you eat fruits or vegetables as snacks?	___
How many servings of fruit do you eat each day?	___
Milk items	
Do you drink milk daily?	___
During the past week, did you have milk as a beverage or on cereal?	___
Fat and cholesterol items	
During the past week, did you have fish? (yes = 2; no = 1)	___
Do you take the skin off chicken?	___
Diet quality	
When shopping, do you use the Nutrition Facts label to choose foods?	___
Do you drink regular soft drinks?	___
Do you buy Kool-Aid, Gatorade, Sunny Delight, or other fruit drink/punch?	___
Would you describe your diet as excellent (5), very good (4), good (3), fair (2), or poor (1)?	___
Food security	
Do you run out of food before the end of the month?	___

Reprinted from *Journal of Nutrition Education and Behavior*, Vol 35, M. S. Townsend, L. L. Kaiser, L. H. Allen, A. Block Joy, and S. P. Murphy. "Selecting Items for a Food Behavior Checklist for a Limited-Resource Audience," pp. 69–82. Copyright 2003, with permission from the Society for Nutrition Education and Behavior.

that you have identified as major concerns for your selected audience or population?

The strength of the evidence linking the behaviors to the issue of concern can be evaluated based on a review of the relevant nutrition science literature. For example, several behaviors have been shown to be strongly linked to cardiovascular risk, such as a diet high in saturated fat and a diet low in fruits and vegetables. Breastfeeding is highly linked with healthy outcomes for the baby, and its low prevalence is problematic. So addressing these behaviors for given audiences may be important.

2. How Modifiable Is the Behavior or Practice by Educational Methods?

For each of the behaviors identified, ask: How modifiable or easy is it to change by educational means? A given behavior may be a very important contributor to the issues of concern that have been identified, but it is not a suitable target for a nutrition education intervention because there is not reasonable evidence that it is changeable by educational means.

Modifiability from Evidence in the Literature

Judgment about modifiability can be based on evidence from scientific and professional nutrition education, health education, and health promotion literature showing that such behaviors have responded previously to interventions.

Modifiability from the Perspective of the Audience

Studies have found that the likelihood of people accepting or adopting an innovation (in this case, a diet- or physical activity–related behavior) is influenced by a number of features of the innovation or behavior (Rogers 2003). See Chapter 6 for details. Use these criteria to judge the modifiability of the problem behaviors you have identified from your assessment from the point of view of the participants:

- *Relative advantage*: How is this behavior better than what I currently do?
- *Complexity*: Is it simple enough for me to understand and do?
- *Compatibility*: How is it relevant to the way I live my life? Recommended behaviors that seem similar enough to current behaviors can be incorporated without too much dislocation and are more likely to be adopted.

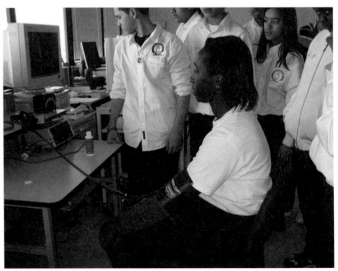

Students learn about their own blood pressure.

Courtesy of Linking Food and the Environment, Teachers College Columbia University.

- *Trialability*: Can I try it first before I make a long-term commitment to act upon it or to adopt it?
- *Observability*: Can I see what happens to me or others when we do it? Clearly visible benefits are more likely to motivate adoption.

3. How Feasible Is It in Practice?

How feasible will it be for you to design an intervention and carry it out? That is, how much time and how many resources will you be able to devote to the intervention? How long a program can you offer? Will that be sufficient to show change?

4. How Desirable Is It to the Intended Audience?

How desirable is it to the intended audience to take this action or to adopt this particular recommended dietary behavior? Do they see the behavior as realistic? Effective? Practical? Easy to do?

5. How Measurable Is Change in This Behavior, Action, or Practice?

Having measurable outcomes will help you to evaluate whether your program or sessions are effective.

NUTRITION EDUCATION IN ACTION 7-1 provides some examples of how the nutrition education issues, audiences, and behaviors have been stated for the Supplemental Nutrition Assistance Program–Education (SNAP-Ed) component and the Team Nutrition program.

NUTRITION EDUCATION IN ACTION 7-1 Examples of Core Behavior Goals of Nutrition Education Programs and Their Rationales

Supplemental Nutrition Assistance Program–Education (SNAP-Ed)

Although there are many important nutrition-related issues that affect the SNAP-eligible audience, the Food and Nutrition Service of the U.S. Department of Agriculture (USDA) encourages states to focus their Supplemental Nutrition Assistance Program–Education (SNAP-Ed) program efforts on the behavior outcomes suggested by the Dietary Guidelines:

Balancing calories:

- Enjoy your food but eat less.
- Avoid oversized portions.

Foods to increase:

- Make half your plate fruits and vegetables.
- Make at least half your grains whole grains.
- Switch to fat-free or low-fat (1%) milk.

Foods to reduce:

- Compare sodium in foods such as soup, bread, and frozen meals and choose foods with lower numbers.
- Drink water instead of sugary drinks.

These behaviors are associated with a reduced risk of some forms of cancer, type 2 diabetes, and coronary heart disease. It is appropriate to focus on these behavior outcomes for SNAP-Ed because low-income individuals often experience a disproportionate share of diet-related problems that are risk factors for the major diseases contributing to poor health, disability, and premature death.

Team Nutrition

The USDA's Team Nutrition promotes comprehensive, behavior-based nutrition education to enable children to make healthy eating and physical activity choices. Social cognitive theory is the foundation of efforts to help children understand how eating and physical activity affect the way they grow, learn, play, and feel today as well as the relationship of their choices to lifelong health. These efforts are designed to increase their understanding that healthy eating and physical activity are fun and that skills developed today will assist them in enjoying healthy eating and physical activity in later years.

All program materials encourage students to make food and physical activity choices for a healthy lifestyle. The focus is on five behavior outcomes:

- Eat a variety of foods.
- Eat more fruits, vegetables, and grains.
- Eat lower-fat foods more often.
- Get your calcium-rich foods.
- Be physically active.

Sources: Food and Nutrition Service, U.S. Department of Agriculture. 2009. Supplemental Nutrition Assistance Program guiding principles. http://www.fns.usda.gov/snap/nutrition_education/default.htm; and Food and Nutrition Service, U.S. Department of Agriculture. n.d. About Team Nutrition. http://www.fns.usda.gov/tn/about.

Decide the Behavior Change Goals of the Program for Your Audience

From the set of behaviors or practices that you have identified, now *decide* on those few that the program or sessions will address and state them in terms of targeted and specific behavior change goals. These goals should state the desired *behavior change outcomes* of your entire program or individual group sessions for your audience. As noted previously, evidence strongly suggests that nutrition education is more likely to be effective if it focuses on specific behaviors or community practices. (And yes, in your educational sessions you can place these behaviors in a larger framework and work with your audience to develop the knowledge, values, and skills to make thoughtful decisions). Thus, you will want to state the program goals in terms of behaviors or practices that the audience members will change or the actions they will take. Remember that these behaviors or actions are based in part on the desires of audience members that you learned about during the assessment process, and your role is to facilitate change.

Examples of behavior change goals are to increase fruit and vegetable consumption among adolescents, increase consumption of calcium-rich foods among women in the

WIC program, increase use of the SNAP Electronic Benefit Transfer (EBT) card at farmers' markets, increase the choice of more healthful snacks by elementary school students, reduce the intake of sweetened beverages by high school students, increase the proportion of women with type 2 diabetes who practice effective food management skills, or increase the number of those who participate in community-supported agriculture.

WORKSHEET FOR PRIORITIZING BEHAVIORS, ACTIONS, OR PRACTICE

You can use the information you have collected to decide on the specific food- and diet-related behavior(s) or action(s) that will be the focus of your nutrition education intervention or program. You can prioritize informally, but it is best to be systematic about selecting priority behaviors to address, using the criteria listed previously.

The Step 1 Decide Behavior Change Worksheet asks you to identify up to four behaviors or practices that are important for addressing the issues of concern that you have stated. For each behavior, think about the five criteria above, and write about them in the boxes provided. Make a judgment based on these criteria regarding which of the behaviors deserves high priority for your sessions for the program. From this reflection, select or decide the specific behaviors that will be the focus of your nutrition education program. We suggest only one or two for any given session, and one overarching theme for the behaviors if it is

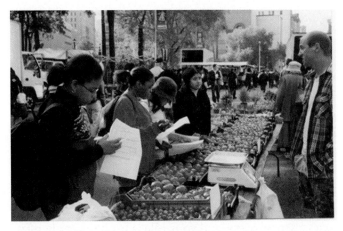

Students can find out the cost of tomatoes as part of a farmers' market scavenger hunt.

Courtesy of Linking Food and the Environment, Teachers College Columbia University.

a series. For example, the behavioral theme for childhood obesity prevention can be "energy-balance–related behaviors" made up of several specific behaviors. For those at risk of diabetes, select specific diabetes-prevention eating and physical activity behaviors; for those with hypertension, the DASH diet. Individual sessions will then address only one or two of the specific behaviors within each of these themes. Write a short justification for your decision.

BEHAVIOR CHANGE GOALS: HOW SPECIFIC IS SPECIFIC?

What does it mean to make the intervention or session behavior change goals very clear? How specific is specific? Remember the example in Chapter 3 about a proposed media campaign that went from a behavioral goal of "eating a healthy diet" to "eating less fat" to "drinking low-fat milk" to finally "purchasing low-fat milk" using the message of "1% or less" (Reger et al. 1998; Booth-Butterfield and Reger 2004)? The final message made the targeted behavior crystal clear.

Here are some more examples. The behavior change goal for sessions can be stated as "adolescents will increase their fruit and vegetable consumption" or as "adolescents will eat two or more cups of fruits and vegetables a day." The latter makes it much clearer what the adolescents should aim for. In another example, the behavior change goal can be stated as "postpartum women will increase breastfeeding," or, more specifically, as "new moms will exclusively breastfeed for at least 3 months." Other behaviors can be related to food safety, diabetes self-care, or resource management.

Sometimes two behaviors can be addressed at the same time if they are related to each other, such as "drink water instead of sweetened drinks" or "eat fruit instead of a packaged high-sugar snack." We are aiming for a clear "take-home" behavioral message for the audience. When there are too many take-home messages, the audience members lose focus and often leave feeling they learned a lot but don't have the time or energy to do all of them, so they won't do any of them.

An important reminder—just because the focus is on specific individual behaviors or community practices does not mean that the sessions should not involve critical thinking or address important values—they should. We are only providing coaching or guidance regarding what to do after that careful thinking and clarification of values.

In this context, the common practice of going through all the food groups of MyPlate in one session is less likely to lead to action because there are too many behaviors to consider all at once. Audience members can see it as good general information but not as truly actionable. Devoting several sessions and activities to each food group, with specific goal-setting or action plans at the end of each, is likely to make this tool more effective. The MyPlate tool *can* be used in one session if, for example, the one behavior to focus on is "eating appropriate portions." That way the audience members can focus on a single behavior without worrying about the details of all the foods in all the groups. This can be followed by individual sessions on the individual food groups, perhaps built around specific behavioral messages, as suggested by the *Choose MyPlate 10 Tips to a Great Plate Nutrition Education Series,* such as: Make half your grains whole; switch to fat-free or low-fat (1%) milk; or drink water instead of sugary drinks (USDA n.d.), or similar guidelines of other countries. Likewise, for behaviors that address ecological or environmental issues of concern, descriptions of the overall state of the food systems and their impacts on the environment with general calls of ecological eating may not be sufficiently helpful to guide audience actions. Recommending specific actions people can take individually or collectively will be more effective.

The U.S. government–sponsored educational programs described in Nutrition Education in Action 7-1 focus on three to five specific behavioral goals. These are still very general and are suitable as the overall behavioral goals of a program. However, individual sessions need to be more specific to be effective.

Some programs or series of sessions may be devoted entirely to one behavior. Squire's Quest for fourth grade students devoted 10 sessions to fruits and vegetables (Baranowski et al. 2003). Choice, Control & Change, an obesity prevention curriculum for middle school students, devoted 24 lessons to six very specific behaviors (eating 2.5 cups of fruit and vegetables each day, reducing sweetened drinks to no more than 8 ounces per day, and so forth) with children setting specific action goals for those behaviors that were relevant to them based on their self-assessment of intake (Contento et al. 2010). The 10 sessions of the People at Work: 5-a-Day Tailgate Program for sawmill workers who ate their lunches from coolers out of their cars in the parking lot were all devoted to increasing fruit and vegetable intakes (see **NUTRITION EDUCATION IN ACTION 2-2** in Chapter 2). Sub-behaviors were: including fruits and vegetables in the sack lunches they brought (they sampled bananas in one session); adding vegetables to main courses (sampled: "Sawmill chili"); breakfast (sampled: sunrise smoothies); fruit desserts (sampled: baked apple); and so forth. Sessions for parents often select as their behavior change goals parenting practices that foster healthy eating in their children, such as eating family meals together or offering appropriate serving sizes of food.

In the case study at the end of this chapter, the overall issue of concern is youth overweight. (Please note that this will never be stated to the youth.) Based on assessment data, four behavior change goals have been selected for the series of 10 sessions, including increasing fruits and vegetables to 2.5 cups or more per day and increasing physical activity to 10,000 steps or more a day. Use the Step 1 Decide Behavior Change Worksheet to state the behavior change goal(s) of your program or session(s).

BEHAVIOR CHANGE GOALS VERSUS BEHAVIORAL OBJECTIVES

The terms *goals* and *objectives* are often used interchangeably. Both are statements of desired outcomes. However, the term *behavioral objectives* has other meanings in the educational field, as described in Chapter 10, including very cognitive outcomes (e.g., being able to "state" that 2 + 2 = 4 is considered a "behavior"). Thus, there may be confusion about what the term means, so it will not be used in this text. Instead we use the term *behavior change goals* whenever we refer to observable actions or behaviors. Both the more general way to state a behavior change goal, such as "to increase fruit and vegetable intake among adolescents," and the more specific way to state it, "adolescents in seventh and eighth grades will increase their fruit and vegetable intake to 2.5 cups or more a day," are described as behavior change goals. The choice of specificity depends on the purposes of your intervention. If you will be measuring specific behavioral outcomes in your evaluation, you need to state your behavioral outcomes in specific, measurable terms. General behaviors, such as eating fruits and vegetables, are often referred to as behavioral categories. These are often made up of more specific actions, such as adding a vegetable to lunch, or eating fruit as a snack mid-morning or mid-afternoon. These can be considered *sub-behavior goals* and are referred to in this book as *action goals* or *action plans.* (See Chapters 5, and 12 for more details.)

BEHAVIOR CHANGE GOALS VERSUS EDUCATIONAL OBJECTIVES

In this book, the term *objectives* will be used only for *educational objectives*. Educational objectives are often confused with behavioral goals. Educational objectives are statements to guide the development of educational activities that will help the audience achieve the behavior change goal(s). For example, with the behavior change goal of "adolescents will eat more fruits and vegetables," educational objectives might be "adolescents will be able to state key reasons (benefits) for eating a variety of fruits and vegetables," ". . . appreciate that fruits and vegetables taste good," ". . . be able to state appropriate serving sizes," and so forth.

BEHAVIOR CHANGE GOALS ACHIEVABLE IN THE SHORT TERM AND LONG TERM

Sometimes a behavior change goal that is the desired long-term outcome is not likely to be achieved in the short term, say after one session. It is still important to state the general behavior change goal, but in each given session, focusing on a sub-behavior through an action plan may have to suffice. For example, the desired long-term goal may be for mothers to encourage their preschool child to eat the required number of fruit and vegetable servings each day. However, for the preschool child to eat one fruit as an afternoon snack may have to suffice as the short-term behavior change goal. For evaluation purposes, a statement of behavioral intention may have to serve as a proxy for behavior, especially if the intervention is short or you will not be seeing the group on an ongoing basis.

BEHAVIOR CHANGE GOALS MAY SERVE LARGER VALUE GOALS

Both short- and long-term behavioral goals may serve long-term non behavioral value goals. For example, a school garden may be initiated for many reasons, one being that students will eat more vegetables (shorter term behavioral goal), thereby contributing to healthy eating (longer term behavioral goal). But the long-term value goal may be for students to be able to understand how food is grown and to appreciate farmers and the agricultural system that brings us our food so that they can become better informed citizens in the future for difficult decisions that society needs to make. From the school's point

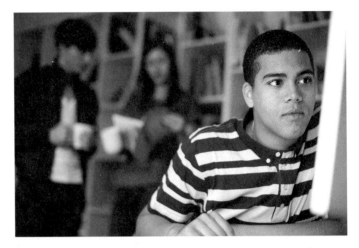

Nutrition education research can be gathered at town or school libraries.

© sturti/iStock.

of view, the garden can also be used to teach science, to provide an outdoor activity for children, build social relationships, increase the attractiveness of the campus, and instill a feeling that the school cares, thus engendering a greater commitment to coming to school and possibly better academic performance.

NUTRITION EDUCATION IN ACTION 7-2 provides some examples of how the nutrition education focus and issues, audiences, and behaviors have been stated for some social marketing and Web-based programs.

Case Study: The DESIGN Procedure in Action

A case study is presented here to illustrate the DESIGN Procedure. This case study is continued throughout the next several chapters for each of the steps in the process. Here it begins with Step 1. Use the completed Step 1 Decide Behavior Change Worksheet for the hypothetical case study shown at the end of the chapter as a guide for how to complete each of the components of Step 1. A blank Step 1 Decide Behavior Change Worksheet is located in the DESIGN Workbook at the end of Chapter 13.

The case involves a university-affiliated organization that works with children and youth. Thus, the general audience is already determined. The mission of the organization is to provide health services to youth and their families in the community. The community is ethnically and economically diverse. The organization has provided

NUTRITION EDUCATION IN ACTION 7-2 Examples of Behavioral Goals of Nutrition Education Programs

Sisters Together: Move More, Eat Better

Sisters Together is a national initiative of the Weight-Control Information Network (WIN) designed to encourage black women aged 18 years and older to maintain a healthy weight by becoming more physically active and eating healthier foods.

Sisters Together works with national and local newspapers, magazines, radio stations, schools, and consumer and professional organizations to raise awareness among black women about the health benefits of regular physical activity and healthy eating. This effort is timely because recent statistics indicate that nearly 80% of black women are overweight or obese.

Pick a Better Snack

Pick a Better Snack is a social marketing campaign in Iowa directed at low-income families and children. The objectives are to:

- Increase awareness of the campaign's logo and supporting messages.
- Improve attitudes about eating fruits and vegetables as snacks.
- Increase fruit and vegetable consumption among low-income children and their families.

We Can!

We Can! (Ways to Enhance Children's Activity and Nutrition) is a national education program designed for parents and caregivers to help children aged 8 to 13 years stay at a healthy weight. Parents and caregivers are the primary influencers for this age group. We Can! offers parents and families tips and fun activities to:

- Encourage healthy eating.
- Increase physical activity.
- Reduce sedentary or screen time.

Sources: Weight-Control Information Network. Sisters Together: Move More, Eat Better. http://win.niddk.nih.gov/sisters/index.htm; Iowa Department of Public Health, Iowa Department of Education. Pick a better snack and act. http://www.idph.state.ia.us/Pickabettersnack; and U.S. Department of Health and Human Services, National Institutes of Health. We Can! http://www.nhlbi.nih.gov/health/public/heart/obesity/wecan.

general health services in schools, but it has not developed a nutrition education program before. Organization directors think that it will be important to use some of its funds to develop a nutrition education program for youth in the schools it serves because they believe, from their experience, that the diets of youth need improving. There is only one middle school in town so they decide to start there. However, they do not have any specific data on their youth in relation to nutrition or what kind of intervention should be developed. Thus, the organization needs to find out the major nutrition-related health issues and problems that face the youth in their community and to develop a nutrition education program that addresses these issues. They hired a nutrition educator to help them with this program. She worked with school personnel to conduct all the assessments for Step 1 as described in this chapter.

The behavior change goals selected as the desired behavioral outcomes for the program are as follows.

STUDENTS WILL ADOPT BEHAVIORS TO ACHIEVE ENERGY BALANCE AND IMPROVE HEALTH

More specifically, the behavior change goals are that students will:

- Increase fruit and vegetable intakes to 2.5 or more cups a day.
- Increase physical activity to 10,000 steps or more per day.
- Decrease intake of highly processed, energy-dense snacks to 150 calories or less per day.
- Decrease intake of sugar-sweetened beverages to less than 8 ounces per day.

The organization decides to call the program "Taking Control: Eating Well and Being Fit." It will consist of the following components:

- *Classroom sessions* for middle school youth. For the classroom component they will use the six-step process to design the 10-session curriculum. This process is described in Chapters 7–13.

- *Parent component* (to support the middle school youth). For the parent component, they will use the same six-step process to design two sessions and two newsletters for parents. This component is described in Chapter 14.
- *School environmental/policy support component.* For the environmental support component they will use the six-step process to design the school-wide activities in support of the student curriculum. This process is described in Chapter 14.

Note that all three components are directed at helping middle school students achieve energy balance, and this outcome will be the basis for the evaluation.

After the specific behavior change goals have been established, the nutrition educator used a variety of sources and interviewed students to find out why they ate the current foods that they did and what would motivate them to adopt the recommended behavior change goals. Remember that we call these motivations the *determinants* of behavior change. They are the precursors of change. The process for conducting this kind of assessment is part of Step 2 and is described in the next chapter. The nutrition educator will use these understandings to develop the group sessions for the middle school students.

Your Turn to Design Nutrition Education: Completing the Step 1 Decide Behavior Change Worksheet

Information needed to complete the Step 1 Decide Behavior Change Worksheet has been provided throughout this chapter. Use the completed worksheet for the case study at the end of this chapter as a guide for how to complete the Step 1 Worksheet for your intervention. A blank Step 1 Worksheet is located in the workbook at the end of Chapter 13 and online at the publisher's website (http://nutrition.jbpub.com/education/3e). The Step 1 Worksheet consists of the following sections:

- Who is your audience?
- What can you learn about issues and behaviors of concern of your audience from general sources?
- What can you learn about the issues and behaviors of concern of your specific audience?
- Decide the behavior change goals of the program for your audience.

Complete the Step 1 Decide Behavior Change Worksheet to gather the assessment information you need as you start the DESIGN Procedure for a hypothetical or real nutrition education program or session(s) that you will create.

Questions and Activities

1. Why is it important to do a thorough assessment of the needs, interests, and concerns of the intended audience?

2. For a female teenage modern dance class in a low-income urban area, what information sources would you use to select health issues or problems to address in a nutrition education program?

3. When we think about nutrition education sessions, in our heads we can organize them based on "topics" (e.g., diet-related diseases, vitamins and minerals, overfishing) *or* behaviors (choose fewer sweetened beverages, chips, and other processed snack foods; choose more fruits, vegetables, whole grains and legumes; and eat fish that has been produced sustainably). What are

the pros and cons of organizing around topics versus organizing around behaviors? Which do you prefer and why?

4. We recommend that you focus on one or two behaviors for a given session or piece of indirect nutrition education and only a few for a series. Why do you think it is important to focus on only a few behaviors?

5. How would you select which behaviors or practices your program should address for your intended audience? That is, what criteria would you use and why?

6. If you have provided nutrition education sessions before, which of the steps from the DESIGN Procedure did you use, whether consciously or unconsciously? Do you think the steps are really needed? Why or why not?

References

American Dietetic Association. 2008. Nutrition Care Process and Model Part I: The 2008 update. *Journal of the American Dietetic Association* 108:1113–1117.

Australian National Health and Medical Research Council. 2013. *Eat for Health: Australian Dietary Guidelines—Providing the scientific evidence of healthier Australian diets.* Canberra, Australia: National Health and Medical Research Council.

Baker, S., G. Auld, C. MacKinnon, A. Ammerman, G. Hanula, B. Lohse, et al. 2014. Best practices in nutrition education for low-income audiences. http://snap.nal.usda.gov/snap/CSUBestPractices.pdf Accessed 1/15/15.

Baranowski, T., J. Baranowski, K. W. Cullen, T. Marsh, N. Islam, I. Zakeri, L. Honess-Morreale, and C. deMoor. 2003. Squire's Quest! Dietary outcome evaluation of a multimedia game. *American Journal of Preventive Medicine* 24(1):52–61.

Baranowski, T., E. Cerin, and J. Baranowski. 2009. Steps in the design, development, and formative evaluation of obesity prevention–related behavior change. *International Journal of Behavioral Nutrition and Physical Activity* 6:6.

Baranowski, T., L. S. Lin, D. W. Wetter, K. Resnicow, and M. D. Hearn. 1997. Theory as mediating variables: Why aren't community interventions working as desired? *Annals of Epidemiology* 7:589–595.

Block, G., C. Gillespie, E. H. Rosenbaum, and C. Jenson. 2000. A rapid food screener to assess fat and fruit and vegetable intake. *American Journal of Preventive Medicine* 18:284–288.

Block, G., F. E. Thompson, A. M. Hartman, F. A. Larkin, and K. E. Guire. 1992. Comparison of two dietary questionnaires validated against multiple dietary records collected during a 1-year period. *Journal of the American Dietetic Association* 92:686–693.

Bonvecchio, A., G. H. Pelto, E. Escalante, E. Monterrubio, J. P. Habicht, F. Navada, et al. 2007. Maternal knowledge and use of a micronutrient supplement was improved with a programmatically feasible intervention in Mexico. *Journal of Nutrition* 137:440–446.

Booth-Butterfield, S., and B. Reger. 2004. The message changes belief and the rest is theory: The "1% or less" milk campaign and reasoned action. *Preventive Medicine* 39:581–588.

Contento I. R., P. A. Koch, H. Lee, and A. Calabrese-Barton. 2010. Adolescents demonstrate improvement in obesity risk behaviors following completion of *Choice, Control & Change*, a curriculum addressing personal agency and autonomous motivation. *Journal of the American Dietetic Association* 110:1830–1839.

Food and Agricultural Organization. 2013. Food-based dietary guidelines by country. http://www.fao.org/ag/humannutrition/nutritioneducation/fbdg/en/ Accessed 12/2/14.

Green, W., and M. W. Kreuter. 2005. *Health education planning: An educational and ecological approach.* 4th ed. New York: McGraw-Hill.

Gussow, J. D., and K. Clancy. 1986. Dietary guidelines for sustainability. *Journal of Nutrition Education* 18(1):1–4.

Hawkes, C. 2013. *Promoting healthy diets through nutrition education and changes in the food environment: An international review of actions and their effectiveness.* Rome, Italy: Nutrition Education and Consumer Awareness Group, Food and Agriculture Organization of the United Nations. Available at http://www.fao.org/docrep/017/i3235e/i3235e.pdf Accessed 6/18/15.

Health Council of the Netherlands. 2011. *Guidelines for a healthy diet: The ecological perspective.* The Hague: Health Council of the Netherlands publication no. 2011/08E.

Heath C., and D. Heath. 2010. *Switch: How to change things when change is hard.* New York: Random House.

Hersey, J., J. Anliker, C. Miller, R.M. Mullis, S. Daugherty, S. Das, et al. 2001. Food shopping practices are associated with dietary quality in low-income households. *Journal of Nutrition Education and Behavior* 33:S16–S26.

Hunsberger M., J. O'Malley, T. Block, and J. C. Norris. 2012. Relative validation of Block Kids Food Screener for dietary assessment in children and adolescents. *Maternal and Child Nutrition.* Sep 24. doi: 10.1111/j.1740-8709.2012.0044.

McClelland, J. W., D. P. Keenan, J. Lewis, S. Foerster, S. Sugerman, P. Mara, et al. 2001. Review of evaluation tools used to assess the impact of nutrition education on dietary intake and quality, weight management practices, and physical activity of low-income audiences. *Journal of Nutrition Education* 33:S35–S48.

Medeiros, L., V. Hillers, P. Kendall, and A. Mason. 2001. Evaluation of food safety education for consumers. *Journal of Nutrition Education* 33:S27–S34.

Ozer, E. J. 2007. The effects of school gardens on students and schools: Conceptualization and considerations for maximizing healthy development. *Health Education & Behavior* 34(6):846–863.

Reger, B., M. Wootan, S. Booth-Butterfield, and H. Smith. 1998. 1% or less: A community-based nutrition campaign. *Public Health Reports* 113:410–419.

Rogers, E. M. 2003. *Diffusion of innovations.* 4th ed. New York: Free Press.

Shannon, J., A. R. Kristal, S. J. Curry, and S. A. Beresford. 1997. Application of a behavioral approach to measuring dietary change: The fat and fiber-related diet behavior questionnaire. *Cancer Epidemiology, Biomarkers and Prevention* 6:355–361.

Thompson, B., and L. Amoroso. 2010. *Combating micronutrient deficiencies: Food-based approaches.* Rome, Italy: Food and Agricultural Organization of the United Nations and CAB International.

Townsend, M. S., L. L. Kaiser, L. H. Allen, A. Block Joy, and S. P. Murphy. 2003. Selecting items for a food behavior checklist for a limited-resources audience. *Journal of Nutrition Education and Behavior* 35:69–82.

U.S. Department of Agriculture. n.d. *Choose MyPlate 10 Tips to a Great Plate Nutrition Education Series.* http://www.choosemyplate.gov/healthy-eating-tips/ten-tips.html Accessed 9/15/14.

U.S. Department of Health and Human Services. 2010. Dietary Guidelines for Americans. www.health.gov/dietaryguidelines/ Accessed 9/20/14.

U.S. Department of Health and Human Services. 2008. Physical Activity Guidelines for Americans. www.health.gov/paguidelines Accessed 9/20/14.

Whitehead, F. 1973. Nutrition education research. *World Review of Nutrition and Dietetics* 17:91–149.

Willett, W. C., R. D. Reynolds, S. Cottrell-Hoehner, L. Sampson, and M. L. Browne. 1987. Validation of a semi-quantitative food frequency questionnaire: Comparison with a 1-year diet record. *Journal of the American Dietetic Association* 87:43–47.

World Health Organization. 2003. *Diet, nutrition and the prevention of chronic diseases.* Report of a joint WHO/FAO expert consultation. WHO Technical Report Series 916. Geneva, Switzerland: WHO.

Yaroch, A. L., K. Resnicow, and L. K. Khan. 2000. Validity and reliability of qualitative dietary fat index questionnaires: A review. *Journal of the American Dietetic Association* 100(2):240–244.

Nutrition Education DESIGN Procedure

Decide behavior(s) ⟩ **E**xplore determinants of change ⟩ **S**elect theory & clarify philosophy ⟩ **I**ndicate general objectives ⟩ **G**enerate plans ⟩ **N**ail down evaluation plan

Step 1   Step 2   Step 3   Step 4   Step 5   Step 6

Step 1: Decide behavior change or action goal(s).

Before you design any nutrition education intervention, whether it is a few sessions or a larger intervention with several components, it is important to learn about your primary audience. From this you will be able to determine the behaviors and issues upon which to focus your intervention.

The Decide Behavior Change Worksheet will help you conduct assessments to obtain the information you will need within a framework that allows for your creativity. Use this worksheet as a guide to help you decide behavioral goals for your educational session. The references (in parentheses) are listed at the end of the case study workbook in Chapter 13.

Who is your audience? For example, moms, teens, older adults, diabetics, Head Start teachers

7th and 8th graders in a public, urban middle school

What can you learn about your audience in general? What do general sources, including the research literature and policy documents, tell you about your audience's issues and behaviors of concern? Consider demographics, eating patterns, and health risks. Remember, issues are health problems such as diabetes and obesity, food system problems such as excessive energy use from over processed food, and societal issues such as unfair wages for food workers. Behaviors include not enough fruits and vegetables, too many energy-dense snacks, etc.

- Overweight and obesity rates are highest and rising the fastest among minority adolescents living in low-income communities [1].
- Childhood overweight is associated with both immediate (e.g., increased cholesterol levels) and long-term consequences (e.g., cardiovascular disease, Type 2 diabetes) [2].
- The Office of the Surgeon General and Healthy People 2020 have named obesity as a priority [3,4].
- NHANES trends show increases in intakes of soft drinks, fruit drinks, and candy and decreases in milk and certain vegetables. Intakes of discretionary fat and added sugars are much higher than recommended [5].
- Youth do not eat the recommended amount of fruits or vegetables [6].
- Soft drink consumption has been linked to excess energy intake and weight gain among adolescents [7]. Adolescents, on average, get 11% of all their calories from sugar-sweetened beverages [8].
- Teens and preteens should typically consume about 1600–2000 calories per day (more for boys than girls). This should include at least 2–2.5 cups of vegetables and 1.5–2 cups of fruits, as well as 3 cups of dairy, 5–5.5 oz. of protein, and 5–6 oz. of whole grains. Adolescents should get 60 minutes of moderate to vigorous physical activity each day [9].
- National data show that by adolescence, children are spending $4 billion per year on foods and snacks for themselves [10].

Nutrition Education DESIGN Procedure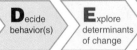

Decide behavior(s)	**E**xplore determinants of change	**S**elect theory & clarify philosophy	**I**ndicate general objectives	**G**enerate plans	**N**ail down evaluation plan
Step 1	Step 2	Step 3	Step 4	Step 5	Step 6

What can you learn about your specific audience? What do you learn from your specific audience about their issues and behaviors of concern through questionnaires, focus groups, interviews, and visiting the neighborhood?

- Overweight and obesity are higher among this group than national rates [11].
- Only 54% attend PE class 1 or more days a week [12].
- Thirty-five percent of adolescents watch 3 or more hours of TV during the school week and do not meet physical activity recommendations. Most adolescents watch TV 3 to 4 hours a day. Those who have computers at home also play video games or surf the Internet for over an hour a day [12].
- Adolescents consider "weight" to be an important issue. Adolescents also think about other health conditions like diabetes, asthma, and food allergies. These issues are most important to students who have the condition or have a close friend or family member with the condition [12].
- On average, the students eat only one serving of fruits and vegetables each day, mostly fruit [12].
- They drink two 16-ounce bottles of sugar-sweetened beverages each day [12].
- They eat an average of three packaged sweet and salty snacks every day, such as cookies, baked goods, or potato chips [12].
- They eat at fast food places four times a week. They eat there with friends or family [12].
- Students walk to school (a few blocks) but do not walk much otherwise. Some do go to the park and play basketball with friends [12].

What could be the behavioral goals for your session? Given the assets and concerns you described on the previous page, list potential behavior change goals for your session(s) or intervention in the left column of the table. Then, in the right column, consider the importance, feasibility, and desirability of each of these potential behavior change goals and think about how modifiable and measurable each would be.

Potential Goal Behaviors	Considerations • How **important** is this behavior in addressing the issues of concern? • How **feasible** is changing this behavior, given the time allotted and resources available? • How **desirable** is changing this behavior from the audience's point of view? • How **modifiable** is this behavior by educational means? • How **measurable** is change in this behavior?
Increase fruit and vegetable consumption	F&V consumption assists weight maintenance. Low F&V consumption is also associated with cardiovascular disease and some cancers. It is feasible to increase F&V consumption through hands-on education with tastings. The students already eat some fruit, but vegetable consumption is not highly desirable. Can be measured with recall or frequency survey data.
Decrease sugar-sweetened beverage consumption	Consuming SSBs is related to excess calorie consumption and overweight/obesity. It is feasible to shock teens about sugar consumption with demonstrations of the amount of sugar in SSBs. Water and fruit-flavored water can be good substitutes for SSB. Teens can be convinced that reducing SSB consumption can help maintain energy and weight, and this is desirable. Can be measured with recall or frequency survey data.
Decrease fast food consumption	Although palatable, the large amount of calories in fast foods can lead to weight gain. Additionally, fast food is highly processed with substances (e.g., added sugars, trans-fats, salt) that are associated with preventable, chronic diseases, including heart disease. This behavior is difficult to change because of the prevalence and accessibility of fast food outlets. Can be measured with recall or frequency survey data.
Increase physical activity	Physical activity helps maintain energy balance and avoid overweight/obesity. Participation in physical activity decreases throughout childhood and adolescence; sedentary lifestyle is related to overweight. Many kids are naturally inclined to like physical activity, but school is not conducive to being active. Video games often take the place of physical activity. Social norms and the desire to attain an attractive appearance can become increasingly important to teens. Can be measured with recall or frequency survey data.

Nutrition Education DESIGN Procedure

Decide behavior(s)	**E**xplore determinants of change	**S**elect theory & clarify philosophy	**I**ndicate general objectives	**G**enerate plans	**N**ail down evaluation plan
Step 1	Step 2	Step 3	Step 4	Step 5	Step 6

What is your behavior change goal? Evaluate the information in the above table and decide on the behavioral goal(s) for your session(s) or progam. This decision will guide you as you complete the DESIGN Procedure.

- *Students will increase fruit and vegetable consumption.
- Students will decrease sugar-sweetened beverage consumption.
- Students will decrease fast food consumption.
- Students will increase physical activity.

*For the purposes of this workbook case study, only this behavior will be addressed. The entire case study intervention involves all four of these behaviors. An intervention with multiple sessions and/or components may address one or more of the potential behavior changes, depending on the audience and the length of the intervention.

How would adopting this behavior benefit your audience? What issues of concern* will be made better if your audience reaches your behavior change goal(s)?

Increasing F&V consumption will address childhood obesity, which has implications for chronic disease reduction, including cancers and heart disease. Furthermore, if students are taught to purchase local, seasonal produce whenever possible, it will support the sustainability of the food system as well as fair wages for food workers.

* Note: You may or may not discuss these issues of concern with your audience.

The Nutrition Education DESIGN Procedure

Audience _____

ASSESSMENT

1: Decide behavior(s) →

Assess issues[a] and behaviors[b] of concern for audience from general sources.	Assess issues[a] and behaviors[b] of concern for your specific audience.
• • •	• • •

Behavior Change Goal[c]

2: Explore determinants of change →

Motivational theory-based determinants for behavior change

What audience said and/or what you learned	Determinant
• • • • • •	• • • • •

Behavioral knowledge & skills theory-based determinants for behavior change

What audience said and/or what you learned	Determinant
• • • • • •	• • • • • •

INTERVENTION

3: Select theory & clarify philosophy →

Theory Model

Educational philosophy	Philosophy about food and nutrition

The Nutrition Education DESIGN Procedure

Audience _____

<table>
<tr>
<td rowspan="2">

4: Indicate general objectives

&

5: Generate plans ⟶
</td>
<td colspan="1">**Objectives for each determinant
in your theory model**</td>
<td>**Activities to
address each objective**</td>
</tr>
<tr>
<td>

Objectives for motivational determinants
Participants will be able to:

•

•

•

•

•

•

•
</td>
<td>

•

•

•

•

•

•

•
</td>
</tr>
</table>

<table>
<tr>
<td>

Objectives for knowledge and behavioral skills determinants
Participants will be able to:

•

•

•

•

•

•

•
</td>
<td>

•

•

•

•

•

•

•
</td>
</tr>
</table>

INTERVENTION

6: Nail down evaluation plan ⟶

EVALUATION

<table>
<tr>
<td>**Outcomes you will measure**</td>
<td>**Tools to measure outcomes**</td>
</tr>
<tr>
<td>

•

•

•

•

•

•
</td>
<td>

•

•

•

•

•

•
</td>
</tr>
<tr>
<td colspan="2">

Process evaluation tools to measure how your session(s) went

•

•

•
</td>
</tr>
</table>

CHAPTER 8

Step 2: Exploring Determinants of Intervention Behavior Change Goals

OVERVIEW

The procedure described in this chapter helps you to get to know your audience, which is crucial for creating engaging, relevant, and effective nutrition education sessions and related activities. It describes how to use Step 2 of the DESIGN Procedure to explore the psychosocial determinants of the behavior change goals targeted by your intervention for the intended audience. Such understanding will be directly used to design your sessions and activities. Chapter 14 describes how to explore policy, systems and environmental determinants that support the behavior change goal(s).

CHAPTER OUTLINE

- Exploring your audience and their environments
- Exploring psychosocial determinants of behavior change
- Case study: the DESIGN Procedure in action—Step 2
- Your turn to design nutrition education: completing the Step 2 Explore Determinants of Change Worksheet

LEARNING OBJECTIVES

After completing this chapter, you should be able to:

- Appreciate the importance of thoroughly understanding the intended audience in the context of their families, community, and culture
- Identify the psychosocial factors that are potential determinants of the intervention's targeted behaviors for this audience
- Compare the advantages and disadvantages of different methods for obtaining the assessment information

Exploring Your Audience and Their Environments

Individuals' food and physical activity behaviors involve many complex, and often conflicting, beliefs and emotions that are embedded in many aspects of their life histories and current life situations. Taking action and making the behavior changes identified in Step 1 may thus be very difficult. The motivations, ability, and opportunities to make these changes will differ for a group of single mothers who are concerned about their children's health, teenagers who are interested in excelling in sports, or adult men who have been told they are at risk for diabetes. Understanding the numerous influences on—or determinants of—change is very challenging. But understand these you must if you are to design learning experiences that are meaningful and effective for the intended audience.

Imagine a nutrition educator who is assigned to provide nutrition education about breastfeeding to a group of expectant moms in a WIC program. She reads up on the scientific literature on the benefits of breastfeeding and makes sure she is very clear on the techniques to make breastfeeding successful. She designs a lesson around why-to and how-to breastfeed, with suitable props. As she embarks on her session, the women soon become restless and interrupt her to talk about their real concerns. It turns out that they knew all about breastfeeding but feel embarrassed to breastfeed except when alone, and their husbands do not like them to breastfeed. These represent psychosocial barriers to breastfeeding in the form of social norms. Clearly the nutrition educator would have been more effective if she had conducted a thorough assessment of her intended audience before she designed her session.

FIGURE 8-1 shows that the focus of Step 2 is exploring the potential psychosocial determinants of action or behavior change. In this step, you will find out as much as possible about why audience members make the food and activity choices they do and what might motivate,

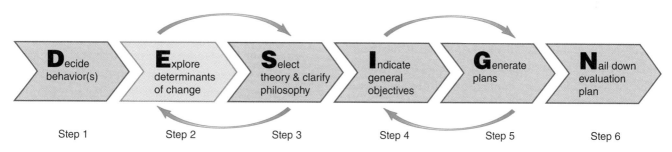

Inputs: Collecting the Assessment Data		Outputs: Designing the Theory-Based Intervention			Outcomes: Evaluation Plan
Tasks: • **Decide** behavior change goal(s) of the intervention based on: • analyzing issues and behaviors of concern for audience	*Tasks:* • **Explore** determinants of behavior change based on a variety of data sources	*Tasks:* • **Select** theory and draw intervention-specific theory model • Clarify educational philosophy • Articulate perspectives on content	*Tasks:* • **Indicate** general objectives for each determinant in your theory model	*Tasks:* • **Generate** educational plans: • Educational activities to address all determinants in theory model • Sequence for implementation using the 4 Es	*Tasks:* • **Nail down** evaluation plan • Select methods and questions to evaluate outcomes • Plan process evaluation • Create questions to measure how implementation went
Products: *Statement of intervention behavior change goal(s)*	*Products:* *List of determinants to address in the intervention*	*Products:* *Theory model for intervention* *Statement of educational philosophy* *Statement of content perspectives*	*Products:* *A general objective for each determinant in the theory model*	*Products:* *Educational plans that link determinants and educational activities to achieve behavior change or action goal(s)*	*Products:* *List of evaluation methods and questions* *Procedures and measures for process evaluation*

FIGURE 8-1 Nutrition education DESIGN procedure: Explore determinants of change—Step 2.

facilitate, and support them to take on the goal behaviors. Think of yourself as a detective, aiming to identify the potential determinants of the behavior change goals that you selected for the intervention in Step 1.

This DESIGN Procedure graphic (Figure 8-1) highlights the tasks and products for Step 2. A blank Step 2 Explore Determinants of Behavior Change worksheet is provided in the workbook at the end of Chapter 13 for you to use to conduct the Step 2 assessment for your nutrition education session or intervention. The completed Step 2 Explore Determinants of Behavior Change Worksheet for the case study is provided at the end of this chapter to help guide you in how to complete the blank Step 2 worksheet.

EXPLORING THE SOCIAL AND CULTURAL CONTEXTS OF YOUR AUDIENCE

The social and cultural contexts of people's lives, their religious beliefs, their ethnic origins, and lifestyles, all influence their perceptions about their current and desired food and activity behaviors. These influences can shape the psychosocial determinants of behavior. (This issue is discussed in greater detail in Chapter 4.) It has been found that psychosocial variables from theory help explain health behavior within the context of culture (Liou and Contento 2001). For example, for those who live in a collectivist culture where the basic social unit is the group or family rather than the individual, perceived benefits of taking action (outcome expectations) might not be stated in terms of impact on personal health, but "by keeping ourselves strong and healthy, we are better able to take care of others in our families and in our communities." In a culture where fatalism is an important underlying factor, perceived control to make behavior changes may be low because it is felt that people will get diabetes if that is their fate or God's will, so there is nothing they can do. Here, increasing their perception of control may be an important determinant of change on which to focus; that is, culture can influence the nature and strength of the role of determinants for taking action or making changes.

Life stage and family situation are also important. For women of young children, the perceived benefits of a dietary behavior may be in terms of the health of their children rather than their own health. For a woman who has teenage children and is also taking care of elderly parents living with them, perceptions of benefits may have to greatly exceed perceived barriers for her to take action.

Consequently, it is important to know about people's perceptions based on their cultural context, life stage, and family situation before you explore the personal psychosocial determinants in depth.

To find out about the beliefs, feelings and motivations, and skills that the intended audience may have as a result of their social situations and cultural context, you might ask some of the following questions:

- *Lifestyle and work style*: How do they perceive their work, family, recreation, and social obligations as influencing their willingness and ability to make healthy food and activity choices?
- *Life stage and life trajectories*: What is their life stage at this time? Are they in their child-rearing stage? Retired? What previous life experiences, life trajectories, or life stage considerations are important to them at this point?
- *General cultural and religious beliefs*: What are some general cultural or religious beliefs that influence their eating and activity patterns? What is the community's sense of time and space?
- *Degree of acculturation*: If they are immigrants, find out about the degree to which they feel comfortable with mainstream language and culture. You can ask about their use of their home language and food and who are in their social circle. See **BOX 8-1** for an example of questions to ask.

EXPLORING RELEVANT INDIVIDUAL AND COMMUNITY STRENGTHS OR ASSETS

The groups and communities with whom nutrition educators work may often already have practices, beliefs, and attitudes that are health promoting. You can build on these to achieve the behavior change goals of your session(s) or intervention. Therefore, it is important to learn about them. Heath and Heath describe this step as "follow the bright spots. Investigate what is working and clone it" (Heath and Heath 2010).

- *Behaviors and practices*: What is the intended audience already doing that is healthy? How can you build on these actions to achieve the health outcomes and behavior change goals of your intervention?
- *Beliefs and attitudes*: What are some beliefs and attitudes that are already assets in terms of the behavior changes targeted by the intervention? What personal

BOX 8-1 Considering Acculturation of Intended Audiences

In the United States, and increasingly so in other countries, audiences of nutrition education programs are very diverse, coming from a variety of ethnic, cultural, and social backgrounds. Many have come from several countries of origin. Some schools report that their students speak as many as 50 or more different languages. In addition, not all individuals from the same country of origin are alike. Indeed, the differences within groups may be as great as between groups.

Individuals may be at different levels of acculturation, including differences in the degree to which they have adopted mainstream American (or British or European) foods and food practices. This is important to find out so that your nutrition education intervention is appropriate for your audience. The following short acculturation questionnaire may help you understand your audience better. You can ask these questions orally and informally.

	(1) Only Spanish/ Chinese/Arabic, etc.	(2) Both equally	(3)	(4) Only English
What language do you speak?				
What language do you think in?				
What types of food do you prefer to eat?				
What foods do you usually eat at home?				
What are your favorite types of restaurants?				
When you select friends, what ethnic background do you prefer?				
When you select health professionals, what ethnic background do you prefer?				

Sources: Liou, D., and I. R. Contento. 2001. Usefulness of psychosocial theory variables in explaining fat-related dietary behavior in Chinese Americans: Associations with degree of acculturation. *Journal of Nutrition Education* 33:322–331; and modified from Suinn, R. F., K. Rickard-Figueroa, S. Lew, and P. Vigil. 1987. The Suinn-Lew Asian self-identity acculturation scale: an initial report. *Educational and Psychological Measurement* 47:401–407.

or cultural beliefs and attitudes does the intended audience possess that make positive contributions to nutritional health or the sustainability of the food system? What do they already know about the health or food issues of concern? What knowledge and skills do they already possess to address the concerns? What community support systems or environmental factors are supportive of healthy eating, active living, and sustainable food systems?

Exploring Psychosocial Determinants of Behavior Change

After understanding some general background factors about your audience, you can seek to understand the audience more specifically. Where, then, to begin? What will you ask about? This is where theory can be of assistance: it provides a framework for asking questions and organizing the answers.

THEORY PROVIDES GUIDANCE

You cannot ask questions about everything in their lives—that would be very time-consuming, intrusive, and unnecessary. Using theory as a tool, you can ask about the potential determinants of current behavior and of behavior change–taking action, such as beliefs, attitudes, feelings, identities, or self-confidence in making changes. This is important because the specific psychosocial determinants that you identify become the primary targets of the educational strategies and learning experiences that you design. Theory can thus provide an important and efficient framework for asking questions and organizing the answers in the needs assessment, just as it does for conducting the nutrition education intervention itself. Knowledge of theory enables you to conduct a more thorough, accurate, and complete assessment of your audience (Baranowski, Cerin, and Baranowski 2009).

If you have chosen more than one behavior change goal or action to target, the potential determinants of each of these may have to be assessed separately. For example, there is evidence that the motivations and barriers may be different for actions involving adding healthy foods to the diet (such as fruits and vegetables) compared with those of reducing the amount of less healthy food in the diet (such as high-fat foods or sweetened beverages). The kinds of determinants may also differ between food-related behaviors and physical activity behaviors. Thus, the determinants of behavior change may be quite different for each of the following target behaviors if they are chosen: eating more fruits and vegetables, eating fewer high-energy snacks, and reducing sedentary behaviors. Clearly, limiting the number of behaviors or practices to address makes the assessments easier to conduct (and the nutrition education sessions or intervention more likely to be feasible and effective).

As mentioned in earlier chapters, behavior change can be seen as involving two functions or components: a *motivational*, usually pre-action component, where the emphasis is on beliefs and feelings, and an *action* component, where the emphasis is on knowledge and skills. Some determinants are more important than others for each component. You can thus ask questions that are related to each of the components of behavior change. The answers are crucial for determining educational objectives in Step 4 and for designing educational strategies in Step 5.

EXPLORING POTENTIAL MOTIVATORS OF BEHAVIOR CHANGE

Theory provides a framework for systematically asking about the potential influences or determinants of change. You might want to consider assessing some or all of the

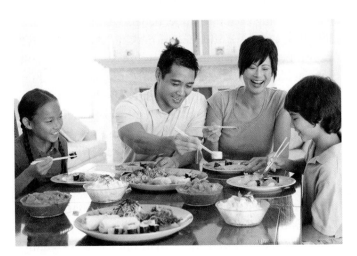

Cultural identity and acculturation are factors in food choice.
© iStockphoto/Thinkstock.

determinants listed below, depending on which theory you use to structure the intervention. They are all described in detail in Chapter 4. The centrality of determinants in nutrition education is emphasized by research evidence (Baranowski et al. 1997; Baranowski et al. 2009).

In Step 3 you will create a theory model to guide your sessions based on what you find in Step 2. If you are not yet sure which theory is appropriate, you should collect the information on a variety of determinants of behavior change or theory constructs such as those listed here. Information on them will be usable for whatever model you create for the intervention (Shaikh et al. 2008). Ask the audience about specific potential factors that would motivate them to take action, even if these factors do not seem to fall into a theory.

However, if you have already chosen an existing theory or have created an intervention model for your behavior change goals and audience based on strong evidence from prior studies, then you need to assess only those determinants or theory constructs that are part of your model in Step 2.

Questions About Potential Determinants of Motivation

We have used the analogy that the names of the determinants or precursors/antecedents of behavior are like names on buckets. What specifically goes into each of the buckets depends on what you find out about your audience. **TABLE 8-1** shows the words used by middle school students to describe their motivations and the names of the buckets into which each of these motivations belong.

Here we provide a list of potential motivation-related determinants of the behavior change goals of your intervention. For each of these determinants, assess potential motivations for the audience to engage in your intervention-specified behavior(s). For the design of your session or sessions, reflect on these. Remember that for each determinant, family practices and cultural and religious beliefs will influence the specific nature and strength of the determinant.

- *Perceived risks (perceived negative outcomes).* What are their beliefs regarding the severity of the health issue identified and their perception of their personal susceptibility or vulnerability to it? For example, how likely do they think it is that they will develop heart disease? Hip fractures? Or that their children will

Table 8-1 Examples of Middle School Youth's Descriptions of Their Motivations and Skills for Choosing Healthful Behavior Change Goals, Mapped onto Determinants from Theory

Youth's Descriptions of Motivations	Determinants from Theory
I want to stay healthy... so I can lose weight. so I can get strong and smarter. because I will have better eyesight and better skin. because all I did was drink soda and I got bumps on my face.	Outcome expectations
I don't walk enough. I eat too much junk food. I usually eat at fast food restaurants. I don't drink a lot of water.	Self-assessment
I want to know how many steps I walk per day. I want to see what would happen to my body.	Self-monitoring
I know I can achieve this goal and be successful. I want to prove that I can stop eating potato chips.	Self-efficacy
The doctor said I should eat healthy food and fruits; she said I don't eat enough. My mom thinks I don't drink enough water.	Perceived social norms
It is important. It is a goal I want to accomplish.	Values
Because it is easier. It is easy to follow.	Perceived barriers
I like to walk. I love vegetables.	Feelings/affective attitudes

Data from Petrillo-Myers, M., H. Lee, P. Koch, and I. R. Contento. 2009. Middle school students' reasons for selecting specific obesity risk reduction goals: Mapping to potential mediators from theory. *Journal of Nutrition Education and Behavior* 41(4S):O38.

become obese? Cultural and religious beliefs may be especially important here. If your sessions or intervention will address food system issues, you can ask about their sense of personal risk from the kinds of food that they buy from the current food supply.

- *Perceived benefits (positive outcome expectations).* What expectations do participants have about how the targeted behavior change(s) may reduce the risk for the health issue or improve health? What would be the benefits (for personal health, for carbon footprint) of the targeted behavior change, such as increasing their intakes of fruits and vegetables?
- *Perceived barriers.* What barriers does the intended audience see for engaging in the behavior? What costs? In social marketing language, what must they exchange or sacrifice for the benefits they will experience?
- *Attitudes (cognitive).* What are the intended audience's attitudes toward the behaviors that are advocated by the session or intervention? What would motivate them to change? Attitudes or motivations depend on beliefs and outcome expectations (listed previously).

- *Attitudes (affective)—feelings or affect.* What feelings do they anticipate they will have by engaging in the targeted behavior? Will they have anticipated regret about not taking action?
- *Values.* What values does the intended audience have that might influence whether they will consider taking action on the needs or issues identified? How do these affect the psychosocial determinants?
- *Food preferences and enjoyment (positive outcome expectations).* What are the participants' food preferences, likes, and dislikes? We know that taste is one of the most important mediators of food choices. How do they judge the intervention's recommended behavior(s) in terms of foods they will eat? Will these foods be enjoyable? Satisfying? Filling?
- *Social norms or felt group pressure.* Do participants believe that specific individuals or social and cultural groups important to them think they should or should not perform the particular behaviors or practices recommended by your session(s) or intervention? How much are they motivated to comply with these expectations of how they should behave?

- *Social roles.* What are participants' conceptions of behaviors that are appropriate or desirable for people holding their particular position in their group or society? For example, what are their perceptions about whether women in their station in life should breastfeed or bottle feed?

- *Self-identities.* What are their self-identities? For example, do they see themselves as health-conscious consumers, "green" consumers, vegetarians, or having other identities?

- *Perceived behavioral control or personal sense of control or agency.* To what extent do participants believe that they have some control over their behaviors, their health, and their environment? That they can take charge? Cultural beliefs may be especially relevant here.

- *Perceived self-efficacy.* What are the participants' perceptions of their ability to carry out desirable health actions? For example, although participants may believe that glucose monitoring will lead to the glucose control that they desire, they may not feel confident that they can prick themselves every day to monitor blood glucose levels.

- *Stage of motivational readiness to take action.* Overall, at what stage are they with respect to motivational readiness to take action—pre-action or ready to take action? More specifically, are they in the precontemplation, contemplation, deciding, action, or maintenance stage?

- *Culture- or religion-specific health and food beliefs.* What are the specific culturally based or religious health beliefs that will influence perceived benefits and barriers to the behavior change goal(s) of your session? Sense of self-efficacy and autonomy? Social norms?

- *Cultural and ethnic identities.* What are participants' ethnic and cultural identities? If they are immigrants, what is their degree of **acculturation**? It has been found that degree of acculturation is a better gauge of attitudes and practices in terms of diet than is length of stay (Liou and Contento 2001) (see Box 8-1). These identities may influence their health beliefs, attitudes, self-efficacy, and so forth. Be sure to explore.

Such information on the motivations of the intended audience is vital for developing sessions, interventions, and media campaigns for helping your audience understand and appreciate why to change their behaviors or to take action. However, such information may not be enough to plan a successful intervention. Participants must also have access to the knowledge and skills needed to carry out the advocated behaviors. Determining whether they do is the next step.

The public does not, of course, use the words from the theory just listed; they use different terms for these determinants. As we noted earlier, Table 8-1 presents an example of the wording used by middle school students to describe why they chose goals to eat more healthfully. The words of the youth are mapped onto theory constructs. In Chapter 3, the words used by Alicia and Ray in the case examples are also mapped onto the terms used in psychosocial theories (see pages 70–71). Similarly, in the Step 2 Worksheet you first record the words of the audience members and then link them to the psychosocial determinants.

EXPLORING POTENTIAL FACILITATORS OF BEHAVIOR CHANGE

Behavioral Capabilities

Behavioral capabilities is the term used by health psychologists for the food- and nutrition-specific knowledge and cognitive, affective, and behavioral skills that people need in order to be able to act on their motivations to eat healthfully. They are all described in detail in Chapter 5. Such knowledge and skills are important for people to act appropriately on their motivations. For example, during earlier decades in the United States, many people thought that eating large quantities of red meat was vital to getting enough protein in the diet. They were motivated to eat healthfully, but their knowledge about what constitutes healthful eating was not correct.

Thus, before conducting an educational intervention, you must find out whether the participants have the necessary nutrition information and food-related skills to act upon their motivations. Assess the following:

- *Food- and nutrition-related knowledge to carry out targeted behavior (factual and procedural or how-to knowledge; nutrition literacy).* For example, do they know how many servings of fruits and vegetables they should eat? Which foods are high in saturated fat? The nutritional value of favorite snacks? What information do they feel they need or would they like to learn about?

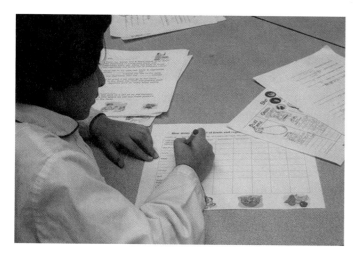

Questionnaires provide an excellent window into a person's motivations for and barriers to nutritious eating.

Courtesy of Linking Food and the Environment, Teachers College Columbia University.

- *Food- and nutrition-related behavioral skills.* Examples are label reading, food safety practices, cooking skills, menu modification skills, breastfeeding, and choosing local foods. What skills do they think they will need to take action? What skills would they like to acquire?
- *Critical thinking skills.* Can they discuss the advantages and disadvantages of different kinds of foods and food practices (e.g., traditional, organic, local, genetically modified)? Breastfeeding versus bottle feeding? Weight-loss diets?
- *Misconceptions.* What are their misconceptions?

Self-Regulation Skills (Skills in Self-Directed Change)

What self-regulation skills or skills in self-directed change do they currently have in order to make voluntary choices and consciously take charge of their behaviors?

- *Ability to make action plans; goal-setting and self-monitoring skills.* How do they usually make changes? Are they able to analyze their own diets and set action plans to achieve behavior change goals of the intervention? Have they made action plans before? How useful were these plans for them? Are they able to monitor their progress toward their action plans and make course corrections or set new, more appropriate goals?
- *Emotion-coping skills.* Do they cope with stress by eating food? Do they have specific difficulties in

certain situations? Do they have the emotion-coping skills to handle stress more appropriately in order not to use food as a stress reducer?

- *Reward structures.* What are the reward structures for the group's behaviors?

It is important to ask the intended audience about potential knowledge and skills they think they will need to overcome barriers and enact the targeted behaviors or practices.

METHODS FOR EXPLORING POTENTIAL PSYCHOSOCIAL DETERMINANTS OF BEHAVIOR CHANGE

Indirect Methods: Information from General Sources

You can find out about the attitudes, beliefs, and other person-related determinants of change listed earlier indirectly through a review of the relevant studies on motivation to take action and the dietary change process; monitoring data for the intended audience or similar population (e.g., adolescents, postmenopausal women, African American men); government and industry opinion surveys of people's beliefs and attitudes; food marketing surveys; studies of population segmentation by psychographic variables; or existing records for the group (e.g., Contento, Randell, and Basch 2002).

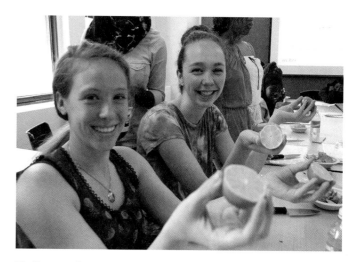

Finding out about people's food preferences is important.

Tania Fuentez. Courtesy of Food Bank For New York City.

Direct Methods: Information from Your Audience

It is best to obtain information directly from the intended audience, if possible. You can administer surveys or brief questionnaires using existing instruments or intervention-specific instruments that you design. **TABLE 8-2** is an example of an instrument that has been validated for use with low-income audiences and assesses motivational readiness to take action. **TABLE 8-3** shows an instrument validated to ask specifically about self-efficacy in relation to the behavior of fat intake. If the audience is low literacy, you can ask these questions orally and informally and record the answers yourself.

Talking personally with the group is highly desirable. You can conduct focus group interviews, in-depth interviews of individuals from the intended audience or key informants, or intercept interviews as individuals leave stores, clinics, or service centers. Use the Step 2 Explore Determinants of Change Worksheet to record your answers.

NUTRITION EDUCATION IN ACTION 8-1 contains examples of open-ended questions for use with young adults, and **NUTRITION EDUCATION IN ACTION 8-2** describes the outcomes of in-depth interviews with community members. **TABLE 8-4** summarizes the advantages and disadvantages of a variety of methods to gather assessment data.

Table 8-2 Tool to Assess Psychosocial Indicators of Fruit and Vegetable Intake in Limited-Resources Audiences	
Determinant/Theory Construct	**Items**
Perceived benefits[a]	I feel that I am helping my body by eating more fruits and vegetables.
	I may develop health problems if I do not eat fruits and vegetables.
Perceived barriers	I feel that fruit is too expensive.
	I feel that fruit is not always available.
	I feel that fruit is time-consuming to prepare.
	I feel that fruit is not liked by my family.
	I feel that fruit is not tasty.
	(Similar items for vegetables)
Perceived control[a]	In your household, who is in charge of what foods to buy?
	In your household, who is in charge of how to prepare the food?
Self-efficacy[a]	I feel that I can plan meals or snacks with more fruit during the next week.
	I feel that I can eat fruits or vegetables as snacks.
	I feel that I can add extra vegetables to casseroles and stews.
	I can eat two or more servings of vegetables at dinner.
Social support[b]	Are there other people encouraging you to buy, prepare, and eat fruits and vegetables?
	(My children, partner, mother, father, other)
Perceived norms[a]	People in my family think I should eat more fruits and vegetables.
	My doctor (or WIC nutritionist) tells me to eat more fruits and vegetables.
Intention: readiness to eat more fruits and vegetables[c]	I am not thinking about eating more fruit (coded as 1, precontemplation).
	I am thinking about eating more fruit (coded as 2, contemplation).
	I am definitely planning to eat more fruit in the next month (coded as 3, preparation).
	I am trying to eat more fruit now (coded as 4, action).
	I am already eating two or more servings of fruit a day (coded as 5, maintenance).
	(Similar items for vegetables)
Diet quality	How would you describe your diet? (5-point scale: Very poor to very good)

Note: Only selected items of this assessment tool are shown.
[a] Scores of 1 to 3: are disagree (1), neither agree nor disagree (2), agree (3).
[b] Instructions to client: "Check as many as apply." Coding: no = 0 = no support; yes = 1 = support by one person; yes = 2 = support by two or more people.
[c] Instructions to client: "Check one."
Townsend, M. S., and L. L. Kaiser. 2005. Development of a tool to assess psychosocial indicators of fruit and vegetables intake for two federal programs. *Journal of Nutrition Education and Behavior* 37:170–184. Used with permission of the Society for Nutrition Education.

Table 8-3 National Cancer Institute's Food Attitudes and Behaviors Survey

Assuming that you want to, how confident are you that you could do each of the following starting this week and continuing for at least 1 month? ("X" ONE BOX ON EACH LINE, USING THE SCALE OF 1, NOT AT ALL CONFIDENT, TO 5, VERY CONFIDENT.)

How confident are you that you could...	NOT AT ALL CONFIDENT 1	2	3	4	VERY CONFIDENT 5	DOES NOT APPLY
Eat a healthy snack, like a fruit or a vegetable, when you're really hungry?	☐	☐	☐	☐	☐	☐
Eat healthy foods, like fruits or vegetables, when you are tired?	☐	☐	☐	☐	☐	☐
Eat healthy foods, like fruits or vegetables, when there are junk foods in your house like chips, cookies, or candy?	☐	☐	☐	☐	☐	☐
Eat fruit instead of cake, cookies, candy, ice cream, or other sweets for dessert?	☐	☐	☐	☐	☐	☐
Eat fruits and vegetables when your family and friends are eating junk foods like chips, cookies, or candy?	☐	☐	☐	☐	☐	☐
Buy or bring fruits and vegetables to eat at work?	☐	☐	☐	☐	☐	☐
Snack on fruits and vegetables rather than on junk foods while watching TV?	☐	☐	☐	☐	☐	☐

Erinsosho, T. O., C. A. Pinard, L. C. Nebeling, R. P. Moser, A. R. Shaikh, K. Resnicow, et al. 2015. Development and implementation of the National Cancer Institute's Food Attitudes and Behaviors Survey to assess correlates of fruit and vegetable intake in adults. *PLoS ONE* 10(2): e0115017. DOI:10.1371. February 23, 2015.

NUTRITION EDUCATION IN ACTION 8-1 Open-Ended Questions

The following questions were used for assessing the opinions regarding fruits and vegetables of ethnically diverse young adults (ages 16–25) in a community college program:

- *How many fruits and vegetables do you believe you need to eat each day? Why or why not?* Responses varied, with a majority indicating between two and five servings per day. "Good for the body" or health-related answers were the top reasons to eat fruits and vegetables each day.

- *If you learned the following facts (list provided) about fruits and vegetables, which would most likely cause you to eat more fruits and vegetables?* The top two facts selected from the list were "eating fruits and vegetables gives me healthy and beautiful teeth, gums, skin, and hair" and "eating fruits and vegetables helps reduce my risk of developing a chronic disease such as cancer, heart disease, or stroke."

- *What would encourage you to eat more fruits and vegetables?* Freshness, increased availability and selection, and health were the top reasons mentioned.

- *How important is it to you to eat fruits and vegetables?* Seventy-one percent said that it was "very important," and 21% said it was "somewhat important."

- *Do you eat fruits and vegetables in the cafeteria? Why or why not?* Seventy-five percent indicated that they ate fruits and vegetables in the cafeteria for reasons of taste or health. Those who did not cited the lack of freshness and availability.

- *When you buy beverages from vending machines, which ones do you usually choose?* Cola, water, and non-cola soda were the more frequent choices. Only 5% indicated usually purchasing fruit juice. Thirty-nine percent indicated that they would purchase 100% fruit juice if it were available in the vending machine.

- *When are you most willing to eat more fruits and vegetables? Breakfast, lunch, between meals, dinner, or dessert?* Responses were divided between all times, with slightly more respondents favoring fruits and vegetables for lunch.

- *How would you prefer to receive nutrition information?* Taste tests, brochures, posters, classes, staff at the campus health clinic, radio, and television were the top preferred methods for the target audience to receive nutrition information.

Source: California Project LEAN, California Department of Health Services. 2004. *Community-based social marketing: The California Project LEAN experience.* Sacramento, CA: Author. http://www.californiaprojectlean.org.

NUTRITION EDUCATION IN ACTION 8-2 Wellness IN the Rockies (WIN the Rockies): A Research, Education, and Outreach Project that Seeks to Address Obesity Innovatively and Effectively

The Focus of the Program

Overall project goals are to enhance the well-being of individuals by improving their attitudes and behaviors related to food, physical activity, and body image, and to help build communities' capacities to foster and sustain these changes.

Assessment

Prior to developing the various nutrition education programs of this project, program staff gathered narratives or life stories related to physical activity, food and eating, and body image from extensive interviews and focus group discussions with 103 adults. The narratives were recorded. Key quotations were identified and grouped into 146 narrative thematic codes using grounded theory.

Values

Values emerged as an important theme. A major finding of relevance here is that being productive, working hard, and not wasting resources were important values. Thus, physical activity should be productive or serve some purpose, such as mowing the lawn or doing other chores. Going to the gym to exercise or just going for a walk was not seen as productive. These activities were a "waste" of time compared with activities in which work was being accomplished or when compared with other things that they might be doing with their families or communities.

In the same way, wasting food was seen as violating an important value of not wasting resources. That value led to the importance of cleaning one's plate and not squandering food.

The Power of Others

The study also found that other people have profound and often lifelong impacts on individuals' feelings about their body and physical abilities. These feelings, in turn, can contribute to their sense of identity and influence their lifestyles and their long-term health. Thus, the interviews suggested that nutrition professionals need to create social environments that nurture others, particularly youth, rather than be critical and hurtful. Respecting diverse body sizes is highly important.

Sources: Pelican, S., F. Vanden Heede, B. Holmes, et al. 2005. The power of others to shape our identity: Body image, physical abilities, and body weight. *Family and Consumer Sciences Research Journal* 34:57–80; Wardlaw, M. K. 2005. New you/health for every body: Helping adults adopt a health-centered approach to well-being. *Journal of Nutrition Education and Behavior* 37:S103–106; and Pelican, S., F. Vanden Heede, and B. Holmes. 2005. *Let their voices be heard: Quotations from life stories related to physical activity, food and eating, and body image.* Chicago, IL: Discovery Association Publishing House.

Case Study: The DESIGN Procedure in Action—Step 2

In the Step 1 assessment for our case study in Chapter 7, the university-based agency chose "Taking Control: Eating Well and Being Fit" as the title of the intervention. The agency identified the following four behavior change goals for their audience of middle school students:

- Increase intake of fruits and vegetables.
- Reduce consumption of sweetened beverages.
- Reduce intake of packaged, highly processed, energy-dense snacks.
- Increase physical activity.

In designing the full intervention, the nutrition educator needs to explore and identify the motivators and facilitators of change separately for all four behaviors because it is unlikely that these would be the same for all behaviors. For example, the motivators and facilitators for eating more fruits and vegetables would likely be different from those for decreasing consumption of sweetened beverages. Therefore, for reasons of space, in Step 2 of the case study we focus on only one of the four behaviors—eating more fruits and vegetables. Thus, we report only the results from the comprehensive assessment conducted by the university-based agency nutrition educator for those determinants that can potentially increase the behavior of eating more fruits and vegetables by these middle school students. The results are shown in the completed Step 2 Explore Determinants of Change Worksheet for the case study at the end of this chapter.

Table 8-4 Advantages and Disadvantages of Various Methods for Finding Out About Your Audience

	Advantages	Disadvantages
Reviews of existing information		
Review of research or survey literature	Quick, inexpensive, nonthreatening	Information not specific to intended audience
National survey and monitoring data, opinion polls	Quick, inexpensive, nonthreatening	Information not specific to intended audience
Review of existing records of intended audience	Information specific to intended audience; quick, inexpensive, nonthreatening to intended group	Limited by quality of data, scope of data
Surveys of intended audience		
Telephone	Information specific to group; chance for detailed insight into perceived and real needs	Expensive; extensive training needed for interviewers; leaves out people with no phones or unlisted numbers
Group administered	Quick, inexpensive; information specific to intended audience	Survey instrument must be designed and tested
Internet administered	Quick, inexpensive; information specific to intended audience; liked by most audiences	Survey instrument must be designed and tested; appropriate online program must be available inexpensively; participants' email addresses must be available; eliminates those with no access to computers
Mailed survey	Information specific to intended audience; chance for more honest answers	Eliminates low-literacy individuals; responses less open-ended than in-person interviews; moderately expensive; time delay in getting information; may get low response rate
Individual interviews		
Informal	Information specific to intended audience; inexpensive	Not systematic
Formal in-person interviews	Information specific to intended audience; comprehensive insight into intended audience	Expensive; extensive training needed for interviewers; time-consuming
Group meetings		
Group discussion	Relatively low cost, quick	People attending may not be representative; not enough time for people to express their thoughts or needs publicly
Focus groups	Provides detailed information on beliefs, emotions, and attitudes	Expensive; training needed for interviewers
Observation	Accurate information on behaviors	Expensive; can be intrusive; can alter the behavior being observed if observation is known

Your Turn to Design Nutrition Education: Completing the Step 2 Explore Determinants of Change Worksheet

Use the completed worksheet for the case study as a guide for how to complete the Step 2 Worksheet for your intervention. A blank Step 2 Explore Determinants of Change Worksheet for you to use is located in the DESIGN Workbook at the end of Chapter 13. This Step 2 Worksheet consists of the following components:

- Description of the sociocultural environment, life stage, and other aspects of the lives of your audience.
- Description of the personal and community assets or strengths of the audience: What are they already doing right?

- List of the specific determinants that would motivate change and facilitate the audience to achieve the intervention's behavior change goals.

After completing Steps 1 and 2 you should have statements regarding the following:

- *High-priority behavior change goals* to be targeted by the intervention. For example, improved food safety behaviors among low-income women.
- *Psychosocial determinants that are potential influencers of the target behavior changes.* This list can, and indeed should, be quite long (e.g., 8 to 10 items). You will prioritize them later, in Step 3, based on evidence and on the theory or model you select to guide the intervention. These determinants will become the basis for writing the educational objectives that guide the development of your intervention.

DETERMINANTS OF CHANGE AS THE BRIDGE BETWEEN THEORY AND NUTRITION EDUCATION PRACTICE

Although a comprehensive process of selecting the behavior change focus of the intervention and identifying the specific determinants of change may seem time-consuming, it is probably the most critical step in creating effective nutrition education learning experiences in practice settings. These determinants become the targets of the educational strategies and activities in your program. In addition to providing you with important data, an audience assessment can be a useful tool in establishing a rapport with audience participants. If done thoughtfully, a good assessment of an audience may reveal preconceptions you may have had about the participants, as well as your own attitudes about teaching and learning. Nutrition education is most successful when both group participants and educators can communicate openly, honestly, and with respect for each other as individuals. A comprehensive assessment process can help to establish this relationship, providing the basis of nutrition education that is both important and responsive to the needs and desires of the audience.

Questions and Activities

1. In the last chapter, you identified issues and behaviors of concern for a given audience. You also identified the behavior change goals that will be the focus of your intervention. Why is it important to identify the potential determinants of change for these behaviors before your create your educational session activities?

2. Before you conduct the assessment of your audience, practice the procedure by finding two or three people who have made changes in their eating or activity patterns. Ask them to explain what motivated them to make these changes. Also ask what made it difficult. Write the answers down. Can you identify from their words what the psychosocial determinants of motivation are for them? Use Table 8-1 as a guide. Now ask them if they feel they have the knowledge and skills to make the changes; if not, what would they need?

3. As you review the several methods for assessing potential psychosocial determinants of behavior change, which methods do you think will be useful for an audience you have in mind or will be working with? Why? Give the relative advantages and disadvantages.

References

Baranowski, T., E. Cerin, and J. Baranowski. 2009. Steps in the design, development, and formative evaluation of obesity prevention–related behavior change. *International Journal of Behavioral Nutrition and Physical Activity* 6:6.

Baranowski, T., L. S. Lin, D. W. Wetter, K. Resnicow, and M. D. Hearn. 1997. Theory as mediating variables: Why aren't community interventions working as desired? *Annals of Epidemiology* 7:589–595.

Contento, I. R., J. S. Randell, and C. E. Basch. 2002. Review and analysis of evaluation measures used in nutrition education intervention research. *Journal of Nutrition Education and Behavior* 34:2–25.

Heath and Heath. 2010. *Switch: How to change when change is hard.* New York: Random House.

Liou, D., and I. R. Contento. 2001. Usefulness of psychosocial variables in explaining fat-related dietary behavior in Chinese Americans: Association with degree of acculturation. *Journal of Nutrition Education and Behavior* 33:322–331.

Shaikh, A. R., A. L. Yaroch, L. Nebeling, M. C. Yeh, and K. Resnicow. 2008. Psychosocial predictors of fruit and vegetable consumption in adults: A review of the literature. *American Journal of Preventive Medicine* 34(6):535–543.

Nutrition Education DESIGN Procedure

| **D**ecide behavior(s) | **E**xplore determinants of change | **S**elect theory & clarify philosophy | **I**ndicate general objectives | **G**enerate plans | **N**ail down evaluation plan |
| Step 1 | Step 2 | Step 3 | Step 4 | Step 5 | Step 6 |

Step 2: Explore determinants of behavior change or action(s).

After deciding on the behavioral goal for your educational session(s), it is important to figure out what might motivate and facilitate your audience in taking on the goal behavior(s). You should always strive to keep in mind what you have learned about your audience as you proceed through the Nutrition Education DESIGN Procedure. By combining these insights with new information about your audience's beliefs and feelings about the goal behavior and their knowledge and skills related to the goal behavior, you will be able to identify the theoretical determinants that will become the framework for your session(s).

Use the Explore Determinants of Change worksheet as a guide to help you identify and select motivations and skills that relate to the behavioral goals of your educational session or intervention. The references (in parentheses) are listed at the end of the case study workbook in Chapter 13.

What can you learn about your audience's sociocultural environment? What do you learn about your audience's interests, as well as their social and cultural context, by talking with them and visiting the neighborhood?

There are approximately 1,750 students in the school. Based on the last census, the community in which the intervention will be taking place is ethnically diverse: 55% of the population is White, 30% Black or African American, 10% Hispanic, and 5% from other races. The median household income is $32,000 and median family income is approximately $40,000. Roughly 20% of the population is below the poverty level. The demographics of the students and their parents mirror those of the community at large. The primary participants are adolescents who are in the 7th and 8th grade. This is an age where students may be experiencing great physical and emotional changes. Additionally, this is an age where they want and are given more individual freedom. They are increasingly influenced by their friends/peers and influenced less by their parents. All of the students live with a parent or other adult caregiver. 60% report having input on household groceries. 60% have regular responsibilities at home ranging from chores to taking care of younger siblings. The students report that they are as busy or busier than the average middle school student. Outside of school, 40% are involved with organized sports, and 50% take part in after school activities associated with the school (e.g., baseball, art club, yearbook). Eating out at local diners and fast food spots with friends after school is a "status symbol." The demographics of the students and the community in which they live is diverse, and no primary cultural or religious belief that influences food choice stands out. [12]

What can you learn about your audience's assets? What can you learn about individual or community strengths by talking with your audience and visiting the neighborhood?

- A number of students (~20%) regularly reach one or more of the behavioral goals. [11]
- By middle school, children are able to integrate motivations and cognitions in a self-regulatory process for a variety of food choice criteria, including not only taste and convenience, but also in terms of health and weight concern issues. [11, 12]
- The school where the intervention will be implemented currently provides healthcare services to the students and their families. There is a clinic within the school that offers basic medical services, such as wellness exams and treatment for common illnesses and conditions. The clinic also has a dental unit that provides dental cleanings and cavity fillings. The clinic is a source of pride for the school and the community, and there has been recent interest in adding nutrition-related programs that would help promote wellness and prevent certain conditions, like obesity. There is a lot of support from faculty, parents, and the general community for this expansion. However, the school does not have the expertise to do it alone, so we will help them conduct a needs assessment, develop an appropriate intervention, and plan the evaluation. [11]
- The program funder's mission is to provide nutrition education and services to the pediatric population and their families in the community. Overweight/obesity prevention has been selected by the agency as its priority area for education and service. Promoting health—physical and mental—and the development of healthy habits is part of the mission of the school.
- The school has a fledgling School Wellness Council. [11]
- There is a tradition of peer leadership (e.g., all conflict mediation includes a peer as one of the mediators), and some of the students that are looked at as leaders already reach one or more of the behavioral goals. [11]

Nutrition Education DESIGN Procedure

Decide behavior(s)	**E**xplore determinants of change	**S**elect theory & clarify philosophy	**I**ndicate general objectives	**G**enerate plans	**N**ail down evaluation plan
Step 1	Step 2	Step 3	Step 4	Step 5	Step 6

Why would your audience want to engage in the behavior change goal(s)? Being mindful of what you learned about your audience's sociocultural environment and community assets, find out your audience's beliefs and feelings about the goal behavior. What would motivate them to change their behavior or take action? If possible, use information from your audience; however, the research literature may be equally helpful in identifying motivators. After you've listed the motivators in the left column of the table, identify the motivational determinants from psychosocial theories to which they correspond in the right column.

Audience-Identified Motivators	Psychosocial Determinant(s)
Teenage girls say they would eat vegetables if they tasted good.	Outcome expectations
Teenage girls say they would eat fruits and vegetables at school if it were perceived as "cool" by their peers.	Perceived social norms
Students say they want to know specific benefits of eating fruits and vegetables—how they keep the body healthy and help you maintain a healthy weight, and which fruits and vegetables have which benefits.	Perceived benefits/ positive outcome expectations*
Students say they had no idea there were health risks associated with eating too few fruits and vegetables.	Perceived risk/ negative outcome expectations*
Students say they would eat more fruits and vegetables if they weren't so expensive, if they were more convenient to carry around in their backpack, if there were more fruit and vegetable choices at school lunch, and if they were tastier.	Perceived barriers (self-efficacy)*; Food preferences*
Students think eating vegetables is something you do just because your parents tell you to. They don't think of it as something they want to do for themselves—the only chance they'll eat them is if they are served on their plate at lunch or dinner and they are expected to eat them.	Perceived behavioral control
Students say the trends for what they and their classmates do are set by their peers.	Perceived social norms*
Students say they are interested in evaluating if they have a good diet or not.	Perceived risk/ negative outcome expectations*

Nutrition Education DESIGN Procedure

Decide behavior(s)	**E**xplore determinants of change	**S**elect theory & clarify philosophy	**I**ndicate general objectives	**G**enerate plans	**N**ail down evaluation plan
Step 1	Step 2	Step 3	Step 4	Step 5	Step 6

What knowledge and skills will enable your audience to change their behavior? Again, being mindful of what you learned about your audience, find out about your audience's knowledge and skills related to the goal behavior. This includes skills needed to choose and prepare foods, as well as goal setting and self-monitoring. If possible, use information from your audience; however, the research literature may be equally helpful in identifying facilitators. After you've listed the facilitators in the left column of the table, identify the facilitating determinants from psychosocial theories to which they correspond in the right column.

Audience-Identified Facilitators	Psychosocial Determinant(s)
Teenage girls say they would eat fruits and vegetables if they knew how to prepare tasty snacks with them.	Food preparation skills
Teenage girls say they would eat fruits and vegetables at school if they received a daily reminder message on their phones.	Self-monitoring
Students indicate that they are not aware of fruit and vegetable serving sizes or recommendations.	Behavioral capability/competence: Cognitive skills*
Students say they don't know where to purchase fruits and vegetables around their school or how to prepare them at home.	Behavioral capability/competence: Behavioral skills*; Self-efficacy*
Students have experience with setting goals and tracking progress in other subject areas and should be able to transfer those skills to a new context.	Goal setting*

Which motivators and facilitators will be useful for your session(s)? Keep your behavior change goal(s) in mind and go back through the two tables to identify which determinants you will use in your session(s). Indicate them with a highlight or a star.

CHAPTER 9

Step 3: Selecting Theory and Clarifying Intervention Philosophy

OVERVIEW

With a thorough understanding of the intended audience in hand, you are now ready to use all you have learned about your audience and the relevant evidence from the research literature to select the theory or create the theory model that will be most appropriate to guide the development of the behavior change strategies and educational activities for your sessions or intervention. This is also the time to reflect on your educational philosophy and other assumptions underlying the intervention.

CHAPTER OUTLINE

- Introduction: preliminary planning
- Selecting a theory or creating an appropriate model
- Clarifying the educational philosophy of the sessions or intervention
- Articulating the intervention's perspectives on how food and nutrition content will be addressed
- Clarifying the intervention's perspectives on use of educational resources from a variety of sources
- Thinking about your needs and approach as a nutrition educator
- Conclusions
- Case study: the DESIGN Procedure in action
- Your turn to design nutrition education: completing the Step 3 Select Theory and Clarify Philosophy Worksheet

LEARNING OBJECTIVES

At the end of the chapter, you should be able to:

- Select an appropriate theory or create a relevant model to design a given set of sessions or intervention
- Appreciate how nutrition educators' own philosophy about educational approach influences the nature of the nutrition education intervention
- Identify your own beliefs and perspectives about how nutrition and food content should be addressed

Introduction: Preliminary Planning

You have now completed your assessment of your audience. For example, you have explored the beliefs, attitudes, and skills already held by a group of low-income single mothers who work full time and you have identified the additional skills they will need to empower themselves to achieve the intervention's goal of developing good parenting practices around food. You have understood the challenges they face in the context of their families, social networks, culture, and communities. You have met with that group of teenagers who seem eager to take on healthier eating patterns if that will help them excel in sports or that group of adult men in the outpatient clinic who tell you that they have very little confidence that they will be able to make the changes they need in order to avoid diabetes. This is an important first step in planning effective nutrition education. However, before rushing to do what you like to do best based on this understanding, such as preparing presentations or creating exciting activities for the group, you still have some preliminary planning to do.

In this preliminary planning step, you will:

- Select the theory or create the theory model that will guide your sessions or intervention.
- Clarify your philosophy about the appropriate educational approach for this audience.
- Clarify your perspectives on nutrition content and related issues.

FIGURE 9-1 reminds us where we are in the design process and summarizes the tasks and products for Step 3. A blank Step 3 Select Theory and Clarify Philosophy worksheet is provided in the DESIGN Workbook at the end of Chapter 13 for you to use as you proceed through this chapter. The completed Step 3 Select Theory and Clarify Philosophy Worksheet for the case study at the end of this chapter serves as an example of how to complete the Step 3 worksheet.

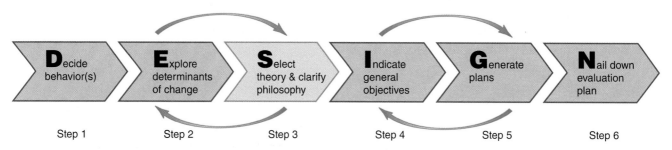

Inputs: Collecting the Assessment Data		**Outputs:** Designing the Theory-Based Intervention			**Outcomes:** Evaluation Plan
Tasks: • **Decide** behavior change goal(s) of the intervention, based on: • analyzing issues and behaviors of concern for audience	*Tasks:* • **Explore** determinants of behavior change based on a variety of data sources	*Tasks:* • **Select** theory and draw intervention-specific theory model • Clarify educational philosophy • Articulate perspectives on content	*Tasks:* • **Indicate** general objectives for each determinant in your theory model	*Tasks:* • **Generate** educational plans: • Educational activities to address all determinants in theory model • Sequence for implementation using the 4 Es	*Tasks:* • **Nail down** evaluation plan • Select methods and questions to evaluate outcomes • Plan process evaluation • Create questions to measure how implementation went
Products: *Statement of intervention behavior change goal(s)*	*Products:* *List of determinants to address in the intervention*	*Products:* *Theory model for intervention* *Statement of educational philosophy* *Statement of content perspectives*	*Products:* *A general objective for each determinant in the theory model*	*Products:* *Educational plans that link determinants and educational activities to achieve behavior change or action goal(s)*	*Products:* *List of evaluation methods and questions* *Procedures and measures for process evaluation*

FIGURE 9-1 Nutrition Education DESIGN Procedure: Select theory and clarify philosophy—Step 3.

After you have completed this preliminary planning step, you will be ready to write educational objectives directed at the relevant modifiable determinants of change that you have identified. You will also be able to design appropriate theory-based behavior change strategies and educational activities directed at these determinants of change.

Selecting a Theory or Creating an Appropriate Model

From Step 2, you now have a long list of people's beliefs, motivations, and skills in relation to the behavioral change goal(s) of your sessions or intervention. These are the potential *determinants of change* for your audience to achieve the behavioral change goals. Consequently, these are the direct targets of your nutrition education activities. However, a list by itself is not sufficient. Theory helps you organize that list into a meaningful set of related predictors of behavior change suitable for nutrition education. It provides a tool, a mental map for what to address and how to do so. Clearly laying out the theory or model for the intervention or sessions before you begin is thus crucial.

Consider the following in choosing your theory:

- *Audience stage of readiness to take action.* Based on what you found out, is the intended audience mostly those who are not yet aware or motivated to take action or are they already motivated and need skills and other resources to empower them to act on their motivations? Thus, will the intervention aim to increase awareness, promote active deliberation, and enhance motivation to take action? Or, will it focus on building skills and the ability to take action? Or, will it aim to do both?

- *Strength of the evidence for the determinants of the behavioral change goals.* How strong is the evidence that the particular psychosocial influences or determinants you identified in Step 2 will serve as the determinants of the behavioral change goals for the intervention or sessions for this audience? Information on the nature of the evidence for various theories was provided in the first part of this book in a general way. It is desirable, however, to have specific evidence for the behavior and audience you have selected. Examples might be evidence from the research literature about specific determinants of change that are

effective for increasing fruit and vegetable consumption among pregnant women or eating more calcium-rich foods among adolescents (Baranowski, Cerin, and Baranowski 2009; Diep et al. 2014).

Because developing behavior change strategies and educational activities directed at each of the determinants of change requires much time, energy, and other resources on your part, as well as time commitment and effort on the part of the intended audience, you want to carefully choose the theory you use and those theory constructs that are most likely to serve as the determinants of change in your intervention. Later we will discuss how theory may be useful in the different phases and components of the nutrition education intervention.

THEORY IN SOCIOCULTURAL CONTEXT

The audiences with whom we work as nutrition educators come from a variety of cultural backgrounds, life-cycle stages, and socioeconomic circumstances. If they are recent immigrants, they may be at different stages of acculturation. How does theory apply in these varied circumstances? As we discuss in greater detail in Chapter 4, external factors such as culture and social situations influence behavior because these factors are internalized and interpreted by each individual. Culture and social situations exist not only "out there" but also "in here," as *subjective culture* and *subjective social situations*. These internalized beliefs and feelings become part of people's psychosocial make-up and thus become the *determinants* of behavior that are captured in the psychosocial theories. For example, in a culture that emphasizes chance, fate, and God as the major influences on health, illness, and healing, these cultural beliefs influence individuals' psychosocial determinants of sense of personal agency, perceived control over the behavior, and self-efficacy, which may be low in these individuals. Or, if the impact of changes in their behaviors on the family is more important than on their own health, this likely will translate into individuals' social norms being high. Consider these cultural influences as you create your theory model.

THEORIES ESPECIALLY USEFUL FOR MOTIVATING OUR AUDIENCES

If your intended audience is mostly unaware or unengaged in the behaviors or actions that are the goals of the intervention, your educational objectives will likely be to increase awareness, promote active contemplation, enhance motivation, assist the audience in understanding and resolving any ambivalences, activate empowered decision making, and facilitate the formation of intentions to take action. Beliefs and attitudes, including feelings and emotions, are at the heart of the motivation to act, as we discuss earlier. This is a *deliberative or contemplation/ thinking* phase for individuals. The function of nutrition education here is to help individuals to see *why-to take action* in the context of family, culture and community. Examples may be motivational sessions, materials, or health communication campaigns. See Chapter 4 for more details.

The following theories can serve as useful tools that provide the most guidance on designing messages and activities that increase awareness for action and enhance motivation. The outcome desired in this phase is that our audience will form an intention to act, based on active contemplation and a deliberative decision-making process. Individuals can, of course, choose not to act, and their decision needs to be respected. They will take action when they choose to do so and are ready.

- *Psychosocial theories that focus on personal decision making and motivational factors* such as the health belief model; the theory of planned behavior/reasoned action approach and its extensions that include considerations of affect or feelings, values, self-identities, and personal norms; model of goal-directed behavior; self-determination theory; attitude-change theories; or health communications using the elaboration likelihood model. (See the figures in Chapter 4.)
- *Models of food choice* that address food preferences and enjoyment, emotions and mood, and the physiological impacts of food on the body.
- *Models from interpretative or qualitative research* with the intended audience or applicable to the audience with an emphasis on personal and cultural meanings and values and self-identities.

THEORIES ESPECIALLY USEFUL FOR FACILITATING THE ABILITY TO TAKE ACTION

Translating motivations and intentions into action is difficult for all people, and assisting individuals to become empowered to take action is a major task of nutrition education. Here, the emphasis is on facilitating individuals' *ability* to take food-related actions or change dietary behaviors that they consciously and deliberatively want. Individuals with strong intentions will form *implementation intentions* or begin making simple *plans of action*. Those with weak intentions may need some reminders and cues to action. Food- and nutrition-specific knowledge and skills are important, including food selection and food preparation skills. Critical evaluation skills may be important, where appropriate. The emphasis is on information and skills for *how-to take action*.

In addition, self-regulation skills or skills in being able to influence their own behaviors and exercise deliberate choice (including goal-setting and self-monitoring skills) are important for individuals to be able to act on their chosen motivations and intentions and to express personal agency. The following theories provide the most guidance in action-planning and self-regulation skills and are described in detail in Chapter 5:

- *Social cognitive theory* with its emphasis on self-efficacy, goal setting/action planning, self-monitoring, and self-regulation (skills in consciously making desired choices and acting on them) (Bandura 1997, 2001, 2004). (See Chapter 5 for more details.)
- *Self-efficacy and self-regulation theories* (including the **health action process approach**, which describe how people set implementation or goal intentions (specific plans for attaining the goals), and maintain goal commitments (Schwarzer and Renner 2000; Gollwitzer 1999; Bagozzi and Edwards 1999; Abraham and Sheeran 2000; Sniehotta 2009). Self-determination theory also draws on the self-regulation processes as a means toward greater autonomy in behavioral choices.

THEORIES USEFUL FOR BOTH MOTIVATING AUDIENCES AND BUILDING SKILLS FOR ACTION

In most instances, nutrition education seeks to include both motivational and action phase activities—both *why-to* and *how-to* education. This can occur at varying levels of depth and breadth; that is, one can begin with motivational activities and conclude with how-to activities in one session. Each of these components would, of course, be brief in this instance. Or, the activities can be spread over several sessions and even between direct and indirect activities so that health communications through the mass media, emphasizing motivational why-to messages, can be accompanied by group sessions that focus on how-to skills.

- *The extended theory of planned behavior* is useful here, with its strong emphasis on motivation and attitudes, accompanied by setting behavioral intentions (goal intentions) and developing specific implementation plans (or action plans) to implement these intentions (goals). (See Figure 4-4.)
- *Social cognitive theory* provides extensive guidance on translating motivation into action through specific action goal-setting and self-regulation or self-direction practices. It also emphasizes that individuals and their environments interact, mutually influencing each other, and so the environment must also be addressed. (See Figure 5-1.) Often nutrition education interventions use social cognitive theory without involving an environmental component. This is not a true use of the theory but is a widespread practice.
- *The health action process approach* also provides guidance for both phases of health education, emphasizing perceived risk and outcome expectations in the motivational phase and planning processes in the action phase, and self-efficacy throughout both phases. (See Figure 5-2.)
- *The transtheoretical model* describes processes of change for all stages and suggests that procedures or strategies for change can be based on these processes. (See Figure 5-3.)

DETERMINANTS IN COMMON AMONG THEORIES

The various social psychological theories have many determinants in common so that they overlap one another. Constructs in common that have been shown to be important motivators of food- and nutrition-related behavior or determinants of dietary change are the following:

- Outcome expectations/beliefs about anticipated outcomes (including perceived benefits and negative outcomes or pros and cons of change)

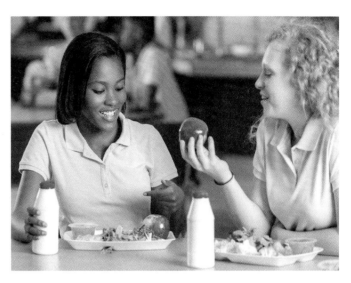

Nutrition education can help change social norms.

© Steve Debenport/Getty Images.

- Attitudes and affect (feelings) (in some theories)
- Perception of risk/threat of current behavior (in some theories)
- Food preferences and enjoyment based on sensory-affective factors
- Perceived social and personal norms (often derived from cultural norms)
- Self-efficacy or perceived control in performing the targeted behaviors

Constructs in common that have been shown in many studies to be important for facilitating the ability to act are as follows:

- Self-efficacy
- Perceived behavioral control or personal agency
- Self-regulation/self-direction skills, including goal setting and self-monitoring
- Behavioral capabilities or food- and nutrition-specific knowledge and skills needed to enact goals, including food preparation or physical activity skills, and critical evaluation skills where relevant (these are described in detail in Chapter 5)

A summary of the determinants of behavior change from various major theories and how they overlap is shown in **FIGURE 9-2**.

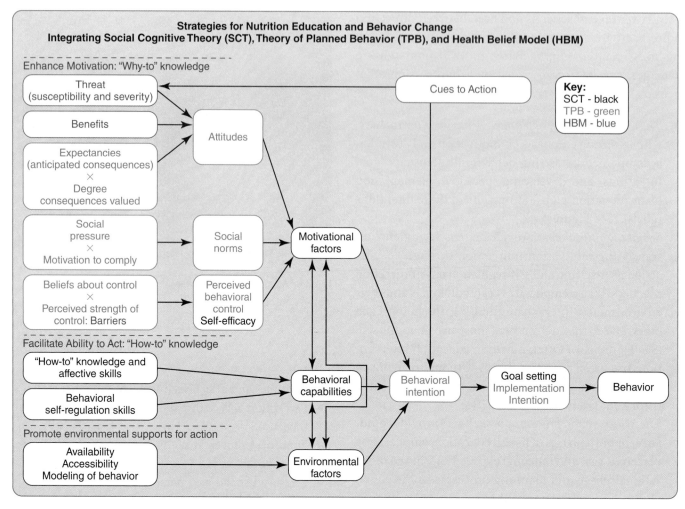

FIGURE 9-2 Summary of relationships among determinants from key psychosocial theories.

EXAMPLES OF MODELS COMBINING DETERMINANTS FROM RELEVANT THEORIES

Some integrated models have been developed that combine constructs or determinants from several theories (Kok et al. 1996; Fishbein 2000; Institute of Medicine [IOM] 2002; Montano and Kasprzyk 2008; Fishbein and Ajzen 2010).

Integrated Model of Determinants of Health Behavior Change

A general or integrated model of the determinants of behavior change is shown in **FIGURE 9-3**. It was developed by a committee of the Institute of Medicine that included the key researchers who originated the health belief model, theory of planned behavior, and social cognitive theory, among others (IOM 2002). It combines the basic constructs of theory of planned behavior (attitudes, social norms, and perceived behavioral control) and perceived risk from the health belief model with the emphasis on skills and environmental constraints from social cognitive theory. The model acknowledges the importance of environmental barriers or supports but does not elaborate on them. This model is very similar to updated versions of the theory of reasoned action approach that incorporates constructs from other theories (Montano and Kasprzyk 2008; Fishbein and Ajzen 2010).

The Health Action Process Approach (HAPA) Model

The HAPA model is shown in Chapter 5, in Figure 5-2 (Schwarzer 2000; Sniehotta 2009). This model incorporates perceived risk from the health belief model with outcome expectations and self-efficacy variables from social cognitive theory that are also in common to many theories.

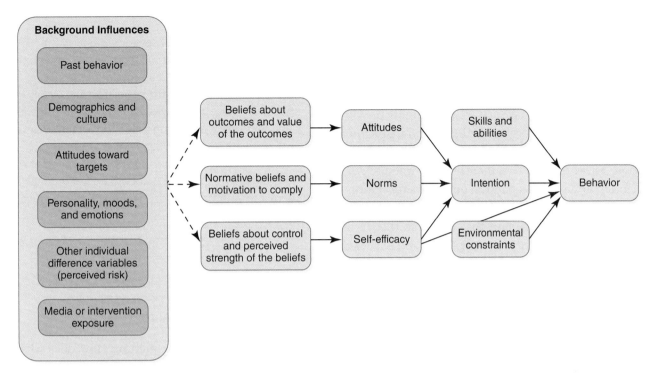

FIGURE 9-3 General model of determinants of health behavior change.

Reprinted with permission from Speaking of health: Assessing health communication strategies for diverse populations. Institute of Medicine 2002 by the National Academy of Sciences, Courtesy of the National Academies Press, Washington, D.C.

It incorporates a time dimension, with a pre-action motivational phase and an action phase, somewhat similar to the stages of change construct of the transtheoretical model. It points out that self-efficacy is needed at all phases of change: making an intention, developing action plans, and initiating and maintaining action. The model also acknowledges the importance of environmental barriers or supports but does not elaborate on how to address them in an intervention.

SELECTING OR CONSTRUCTING YOUR INTERVENTION THEORY MODEL

Look over the information about the determinants of behavior change that you collected in Step 2 and recorded on your Step 2 Explore Determinants Worksheet (located at the end of Chapter 13). Are audience members mainly in the contemplating, pre-action phase with respect to the behaviors you are recommending in your intervention? If so, one of the motivational theories will be appropriate, such as the health belief model, reasoned action approach, or model of goal directed behavior. Are audience members already highly motivated and are only awaiting needed

knowledge and skills? If so, using one of the theories that focus on behavior change strategies or techniques may be appropriate. Note that if the participants show up in your sessions, they are probably motivated to some degree. However, in many cases they are recommended or required to attend, and while they are moderately motivated, they will need some motivational boosters. Thus, most sessions will need to focus on both motivational and skills activities. Social cognitive theory is the most commonly used for such purposes. The transtheoretical model may also be useful (Prochaska and Velicer 1997).

You will then need to operationalize the theory for your particular audience; that is, decide whether you will be able to address all the determinants of change in your chosen theory or only some. Evidence from ongoing research will provide guidance regarding which specific theory constructs are most likely to serve as determinants of behavior change in an educational intervention for your particular audience. Also consider the length of your intervention or the number of sessions you will provide and the resources available to determine how many and which determinants of change you will address.

Based on your assessments in Step 2, you may find it most useful to combine theory constructs (determinants of behavior change) from several compatible theories to create an intervention theory model specific to your particular audience. For example, it may be that *outcome expectations* related to health and *self-efficacy* are most highly predictive of behavior change for your audience and that *action goal setting, planning, and self-regulation skills* are needed for action. These three determinants are common to several theories. For example, physical outcome expectations related to health are included in social cognitive theory. This is the same determinant that is in the theory of planned behavior/reasoned action approach, and is labeled perceived benefits in the health belief model. You do not need to say you will use all these theories because that would be redundant. Stating one of these theories will do, probably social cognitive theory because that is the most comprehensive. Likewise, perhaps for your audience *social norms* of the theory of planned behavior/reasoned action approach are also important. These are the same as social outcome expectations of social cognitive theory. If you address social norms, you do not need to list both theories: social cognitive theory will do. Let's say your data from Step 2 suggest that you should also address self-identity and moral obligation. These are unique to the extended theory of planned behavior. You can then say, for example, that your theory model is based on the following determinants from social cognitive theory: the physical outcome expectations/perceived benefits, social outcome expectations, self-efficacy, and action goal-setting with the addition of self-identity and moral obligation from the extended theory of planned behavior/reasoned action approach.

In creating your intervention model, you must specify the exact outcome expectations, values, attitudes, affect, and self-efficacy issues (or other constructs you intend to address) for your audience based on your assessment. In other words, do not just state "outcome expectations" as a determinant but "pregnant women expect/believe that breastfeeding will be good for their newborn's health." Drawing a diagram to illustrate the relationships among constructs can be very helpful. An example of a diagram for the theory model for a specific intervention is shown in the case study at the end of this chapter.

Consequently, state your theory model and draw a diagram of your model in the Step 3 Select Theory and Clarify Philosophy Worksheet (located in the workbook at the end of Chapter 13).

> For your session, series of sessions, or intervention, start with the theory that most closely aligns with the information you gathered about your audience in Step 2 and the evidence from the literature. Apply it specifically to your behavior change goal(s) and audience. This may mean using only those determinants that will be predictive of behavior change for your audience and/or selecting specific complementary determinants from other theories and integrating them into your basic model. This is the *theory model* for your intervention.

OVERALL CONCEPTUAL FRAMEWORK FOR LINKING DETERMINANTS AND THEORY TO NUTRITION EDUCATION PRACTICE

Let's take a look at the big picture. How does what you learned about the motivators and facilitators of behavior change and the theory model you developed from that understanding relate to nutrition education practice? A conceptual framework for showing these linkages is shown in **FIGURE 9-4**. It focuses on the use of theory as a tool to design the intervention or "outputs" section of the logic model. It translates behavioral theory into a format that is suitable for conducting nutrition education in practice settings.

The constructs in common among several theories have been used to build this integrated conceptual framework for nutrition education interventions. The framework suggests that dietary change can be thought of as occurring in two phases and four sub phases: considering action, deciding on action, initiating action, and maintaining action. It proposes that nutrition education intervention objectives are different for each phase. The conceptual framework links determinants of change from theory, phases of change, and nutrition education objectives for intervention. An environmental support component is also very important. Useful theories for each phase are also listed.

- *Considering action* involves determinants of motivation for dietary change from theory, such as perception of risk, outcome expectations, attitudes based on beliefs and feelings about taking action, sensory affective aspects of food, social norms, and self-efficacy. *The objective of the nutrition education intervention in this motivational phase is to increase awareness and enhance motivation.*

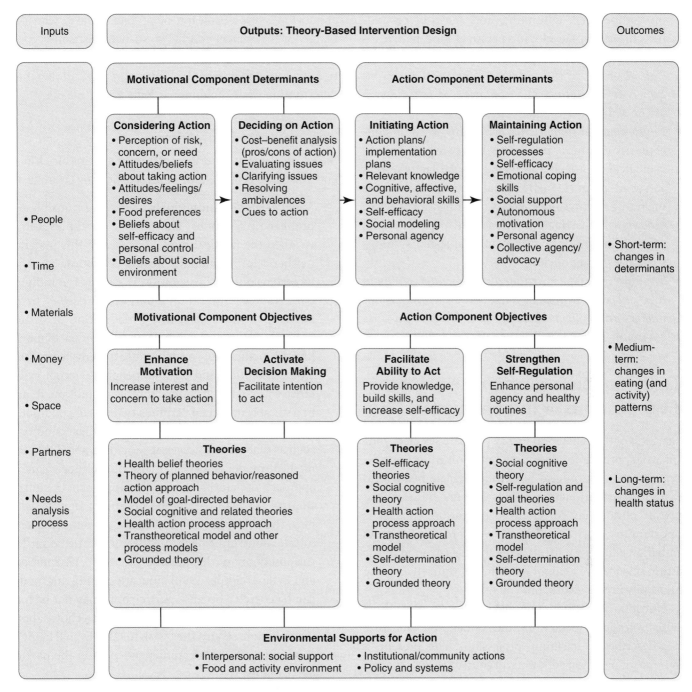

FIGURE 9-4 Conceptual framework for translating behavioral theory into effective nutrition education practice.

- *Deciding on action* involves cost–benefit analyses, resolving ambivalences, and experiencing cues to action.
  The objective of the nutrition education intervention is to activate and empower decision making.
- *Initiating action* involves several determinants or procedures of change from theory: stating action plans or implementation plans, behavioral capabilities

  (learning relevant diet-related knowledge and skills), social modeling, and self-efficacy.
  The objective of the nutrition education intervention is to facilitate the ability to act.
- *Maintaining action* requires self-regulation (self-direction) skills including planning and self-monitoring skills, emotion-coping skills, and perceived personal agency or autonomous motivation based

on competence, autonomy, and sense of related-ness to others. Developing personal food policies is very helpful.

The objective of the nutrition education interven-tion is to strengthen self-regulation or self-directed action skills.

- *Environmental supports for action* are based on con-cepts in common from research using the social ecological approach and include social factors, such as social support, institutional/community actions including community capacity building for collective efficacy; physical factors such as food availability and accessibility/built environment; and social systems, structures, and policies.

  The objective of the nutrition education intervention in this context is to work in collaboration with decision-makers and policymakers at many levels to increase environmental and policy supports for action.

Clarifying the Educational Philosophy of the Sessions or Intervention

Regardless of the behavioral theory you have selected, your choice of approach for designing nutrition education ses-sions or intervention and how you translate behavioral theory into educational practice is very much influenced by your philosophy of nutrition education; thus, it is important to clarify this philosophy before you begin. As a nutrition educator with considerable background in the natural sciences, you might not think of yourself as using philosophy in your work, but you do.

Nutrition education, along with health education, allied health professions, social work, and similar professions, are often described as "helping" professions. This presents a dilemma for nutrition educators, of course, because there is a tension between the desire to "help" on the part of nutri-tion educators and the need for a sense of human agency or self-determination on the part of participants. For those in the nutrition professions, having a philosophy about whether and how to help is particularly important.

HELPING AND EDUCATING: WHO IS RESPONSIBLE FOR THE PROBLEM AND WHO THE SOLUTION?

One way to approach these issues, proposed by Brickman and colleagues (1982) and elaborated by Achterberg and Lytle-Trenkner (1990) for nutrition education, is to think about who is responsible for the problem (that is, who is to blame for the current condition, such as a person's type 2 diabetes or obesity) and who is responsible for the solu-tion (that is, who is to control future events) and therefore determining what "helping" or "educating" means.

Brickman's Model of Helping

Based on these attributions of responsibility, Brickman and associates propose four models of helping (**TABLE 9-1**):

- *Medical model.* Individuals are not responsible for problems or solutions. This philosophical perspective is called the medical model because in this instance neither the individual's health condition, such as hypertension, nor its solution is seen as the individ-ual's responsibility. Individuals are *in need of treat-ment* by professionals, using medication or drugs, perhaps. Many professionals and group participants like the medical approach because it seems to promise a quick solution and permits people to accept assis-tance without being blamed for their condition. It may be a suitable model for certain situations or conditions, especially emergencies related to a medical condition such as diabetes. However, it should be noted that the medical model is a special case of the more general approach of paternalism. In this approach, the nutri-tionists are the experts, the dominant figures, who have the information—and hence power—and tend to take control of decisions, leaving little room for the autonomy of the audience members (Achterberg and Lytle-Trenkner 1990). Education using this model can be coercive because participants may not be told about acceptable alternatives and given a choice about which actions, if any, they wish to take. Even if benign, this approach can create dependency on the part of participants.
- *Moral model.* Individuals are responsible for both problems and solutions. This philosophical perspec-tive is at the other end of the spectrum from the med-ical model. Here, the individuals are considered to have full personal responsibility for having created their problems and also for solving them. They are considered to have considerable personal control. They are primarily *in need of motivation.* This is a widely accepted perspective. In a free society with freedom of choice, and in a food system that offers many food items in the typical supermarket, individuals are

considered to have control over their own food intake. Hence, their health conditions are the result of their own choices and actions. The role of nutrition educators in this model is to increase interest and enhance motivation. However, this approach can result in "person blame," in which people are blamed for their conditions, such as heart disease. It becomes easy to ignore the fact that genetic factors affect health, as do powerful environmental forces related to the food marketing system and social conditions that shape and reinforce behavior, and resource considerations that limit choices for many.

- *Enlightenment model.* Individuals are responsible for problems but are not responsible for solutions. In this philosophical perspective, individuals recognize and accept that their lifestyles and health behaviors have led to problematic consequences (weight gain, hypertension, or type 2 diabetes) but feel that they cannot do much about it. They need to be enlightened about the true nature of their problem(s) and are primarily *in need of enlightenment and discipline,* which can often be supplied by some outside force. Thus, people in Overeaters Anonymous believe that they are responsible for their overeating or weight problems but need an outside authority or support group to help them gain control over their behavior and their lives.

- *Compensatory model.* Individuals are not responsible for problems but are responsible for solutions. Here, individuals are not blamed for their current condition or problems but are held responsible for solving these problems. They have to compensate or cope with the particular problems they have. In this philosophical perspective, individuals are seen as suffering from problems that are not of their own making, but which instead result from the failure of their social environment to provide them with the goods and services to which they are entitled, such as accessibility to nutritious, wholesome food or to education. Individuals are thus primarily *in need of power.* The role of the nutrition educator is to mobilize resources for them and/or to assist them to acquire the skills of personal and collective efficacy or empowerment to deal effectively with the environment to obtain what they need.

Of these perspectives, Brickman and colleagues prefer the compensatory model because it is the only one that resolves the dilemma faced by nutrition educators: it

Table 9-1 Models of Helping

Self Responsible for the Problem	Self Responsible for the Solution	
	High	**Low**
High	Moral model (need motivation)	Enlightenment model (need discipline)
High	Compensatory model (need power)	Medical model (need treatment)

Data from Brickman, P., V. C. Rabinowitz, J. Karuza, D. Coates, E. Cohn, and L. Kidder. 1982. Models of helping and coping. *American Psychologist* 37:368–384.

justifies the act of helping or assisting (because individuals are not responsible for their problems) but still leaves the individuals with active control over their lives (because they are responsible for using this help to find a solution if they wish). They also point out that it is important that the health professional (nutrition educator) and the intended audience have the same expectations and subscribe to the same philosophical perspective in terms of the particular intervention. At the least, they should be aware of each other's philosophical perspectives and resolve any differences in expectations.

Humans Have Free Will

Others emphasize the fact that humans have agency or free will. People act, not just react (Bandura 2001). This free will, or the capacity to choose, gives human beings their unique place in the world and their human dignity. This makes behavior change hard to predict because behaviors have many rational and irrational determinants. Individuals should have "the freedom to choose their own motivations, beliefs and objectives in living; and the freedom to select among alternatives that can, or might, bring about those objectives" (Achterberg and Lytle-Trenkner 1990). Nutrition educators can engage in a dialogue with individuals about ways of living that they find most worthwhile for themselves, their families, or their communities, exploring questions such as, "Will losing weight really help me to achieve the goals that I have set for myself?" and "How will it affect my family?" or "Is being physically fit an important purpose in my life?" Buchanan proposes that the nutrition educator and participants should be "fully engaged in mutual dialogue, deliberation, and debate with the aim of finding ways that we can work together to make this a better world" (Buchanan 2004, p. 152).

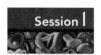

Session 1
Set Your Goals

Recommended Goals

① Eat at least 3 ½ cups of fruits and vegetables every day.

② Participate in at least 30 minutes of moderate-intensity physical activity most days.

My Personal Goals

I will eat _____ cup(s) of **fruits** and _____ cup(s) of **vegetables** every day.

I will get at least _____ minutes of **moderate-intensity physical activity** on _____ days next week.

My Weekly Log

In the space provided, write the cups of fruits and vegetables you ate and the minutes of physical activity you completed each day.

	Sunday	Monday	Tuesday	Wednesday	Thursday	Friday	Saturday
Cups of fruits	# of cup(s)	# of cup(s)	# of cup(s)	# of cup(s)	# of cup(s)	# of cup(s)	# of cup(s)
Cups of vegetables	# of cup(s)	# of cup(s)	# of cup(s)	# of cup(s)	# of cup(s)	# of cup(s)	# of cup(s)
Minutes of physical activity	# of minutes	# of minutes	# of minutes	# of minutes	# of minutes	# of minutes	# of minutes

Handout 1a: *Eat Smart, Live Strong*
Revised November 2012

Planning and setting goals is important to translate motivations to action. Eat Smart, Live Strong. Nutrition Education for Older Adults.

http://snap.nal.usda.gov/snap/ESLS.

Self-Determination

Self-determination theory suggests a similar approach (Deci and Ryan 2000, 2008). This theory proposes that psychological development and well-being and indeed, achievement of goal-directed behavior, is very much dependent on people's ability to satisfy their inherent need for autonomy, competence, and relatedness. Nutrition education that provides support for individuals' experience of autonomy, positive feedback in situations where individuals feel they are responsible for their competent actions, and a secure base of relatedness between educator and participants can lead to autonomous motivation and self-determination.

"Helping" in Practice

In practice, groups include those who need motivation, those who need power or skills, and those who need both. Thus, mutual participation in the process of change proceeds best through a two-phase sequence in which motivation is first facilitated and supported by the nutrition educator or nutrition education intervention, in the context of family, culture, and community. This is a time to build trust, whereby feelings and expectations are expressed and motivations are developed. In the second phase, skills are provided at a time when they are helpful so that individuals can choose actions for change, internalize them, and then maintain the actions by themselves

(Kolbe et al. 1981; Achterberg and Lytle-Trenkner 1990; Miller and Rollnick 2013; Laidsaar-Powell et al. 2013). Although the model of joint decision making and active participation was developed to describe one-on-one interactions, it can, and should, be applied to groups. In this case, joint decision making comes from: (1) a thorough understanding of the group as the intervention is being designed that involves the group in the assessment process, and (2) designing session activities—*with* the group if possible—that are interactive so that the audience's prior knowledge, feelings, and expectations can be incorporated and onsite corrections can be made to the education or lesson plan, if necessary, to suit the situation on the ground.

Two-Phase Process

This two-phase process for counseling is similar to the two phases for conducting group nutrition education proposed in this text, whereby in the early phase the emphasis is on encouraging active deliberation and motivation, and in the later phase the emphasis is on empowerment through acquisition of relevant food and nutrition knowledge and skills and behavioral self-regulation skills, accompanied, where appropriate, by collective efficacy and advocacy skills to inform policy-making and to take action on the environment. Nutrition education provides the structure and educational resources to assist individuals as they seek to become motivated, willing, and able to take action, but individuals choose the goals that are important for them at any given time and ways to achieve the goals. That is, the nutrition educator has a role, and the individuals have a role.

OTHER CONSIDERATIONS

"Life Is Open-Ended"

Achterberg and Lytle-Trenkner (1990) provide thoughtful perspectives about nutrition education that are useful to consider at this time. One is that "life is open-ended," meaning that change is always possible. Thus, nutrition educators should not give up on any group or individual. Maybe not now, but perhaps sometime later, the nutrition education messages and activities you have provided will become meaningful and be acted upon. This also means that you can encourage the intended audience members to view change as being always possible, if and when they choose to change. Maybe not now, but sometime in the

future they may be in a better place to take action given considerations of their family, culture and community. This approach also is a central tenet of chaos theory (described in Chapter 3); nutrition educators thus should still design theory-based interventions, recognizing that they cannot tell when the messages and activities will coalesce in the minds and hearts of group participants and they will take action.

"Life Is Difficult"

Life can be difficult, both for the intended audience and for you. You have to accept that your intended audience members have many issues and concerns in life, and healthy eating and physical activity may not be a high priority at the time of your nutrition education activity. You also have to accept that nutrition education is a difficult venture and that you may experience many professional dilemmas in practice for which there are no easy solutions.

NUTRITION EDUCATION IN ACTION 9-1 provides the statements of the philosophies and perspectives of one particular intervention as an illustration. The philosophy and perspectives of the case study intervention are shown in the Step 3 Select Theory and Clarify Philosophy Worksheet at the end of the chapter.

Articulating the Intervention's Perspectives on How Food and Nutrition Content Will Be Addressed

All nutrition educators have a point of view about the content of nutrition education. Your perspective will influence how you present food- and nutrition-related content to your audience. Thus, you, or the nutrition education planning team, will need to clarify your own or the organization's stand on substantive issues related to the scope and nature of the content of the educational intervention that you are designing, both in broad terms and in specific ones. Now is the time to consider how the intervention will treat issues in your sessions or intervention, given the nature, concerns, and life contexts of the audience, such as the following:

- *Weight.* Will you encourage health at every size or will you encourage weight control or weight loss along with healthy eating?

NUTRITION EDUCATION IN ACTION 9-1   The Wellness IN the Rockies (WIN the Rockies) Project

Project Description and Philosophy

Project: WIN the Rockies is a research, education, and outreach project that seeks to address obesity innovatively and effectively.

Philosophy: People have responsibility for their own health, but communities need to create environments that foster good health and provide healthy options.

Mission: To assist communities in educating people to:

- Value health.
- Respect body-size differences.
- Enjoy the benefits of self-acceptance.
- Enjoy healthful and pleasurable eating.

Components for Adults, Children, and Patients

Adults

- *A New You: Health for Every Body:* Ten 1-hour sessions for small groups that can be mixed, combined, or taught independently

- *Cook Once: Eat for Two Weeks*: A family mealtime program that can be used in a class setting or as a do-it-yourself program that involves recipes and food purchasing directions
- *WIN Steps:* A community walking program

Children

- *WIN Kids Lessons:* Thirteen lessons for youth that address food and eating, physical activity, and respect for body-size differences
- *WIN Kids Fun Days:* A collection of 40 activities for youth
- *WIN the Rockies Jeopardy:* A question and answer game for youth

Patients

- *Goal-setting forms:* Health improvement goals for adult patients in consultation with their healthcare providers

Data from University of Idaho, Montana State University, and University of Wyoming. 2005. A community-based research, intervention, and outreach project to improve health in Idaho, Montana, and Wyoming. http://www.uwyo.edu/wintherockies.

- *Breastfeeding.* Will you favor breastfeeding or bottle feeding, or will you promote both as equally acceptable nutritional alternatives? This will influence your design of educational activities.

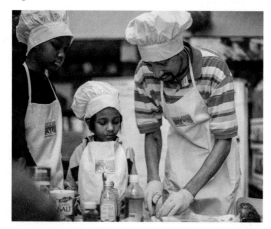

Food preparation can be an important feature in nutrition education for young children, such as those seen here at a CookShop program.

Tim Reiter. Courtesy of Food Bank For New York City.

- *Supplements.* Will you recommend vitamin supplements or not to your audience?
- *All foods fit.* Will you take the stance that there are no "good foods" or "bad foods," that is, that all foods are equally good and can fit into a healthful diet? Or will you take the stance that although all foods fit, some foods are more nutritious than others and use a "sometimes foods" and "anytime foods" approach; green-, red-, and yellow-light foods; or some other approach? The U.S. Dietary Guidelines (2010) now provide recommendations for "foods to increase" and "foods to reduce." Will you use such a system as you make your recommendations?
- *Whole foods versus fortified highly processed foods.* What will be your stance on using fortified foods (e.g., highly processed cereal fortified with vitamins) to obtain nutrients or on eating whole foods (e.g., minimally processed whole grain cereals)? What about calcium tablets or calcium-containing foods?

This is very important to clarify if you are working with others to plan and deliver nutrition education. An example illustrates this point: a team of two nutrition educators who were planning a session for upper elementary students were doing well until they came to the point of designing the specific activities. One thought it would be important to teach students label reading skills to select among highly processed packaged food products those highest in whole grains, while the other thought that the youth should be encouraged to eat minimally processed whole foods that come as close as possible to being directly from nature. It took some time to resolve how they would handle this in the session.

■ *Food system sustainability issues.* Increasingly, government dietary guidance documents are incorporating considerations of food sustainability or eco-friendly eating as criteria for recommendations (World Health Organization 2003; Australia National Health and Medical Research Council 2013). Will you? Will you consider how food is grown, processed, and transported in your recommendations regarding foods to eat? When you encourage a group to increase their fruit and vegetable intake, will you suggest any particular source such as organic or local, or will all sources be recommended, such as fresh, frozen, canned, local, or flown in from another country? How will you resolve these issues when your audience is low-income? These considerations influence your selection of nutrition content and messages.

Clarifying the Intervention's Perspectives on Use of Educational Resources from a Variety of Sources

Nutrition education interventions are often not well funded and therefore cannot afford to develop and print their own high-quality educational materials or visual media or develop high-tech websites. Instead, they use educational materials and visual and other resources from a variety of sources. These are often high quality and visually appealing, whether in print format or online. These sources may be from nonprofit voluntary organizations,

such as heart associations or cancer societies, or from the food industry or other businesses. You and your team will want to carefully discuss the pros and cons of using resources from other sources that carry their logos or promote their brands and decide your policy regarding the use of such resources. You might want to consider the following guidelines for good practice that were established by the International Organization of Consumers Unions (1990):

■ *Accuracy.* Information must be consistent with established fact or best evidence. It should be appropriately referenced so that it can be easily verified.

■ *Objectivity.* All major or relevant points of view are fairly presented. If the issue is controversial, arguments in favor must be balanced by arguments against. The sponsor bias should be clearly stated, and reference to opposing views should be made.

■ *Completeness.* The materials contain all relevant information and do not deceive or mislead by omission—and not just by commission.

■ *Nondiscriminatory.* The text and illustrations are free of any reference or characteristics that could be considered derogatory or that stereotype a particular group.

■ *Noncommercial.* Sponsored material that is specifically designated as being for educational use should be clearly presented as such. Promotional materials should not be presented as "educational." There should be no implied or explicit sales message or exhortation to buy a product or service. Corporate identification should be used to identify the sponsor of the material and provide contacts for further information, but text and illustrations should be free of the sponsor's brand names, trademarks, and so forth.

Thinking About Your Needs and Approach as a Nutrition Educator

You may also want to think about the following about yourself:

■ *Your skill level and experience* in teaching, conducting workshops, designing health fairs, developing materials, and so forth; professional experience, such as in Cooperative Extension Service; and level of understanding of nutrition and food and food systems issues (one or several courses in nutrition, nutrition degree, graduate work?).

- *Preferred style of providing sessions* for groups, such as lectures, discussion, hands-on activities, group work, field projects, food demonstrations, or cooking with groups. (Learning and teaching styles are described more fully in Chapter 15.)

- *Personal priorities and motivations* for being a nutrition educator. Why do you want to educate people about nutrition? What made you want to enter the field?

If you will be designing and/or delivering the nutrition education as a team, you may want to discuss these issues openly so that you can integrate team members' individual preferences and skills into the educational plan and create activities that use your complementary skills.

Conclusions

Creating a theory model using the determinants of behavior change that you identified in Step 2 provides a framework for designing nutrition education that is effective for achieving the behavior change or action goals of your sessions or intervention as stated in Step 1. This is crucial, whether the intervention consists of direct education with groups or indirect education using a variety of non-personal channels.

Clarifying your educational philosophy and the assumptions about your approach to nutrition content are extremely important because they will influence all that you do.

BOX 9-1 summarizes the key elements that contribute to the effectiveness of nutrition education interventions, as determined by reviews of studies. Consider these as you reflect on the theoretical underpinnings of your intervention and begin the process of designing sessions in the next few steps.

BOX 9-1 Elements of Effectiveness for Nutrition Education

General

- Nutrition education is more likely to be effective when it focuses on specific food-choice behaviors or diet-related practices for our audiences.

- Nutrition education interventions are more likely to be effective when they employ behavior change strategies and educational activities that are directly relevant to the behavior change focus and are derived from appropriate theory and prior research evidence.

Communications and Educational Activities for Enhancing Motivation

Most nutrition education involves information in some form. The manner in which it is communicated influences its role. For information to enhance motivation, the following elements are likely to be effective:

- Addressing the motivators that have personal meaning for the particular population group is of primary importance.

- Taking into account the group's stage of motivational readiness to take action and adopt dietary change may improve effectiveness.

- Cultural appropriateness or sensitivity, in the context of family and community, along with behavioral theory, can enhance effectiveness.

- Use of personalized self-assessment of food-related behaviors in terms of impact on health or on food system sustainability (e.g., carbon or water footprint) and feedback in comparison with recommendations can enhance motivation.

- Direct experience with food can enhance enjoyment of healthy food, motivation to act, and self-efficacy.

- Active participation is important.

- The effectiveness of communications through non-personal media such as newsletters and Web-based approaches is enhanced when they are based on appropriate theory and evidence.

- Mass media health campaigns can increase awareness of issues, affect beliefs and attitudes, and increase knowledge of targeted behaviors.

- Use of new technologies such as smartphones, tablets, personal digital assistants (PDAs), electronic and digital games, websites and social media show promise.

Strategies for Facilitating the Ability to Take Action and Maintain Behavioral Change

For information to facilitate knowledge and skill building, the following elements are likely to be effective:

- Use of a systematic goal-setting and self-regulation (or self-directed change) process that fosters people's agency is most likely to be effective in facilitating individuals' ability to take action and maintain change. In this process, individuals are provided with opportunities to conduct accurate self-assessments and compare them with recommendations; learn effective behaviors for healthful and enjoyable eating (and physical activity); choose among alternatives to set their own goals; learn the cognitive, affective, and behavioral skills needed to achieve their goals; monitor their progress toward goal attainment; and experience a sense of agency, empowerment, and control, all in the context of practical realities related to family, community, and culture.

- Sufficient attention to the complexity of food-specific issues is important.

- Adequate duration and intensity of the intervention are needed for changes in health actions to take place.

- Use of small groups is likely to improve the effectiveness of nutrition education interventions.

- Consideration of cultural context and available resources of the audience is essential.

- Long-term maintenance of behavior change is enhanced with continued experience of the new way of eating to increase familiarity and enjoyment and opportunity to develop personal food-related routines or policies.

Policy and Environmental Interventions (Chapter 14)

- Social support such as family and peer involvement is important in all population groups and should be incorporated.

- Collaborating with policymakers, service providers, organizations, community leaders, and agencies is important for promoting healthful food environments in schools, workplaces, and communities.

- Enhancing community capacity and facilitating collective efficacy or agency to create environments and policies that provide healthy options are likely to enhance individuals' ability to take action.

- Delivering nutrition education through multiple venues and directed at multiple levels of influence enhances dietary change.

Nutrition Educator Factors

- The enthusiasm and passion of the nutrition educator are crucial for success.

- Educator engagement with, and respect for, the audience increases audience responsiveness.

- The credibility and trustworthiness of the nutrition educator enhance audiences' willingness to respond to, and accept, the message. Open-mindedness and fairness engender a safe learning environment.

- Being organized is key to being effective. This allows for wise use of time and increased participant interest and engagement as well as enhanced credibility for the nutrition educator.

- The educator's ability to adapt to the situation on the ground is important for implementation of the intervention.

- Sensitivity to the audience is crucial to the effectiveness of nutrition education. This includes being appropriate in terms of developmental level, age-related concerns, and learning styles as well as sensitivity in terms of the culture and resources of the audience.

Sources: Contento, I. R., G. I. Balch, S. K. Maloney, et al. 1995. The effectiveness of nutrition education and implications for nutrition education policy, programs, and research. *Journal of Nutrition Education* 127:279–418; Waters, de Silva-Sanigorski, Hall, et al. 2010. Intervention for preventing obesity in children. *Cochrane Data base of Systematic Reviews* (12):CD001871; and Johnson, Scott-Sheldon, and Carey. 2010. Meta-synthesis of health behavior change meta-analyses. *American Journal of Public Health* 100(11):2193–2198.

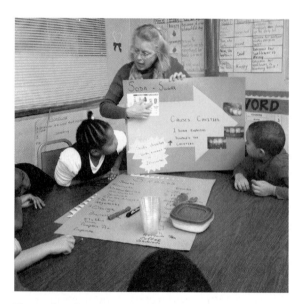

Theory-based sessions are suitable even for young children: health risk from drinking soda.

Courtesy of the Program in Nutrition, Teachers College Columbia University.

Case Study: The DESIGN Procedure in Action

The Step 3 Select Theory and Clarify Philosophy Worksheet is shown at the end of this chapter for the case study of the ongoing hypothetical intervention to promote more healthful eating and physical activity by middle school adolescents. The worksheet records the theory, educational philosophy, and approach to food and nutrition content for "Taking Control: Eating Well and Being Fit." Use it as an example to help you select your theory model and think through your philosophy to design your own nutrition education sessions or intervention.

Recall that four behavioral goals were chosen for the intervention "Taking Control: Eating Well and Being Fit": increase intake of fruits and vegetables; reduce consumption of sweetened beverages; reduce intake of packaged, highly processed, energy-dense snacks; and increase physical activity.

Social cognitive theory was considered the most suitable theory based on the issues identified and the modifiable determinants of change explored. It is shown as a diagram on the worksheet. The case study also lays out the educational philosophy, which takes a compensatory approach to helping the youth make changes. The approach to how food and nutrition content will be addressed is that the intervention will recommend eating whole, minimally processed foods obtained from local sources to the extent possible and consistent with youth's resources and access. The intervention will not focus on weight but instead focus on eating healthfully and being active.

Based on the findings from Steps 1 and 2, the university-related agency chose three components to achieve these behavioral goals: a classroom curriculum; a parent component; and a policy, systems, and environmental change component involving changes in school meals, food policies, and the school food and information environment. The educational philosophy and perspective on food and nutrition content applies to all three components. The case study in this chapter presents the theory model for the *classroom component* of the case study intervention only. The other two components are described in Chapter 14.

The classroom curriculum component consists of 10 sessions: an introductory lesson, two lessons on each of the behavior change goals, and a concluding lesson.

Your Turn to Design Nutrition Education: Completing the Step 3 Select Theory and Clarify Philosophy Worksheet

Review the information on determinants of change that you obtained in Step 2. You and/or your planning team should now select the theory you will use to design the nutrition education intervention or create the specific intervention model based on the discussion in this chapter. Now is also the time to clarify the philosophical perspectives of the intervention in terms of educational approach and food and nutrition content. Record your decisions on the Step 3 Select Theory and Clarify Philosophy Worksheet in the DESIGN workbook (located at the end of Chapter 13).

© Africa Studio/Shutterstock

Questions and Activities

1. Describe at least three criteria that nutrition educators can use to select which theory to use for a given nutrition education intervention or session(s). Describe how you would use these criteria to select a theory (or theories) or create the theory model for your intervention.

2. What are the advantages and disadvantages of using combined theory models for intervention purposes?

3. List and briefly describe three theory constructs (determinants) in common to at least two theories that are useful in interventions that focus on increasing awareness and enhancing motivation. How might you use these constructs in developing your intervention model?

4. List and briefly describe three constructs (determinants) in common to at least two theories that are useful in interventions that focus on facilitating the ability to take action. How might you use these constructs in developing your intervention model?

5. Compare, contrast, and critique the medical, moral, enlightenment, and compensatory models for helping people, indicating when and how each of them might be used in nutrition education, or if they even should be used. Use an example of each type of model from your experience in education—as an educator or a learner.

6. Think carefully through your intervention for your intended audience: which philosophical model of helping will guide your approach, and why?

References

Abraham, C., and P. Sheeran. 2000. Understanding and changing health behavior: From health beliefs to self-regulation. In *Understanding and changing health behavior: From health beliefs to self-regulation*, edited by P. Norman, C. Abraham, and M. Conner. Amsterdam: Harwood Academic Publishers.

Achterberg, C., and L. Lytle-Trenkner. 1990. Developing a working philosophy of nutrition education. *Journal of Nutrition Education* 22:189–193.

Australian National Health and Medical Research Council. 2013. *Eat for Health: Australian Dietary Guidelines—Providing the scientific evidence of healthier Australian diets.* Canberra, Australia: National Health and Medical Research Council.

Bagozzi, R. P., and E. A. Edwards. 1999. Goal striving and the implementation of goal intentions in the regulation of body weight. *Psychology and Health* 13:593–621.

Bandura, A. 1997. *Self-efficacy: The exercise of control.* New York: WH Freeman.

———. 2001. Social cognitive theory: An agentic perspective. *Annual Review of Psychology* 51:1–26.

———. 2004. Health promotion by social cognitive means. *Health Education and Behavior* 31 (2):143–164.

Baranowski, T., E. Cerin, and J. Baranowski. 2009. Steps in the design, development and formative evaluation of obesity prevention-related behavior change trials. *International Journal of Behavioral Nutrition and Physical Activity* 6:6.

Brickman, P., V. C. Rabinowitz, J. Karuza, D. Coates, E. Cohn, and L. Kidder. 1982. Models of helping and coping. *American Psychologist* 37:368–385.

Buchanan, D. 2004. Two models for defining the relationship between theory and practice in nutrition education: Is the scientific method meeting our needs? *Journal of Nutrition Education and Behavior* 36:146–154.

Deci, E. L., and R. M. Ryan. 2000. The "what" and "why" of goal pursuits: Human needs and the self-determination of behavior. *Psychological Inquiry* 11(4):227–268.

———. 2008. Facilitating optimal motivation and psychological well-being across life's domains. *Canadian Psychology* 49:14–23.

Diep, C. S., T. A. Chen, V. F. Davies, J. C. Baranowski, and T. Baranowski. 2014. Influence of behavioral theory on fruit and vegetable intervention effectiveness among children: A meta-analysis. *Journal of Nutrition Education and Behavior* 46(6):506–546.

Fishbein, M. 2000. The role of theory in HIV prevention. *AIDS Care* 12(3):273–278.

Fishbein, M., and I. Ajzen. 2010. *Predicting and changing behavior: The reasoned approach.* New York: Psychology Press.

Gollwitzer, P. M. 1999. Implementation intentions—strong effects of simple plans. *American Psychologist* 54:493–503.

Institute of Medicine. 2002. *Speaking of health: Assessing health communication strategies for diverse populations.* Washington, DC: National Academies Press.

International Organization of Consumers Unions. 1990. Code of good practice. In *IOCU code of good practice and guidelines for business sponsored educational materials used in schools*. Policy statement. London: Author.

Kok, G., H. Schaalma, H. De Vries, G. Parcel, and T. Paulussen. 1996. Social psychology and health. *European Review of Social Psychology* 7:241–282.

Kolbe, L. J., D. C. Iverson, W. K. Marshal, G. Hochbaum, and G. Christensen. 1981. Propositions for an alternate and complementary health education paradigm. *Health Education* 12(3):24–30.

Laidsaar-Powell, R. C., P. N. Butow, S. Bu, C. Charles, W. W. Lam, J. Jansen, et al. 2013. Physician-patient-companion communication and decision-making: A systematic review of triadic medical consultations. *Patient Education and Counseling* 91(1):3013.

Miller, R. W., and S. Rollnick. 2013. *Motivational interviewing: Helping people change*, 3rd edition. New York: Guilford Press.

Montano, D. E., and D. Kasprzyk. 2008. Theory of reasoned action, theory of planned behavior, and the integrated behavioral model. In *Health Behavior and Health Education: theory, research, and practice*, edited by K. Glanz, B. K. Rimer, and K. Viswanath. San Francisco: Wiley.

Prochaska, J. O., and W. F. Velicer. 1997. The transtheoretical model of health behavior change. *American Journal of Health Promotion* 12:38–48.

Schwarzer, R., and B. Renner. 2000. Social-cognitive predictors of health behavior: Action self-efficacy and coping self-efficacy. *Health Psychology* 19(5):487–495.

Sniehotta, F. F. 2009. Towards a theory of intentional behavior change: Plans, planning, and self-regulation. *British Journal of Health Psychology* 14:261–273.

World Health Organization. 2003. *Diet, nutrition and the prevention of chronic diseases*. Report of a joint WHO/FAO expert consultation. WHO Technical Report Series 916. Geneva: Author.

Nutrition Education DESIGN Procedure

Decide behavior(s) — Step 1
Explore determinants of change — Step 2
Select theory & clarify philosophy — Step 3
Indicate general objectives — Step 4
Generate plans — Step 5
Nail down evaluation plan — Step 6

Step 3: Select theory and clarify philosophy.

Now that you have identified the psychosocial determinants that will motivate and facilitate your audience's achieving the behavioral goal, it is time to put them together in a theoretical framework that will guide your planning and evaluation. It is also important to reflect on your personal philosophy of nutrition education and see how it meshes with any other nutrition educators you may be collaborating with during your session(s).

Use the Select Theory and Clarify Philosophy Worksheet to help you select a theory model for your session(s) or intervention and describe your personal philosophies related to nutrition education in general as well as the goals of your session(s) or intervention.

What theory (or combination of theories) will guide your educational session(s)? Compare the determinants you identified from your audience in Step 2 to the theories in Chapters 4 and 5 and choose the one(s) most representative of the determinants you highlighted in Step 2.

Social cognitive theory

How can your theoretical framework be visually represented? Modify the theory or theories you chose to be suitable for your audience based on your determinants from Step 2 in order to create a theory model. Below draw a visual of the theory model to show the flow of how your determinants relate to each other to help your audience achieve your behavior change goal(s).

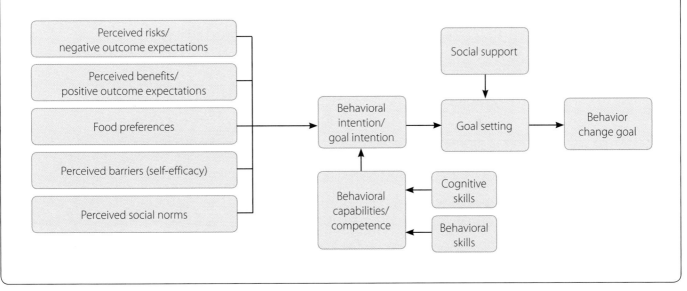

SOCIAL COGNITIVE THEORY (applied to intervention)

Nutrition Education DESIGN Procedure

| **D**ecide behavior(s) | **E**xplore determinants of change | **S**elect theory & clarify philosophy | **I**ndicate general objectives | **G**enerate plans | **N**ail down evaluation plan |
| Step 1 | Step 2 | Step 3 | Step 4 | Step 5 | Step 6 |

What is your educational philosophy? How do you view your approach as an educator? Look at Table 9-1 and decide which of Brickman's models is appropriate for your audience and your behavior change focus. State the model, and then describe why it is appropriate and what you will do to apply the model in your session or intervention.

We, as nutrition educators, believe that youth are responsible for their health and have the power to make healthful food and activity choices, but that they need the necessary understanding, motivation, and tools to take charge in today's difficult environment. We also believe that it is the responsibility of the school and home to provide an environment that is supportive and makes healthful options available. Our philosophy is that regardless of how the teens acquired their eating patterns, they need motivation to act and a sense of agency. We also recognize that individuals need skills and environmental support, thus suggesting a compensatory model. The intervention is designed to assist youth to increase awareness of their own behaviors and of environmental forces influencing their choices and to enhance their ability to make healthful food choices and overcome environmental barriers. Activities will provide them with tools to take charge of their own eating and activity patterns through goal setting and self-regulation processes. The aim will be carried out through an intervention directed at psychosocial mediators that includes two components: one that encourages analysis of self and environment, understanding, deliberation, and motivation and one that focuses on skills to take action. The intervention will also include an environmental component to provide support and increase options for the behaviors identified.

What is your perspective on how food and nutrition content will be addressed? Look at the section in Chapter 9 titled "Articulating the Intervention's Perspectives on How Nutrition Content Will Be Addressed," and in this section write about your perspectives on the food and nutrition content issues you will need to consider in your session(s) or intervention.

We believe kids should be taught to eat foods that are minimally processed, naturally nutrient dense, and fresh and local to the extent feasible given resource and availability constraints. Also, the issue of weight will not be addressed directly; instead, healthful eating and activity patterns will be emphasized.

CHAPTER 10

Step 4: Indicating Objectives: Translating Behavioral Theory into Educational Objectives

OVERVIEW

This chapter describes why we need nutrition education objectives, what they are, and key issues in translating behavioral theory into educational objectives. It also describes how to write educational objectives to help you create activities directed at determinants of behavior change and theory-based behavior change strategies in order to achieve the behavior change goals of your intervention.

CHAPTER OUTLINE

- Translating behavioral theory into nutrition education activities through objectives
- Writing educational objectives for determinants of behavior change goals
- Ensuring educational objectives engage participant thinking, feeling, and doing

- Case study: the DESIGN Procedure in action
- Your turn to design nutrition education: completing the Step 4 Indicate General Objectives Worksheet

LEARNING OBJECTIVES

At the end of the chapter, you should be able to:

- Value the importance of writing educational objectives for nutrition education sessions and interventions
- Describe how to translate determinants of behavior change into educational objectives
- Describe educational objectives for the thinking (cognitive), feeling (affective), and doing (psychomotor) domains of human experience and the levels of complexity of the learning experiences within the domains

- Write general educational objectives for learning outcomes to achieve the behavior change goals of the session or intervention, based on the identified determinants
- Write specific educational objectives to guide creation of specific engaging learning experiences or activities within each session or component, based on identified determinants and behavior change strategies

Translating Behavioral Theory into Nutrition Education Activities Through Objectives

You have spent some time getting to know your audience: the issues they face, the food and activity behaviors and practices they could take that would help to address these issues, and their potential motivations for making these changes as well as the skills they need. You have organized the specific potential determinants of change involving motivators and skills into a theory model to guide your session(s). These are important preliminary steps. The question is now: how exactly will you structure the educational sessions or intervention to assist the intended audience in achieving the changes in the determinants and skills so that audience members can accomplish the behavior change goals of your session(s) or intervention?

The mechanism for translating your theory model into effective educational sessions is to write **educational objectives** (that is, intended outcomes) for each of the determinants and then select the appropriate behavior change strategies and create exciting and relevant activities to achieve these objectives. These objectives and the activities to achieve them become your *educational plan*(s), or *lesson plan*(s), ready for you to use with your selected audience. This is the whole purpose of the DESIGN Procedure. Articulating your objectives is thus crucial. **FIGURE 10-1** shows where we are in the design process.

Educational objectives can be written for the *entire intervention*, which may consist of a series of sessions with or without additional indirect educational channels, such as newsletters, blogs, and so forth. These are your *general educational objectives*. Educational objectives can also be written for *each individual session*; these are the *specific objectives* and guide the development of specific activities in that session.

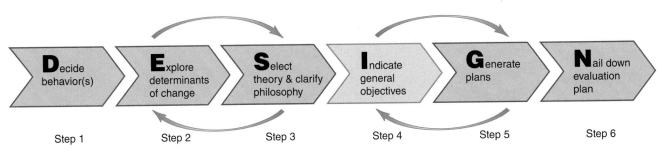

Inputs: Collecting the Assessment Data		Outputs: Designing the Theory-Based Intervention			Outcomes: Evaluation Plan
Tasks: • **Decide** behavior change goal(s) of the intervention, based on: • analyzing issues and behaviors of concern for audience	*Tasks:* • **Explore** determinants of behavior change based on a variety of data sources	*Tasks:* • **Select** theory and draw intervention-specific theory model • Clarify educational philosophy • Articulate perspectives on content	*Tasks:* • **Indicate** general objectives for each determinant in your theory model	*Tasks:* • **Generate** educational plans: • Educational activities to address all determinants in theory model • Sequence for implementation using the 4 Es	*Tasks:* • **Nail down** evaluation plan • Select methods and questions to evaluate outcomes • Plan process evaluation • Create questions to measure how implementation went
Products: *Statement of intervention behavior change goal(s)*	*Products:* *List of determinants to address in the intervention*	*Products:* *Theory model for intervention* *Statement of educational philosophy* *Statement of content perspectives*	*Products:* *A general objective for each determinant in the theory model*	*Products:* *Educational plans that link determinants and educational activities to achieve behavior change or action goal(s)*	*Products:* *List of evaluation methods and questions* *Procedures and measures for process evaluation*

FIGURE 10-1 Stepwise Nutrition Education DESIGN Procedure for planning theory-based nutrition education: tasks and products of Step 4.

Consider the following scenario. A middle school has invited a nutrition educator to speak at a school assembly of several health classes (about 100 students) about "the importance of good nutrition." The nutrition educator designs a 45-minute presentation using slides. Starting with a description of what teens typically eat, she discusses the components of a healthy diet, covering the major recommendations of the government's guidelines, and then talks about the importance of eating more fruits and vegetables and how to add them to the diet; eating fewer energy-dense, high-fat, high-sugar foods; the importance of regular meals during the day; label reading so as to be able to select healthy snacks; the importance of calcium-rich foods for good bone health; and how to make food choices that are good for the environment.

She begins to notice that the teens are getting restless. When she ends, one teen approaches, very worried, and says, "This isn't going to be on the final exam, is it? That was a lot of information and I couldn't write it all down." Another says, "You talked about a lot of different things and I couldn't follow everything you said, so I'm not sure what I should be eating."

Later she tells a colleague about her experience. Her colleague asks her, "What was the overall objective of your talk? What did you hope to accomplish?" The nutrition educator is rather surprised. "I didn't have a specific objective," she says. "This was the only time they were going to hear about nutrition in their health class this year, so I just wanted to make sure they got lots of information so that they could make wise choices." What is going on here? The nutrition educator did not have a clear behavior change goal for the session (or set of closely related behavior change goals): she discussed several behaviors that were unrelated to each other and that did not add up to some coherent, overarching behavior change goals. This made it hard for the audience to know what exactly they should be doing. Nor did she explore the determinants (motivators and skills) needed to act on the behavior change goal(s). If she could not ask the audience directly ahead of time, she could have obtained information from more general sources and from talking with the teachers in the school. Likewise, she did not create a theory model to organize the various determinants of behavior change. Finally, she did not write specific educational objectives directed at each of the key relevant determinants of change. She rambled on, providing a good deal of interesting information but no clear,

identifiable message. So it is not surprising that the teens would leave with no clear understanding of what to do to eat well. A clear behavior change goal and several general educational objectives based on the determinants of change would have helped to focus the presentation and enhance the ability of the youth to make healthy choices. Often less is more—when it is well focused.

Even in situations where you think objectives are not needed, such as in facilitated group discussions where the sessions are conducted in a flexible way in order to allow you to follow group interests to some degree, behavior change goals, educational objectives, and educational plans are still important for providing a map for how to proceed. Without a clear plan, discussions can ramble and no clear message comes through. Participants often leave such sessions frustrated.

In Step 4, you convert the information you have collected and the theory model you created in Step 3 based on behavioral theory into specific objectives—clear statements of intended outcomes for the determinants of the behavior change goals of your intervention to be achieved through educational means. As part of the process, you will go back and forth between this step and the next because in the next step you select behavior change strategies and design practical educational activities to achieve these objectives. The tasks and products for Step 4 are highlighted in the logic model graphic in Figure 10-1.

Many different terms are used that have somewhat similar meanings: goals, objectives, performance objectives, performance indicators, behavioral objectives, educational standards, nutrition competencies, and so forth. They are all about intended outcomes to be accomplished by a given program. Nutrition educators need not be rigid about which terms to use. This text uses the term *goals* to refer *only* to the *behavior change* goals for the intervention that you established in Step 1. The term *objectives* in this text has meanings that are explored below.

Writing Educational Objectives for Determinants of Behavior Change Goals

Educational objectives in the context of nutrition education are ways to convert and operationalize determinants of health behavior change into educational activities.

Educational objectives are needed for both *direct education activities*, such as education sessions and activities delivered to groups, and *indirect education activities*, such as educational materials, computer- or Internet-based nutrition education, or education provided through other channels.

EDUCATIONAL OBJECTIVES ARE BASED ON DETERMINANTS FROM THEORY

Educational objectives are based on the specific determinants that are part of the theory model that you created in Step 3 to guide your intervention. These are the determinants that you have identified as important for achieving the behavior change goals you set for your intervention or sessions, such as perceived risk, attitudes, affect/feelings, perceived benefits and barriers, outcome expectations, values, perceived responsibility, self-identify, self-efficacy, social norms, and goal setting skills.

Select only those determinants that can be realistically addressed in the sessions or intervention to enhance motivation or increase behavioral skills, or both, given the time and resources you have available and the evidence for their effectiveness. Remember, most nutrition educators have a tendency to try to cover too much, so select carefully.

CONSIDERATIONS IN WRITING EDUCATIONAL OBJECTIVES

For each determinant of behavior change in your theory, write one or more educational objectives to guide the design of practical educational activities to address that determinant. These objectives provide ways to convert determinants into a form that is useful for guiding the design of learning activities. They are statements of intended learning outcomes. They are stated in learner terms; that is, in terms of what the learner gets out of the intervention or what the learner can think, feel, or be able to do as a result of the educational experience.

- *General educational objectives* provide *overall guidance* for the development of activities for a given session or a series of sessions or intervention on the same set of behaviors.
- *Specific educational objectives* guide the development of *each of the activities* within a given session.

Learning Objectives and Educational Objectives: A Clarification of Terms

The objectives are expressed in terms of the learner or participant and are thus often called learning objectives. This term is often used interchangeably with educational objectives because learning is what the participant does, and educating is what you do to encourage learning. Both terms refer to the same activity with the same desired outcomes. Both terms are used in this text, but educational objectives is favored, to remind you of what you must do as a nutrition educator to facilitate learning and that "learning" is not all about information or knowledge.

Objectives Are About Ends, Not Means

Objectives are used to describe ends or outcomes intended by the intervention or program, not the means to get there. They state what the intervention or individual will have achieved at the end of the intervention. They should *not* be a statement of what the nutrition educator will do, such as "demonstrate a food preparation technique" or "show a film," or even what the intended audience member will do, such as "discuss" or "make a salad." Instead, learning objectives are statements of what the participant will know, feel, or be able to do differently in terms of the specific determinants of behavior change in order to achieve the behavior change goals.

Educational/Learning Objectives Use Concrete Verbs

Educational objectives state exactly what the learner will be able to do; are measurable; and are related to achievement in terms of a particular personal *determinant* of action or behavior change, such as self-efficacy, perceived benefits, perceived behavior control, goal setting, and so forth. Specific educational objectives have the following form: "At the end of the session/intervention, participants will be able to . . ." followed by a verb such as describe, state, identify, translate, judge, and so forth.

GENERAL EDUCATIONAL OBJECTIVES

Based on the theory you have chosen, identify the three to six major determinants that you think you have time to cover and that evidence suggests will contribute to increasing the group's motivation and ability to enact

Potential Determinants	General Educational Objectives
	At the end of the sessions, youth will be able to:
Outcome expectations (perceived benefits)	Demonstrate understanding and appreciation of the importance of eating a variety of fruits and vegetables (F&V).
Perceived threats	Evaluate own intake of F&V compared to recommendations.
Self-efficacy	Demonstrate increased self-efficacy (confidence) in eating a variety of F&V each day.
Knowledge and skills	Demonstrate increased knowledge and skills in incorporating F&V into their daily food patterns.
Goal setting skills	Prepare action plans using goal setting and decision-making skills to increase their consumption of F&V.

the behavior change goals. Write a general educational objective for each of these determinants. Record them on the Step 4 Indicate General Objectives Worksheet in the workbook at the end of Chapter 13.

Case Study Example

Above is an example of general educational objectives from the case study, where the behavior change goal is that youth will increase their consumption of fruits and vegetables. These objectives will guide educational activities across two sessions.

SPECIFIC EDUCATIONAL OBJECTIVES

You then write specific educational objectives that will guide the development of specific learning/educational activities within each session to achieve the overall general educational objectives. These specific objectives about intended learning outcomes guide the design of each of the specific educational activities or learning experiences within individual sessions; that is, each of these specific objectives is directed to one of the determinants in your theory model and guides you to develop one or two activities directed at that one specific determinant of behavior change. There will be many of these, depending on the length of each session. Sometimes one activity serves two or more specific objectives. On the other hand, sometimes it requires two or more activities to accomplish one specific objective.

Case Study Example

Specific educational objectives in the case study are written to guide the learning experiences within each session. They are linked to the determinants that are part of the theory selected in Step 3 based on the information obtained in Step 2. They are also linked to the general objectives. See the case study at the end of this chapter for details. They take the following format:

Potential Determinants of Behavior from Theory	Potential Determinants of Change: Findings from Step 2	Specific Learning Objectives for Each Personal Determinant
	Audiences' thoughts and feelings for each determinant (from Step 2):	At the end of the session, participants will be able to:
Outcome expectations (perceived benefits)	Students will eat F&V if they taste good, make them look good, and help them build strong bones.	State specific benefits of eating F&V.
Barriers/self-efficacy	Students will eat F&V if the are easy to prepare or to carry for lunch.	Identify barriers to eating F&V and ways to overcome barriers.

Objectives in Practice

In practice, you will probably go back and forth between general and specific objectives and between objectives and educational activities. (See Step 5, Chapters 11 and 12.) As you come up with exciting and relevant activities, you should think carefully about their purpose (specific objectives) in achieving the behavior change goals of the intervention and how they relate to the general educational objectives. If they do not serve any of the identified larger purposes, you should drop the activities, no matter how exciting. However, at this point you may want to rethink your general objectives. Perhaps they need to be changed to accommodate the specific objectives and activities because you consider them important to achieving the behavior change goal.

Objectives in Practice: Example of Food, Health & Choices Program

The development of an obesity prevention intervention program for elementary school students, called Food, Health & Choices (FHC), illustrates how psychosocial determinants or precursors of behavior can be used to generate general objectives for a curriculum.

Detailed assessments, as described in Steps 1 to 3, led to the decision that the behavior change goals of the FHC curriculum would focus on energy-balance behaviors, and the theory model would consist of complementary determinants of change from social cognitive theory and self-determination theory. The general objectives are derived from this theory model, as shown in **NUTRITION EDUCATION IN ACTION 10-1**.

NUTRITION EDUCATION IN ACTION 10-1 **Food, Health & Choices: An Obesity Prevention Intervention for Upper Elementary Schools**

Food, Health & Choices (FHC) is an obesity prevention curriculum intervention that focuses on energy-balance–related behaviors. It consists of two components: a 23-lesson FHC classroom curriculum and a classroom wellness policy component called Positively Healthful Classrooms where students participate in daily short bouts of exercise in the classroom called Dance Breaks, and implement a healthy classroom food policy.

Behavior Change Goals

Choose more fruits and vegetables and physical activity.

Choose less sweetened beverages, processed packaged snacks, fast food, and leisure screen time.

Theory Model

FHC is based on a combination of determinants of behavior change from social cognitive and self-determination theories.

Linking Educational Objectives to Behavioral Theory

Here is how the general educational objectives are stated for the determinants of change from the theory model. Note that there are many general objectives because these are for all 23 lessons combined.

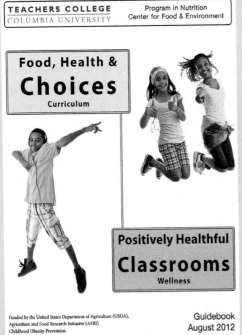

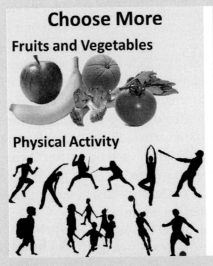

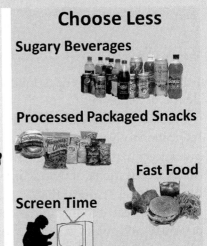

Funded by the United States Department of Agriculture (USDA), Agriculture and Food Research Initiative (AFRI), and Childhood and Obesity Prevention.

Determinants from Theory Model	General Educational Objectives
	At the end of the sessions, students will be able to:
Outcome expectations	■ Articulate why maintaining energy balance is important.
	■ Demonstrate an understanding and appreciation of the importance of eating a variety of fruits and vegetables (F&V) and getting enough physical activity (PA).
	■ Demonstrate an increased awareness of negative health consequences related to excessive consumption of sweetened beverages (SB), processed packaged snacks (PPS), and fast food (FF), and excessive time spent on recreational screen time (RST).
Self-efficacy	■ Demonstrate increased self-efficacy (confidence) in eating more F&V and fewer SB, PPS, and FF.
	■ Demonstrate increased self-efficacy (confidence) in doing more daily PA and spending less time in sedentary behavior.
Intention	■ State intention to increase F&V intake and time in PA.
	■ State intention to decrease consumption of SB, PPS, and FF and time spent engaging in sedentary behavior.
Behavioral capability (factual knowledge)	■ Explain the concept of energy balance.
	■ State the recommendations for daily intakes of FV and water.
	■ State the recommendations for maximum daily intakes of SB, PPS, and FF.
	■ State recommendations for daily PA and maximum daily RST.
Goal setting skills/self-regulation	■ Analyze their current dietary and PA behaviors and choose individual goals for each target behavior.
	■ Demonstrate ability to monitor their progress in achieving behavior change goals.
Competence	■ Express an increased confidence in their skills for choosing more healthful foods and engaging in more PA.
PA. Autonomy	■ State an increased sense of autonomy in choosing more healthful foods and engaging in more PA.
PA. Relatedness	■ Express feeling understood because of connection to similar lead characters in the curriculum case study drama.

F&V = fruits and vegetables, PA = physical activity, SB = sweetened beverages, PPS = processed packaged snacks, FF = fast food, and RST = recreational screen time.
Source: Abrams, E., M. Burgermaster, P. A. Koch, I. R. Contento, and H. L. Gray. 2014. Food, Health & Choices: Importance of formative evaluation to create a well-delivered and well-received intervention. *Journal of Nutrition Education and Behavior* 46(4S):S137.

Ensuring Educational Objectives Engage Participant Thinking, Feeling, and Doing

People are more likely to take action or make changes in their lives if they participate in activities that engage their heads, hearts, and hands. Thus, the effectiveness of nutrition education is improved if nutrition educators design learning experiences that fully engage participants by providing opportunities for knowing/thinking (head), feeling (hearts), and doing (hands) by providing manipulative skills, where needed or appropriate. These three areas of human functioning are also referred to as the mental, emotional, and physical.

Consequently, educators intentionally create educational objectives to guide the development of specific activities that will involve these three areas of the human experience, calling them the cognitive, affective, and psychomotor domains (Bloom et al. 1956; Marzano and Kendall 2007; Gronland and Brookhart 2008):

■ **Cognitive domain** objectives guide the development of activities to promote abilities in thought, understanding, and cognitive skills.

- Affective domain objectives guide the development of activities to promote changes in attitude, feeling, or emotion.
- Psychomotor domain objectives guide the development of activities to promote improvement in physical or manipulative skills.

Thus, it is important to write educational objectives for any given session in such a way as to ensure that they guide the creation of activities that engage all three domains of learning in your audience.

WRITING EDUCATIONAL OBJECTIVES THAT REFLECT THE DESIRED COMPLEXITY OF LEARNING

In addition, within each domain—thinking, feeling, and doing—how difficult or complex do you want your activities be? Educational activities can be directed at intended learning outcomes that range in a graded sequence from simple to complex. Depending on your audience and the behavior change goals of your session(s), the activities may involve fairly simple learning tasks or more complex tasks. You should ensure that your objectives for any given learning task are at the appropriate level of difficulty for that task. It is also very important that any given session or intervention includes objectives for more complex understandings and attitudes, as well as for simple ones. Even young children can do complex learning tasks, such as compare or analyze, when framed to be appropriate for their developmental level.

TABLE 10-1, TABLE 10-2, and TABLE 10-3 provide detailed outlines of the intended learning outcomes in the cognitive, affective, and psychomotor domains and a list of verbs that you can use as you write educational objectives in each of these domains.

Cognitive (Knowing or Thinking) Domain

Human beings are thinking beings. Just about everything people do involves them thinking about it and interpreting it in some way. Educational objectives can be set for activities that range from simple recall of facts to highly original and creative ways of combining and synthesizing new ideas. A group of education and assessment researchers in the 1950s developed a system to classify cognitive domain objectives commonly used in education. They referred to the classification system as a "taxonomy." The handbook describing the taxonomy became known informally as "Bloom's taxonomy" (Bloom et al. 1956). The taxonomy was updated and revised by education researchers in 2000 led by Krathwohl of the original group (Anderson and Krathwohl 2000). Among the changes was a change from nouns for the categories to verbs. The verbs are used here. Also, the category of synthesis was considered to come after evaluation, not before it, and includes the notion of creating.

The cognitive taxonomy describes six levels of understandings that an educational experience or strategy can aim to develop in learners, beginning with *remembering* and then moving through *understanding* to the ability to

Table 10-1 Cognitive Domain: Levels of Thinking

Levels of Thinking (Levels of Complexity of Intended Learning Outcomes)	Description	Useful Verbs
Remember	Recalling information as it is learned	List, recall, name, define, state, label, tell, record
Understand	Reporting information in a way other than how it was learned to show understanding	Describe, explain, summarize, compare, discuss, identify, classify, review, locate
Apply	Applying learned information to a new context	Apply, demonstrate, use, interpret, illustrate, modify, operate, predict, dramatize, sketch, solve
Analyze	Taking learned information apart into components so that its organizational structure may be understood	Analyze, calculate, test, compare, contrast, criticize, diagram, distinguish, differentiate, appraise, debate, relate, examine, inspect, categorize
Evaluate	Making judgments about the value of something using appropriate criteria	Evaluate, rate, compare, value, revise, judge, select, measure, estimate, conclude, justify, criticize
Synthesize or create	Putting together parts and elements into a unified organization or whole, with emphasis on creating new meaning or structure	Compose, create, plan, propose, design, formulate, arrange, construct, organize, manage, prepare, relate

Data from Bloom B. S., et al. 1956. *Taxonomy of educational objectives. Handbook I: Cognitive domain*. New York: David McKay; and Anderson, L. W., and D. R. Krathwohl (Editors). 2000. *A taxonomy for learning, teaching, and assessing: A revision of Bloom's taxonomy of educational objectives*. Boston: Pearson.

apply information to new decision-making situations and the ability to *analyze* and *evaluate* information, and finally ending with the ability to *synthesize or create*. Table 10-1 describes these levels of intended learning outcomes.

The Cognitive Domain and Nutrition Education

In terms of theory-based nutrition education, every *determinant* you select for your sessions can be presented in such a way as to engage the participants at any of these levels of understanding. Do you want the group participants to *recall* something or *understand* something? Do you want them to be able to *apply* the information or to *analyze* it? Do you want them to be able to *evaluate* the information? Depending on the findings of your assessment in Step 2 with respect to the difficulty of the behavior change and the motivations and skills of the target group, you may seek to bring about measurable changes in understanding at different levels of difficulty or complexity. It is recommended that you may also set the objectives at increasingly higher levels, beginning with the simple and moving to the more complex, during a session or over several sessions. See Table 10-1 for details. Also see Chapter 5 for the different kinds of knowledge and cognitive skills.

- *Remember*: Recalling information very much as it was learned. This is also referred to as factual knowledge. At the lowest level of learning, this involves recall and memory. When you set objectives at this level, it means that you will design learning activities that will result in group participants being able to remember or recall specific pieces of information, terminology, and facts, such as which foods are in which food groups, which foods are sources of which nutrients, or how many servings of fruits and vegetables we should be eating.
- *Understand*: Reporting the information in a way other than how it was learned to show that is has been understood. Also referred to as factual knowledge. This level represents the beginnings of understanding. It means that individuals are able to make sense of the information and to paraphrase it in their own words. The individuals may even be able to extrapolate the information to new but related ideas and implications, making simple inferences. For example, when you set educational objectives at this level, you are aiming for group participants to be able to understand general

information about the risk of a health condition and apply it to themselves or to understand the benefits of eating fruits and vegetables for reducing risk of disease.

- *Apply*: Use of learned information in new and concrete situations or to solve a problem. Also called procedural knowledge. At this level of learning, individuals are able to carry over information, principles, concepts, or theories learned in one context to a completely new one. When you set objectives for the session at this level, you are aiming for group participants, after learning how to set goals (a procedure) to increase their consumption of fruits and vegetables, to be able to apply goal setting principles to a new behavior, such as eating more foods high in calcium.
- *Analyze*: Taking information apart so that its organizational structure can be understood. Also referred to as part of higher order or critical thinking skills. This level involves breaking information into its components to identify the elements, the interactions between them, and the organizing principles or structures. It also involves distinguishing fact from opinion, and relevant from extraneous issues or events. For example, when you set educational objectives at this level you may be aiming for group participants to be able to compare and contrast the impacts of low-fat and low-carbohydrate diets on weight and health or to debate the pros and cons of breastfeeding versus bottle feeding.

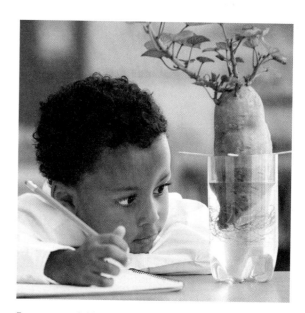

Even young children are capable of objectives and activities involving analysis.

© Jose Luis Pelaez/Getty Images.

- *Evaluate:* Judging the value of something for a particular purpose. Also referred to as part of higher order or critical thinking skills. Here individuals are able to make judgments about the worth of information and experiences based on well-accepted external criteria (such as relevance to stated purposes) or on internal criteria (organization and meaning). These criteria may be given to or created by individuals themselves. Objectives at this level include elements of all the previous levels, as well as conscious value judgments based on the criteria. Setting the objectives at this level means that you are expecting the intended nutrition education audience to be able to evaluate the merits of different ways to assist children to learn good eating habits or to reach sound judgment regarding food and nutrition matters based on evidence.

- *Synthesize or create:* Putting information together in a unique or novel way. Also referred to as part of higher order or critical thinking skills. At this level, individuals are able to reassemble information and experiences into a unified framework to create new meaning or to think about the situation in a new way. When you set objectives at this level, you are expecting the intended audience to be able to use what they are learning and experiencing in the intervention in a new way to affect their food practices and eating experiences. They can plan an investigation or generate hypotheses in order to test out food-related ideas.

Nutrition Literacy, Behavioral Capability, and the Cognitive Domain

Nutrition educators speak about *nutrition literary* as skills in being able to take action about nutrition- or food-related matters, such as being able to read food labels, knowing how to store and prepare foods, shopping wisely, or managing food budgets. These learning outcomes in the cognitive domain span the remembering, understanding, or applying levels. These very same skills are referred to in the social psychological literature as *behavioral capabilities.* Thus you can see that the behavioral capability determinant within social cognitive theory is easily converted to an activity in your session by stating a cognitive objective. These skills, or behavioral capabilities, can vary in difficulty. As noted before, you can gear the educational objective, and hence the activity, toward varying levels of the cognitive taxonomy. An objective at the lowest level might be: "Children will be able to *recall* the number of

servings of fruits and vegetables they should eat each day." (The activity you create will teach them that—factual knowledge). Or it could be: "Diabetes patients will be able to *apply* what they learned about carbohydrate counting in the session to a meal they eat at home." (Your activity will thus provide practice in applying information to new situations—procedural knowledge). Or you may set the educational objective as: "Participants will be able to *evaluate* the data on the carbon footprints for producing and using various foods and products and to select the one with the lowest footprint." (Your activity will provide the group with data in the form of bar graphs, numbers, or other formats showing the carbon footprints of various foods and have the group calculate which ones have the least impact on the environment.)

Affective (Feelings) Domain

Humans are not only thinking beings, but also feeling and emotional beings. Our feelings, attitudes, values, appreciation, and interests contribute to our motivations and are collectively referred to as affect. All educational activities involve feelings and attitudes as well as cognitive learning. We have probably all experienced that at some time—we came to like certain subjects in school cognitively because we felt good about the way the teacher respected us or made learning the subject fun, or we felt we had really accomplished something through the experience. Similarly, we may have been turned off of a subject because of a negative learning environment. Educators recognize the need to create activities that are directed at the affective or emotional side of people or the affective domain in order to assist people to take action. The group of education researchers that developed the cognitive domain taxonomy recognized that educational objectives could also be placed into categories based on the degree to which they encourage affective engagement and internalization of intended outcomes. For this reason, they also came up with a classification system or taxonomy for outcomes in the affective or feeling domain that influence learning (Krathwohl, Bloom, and Maisa 1964).

The affective taxonomy describes five levels of engagement or internalization that an educational experience or strategy can aim to develop in learners, beginning at the lowest level, with awareness or *willingness to receive* or attend to a message, and moving through *responding* to it, *valuing* the message to the point of commitment to it, *organizing* their life around the message (e.g., developing

Table 10-2 The Affective Domain: Levels of Affective Engagement

Levels of Engagement and Integration	Description: Stages Within Level	Useful Verbs
Receiving (paying attention)	1. Awareness with no position taken 2. Willingness to receive or attend to information 3. Will not avoid stimulus	Answers, chooses, describes, follows, locates, names, points to, selects
Responding (active participation)	1. Complying with expectations of educator 2. Stating or defending own position 3. Beginning of own emotional response with satisfaction (opinions/position formation)	Answers, assists, aids, helps, complies, conforms, discusses, labels, tells, reads, performs, reports, writes, recites, selects
Valuing (behavior based on positive regard for something)	1. Tentative acceptance with readiness to reevaluate 2. Conviction 3. Commitment to the behavior or action; beginning to internalize own viewpoint (no longer motivated primarily by value to comply with others; beginning to internalize own viewpoint)	Completes, demonstrates, explains, initiates, joins, proposes, reports, shares, studies, works
Organization (behaving according to a set of principles)	1. Conceptualizing one's important values and understanding that they may be different from those of others 2. Building an internally consistent value system for guiding behavior by resolving conflicts and creating a unique value system (developing one's own values or policies to guide action)	Adheres, alters, arranges, combines, defends, explains, generalizes, integrates, modifies, orders, organizes, relates, synthesizes
Internalizing values (behaving according to a consistent worldview)	1. Integration of values into one's consistent, total worldview that guides behavior 2. Person's behavior is consistent, predictable, and characterized by the values (person has developed a consistent and recognizable way of life guided by a set of values)	Acts, discriminates, displays, influences, modifies, performs, practices, proposes, qualifies, questions, revises, solves, verifies

Data from Krathwohl, D. R., B. S. Bloom, and B. B. Masia. 1964. *Taxonomy of educational objectives. Handbook II: Affective domain*. New York: Longman; and Gronland, N. E., and S. M. Brookhart. 2008. *Gronland's writing instructional objectives* (8th ed.). Upper Saddle River, NJ: Prentice Hall.

a personal food policy to eat only organic vegetables), and finally to *characterization* of themselves by their commitment to the value system (e.g., becoming known as a vegetarian). Table 10-2 describes these levels of active engagement with, and internalization of, the intended learning outcomes.

The Affective Domain in Nutrition Education

For nutrition education to be effective, the intended audience must not only understand the message or information, but also value it, feel actively engaged with it, believe it to be relevant, and feel it is important to them. The affective domain objectives focus on a process of ever greater affective engagement and internalization. It categorizes into levels the inner growth and change that occurs as individuals become aware of, get excited about, come to value, and later adopt the attitudes, behaviors, and principles that guide their actions.

In terms of theory-based nutrition education, every determinant you select for your sessions can be addressed at any of these levels of engagement, as you choose, based on your assessments. Participants will always have feelings during a session regardless. Therefore, it is helpful to make explicit how you will handle these feelings. As you design your sessions, think about the level of affective engagement you wish for your audience. For example, do you want the group to just passively receive your message, or do you want the group to be actively engaged and to value it? Do you want them to value the message enough to make a commitment to adopting a behavior or making a change in their behavior? A general strategy is for the session (or sessions) to provide opportunities for the group to move from lesser degrees of affective engagement and commitment to greater degrees of commitment. Therefore, the objectives will be set at ever-higher levels, during a session or over several sessions, in the classification scheme described here. See Table 10-2 for details.

■ *Receiving: Paying attention.* At this level, the participants are willing to listen to the nutrition educator or other forms of communication and become aware of the ideas communicated. From a purely passive role, they may advance to willingness to attend to the communication despite distractions or competing stimuli.

When you set objectives at this level, it means that you expect participants to be willing to listen to your message, such as the importance of eating fruits and vegetables, but that is about all.

■ *Responding: Active participation.* This level involves willingness to participate in something, although not necessarily with enthusiasm at first. From obedient participation (perhaps a health professional has insisted that participants attend these nutrition education sessions), individuals may advance to voluntary response and, indeed, to a pleasurable feeling or satisfaction in participation.

When you set educational objectives at this level, it means you expect that individuals will move from being onlookers during group nutrition education activities to participating in these activities and finding that they enjoy them. Or objectives may be set even higher, expecting individuals to move from complying with the expectations of the educator to starting to develop their own positions and taking responsibility for themselves. Objectives at this level take the form of aiming for changes in *attitudes, motivations,* and *self-efficacy.*

■ *Valuing: Consistent behavior reflecting positive regard for something.* At this level, the issue or behavior is considered to have worth. This sense of worth ranges from acceptance of the value to a deep enough commitment to the value that it is reflected in observable behavior. Behavior reflects a belief or an attitude. Thus, this level is characterized by motivated behavior in which individuals' commitments guide their behaviors. This is the level that is most appropriate for nutrition education.

When you set objectives at this level, it means that you aim for the learning activities that you design to increase participants' value for the targeted behavior goal or issue so much that they are willing to take action. At the lower end, this may mean tentatively doing the behavior in keeping with advice from others, with readiness to reevaluate. At the upper end, individuals develop conviction about the behavior or issue, resulting in commitment or *behavioral intention.* They have less need to be motivated by the need to comply

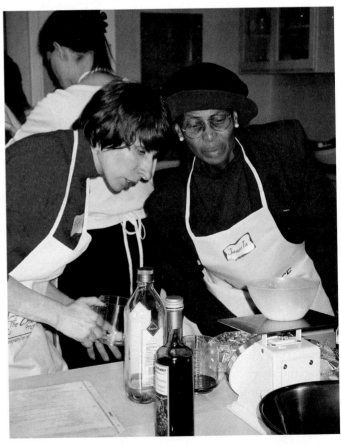

Cooking classes can engage participants in the cognitive, affective, and psychomotor domains of learning all at the same time.

Courtesy of Fredi Kronenberg.

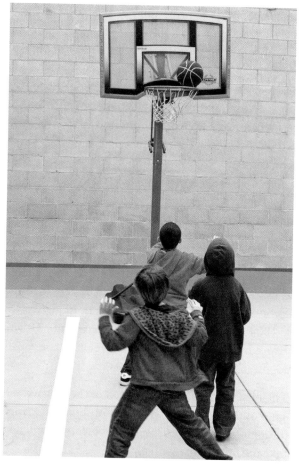

School-sponsored physical activity, such as an informal basketball game, is a fun way for students to develop their psychomotor skills.

© Gennadiy Titkov/ShutterStock.

with others and have begun to internalize their own viewpoints and values as a basis of action. For example, stating your educational objective at this level means that you intend for individuals to move from ambivalence to deciding to eat more fruits and vegetables each day, and then to actually doing so.

■ *Organization: Behaving according to a set of principles.* Here individuals have established a conscious basis for making choices. They understand that there are other values besides their own. Objectives at the organization level are concerned with assisting individuals to bring together different values, resolve conflicts among them, and begin to build an internally consistent value system—a set of criteria—for guiding behavior. Individuals are aware of the basis of their own attitudes and values and are able to defend them. They begin to develop their own personal food policies.

If you set educational objectives at this level, it means that you intend for your learning experiences or activities to lead individuals to use health or food system sustainability concerns; social justice issues; or personal, social, or cultural values as a consistent criterion for making choices about food- and nutrition-related issues now. They may develop *personal food (and activity) policies* to guide their choices.

■ *Internalizing values: Behaving according to a consistent worldview.* At this level, values are integrated into some kind of internally consistent worldview so that the person is recognized by these values. The individual has developed a characteristic lifestyle.

If you set objectives at this level, it means that you expect that the educational activities or learning experiences you design will lead participants to a change in worldview and a lifestyle consistent with that worldview. For example, you expect that as a result of your educational activities, the individual will practice a new way of eating so consistently that he or she becomes known as a vegetarian, as an ecologically conscious or "green" consumer, or as a health-conscious parent.

Psychomotor Domain

The emphasis in the psychomotor domain is on the development of psychomotor skills, even though some degree of understanding and varying degrees of emotion may also be involved. This domain involves a graded sequence from simple to complex (University of Michigan 1976). At the lowest level, participants observe a more experienced person performing the activity (e.g., preparing a recipe)

Table 10-3 Psychomotor Domain: Levels of Psychomotor Skills		
Levels of Performance and Skill	**Description**	**Verbs to Use**
Observing	Observes skilled performance	Observes, watches
Imitating	Follows instructions under supervision	Imitates, mimics
Practicing	Completes entire sequence repeatedly until routine	Practices, carries out
Adopting	Adapts or modifies to further improve outcome	Adapts, modifies, revises

and then are able to imitate it and then practice it, so that conscious effort is no longer necessary and it has become somewhat habitual in nature. Eventually, individuals may be able to adapt the activity. See Table 10-3 for details.

1. *Observing.* When objectives are set at this level, individuals observe a more experienced person performing the skill. Sometimes the reading of directions, as in a recipe, can substitute for this experience. However, usually reading is supplemented with direct observation, such as watching someone preparing a salad or recipe.

2. *Imitating.* When objectives are set at this level, you provide opportunities for individuals to follow directions and sequences under close supervision. It may require conscious effort on the part of individuals to carry out the actions in sequence.

3. *Practicing.* When objectives are set at this level, you provide opportunities for the entire sequence to be performed repeatedly so that conscious effort is no longer required. The actions become more or less habitual, and you can say that the individuals have acquired the skill. Perhaps the individuals have learned to prepare recipes with vegetables in them or to modify recipes to make them lower in fat.

4. *Adapting.* Objectives at this level involve the ability to adapt or modify the actions to improve the outcome even further. This may mean the ability to adapt learned recipes to individual or family tastes.

Overall

Educational objectives help specify which kinds of activities you will design to bring about behavior change. Educational objectives and activities can and should be directed at both the cognitive and affective side of people at the same time to encourage maximum learning, growth, and change; that is, it is best if any given session has clearly articulated cognitive (thinking) and affective (feeling) objectives and activities. Often the same objective and activity can serve both cognitive and affective functions. It may be possible to address the psychomotor domain by including food preparation.

In the cognitive/knowing domain, educational activities should attempt to assist the intended audience to achieve more difficult learning tasks, such as application or evaluation (procedural knowledge or critical thinking skills), and not just the easier tasks, such as recalling information (factual knowledge). In the affective/

feeling domain, it is preferable to design activities that actively engage participants and assist them to contemplate and value the message to the point of being willing to try the recommendations. Too often, objectives are set to achieve the lower levels of audience engagement, such as just listening and receiving the message (through lectures, for example). **BOX 10-1** contains examples of learning objectives directed at determinants of behavior within the three domains.

Note on Writing Detailed, Specific Objectives

In the educational world, educational objectives are often referred to as "behavioral objectives," based on the premise that learning results in an observable response to a specific stimulus; that is, the achievement of each objective, whether cognitive or affective, needs to be demonstrated by a specific observable action (Bloom et al. 1956; Krathwohl et al. 1964; Anderson and Krathwohl 2000; Gronland and Brookhart 2008). The following elements are usually included:

1. The observable action expected of the learner.

2. The conditions under which the observable action is to be demonstrated. Thus, specific objectives will usually take the following form: Given _____ [name of the condition or stimulus], the learner (participant) will _____ [name of the desired observable action]. For example, "Given information on the government's MyPlate graphic for healthy eating, the participant will be able to place foods into the correct food groups."

3. The degree of mastery required is often added as a third element. In this case, the objective might be "Given information on the government's MyPlate graphic for healthy eating, the participant will be able to place 12 foods into the correct food groups with 80% accuracy."

You can follow this format and write detailed objectives if you wish. However, for nutrition education purposes, it is generally not necessary to follow this format slavishly. In addition, in practice, you may not need to specify the learning domains and levels within each domain for *each* educational objective. While it is desirable to do so, this process does take time and effort. You will need to judge to what degree this is necessary for your given session or intervention. However, it is very important to be aware of and to target the different domains and

---

BOX 10-1 Examples of Learning Objectives Directed at Determinants of Behavior Within the Three Domains

....

In each example, the objective is preceded by the following phrase: "At the end of the intervention (or session), the participants will be able to . . .". The way to measure the outcome is shown in parentheses for each objective.

Motivational Determinants

1. *Perceived risk*. Demonstrate understanding that a diet high in processed packaged snacks increases risk of heart disease (by correctly answering a questionnaire at the end of the intervention or session).
   Cognitive domain: Understanding level. *Affective domain:* Responding level.

2. *Concern for the problem or issue*. Demonstrate appreciation of their own susceptibility to heart disease (by naming people in their family who have died of heart disease and discussing how that made them feel).
   Affective domain: Responding level.

3. *Outcome expectations/perceived benefits*. Demonstrate the understanding that a diet high in fruits and vegetables reduces their risk of heart disease and cancer (by correctly answering a questionnaire at the end of the intervention or session).
   Cognitive domain: Understanding level. *Affective domain:* Responding level.

4. *Values*. Appreciate the importance of overcoming psychological barriers to reducing the number of highly processed, packaged snacks (by orally describing one barrier and listing one action the learner will take in the next week to overcome that barrier).
   Cognitive domain: Understanding level. *Affective domain:* Valuing level.

5. *Self-efficacy*. Demonstrate belief in their ability to prepare foods lower in fat (by proposing to bring in a lower-fat recipe to share with the group at the next session).
   Cognitive domain: Understanding level. *Affective domain:* Valuing level.

6. *Social influence*. Appreciate the role of peers in influencing food choices (by noting one instance in which the participant did not eat what peers ate and describing how that made the participant feel).
   Cognitive domain: Understanding level. *Affective domain:* Valuing level.

Facilitating Determinants: Facilitating the Ability to Take Action

1. *Knowledge*. Understand the dietary advice for reducing risk of cancer (by listing three of the relevant dietary guidelines without looking at materials).
   Cognitive domain: Remembering level.

2. *Skills*.

   a. *Cognitive*. Demonstrate ability to apply the recommendations from MyPlate or other national graphic (by comparing own 24-hour dietary intake to recommendations and describing implications for self).
      Cognitive domain: Application level.

   b. *Affective*. Demonstrate resistance to peer pressure to eat high-fat, high-calorie foods (by eating a salad at lunch and not the high-fat choice of peers and appropriately explaining/defending own choice).
      Cognitive domain: Evaluation level. *Affective domain:* Organization level.

   c. *Behavioral capability*. Demonstrate ability to stir-fry vegetables (by imitating demonstration in class by preparing identical dish at home).
      Cognitive domain: Understanding level. *Psychomotor domain:* Imitation level.

   d. *Self-regulation skills*. Engage in systematic planning to change their diet (by identifying a behavior that they wish to change, developing an action plan to make the change, self-monitoring the change, and sharing with the group their progress in attaining the goal).
      Cognitive domain: Evaluation level. *Affective domain:* Valuing level.

   e. Demonstrate satisfaction in achieving a personal dietary change goal (by rewarding self with seeing a movie).
      Affective domain: Valuing level.

3. *Social support*. Demonstrate ability to share feelings about chosen diet with friends and family and to seek support from them (by asking family to support their own vegetarian eating pattern).
   Cognitive domain: Comprehension level. *Affective domain:* Valuing level.

levels in each session and throughout the intervention to ensure that nutrition education activities are directed at a range of levels of difficulty, preferably going from the easiest to the most difficult, and that head, heart, and hands are all engaged.

Case Study: The DESIGN Procedure in Action

This chapter continues the case study of nutrition education for adolescents as an example for you to use as you complete your worksheets. Recall that although four behavior-change goals were chosen for the intervention, because of limited space, we have been focusing on only one behavior: encouraging youth to eat more fruits and vegetables. The intervention devotes two sessions to this behavior.

- *The general educational objectives* for the two sessions are shown in the Step 4 Indicate General Objectives case study worksheet at the end of this chapter. These general educational objectives address potential psychosocial determinants of the behavior changes targeted by the program, based on the theory model created for the intervention in Step 3.
- *The specific educational objectives* for each session or lesson are shown at the same time as the activities they generated in the Step 5 worksheets for the case study (located at the end of Chapters 11 and 12).

These objectives are based on each of the potential determinants of change from theory. For each of these specific educational objectives, the nutrition educator added information on the domain in which the educational activities should occur and the anticipated level of cognitive difficulty or affective engagement for the group for each activity within each domain.

Your Turn to Design Nutrition Education: Completing the Step 4 Indicate General Objectives Worksheet

Carefully review the theory model you created in Step 3. Use the Step 4 Indicate General Objectives Worksheet located at the end of Chapter 13 to write the general educational objectives directed at the key determinants of your model. If you are planning only one session, then you will have three to five general educational objectives. If you are planning a series of sessions on the same or related behaviors, with or without some ancillary activities such as newsletters, then you may have more. In Step 5, you will write specific objectives at the same time that you design appropriate activities based on these objectives. The same principles apply. These specific objectives will guide the selection or creation of each of the activities in your session(s).

Questions and Activities

1. Describe briefly three reasons why it is important to write educational objectives for nutrition education, no matter how brief.
2. For a given session or intervention, describe carefully the relationship between general educational objectives for an intervention or session and the potential determinants of behavior change.
3. Objectives are often described as being written in the cognitive, affective, and psychomotor domains of learning. Carefully summarize what these terms mean. Describe the differences between these domains. How do they guide what you do as a nutrition educator?
4. For practice, write general educational objectives for the following potential determinants of the behavior of increasing the intake of calcium-rich foods among teenage girls. For each objective, indicate the learning domain and level that you think is important to achieve to bring about the behavioral goal:
   - Outcome expectations/perceived benefits
   - Perceived self-efficacy
   - Personal action goals

References

Anderson, L. W., and D. R. Krathwohl, Eds. 2000. *A taxonomy for learning, teaching, and assessing: A revision of Bloom's taxonomy of educational objectives*. Boston: Pearson.

Bloom, B. S., M. D. Engelhart, E. J. Furst, W. H. Hill, and D. R. Krathwohl. 1956. *Taxonomy of educational objectives. Handbook I: Cognitive domain*. New York: David McKay.

Gronland, N. E., and S. M. Brookhart. 2008. *Gronland's writing instructional objectives*. 8th ed. Upper Saddle River, NJ: Prentice Hall.

Krathwohl, D. R., B. S. Bloom, and B. B. Masia. 1964. *Taxonomy of educational objectives: The classification of educational goals. Handbook II: Affective domain*. New York: David McKay.

Marzano, R. J., and J. S. Kendall. 2007. *The new taxonomy of educational objectives*. 2nd ed. Thousand Oaks, CA: Sage Publications.

University of Michigan. 1976. *The professional teachers handbook*. Ann Arbor: University of Michigan.

Nutrition Education DESIGN Procedure

D	E	S	I	G	N
Decide behavior(s)	**E**xplore determinants of change	**S**elect theory & clarify philosophy	**I**ndicate general objectives	**G**enerate plans	**N**ail down evaluation plan
Step 1	Step 2	Step 3	Step 4	Step 5	Step 6

Step 4: Indicate general objectives.

Translating your behavioral theory into educational objectives to guide your session planning is essential. Remind yourself of your behavior change goal(s) and use your theoretical framework as a guide to work through this step and develop general objectives for your session(s). These objectives will also guide your evaluation plan.

Note that you need one set of general objectives for each behavior change goal. If you are planning only one behavior change goal (e.g., to increase fruit and vegetable consumption) you will have only one set of general motivating and facilitating objectives, whether you devote one or several sessions to the same goal.

Use the Step 4 Indicate General Objectives worksheet to help you develop the overarching educational objectives for your one session or several sessions devoted to the same behavior as well as the practical considerations necessary for it to be a success.

> **Which of the behavior change goals from Step 1 do these general educational objectives address?**
>
> Students will increase fruit and vegetable consumption.

What general motivational objectives will guide your session(s) or intervention? First, list the motivational theoretical determinants you identified in Step 3 in the left column of the table, below. Then, in the right column, use the stem provided to write a general objective for each of the motivational determinants. Carefully consider which verb appropriately expresses your objective. Use the word banks provided on the following page to help you write your objectives.

Motivational Psychosocial Determinant	General Educational Objective Participants will be able to [verb]...
Perceived social norms	Participants will be able to persuasively argue to their peer group why they should eat more fruits and vegetables.
Perceived benefits/ positive outcome expectations	Participants will be able to describe the importance of eating a variety of fruits and vegetables.
Perceived risk/ negative outcome expectations	Participants will be able to recognize how far their fruit and vegetable intake is from recommendations.
Food preferences	Participants will be able to appreciate the taste of various fruits and vegetables.
Perceived barriers (self-efficacy)	Participants will be able to identify strategies to overcome perceived barriers to fruit and vegetable consumption.
Perceived social norms	Participants will be able to recognize the influence of peers in their snacking choices.

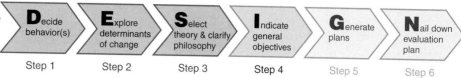

Nutrition Education DESIGN Procedure

Decide behavior(s) — Step 1
Explore determinants of change — Step 2
Select theory & clarify philosophy — Step 3
Indicate general objectives — Step 4
Generate plans — Step 5
Nail down evaluation plan — Step 6

What general facilitating objectives will guide your session(s) or intervention?

Now list the facilitating theoretical determinants and write a general objective for each. Continue to use the word banks to help you consider which verb appropriately expresses your objective.

Facilitating Psychosocial Determinant	General Educational Objective Participants will be able to [verb]...
Food and nutrition skills	Students will be able to prepare appealing fruit and vegetable snacks.
Behavioral capability/competence: Cognitive skills	Participants will be able to describe how to increase their fruit and vegetable consumption and variety.
Behavioral capability/competence: Behavioral skills	Participants will be able to prepare fruit and vegetable snacks.
Goal setting	Participants will be able to set and monitor goals to eat more and/or a greater variety of fruits and vegetables.
Self-efficacy	Participants will be able to have increased confidence in their ability to eat more and/or a greater variety of fruits and vegetables.

Cognitive Verbs	
Remember	List, record, state, define, name, describe, tell, recall
Understand	Explain, describe, summarize, classify, discuss, compare, illustrate
Apply	Sketch, perform, use, solve, construct, role-play, demonstrate, conduct
Analyze	Test, distinguish, critique, appraise, calculate, measure, debate
Evaluate	Review, appraise, justify, argue, conclude, assess, rate, defend
Create	Develop, plan, collect, build, construct, create, design, integrate

Affective Verbs
Express, value, feel, appreciate, care, defend, challenge, judge, question, adopt, advocate, justify, cooperate, persuade, approve, choose, endorse, dispute

Psychomotor Verbs
Cut, prepare, cook, choose, measure, demonstrate, assemble, produce, adjust, locate, arrange, conduct, manipulate, perform, sort, draw, construct

Step 5: Generating Educational Plans: A Focus on Enhancing Motivation for Behavior Change and Taking Action

OVERVIEW

This chapter and the next provide guidance on how to create motivating and effective educational activities from determinants and behavior change strategies and to sequence them appropriately to generate educational plans ready for use with groups or through other channels. The focus of this chapter is on creating and sequencing activities that increase awareness, promote contemplation, and enhance motivation to take action or make changes in behavior. The information in Chapters 3 and 4 will help you with this step in the design process. The next chapter focuses on creating activities to increase knowledge and build skills.

CHAPTER OUTLINE

- Framework for creating theory-based nutrition education activities
- Translating behavioral theory into educational practice: determinants, behavior change strategies, educational activities, and educational plans
- Gaining audience interest and engagement
- Using behavior change strategies to create educational activities to enhance motivation for behavior change
- Organizing and sequencing educational activities

- for delivery with the "4 Es": The educational or lesson plan
- Exploring other audience characteristics and intervention resource considerations
- Generating the educational plan: the nuts and bolts
- Case study: the DESIGN Procedure in practice
- Your turn to design nutrition education: completing the Step 5 Generate Educational Plans worksheet

LEARNING OBJECTIVES

At the end of the chapter, you should be able to:

- Recognize the importance of using a systematic instructional design process for designing and sequencing behavior change strategies and educational activities
- Describe the kinds of theory-based behavior change strategies to address potential determinants of target behaviors that focus on

increasing awareness, promoting contemplation, and enhancing motivation
- Design specific educational activities or learning experiences to make practical the theory-based educational strategies
- Sequence the educational objectives and activities to create an educational plan using the 4 Es

Framework for Creating Theory-Based Nutrition Education Activities

Step 5 in the DESIGN Procedure brings us to the heart of nutrition education: designing messages and activities that are engaging, fun, relevant to the intended audience, and designed to achieve your intervention's behavior change goals. Many nutrition educators find this step to be the most creative and enjoyable part of nutrition education planning. The DESIGN Procedure provides a framework for planning, which then allows you the freedom to express your creativity as a nutrition educator.

Imagine you arrive in the middle of a parent association nutrition education session requested by parents of children in a school in a low-income neighborhood. The parents are all very busily engaged at different tables measuring out how much sugar is in various drinks that are common in their neighborhood. The nutrition educator has supplied empty bottles with labels on them. This generates expressions of surprise about the amount of sugar in these drinks. The parents discuss why they like the drinks. The educator then has parents at each table calculate the cost of these drinks, per drink, then per day, week, and year of consuming them. Again, there are expressions of surprise from all over, and exclamations of "I'm not going to drink that anymore—only on special occasions," and "I am going to drink water instead," and so forth. The session, of course, continues. But what have you witnessed? You have seen considerable engagement of the audience, high motivation, and expressions of intention to act on their motivations. We wish for all our educational sessions to be so well received!

Step 5 is the time to brainstorm numerous ideas for translating the objectives you stated in Step 4 into specific objectives and exciting and meaningful activities. This is the time to choose ways to communicate food and nutrition content that will enhance the motivation of your audience to want to take action on the behavioral goals of your sessions. For these activities to be appropriate, you will base them on the thorough understanding of the audience you acquired in Steps 1 and 2. Keep in mind, of course, the context of their lives in terms of family resources, community, and culture. To the extent possible, involve the audience in the process of developing the activities.

From these activities you will generate an **educational plan** (or **lesson plan**) for each session, which is a plan for arranging into an appropriate sequence the educational activities that you will conduct with any group, in both non-formal settings such as community centers or outpatient clinics and formal settings such as schools. Educational plans, in modified form, also guide educational content and activities conducted through other channels (e.g., newsletters, Internet postings, posters). As you can see in **FIGURE 11-1**, the products of this step are a series of educational plans for group sessions or other indirect educational activities with your intended audience linking determinants, objectives, and activities.

In **FIGURE 11-2**, we present an overview framework for how to link determinants of behavior change to educational objectives and **educational strategies** when designing nutrition education. During the *motivational component or phase*, your audience members may be considering action, or they may be in the process of deciding on taking action. The most prominent influences or determinants of their decision are shown in Figure 11-2. The main *motivational educational objectives* are to enhance motivation and activate decision-making. The **behavior change strategies** that you will employ to achieve these objectives are shown in the two darker boxes. You can see that these strategies are based on determinants that help the audience understand why-to take action, such as perceptions of risks and benefits, barriers to taking action, or self-efficacy. During the *action component or phase*, your audience members are likely to be either initiating action or maintaining their behavior changes. The main *educational objectives* for this component are to facilitate the ability to take action or to strengthen self-regulation or self-direction skills for taking charge of their lives. The *behavior change strategies* that you employ to achieve these objectives are shown in the two lighter strategy boxes and include such how-to procedures as goal setting and knowledge acquisition.

To cover the large number of useful behavior change strategies available to nutrition educators, and the numerous practical educational activities that can be created, as shown in Figure 11-2, we devote two chapters to them. In this chapter we focus on designing activities, based on determinants of motivation, that are engaging and meaningful to the intended audience and increase their interest in and commitment to taking action on the

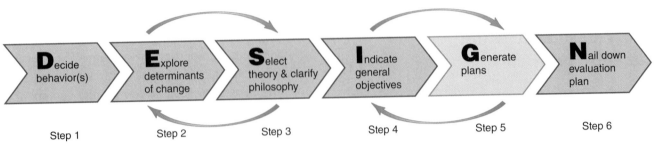

Inputs: Collecting the Assessment Data		Outputs: Designing the Theory-Based Intervention			Outcomes: Evaluation Plan
Tasks: • **Decide** behavior change goal(s) of the intervention, based on: • analyzing issues and behaviors of concern for audience	*Tasks:* • **Explore** determinants of behavior change based on a variety of data sources	*Tasks:* • **Select** theory and draw intervention-specific theory model • Clarify educational philosophy • Articulate perspectives on content	*Tasks:* • **Indicate** general objectives for each determinant in your theory model	*Tasks:* • **Generate** educational plans: • Educational activities to address all determinants in theory model • Sequence for implementation using the 4 Es	*Tasks:* • **Nail down** evaluation plan • Select methods and questions to evaluate outcomes • Plan process evaluation • Create questions to measure how implementation went
Products: Statement of intervention behavior change goal(s)	*Products:* List of determinants to address in the intervention	*Products:* Theory model for intervention Statement of educational philosophy Statement of content perspectives	*Products:* A general objective for each determinant in the theory model	*Products:* Educational plans that link determinants and educational activities to achieve behavior change or action goal(s)	*Products:* List of evaluation methods and questions Procedures and measures for process evaluation

FIGURE 11-1 Nutrition Education DESIGN Procedure: Generate plans—Step 5: Motivational.

behaviors targeted by your intervention. These are the catalysts of action. In Chapter 12 we focus on designing activities that will facilitate the ability of group participants to take action or maintain the behavior changes they have chosen to make. *Numerous behavior change strategies and potential meaningful activities are provided as a reference; you will choose from this universe those that are relevant to your intervention.*

Any given educational plan for groups or related indirect venues, such as printed or visual materials or computer or Internet activities, can consist of activities that are either primarily motivational, primarily skill-building, or both, depending on the objectives that you select. In most cases, however, a given educational plan for group sessions or related materials will address both motivational objectives and skill-building objectives.

Examples of lesson plans for our case study are shown at the end of this chapter.

LOW-INCOME AUDIENCES

Special consideration should be given to low-income audiences when you design activities, given the challenges facing them (described in **BOX 11-1**). They often experience financial limitations caused by low resources, lack of time because many work long hours, and lack of availability of quality healthful foods at affordable prices in their neighborhoods. All of these factors will influence what they will be able to do. In addition, they are also often low in literacy. Thus, it is important in Step 2 to find out their preferences in terms of learning activities.

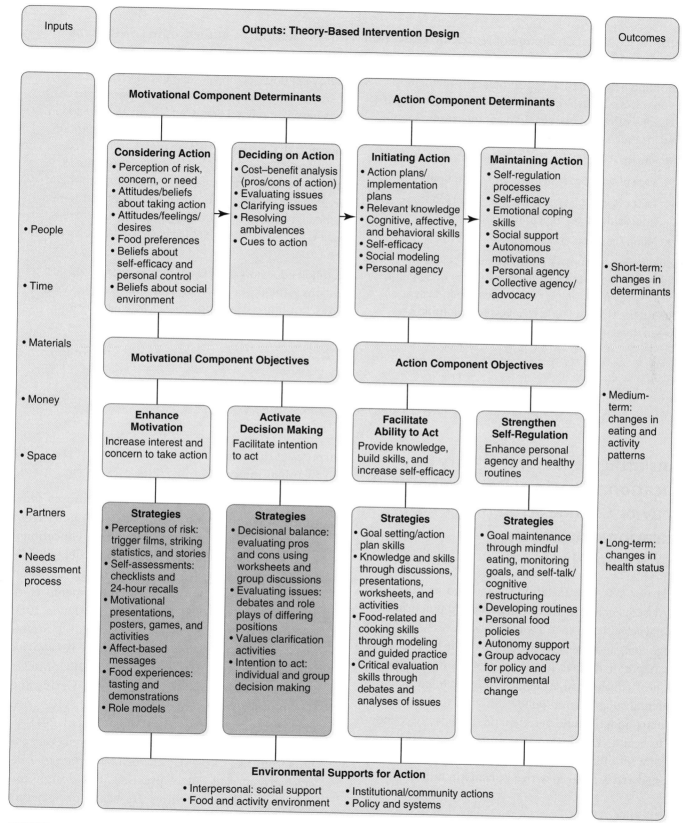

FIGURE 11-2 Conceptual framework for translating behavioral theory into behavior change strategies: Motivational phase educational strategies.

BOX 11-1 **Special Challenge of Nutrition Education with Low-Resources Audiences in Low-Income Neighborhoods**

Adopting healthful eating patterns is difficult for most people. It is especially difficult for low-resources individuals for a variety of reasons. Some of the reasons identified in studies include the following:

- Financial limitations caused by low resources
- Lack of time because many work long hours
- Lack of availability of quality healthful foods at affordable prices in neighborhood
- Family customs and habits

Low-income consumers want to ensure that no one in the family goes hungry. They thus strive to get enough food energy for all at low cost. An economic analysis of diets in the U.S. has found an inverse relationship between the energy density of foods, defined as available energy per unit weight (kilocalories per gram) and energy cost (dollars per kilocalorie). This means that diets based on refined grains, added sugars, and added fats cost less than the diets recommended by nutrition educators that are based on lean meats, fish, fresh vegetables, and fruits. On a *calorie per dollar* basis, bread, cookies, and even chocolate are cheaper than fruits and vegetables. One study found that adding fat and sweets to the diet *lowered* overall adjusted diet costs, whereas adding fruits and vegetables *increased* overall adjusted diet costs.

Nutrition educators must keep these economic considerations in mind when working with low-resources audiences. Institutional- and policy-level activities are also essential to complement group-level activities.

Sources: MacKinnon, C., G. W. Auld, and S. Baker. 2014. Best practices in direct nutrition education for low-income audiences: Program design and delivery. *FASEB Journal* 28:625.1; and Drewnowski, A. 2004. Obesity and the food environment: Dietary energy density and diet costs. *American Journal of Preventive Medicine* 27(3, Suppl. 1):154–162.

Translating Behavioral Theory into Educational Practice: Determinants, Behavior Change Strategies, Educational Activities, and Educational Plans

The major task in translating theory into practice is to design, sequence, and deliver theory-based practical educational activities in such a way as to achieve the behavior change goals and educational objectives you have selected.

Chapter 1 defines nutrition education as a combination of educational strategies, accompanied by environmental supports and policy, designed to facilitate the voluntary adoption and maintenance of behaviors conducive to health. This means that nutrition education consists of a set of learning activities that are systematically designed and organized with a purpose in mind.

CLARIFYING TERMS

The terms *strategies, activities, learning experiences, methods, procedures,* and *techniques* are often used interchangeably in the health education literature. For the purposes of this book, the following terms are used with the meanings indicated:

- *Behavior change strategies* are brief phrases indicating ways to operationalize determinants from theory (i.e., theory constructs) so that educational means can be used to address them in order to facilitate behavior change. These strategies are based on evidence and on ongoing research (Contento et al. 1995; Katz et al. 2008; Thompson and Ravia 2011; Waters et al. 2011; Wong and Stewart 2013). Strategies are similar to what are referred to as *behavior change techniques (BCTs)* (Michie et al. 2011; Michie et al. 2013), *procedures* (Baranowski, Cerin, and Baranowski 2009; Baranowski et al. 2010; Diep et al. 2014), or *methods* (Bartholomew et al. 2011)
- *Educational activities* or *learning experiences* are the numerous ways in which the *behavior change strategies* are carried out in practice. The design and delivery of these activities are based on learning theory and instructional design or teaching theory from the field of education. These are described in detail in Chapter 15; please read in order to help you with this step of the DESIGN Procedure. To provide

an example: the psychosocial determinant of *perceived risk* for osteoporosis may be a determinant (motivator) of eating more calcium-rich foods to reduce its risk. The *behavior change strategy* chosen may be "provide information about risks." The practical *educational activities* or learning experiences might involve showing trigger films, pictures, charts, and striking national or local statistics; telling personal stories; or having the audience identify those in their families who have osteoporosis and describe their experiences.

■ *The educational plan (or lesson plan)* is an outline or description of the step-by-step procedure showing how the educational activities or learning experiences are arranged in an appropriate and logical sequence for use in delivering the intervention to the group or through some other venue.

THE RELATIONSHIP OF BEHAVIOR CHANGE STRATEGIES TO DETERMINANTS AND BEHAVIOR CHANGE

As noted before, behavior change strategies are broad statements of the techniques or procedures that can be used to bring about changes in theory-based determinants, which, in turn, lead to changes in behavior. Behavior change strategies are used in group settings or through other indirect educational methods to facilitate behavior change. **FIGURE 11-3** shows the relationships among these terms.

SELECTING BEHAVIOR CHANGE STRATEGIES

Many behavior change strategies are provided in this chapter as a reference. You will select from among them only those strategies that address the determinants of change from the theory model you created for the

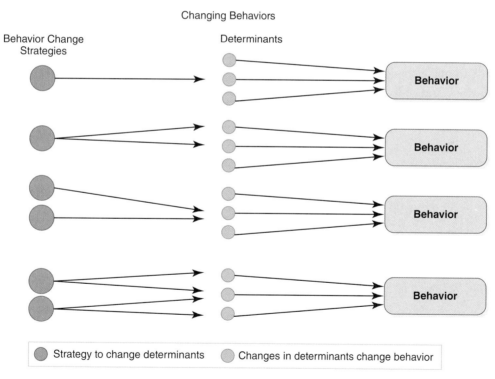

Changing Behaviors

- Changes in determinants change behavior
- Behavior change strategies change determinants
- One strategy may change one or more determinants
- Two strategies may change one or more determinants
- Educational activities are based on behavior change strategies

FIGURE 11-3 Using behavior change strategies (and nutrition education activities based on them) to change determinants, which then leads to behavior change.

intervention in Step 3. There are many overlaps among theories, and many of these strategies will operationalize determinants from several theories.

Kinds of Behavior Change Strategies

The behavior change strategies from theory that are most useful for the motivational component of nutrition education are described in this chapter. Those most useful for the action component are described in the next chapter.

People, of course, are integrated wholes—thinking, feeling, and action are not linearly organized but closely interconnected. For example, learning new skills, such as cooking, may help people act on their motivations; at the same time, the new skills may increase sense of self-efficacy, which is likely to enhance motivation. Furthermore, the immediate social environment, such as family and friends, may provide social support for change but may also prove to be a barrier to change. In addition, individuals who attend your sessions are probably those who are more interested and concerned. However, it is often the case that individuals attend sessions because others have suggested or required that they attend or because they think they are ready to make changes but are not. Hence, assisting them to review and reflect on their motivations and values is still useful and important.

THE RELATIONSHIP OF BEHAVIOR CHANGE STRATEGIES TO EDUCATIONAL ACTIVITIES

We use principles from learning theory and instructional design theory in the field of education to actually create activities to deliver nutrition education that is based on social psychological strategies for motivating and facilitating dietary change. (See Chapter 15.) Stated another way, we use learning theory and the principles of good instruction and apply them to all three domains of human learning to convert strategies into educational activities to deliver our nutrition education. (See description in Chapter 10.) The sequence of developing and delivering our nutrition education sessions can be summarized as follows and is shown in the diagram below:

Choose behavioral change goal → Identify psychosocial theory-based determinants of behavior change → Select behavior change strategies → Create educational objectives and activities based on learning theory and instructional theory from education.

Gaining Audience Interest and Engagement

Designing activities to enhance motivation involves thinking about how to engage the audience with whom

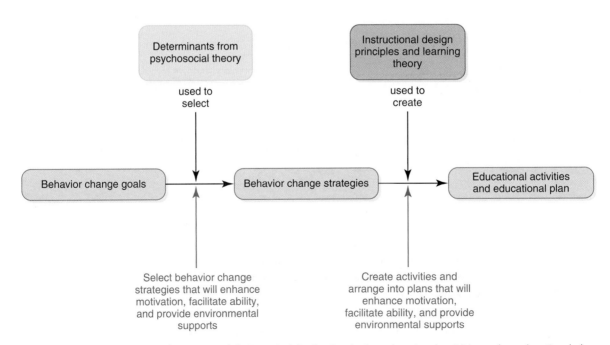

Roles of psychosocial theory and instructional design principles for developing educational activities and an educational plan.

you work; that is, how to engage their interest, passion, and willingness to consider and take action on the behavior change goals that have been selected for your sessions or intervention. You may recall the metaphor that Haidt (2006) and Heath and Heath (2010) use about making changes in our lives: our emotional side is like a 6-ton elephant, on top of which sits our analytical side like a rider. (See Chapter 3 for more detail.) The rider in us knows the direction to go, but we need to engage the elephant in us, where our motivation and power resides, if we are going to get anywhere. How to do that is the subject of this chapter.

INFORMATION VERSUS LEARNING EXPERIENCES

Before we plunge into designing the activities, let us examine what we mean by activities that you will create, intended to *increase learning* and *change behaviors*. Influential educators such as Dewey (1929) and Tyler (1949) make a clear distinction between *presentations of content* and actual *learning experiences*. A learning experience is the interaction between learners and external conditions through which learning takes place. Learning takes place through the active behavior of learners. Education is what nutrition educators do; learning is what the program participants experience and accomplish. Mere educator intentions, however, will not result in learning, just as mere presentation of information may not result in learning. The dynamic engagement of the participants with the content is essential. This is the basis of all good education and is emphasized in learner-centered education.

What Do We Mean By a Learning Experience?

Learning does not mean simply memorizing facts and figures or cognitive information and skills such as the number of calories in a teaspoon of sugar or how to read a food label. Learning is about an interaction between intervention participants and the activities educators have designed. The desired result is active contemplation about issues, change in how participants view the world, examination of their values, and altering of their expectations, attitudes, and feelings about food and nutrition, and, indeed, their actions. Learning takes place through many venues—formal, non-formal, and informal.

This is where the true challenge of nutrition education design rests. It calls on you not only to have a firm grasp of food and nutrition content and psychosocial theory, but also an understanding of educational principles to design creative, productive, and meaningful experiences to address determinants of behavior change in order to bring about specified behavior change goals and educational objectives. This involves creative risk taking on the one hand and careful organization on the other hand.

CREATING OPPORTUNITIES FOR ACTIVE PARTICIPATION AND LEARNING

When designing different activities, keep in mind the importance of creating opportunities for hands-on, active participation within all of your activities. This is because generally people remember:

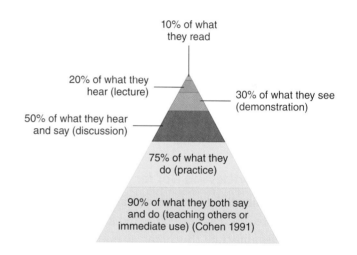

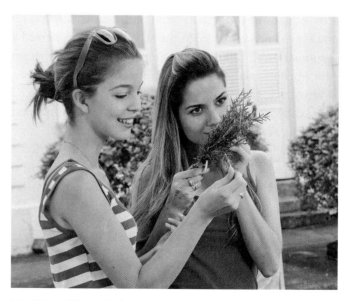

Identifying different herbs is an engaging, hands-on activity.
© Cultura Creative/Alamy.

Activities for Participants Should Be Minds-On as Well as Hands-On

A major way to encourage active participation is with the use of *hands-on* activities. Hands-on activities enhance motivation by giving participants a sense of involvement with the learning. For example, have members of the audience spoon out the amount of fat in various fast foods or the amount of sugar in beverages, rather than tell them. Have teens calculate the amount of money they spend on snacks, and so forth. They will remember the information more vividly.

However, you must be careful to ensure that these activities are also *minds-on* activities; that is, they serve an educational purpose that is clearly relevant for your educational objectives. Thus, if you think you have created a wonderful activity that will be great for your audience, ask yourself: which of my stated objective does it serve? If none, then drop the activity. On the other hand, if you still believe it will provide a truly important learning experience for your group in relation to your behavior change goal(s), then take another look at your educational objectives and perhaps your theory model. Maybe the objectives need to be revised and the determinants of behavior carefully re-analyzed.

Hands-On Activities Are Not for Everyone

Your assessment will let you know what kinds of learning experiences are appropriate or preferred for your audience. Two examples illustrate this point. A nutrition educator who had used a particular hands-on activity with considerable effectiveness was surprised and dismayed when, after explaining the activity to an immigrant audience, no one moved or wanted to do the activity. They preferred a demonstration. In another example, a team of nutrition educators planned a set of activities for a lunchtime session at a worksite. These were theory-based and had worked well with other audiences. This group of businessmen hated the activities. They had been diagnosed with high serum cholesterol, were highly motivated, and wanted a brief presentation and tip sheets so they could return to their desks in 20 minutes. Thus while hands-on activities are good in principle, you must check with your audience for their preferred learning styles.

Discussions and Facilitated Dialogues: Participants Both Hear and Say

You can also engage learners in *discussion* among themselves in pairs, triads, or small groups about such concerns

as why it is so hard to get their children to eat vegetables, why it is so hard to carry out their intentions to eat more healthfully on a low budget, or how to make food choices in a manner that promotes local agriculture. Such an approach encourages cooperative learning, which research shows is more likely to result in people deliberating the issues in light of their life circumstances, examining their own attitudes, and desiring to learn more (Johnson and Johnson 1987). However, note that educational objectives and plans are still needed to guide the learning activities. Without structure and purpose, audience members are likely to leave frustrated.

Facilitated dialogue is based on active exchange between the nutrition educator as facilitator of the group and group participants. It avoids lecturing, instead focusing on open-ended questions, active listening, and respect for the ideas of everyone in the group to promote active participation and to weave a meaningful learning experience for all. Educational plans are still needed to provide focus. Here, structure and a clear purpose are essential, too. All of these methods are described in greater detail in Chapters 15 and 17.

> Many behavior change strategies and educational activities based on learning theory and instructional design/teaching theory used to deliver them are provided here as a reference. You will select from among them only those strategies that address the determinants of change from the theory model you created for the intervention in Step 3.

Using Behavior Change Strategies to Create Educational Activities to Enhance Motivation for Behavior Change

Strategies designed to enhance motivation focus on stimulating interest, enthusiasm, or concern and on provoking thought. These strategies assist individuals to become aware of critical nutrition or food-system–related issues; better understand their own needs, wants, feelings, motivations, and factors that seem to control their behaviors; reflect on the important role of their families, communities and culture on their food-related behaviors; actively contemplate the issues; resolve ambivalences; and then choose to take action—or not to do so—given their life circumstances, which are important for everyone (Blake et al. 2011; Sobal and Bisogni, 2009; Sobal et al. 2012).

SUMMARY TABLE OF BEHAVIOR CHANGE STRATEGIES AND EDUCATIONAL ACTIVITIES

TABLE 11-1 lists the theory-based behavior change strategies derived from determinants of change that are related to motivation and provides examples of possible practical

Table 11-1 Linking Theory Determinants, Behavior Change Strategies, and Practical Educational Activities

Determinants of Behavior Change (Theory Constructs)	Behavior Change Strategies*	Practical Educational Activities, Learning Experiences, Content, or Messages
Perceived risk/negative outcome expectations HBM SCT HAPA	■ Provide information about negative outcomes/risks of behavior (TTM: Consciousness-raising and dramatic relief)	Trigger films, pictures, charts, striking national or local statistics, personal stories, role plays, demonstrations; clear image of threat (e.g., film clips on effect of high–saturated-fat diet in clogging arteries); demonstration using plastic tube clogged with fat and colored water to show blockage
	■ Provide opportunity for personalized self-assessments compared to recommendations (personalize risk) (TTM: Self-reevaluation)	Participants complete self-assessment checklists, food or activity records, or recalls, and then compare to recommendations such as Dietary Guidelines
Outcome expectations/ perceived benefits HBM SCT HAPA TRA Goal	■ Provide information about positive outcomes or consequences of behavior/ perceived benefits (general) ■ Provide information about positive outcomes or consequences of behavior/ perceived benefits (personal)	Presentations, visuals, messages, activities, or demonstrations of scientific evidence regarding diet–health relationships or diet-food system/environment relationships Discussion of benefits of personal behavior change to personal health, family welfare, or community, and benefits to food system/environment
Perceived barriers/self-efficacy HBM SCT TRA	■ Prompt identification of perceived barriers ■ Reframe perception of barriers	Brainstorming; discussion of barriers and ways to overcome them; decrease perceived difficulty of doing behavior
	■ Reframe perception of confidence to carry out behavior	Discussions of successes to increase confidence in being able to do behavior
Perceived behavioral control SCT HAPA TRA Goal SDT	■ Reframe perception of control	Reflection questions, visuals, discussions of degree of control over behavior: correction of misperceptions
Affective attitudes/emotions SCT TRA Goal	■ Promote reflection on anticipated emotions/feelings	Attitude clarification activity—provide attitude statements for participants to select and discuss; explore feelings related to food, breastfeeding, or a recent diagnosis of diabetes; emotion-based messaging
	■ Build on personal meanings	Group discussion or written activity to explore special meanings of food to individuals (these are often desired outcomes); link to intervention behavior change goals
	■ Promote reflection on potential anticipated regret	Explore consequences of not taking action through discussion, visuals
Food preferences TRA SCT Goal	■ Provide direct experience with healthful food ■ Provide repeated exposure	Food tastings, demonstrations, cooking
Perceived social norms and expectations TRA SCT Goal	■ Stimulate reflection on others' expectations and approval ■ Reframe perceived norms	View and analyze print, TV, and online ads, and messages of videos and films; analyze important others' expectations and approval or disapproval of how person should behave Reframe the importance of these norms

(Continues)

Table 11-1 Linking Theory Determinants, Behavior Change Strategies, and Practical Educational Activities (Continued)

Determinants of Behavior Change (Theory Constructs)	Behavior Change Strategies*	Practical Educational Activities, Learning Experiences, Content, or Messages
Descriptive norms TRA SCT Goal	■ Promote exploration of beliefs about others' behaviors and attitudes ■ Promote exploration of cultural practices	Provide statistics, video clips, and activities to explore whether the behavior in question is or is not common Activities, films, and discussion questions to explore cultural practices
Self-identity TRA SCT	■ Stimulate reflection on self-identity (TTM: Self-reevaluation)	Written activities, with sharing where appropriate; provocative statements or scenarios: to prompt exploration of self-identity in terms of health, environmental sustainability, culture, etc. Also explore discrepancies between ideal self and ought-to-be self versus actual self in relation to food and eating.
Personal and moral norms TRA	■ Prompt reflection on personal and moral norms	Provocative scenarios and discussion questions about personal responsibilities and moral obligations
Habit TRA SCT	■ Provide confrontation with automatic behaviors	Checklists of current practices; self-observation tool to bring to consciousness automatic behaviors, habits, or routines
	■ Provide cues to action	Physical cues (refrigerator magnets), mass media cues (cafeteria signage), or digital technology reminders
Behavioral intention/goal intention SCT HAPA TRA Goal	■ Initiate analysis of decisional balance/ pros and cons of action or change	Worksheets or discussions to analyze pros and cons of behavior change and action; provide choice opportunities
	■ Promote values clarification	Values clarification worksheets for individuals or group activities in deciding whether or not to take action
	■ Encourage resolving resistance and ambivalences	Imagery activities, authentic discussion to resolve resistance and ambivalences
	■ Assist intention formation	Create easy-to-use check-off action plans, or have individuals create behavior change intention statements
	■ Create forum for group decision and public commitment (TTM: Self-liberation)	Group discussion followed by group decision on specific goals for action; stimulate pledging and public commitment

Note: HBM = health belief model; TRA = the reasoned action approach/theory of planned behavior and extensions; SCT = social cognitive theory; SDT = self-determination theory; HAPA = health action process approach model; Goal = goal model of goal-directed behavior; SR = self-regulation models; TTM = transtheoretical model

Behavior change strategies are similar to *behavior change techniques* (Michie et al. 2013), and *intervention procedures* (Baranowski et al. 2010).

educational activities or learning experiences that derive from them. From among the strategies, choose those that are part of the theory model you created in Step 3 and are appropriate for your targeted behavior and intended audience.

The following text describes these strategies and activities in greater detail. For example, for the *determinant* "risk perception," a *behavior change strategy* is "provide information about negative outcomes of behavior/risks" and the *practical educational activities* that help the audience confront the risks might include trigger films, striking national or local statistics, or personal stories.

BEHAVIOR CHANGE STRATEGIES AND EDUCATIONAL ACTIVITIES FOR THE THEORY DETERMINANT OF RISK PERCEPTIONS

Several theories propose that a sense of concern about an issue, a perception of personal risk, or understandings about the negative impact of current behaviors is important for individuals to be in a state of readiness to act. Theories described in this book include the health belief model, social cognitive theory, and the health action process approach. Research suggests that although such perceived risk or concern may not be the most immediate or direct determinant of behavior change in many cases, it is often a necessary and important first step. It has been suggested that threat or fear may be more useful for taking precautions against future problems than for dealing with existing problems. The strategies discussed here are similar to those designed to address the consciousness-raising and dramatic relief/emotional arousal processes of change in the transtheoretical model.

Behavior Change Strategy: Provide Information About Negative Outcomes of Behavior or Risk

When using the risk perception approach, the first part of the message is designed to create a motivation to avoid risk or danger.

Practical educational activities might include:

- *Stimulating information*: Trigger films, pictures, charts, striking national or local statistics, personal stories, and other confrontation or consciousness-raising strategies can be used to bring to life and make relevant issues of concern based on scientific evidence, such as the increase in obesity rates or breastfeeding rates, increasing portion sizes, bone loss, and metabolic syndrome in adolescents. Such activities can also be used to bring other issues to awareness, such as the rate of loss of farm land, how much school lunch food is thrown away daily, or the amount of disposable service materials (e.g., paper plates, sporks) that is thrown away each day from the school. (Students could also do a study to find out.) Visuals are especially powerful, such as pictures or actual food products (packages only), to show the portion sizes of various food products and beverages served in movie theaters, fast food outlets, and elsewhere. Media campaigns are especially useful here.
- *Messages about actions*: The second part of the message should be designed to show that people can take specific actions that will reduce the threat or danger and should provide exact instructions for when, how, and where to take action.

Behavior Change Strategy: Provide Opportunity for Personalized Self-Assessments Compared to Recommendations

Self-assessment of food-related behaviors that is personalized and compared with recommendations can be an effective motivational activity as a starting point for nutrition education. People love to find out about themselves!

Accurate self-assessment of risk is key: people are often not aware of their own dietary intake status and do not perceive a need to change. They often have an optimistic bias. Knowing about their actual behaviors can help them become more interested in deliberation of issues and more motivated. Such personalized feedback may also counteract the tendency to be optimistically biased and encourage individuals to consider changes in their dietary behaviors based on their true risk.

Practical educational activities might include:

- *Checklists*: Individuals can complete checklists that provide information specific to the intervention's behavior change goals, such as how many fruits and vegetables they are actually consuming, the number of sweetened beverages or milk products consumed in a day, or how many times they eat breakfast in a week.

  In the Best Bones Forever! campaign from the Office on Women's Health, U.S. Department of Health and Human Services (http://www.bestbonesforever.gov), girls can complete a "How strong are your bone health habits?" quiz online to find out how they are doing in terms of diet and physical activity related to bone health, or a "Are you building your best bones forever?" quiz to find out how much they know about bone health. The website is colorful and motivating, and the quizzes are engaging. The participant gets a score and action recommendations. **NUTRITION EDUCATION IN ACTION 11-1** shows some of the questions in the "Are you building your best bones forever?" quiz.

  Checklists can also be devised to see how "green" individuals' food shopping practices are (based on where the food comes from or its degree of packaging). Or a checklist, with a scoring system, can be devised for positive behaviors that contribute to nutritional well-being. Group members can also complete short instruments that provide them with information on their own stage of readiness to make changes in their diet.
- *Health risk appraisals*: Health risk appraisals are examples of self-assessments. As noted before, personal feedback must be accompanied by information on effective actions that individuals can take to deal with the threat or by information on potentially better alternative behaviors.
- *24-hour food recalls as an educational activity*: Here, ask the group to complete a 24-hour food intake

NUTRITION EDUCATION IN ACTION 11-1 **The Best Bones Forever Quiz: A Motivational Self-Assessment**

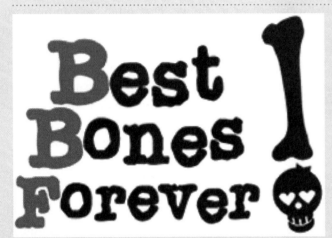

Office on Women's Health, U.S. Department of Health and Human Services. Best Bones Forever! http://www.bestbonesforever.gov.

Are you building your Best Bones Forever?

Is your relationship with your Mom amazing, so-so, or a never-ending tug of war? Take this quiz to find out.

1. You're having a sleepover with your BFFs. What snacks do you have on hand?
   a. Chips and sodas of course!
   b. Ice cream with your favorite toppings.
   c. Chocolate milk and calcium-fortified tortillas stuffed with melted cheese.

2. Where do you head after school?
   a. Straight to the computer to IM all your friends.
   b. Ugh, too much homework! You walk the dog then get to work.
   c. Depends on the season—soccer in the fall and track in the spring.

3. It's a gorgeous Saturday afternoon. How do you spend it with your family?

   a. Shopping! Those killer boots are on sale, and you have to have them.
   b. You agree to a quick game of basketball while your computer is downloading your fave band's latest CD.
   c. Going on a long hike.

4. You're in the lunch line. What do you pick?
   a. Nothing. You and your friends always go to the vending machines.
   b. Just low-fat milk. You brought your lunch.
   c. A healthy salad, baked potato with cheese, and chocolate milk for dessert.

5. Drinking milk gives you a stomachache. What do you eat or drink for the calcium your bones need to grow strong?
   a. You don't worry about it. Who cares about bones, anyway?
   b. You eat ice cream . . . a lot.
   c. Your mom buys lactose-reduced milk and makes sure you get lots of other yummy foods with calcium, like fortified orange juice and broccoli.

6. You're running late for school. What do you do for breakfast?
   a. Nothing. You skip it as usual.
   b. Breakfast is a must to keep you awake, so you grab a cereal bar and a banana for the road.
   c. You know breakfast is the best time to get the calcium and vitamin D your bones need, so you make a quick smoothie with low-fat milk and yogurt and berries.

Office on Women's Health, U.S. Department of Health and Human Services. Best Bones Forever! http://www.bestbonesforever.gov/fun/quizzes_building.htm

recall, and then have members individually compare their intakes with the MyPlate recommendations. Or, you can analyze the intakes of the group and use the average data as the starting point for nutrition education. For example, you can collect such data during your needs analysis process in Step 1, calculate the averages, and display them in a handout or slide when you meet with the group. This is particularly useful if the group is a low-literacy audience. When time permits and the level of education enables people to do so, have people analyze their own data: self-analysis is preferable.

- *Pedometers*: In the area of physical activity, information from pedometers or physical activity monitors can be very motivating. Inexpensive models can be used for this purpose.

■ *Community self-assessments*: Self-assessments can be modified to involve assessment of relevant community or organizational behaviors and practices. Members of an organization or community can do an assessment about food-related practices and resources to provide themselves with a true picture of the extent of risk or the severity of an issue in the community. For example, children can first do a 24-hour food recall on themselves in terms of the packaging they disposed of at each eating occasion. Then, they can investigate how much packaging their school throws out after each lunch, from which they can calculate the amount disposed of by all schools in their city or in the United States.

BEHAVIOR CHANGE STRATEGIES AND EDUCATIONAL ACTIVITIES FOR THEORY DETERMINANT OF POSITIVE OUTCOME EXPECTATIONS OR PERCEIVED BENEFITS

Behavior Change Strategy: Provide Information About Positive Outcomes of Behavior or Perceived Benefits (General and Personal)

Motivational communication focuses on making the case for the positive outcomes or benefits of given behaviors, which are powerful motivators of behavior because they are the basis of cognitive or injunctive attitudes, and thus have an impact on intentions and the formation of goals. (See Chapter 4.) This determinant is common to most theories.

Positive Outcomes or Benefits Are Reasons for Taking Action Based on Evidence and Are Personally Meaningful

Information about desirable outcomes is usually stated in the form of reasons for the behavior change or action; hence this book refers to it as *why-to* knowledge. The reasons can be based on:

■ Health benefits based on scientific or other kinds of evidence for the effectiveness of the behavior change or action
■ Food system–related benefits, also based on data or evidence
■ Benefits that are of personal importance to individuals
■ Other benefits for taking action

Your role is to make a strong case for the reasons your audience might want to consider as they contemplate making changes. It is important for the reasons to be accurate, evidence-based where appropriate, and personally meaningful to the audience.

Developing Effective Activities and Messages Using the Elaboration Likelihood Model

A focus on positive outcomes for taking action is useful not only for group sessions, but also for other related channels such as printed materials, visuals, and mass media campaigns. Here the elaboration likelihood model (ELM) of communication can be especially useful (Petty and Cacioppo 1986; Petty et al. 2009). This model proposes that individuals differ in their ability and motivation to process educational messages thoughtfully. (See discussion in Chapter 4.) Hence, nutrition education messages need to take into account the recipients' *ability* to process the messages and their *motivation* to do so. While simply providing arguments or reasons for taking action is important, the quality of the arguments is likely to increase effectiveness. The way you express the positive outcomes or benefits of change is as important as the content if your message is to be convincing or persuasive.

You can conduct these activities as an attention-getter at the beginning of a session or series of sessions, or as part of a media campaign, where you would present the benefits of action in a way that is brief, catchy, and memorable. When benefits are explored in greater detail later in the instructional sequence, more food and nutrition data can be presented and explored.

Practical educational activities might include the following to increase participants' motivation and ability to process your nutrition education message about behavior change:

■ *Use language that is straightforward, clear, easily understandable by your audience, and feels personally relevant.* This is likely to increase participants' *ability* to process the content of your session. Repeat and reinforce the message with a minimum of distractions.
■ *Present striking information about scientific or other evidence for the effectiveness of taking action.* Perceived benefits are more effective when presented through striking statistics about outcomes.
■ *Use attention-getting graphics.* Communicate the anticipated benefits or positive outcomes of recommended skills and behaviors by using video clips, posters, games, or Internet visuals, or showing excerpts from magazines popular with the intended audience. This is likely to increase participants' *motivation* to process key messages of your session.
■ *Present the benefits* in ways that are memorable, unexpected, or novel; culturally appropriate; and most

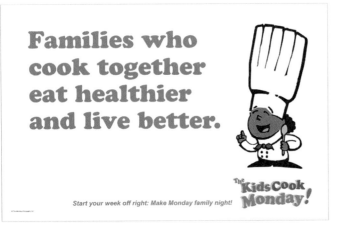

Motivational messages based on outcome expectations.

Kids Cook Monday.

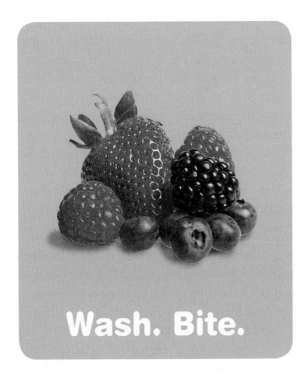

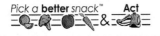

Motivational messages based on outcome expectations.

Iowa's Pick a Better Snack.

important, personally relevant, stressing positive outcomes important to the intended audience. Use humor where appropriate for a given audience.

- *Cite gains and losses.* Provide information on what participants will gain from taking action as well as what they will lose by not taking action.

- *Encourage active participation.* Design activities that are fun, are engaging, and involve active participation to the extent possible. In one intervention, an "Eat the Rainbow" puzzle was developed that showed that "nutrients" from vegetables make connections within the body possible so that it is much quicker to assemble than one lacking the "nutrients" to facilitate essential metabolic functions (Abrams et al. 2013). Participants became very engaged in racing against the clock and learned about the importance of vegetables for healthful functioning of the body.

Benefits Differ for Diverse Groups

Note that the relative importance of different perceived benefits, or reasons for action, may differ depending on the behavior and the group or audience. For example, for the behavior of eating fruits and vegetables, being cool may be important for teenagers, whereas creating clear skin may be important for young women, improving the health of the baby may be important for pregnant women, and reducing cancer risk may be important for men. Immediate benefits usually carry more weight than benefits in the future, particularly for teenagers. Thus, the messages about benefits or positive anticipated outcomes of action must be based on those that are personally meaningful to the specific group, derived from your careful assessment in Step 2.

The VERB Campaign

The VERB campaign, created by the Centers for Disease Control and Prevention (CDC) for children ages 9 to 13, was designed to increase physical activity through targeted advertising, promotions, and events for tweens. The CDC developed a variety of VERB materials to help organizations that work with children connect VERB to their programs, classes, and activities. It is an excellent example of a campaign that was based on making the outcomes meaningful for tweens, based on research regarding potential motivators (see **NUTRITION EDUCATION IN ACTION 11-2**). So, although the rationale for the program was that there are health risks to inactivity and health benefits to being active,

NUTRITION EDUCATION IN ACTION 11-2 VERB: A Physical Activity Campaign for Tweens

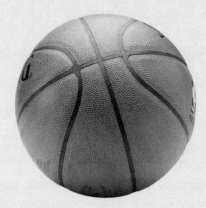

© PhotoDisc

The VERB campaign, created by the Centers for Disease Control and Prevention (CDC 2006), worked to increase physical activity through targeted advertising, promotions, and events for tweens. The CDC also developed a variety of VERB materials to help organizations that work with children connect VERB to their programs, classes, and activities.

- *The VERB vision*: All youth leading healthy lifestyles.
- *The VERB mission*: To increase and maintain physical activity among tweens (youth ages 9–13 years).
- *Campaign audiences*: The main audience for the campaign was tweens. Other important audiences were parents and adult influencers, including teachers, youth leaders, physical education and health professionals, pediatricians, healthcare providers, and coaches.

Tweens could go on the website for ideas for physical activity and participate in all kinds of online activities with other tweens. Parents were also urged to participate.

Rationale for Campaign

The underlying rationale for the campaign had to do with risks to children of inactivity and the benefits of being physically active, such as strengthening muscles, bones, and joints; controlling weight; and improving overall health. Physical activity also helps to develop skills that can benefit children for life, including goal setting and achievement, getting along with others, leadership, and teamwork. Other research shows that physical activity can help increase concentration, reduce anxiety and stress, and increase self-esteem—all of which may have a positive effect on students' scholastic achievement. These important benefits of being physically active are *not,* of course, particularly meaningful to the tween audience.

What Moves Tweens

Meaningful motivators for this age group were based on VERB research findings: children this age respond to the spirit of adventure, discovery, and finding their own thing. So, adults can help tweens discover new activities that they enjoy:

- Give away small prizes such as stickers, pins, or water bottles to reward tweens for being active. Prizes serve as great incentives for kids.
- Design activities with input from the kids. They will be more inclined to participate because they want to, not because they have to, do something.
- Some tweens prefer activities with a competitive edge, whereas others simply like playing a game with friends. Find out their preferences. All tweens will experience the rewards of being active if it is enjoyable for them.
- Tweens, especially girls, like social interaction with friends. It makes playing actively more fun and offers opportunities for peer recognition and praise.
- Praise kids just for trying something new and getting active. Your encouragement means a lot to them.

Campaign Outcomes

After 1 year, the VERB campaign had:

- Narrowed the gap in physical activity between girls and boys
- Resulted in lower-income tweens becoming more physically active, despite greater barriers to being active

(Continues)

NUTRITION EDUCATION IN ACTION 11-2 VERB: A Physical Activity Campaign for Tweens (Continued)

- Reached extraordinarily high awareness levels among tweens (74% nationally and 84% in high-dose communities) and very high understanding (90% nationally) of the campaign's core messages to be physically active and have fun

More specifically, evaluation measures demonstrated significant increases in physical activity as a direct result of VERB in the following key groups (Huhman et al. 2005):

Children 9–10 Years Old (8.6 million national population)

- 34% increase in free-time physical activity sessions nationally

- 32% decline in the number of sedentary 9- to 10-year-olds in high-dose communities

Girls (10 million national population)

- 27% increase in free-time physical activity sessions nationally

- 37% decline among least active in high-dose communities

Tweens from Lower- (<$25,000; 4.5 million national population) to Lower-Middle-Income ($25,000–50,000; 6 million national population) Households

- 25% increase in free-time physical activity sessions nationally among lower-middle-income households

- 31% decline among least active from lower-income households in high-dose markets

- 38% decline among least active from lower-middle-income households in high-dose communities

These analyses included children from all racial/ethnic groups. Older tweens, boys, and tweens from middle- to higher-income households also showed some increases in physical activity, but those increases were not statistically significant.

The active campaign ended, but the materials are still available.

Sources: Centers for Disease Control and Prevention (CDC). 2006. Youth media campaign: VERB. http://www.cdc.gov/youthcampaign; Huhman, M., L. D. Potter, F. L. Wong, et al. 2005. Effects of a mass media campaign to increase physical activity among children: Year 1 results of the VERB campaign. *Pediatrics* 116:277–284; and Wong F. L., M. Greenwell, S. Gates, and J. M. Berkowitz. 2008. It's what you do! Reflections on the VERB campaign. *American Journal of Preventive Medicine* 34(6S):S175–S182.

---

those were not the motivators (or expected outcomes) used with participating youth.

> Your effectiveness as a nutrition educator is greatly enhanced by your enthusiasm, passion about what you are conveying, and respectfulness toward the audience.

BEHAVIOR CHANGE STRATEGIES AND PRACTICAL EDUCATIONAL ACTIVITIES FOR THE THEORY DETERMINANTS OF PERCEIVED BARRIERS AND SELF-EFFICACY

Behavior Change Strategy: Identifying and Reframing Perception of Barriers

Self-efficacy is important for both motivation and taking action. Perceived barriers are closely related to, and often mirror, self-efficacy and perceived behavioral control. That is, as barriers are overcome, self-efficacy increases, and as self-efficacy increases, perceived barriers decrease. In the motivational component of nutrition education, therefore, increasing self-efficacy is about reducing the perceived difficulty of taking action.

Here, the focus is on making the behavior that is the target of the intervention easy to understand and carry out. The determinants of perceived barriers and self-efficacy are common to almost all psychosocial models of health behavior.

Practical educational activities might include:

- *Group identification of barriers and ways to overcome them.* You can assist the group to share and understand the difficulties and identify their (or their family members') barriers to healthful eating practices. You can record them on newsprint. Then ask the group to brainstorm ways of overcoming these barriers. Individuals who have been successful in engaging in the targeted behavior can share their experiences. This is a useful strategy for all age groups.

In one example with inner-city teens, nutrition educators led the group through calculations that showed that packaged snacks from vending machines and their local stores actually cost much more than making their own simple snacks or even fruit that could easily be carried around. They then had the teens assemble simple snacks from basic ingredients that they liked, such as raisins and nuts. The nutrition educators also calculated the time it took to make or assemble the snacks, showing how time did not have to be a barrier.

- *Use of examples of valued social models enacting the behavior,* such as sports figures or successful breast-feeding moms, is also an effective strategy. In using social models, the audience must see that the outcomes of the behavior are clearly beneficial to the model.

- *Correct misconceptions that are barriers.* This is the time to address and, if appropriate, correct individuals' misconceptions about their ability to act. For example, if fruits and vegetables can easily go bad is stated as a barrier, give participants tips on how to store them to reduce spoilage, or to buy other forms, such as frozen or canned.

- *Media messages to decrease barriers and enhance self-efficacy.* An interesting mass media campaign to increase fruit and vegetable intake involves billboards in the community, along with flyers, that had on them a drawing of a specific fruit or vegetable accompanied by a relevant message. For example, a photo of berries is accompanied by the message "Wash. Eat. How easy is that?" (Iowa Department of Health 2015).

- *Cooking demonstrations.* Cooking demonstrations of simple recipes can decrease perceived barriers that healthy foods are time-consuming and difficult to prepare. Recipes that require no cooking are easy to demonstrate. For recipes that require some cooking, nutrition educators often use a rolling suitcase to bring with them a portable electric or butane gas stove (the latter does not require even electricity) as well as the ingredients.

> The information in Chapters 15 and 17 about practical tips for working with diverse groups is very helpful as you design your educational sessions.

BEHAVIOR CHANGE STRATEGIES AND PRACTICAL EDUCATIONAL ACTIVITIES FOR THE THEORY DETERMINANT OF AFFECTIVE ATTITUDES/EMOTIONS

Behavior Change Strategy: Promote Reflection on Anticipated Emotions and Feelings

Beliefs about the outcomes of behavior constitute the cognitive component of attitudes and are a major motivator of behavioral intention, as we have seen. However, the affective component of attitudes, reflecting feelings, is also a powerful motivator, if not a more powerful one when it comes to food and physical activity. Nutrition education can assist individuals to understand their own feelings and emotions about food- and nutrition-related behaviors so that they can make changes where necessary to serve their own interests in improving health.

Practical educational activities can include:

- *Experiences to explore preferences and feelings.* Positive attitudes and feelings often come about from positive educational experiences such as tasting and preparing food. They can also arise from having group members explore their feelings, not just their thoughts, about the behaviors central to your intervention, for example about the behavior changes that will be needed in light of a new diagnosis of diabetes. This can be done through a process of attitudes clarification.

- *Attitudes clarification activity.* Present some attitude statements and ask the group to discuss them or to explore them individually. You can also use the strategy of forming an attitude line. For example, you can verbalize an attitude statement such as the following ones and have participants line up from "strongly agree" to "strongly disagree." Alternatively, the four corners of the room can be used as "attitude corners"—strongly agree, agree, disagree, and strongly disagree. Whatever the format, individuals should be encouraged to discuss their response with their peers. Examples of attitude statements are as follows:

  - Exclusively breastfeeding my baby is a satisfying experience.
  - Healthful foods take too long to prepare.
  - People should have more willpower when they make food choices.
  - I feel good about myself when I eat foods from local farms.

Behavior Change Strategy: Build on Personal Meanings

Personal meanings are important. For example, it has been found that adolescents often use eating certain foods, such as junk foods, as a way to express their independence and personal will, challenge parental authority, and test boundaries. Many women see food as an enemy. Help participants examine and build on their personal meanings.

Practical educational activities can include:

- *Group discussion.* Lead a facilitated dialogue or a set of learner-centered activities to explore the personal and functional meanings that individuals give to food and eating.
- *Written activity.* Use worksheets with engaging and challenging questions to allow participants to explore their feelings individually and privately. Provide opportunities to share, if appropriate for your group. If not, ask them to take home and think about what they wrote and what they might want to do with it.

Behavior Change Strategy: Promote Reflection on Potential Anticipated Regret

Anticipated regret or worry about the consequences of acting or failing to act has been shown to be a motivator of preventive health behavior.

Practical educational activities can include:

- *Visualization activity.* Individuals can be stimulated to visualize or imagine how they will feel about themselves after they have made the decision to act or not to act. Will they regret their choice?

BEHAVIOR CHANGE STRATEGIES AND PRACTICAL EDUCATIONAL ACTIVITIES FOR THE THEORY DETERMINANT FOOD PREFERENCES

Study after study shows that taste is a powerful determinant of food choice. Taste is in some ways an anticipated outcome of eating a food, but it also has an important physiological component. To emphasize the tastiness of healthful foods and to increase the audience's familiarity with and enjoyment of healthful food, nutrition educators should design activities that include tasting foods prepared in a healthful and delicious way.

Behavior Change Strategy: Provide Direct Experience with Healthful Food

Practical educational activities can include:

- *Food tastings.* People often will not eat foods that are unfamiliar or they think will taste bad, even if they have never tasted them. Thus, providing opportunities to taste foods familiar to, or at least similar to, their culture prepared in different ways that are more healthful can increase their motivation to eat the foods that are the target of your intervention. Provide repeated exposure to these healthful foods.
- *Food preparation and cooking.* Although active participation in general (such as group activities, checklists, or self-appraisals) is important in enhancing motivation and self-efficacy, hands-on food-related activities are important enough to be considered a special category (Liquori et al. 1998; Reicks et al. 2014). Cooking or food preparation can provide vivid and motivating experiences when participants are physically involved in the activities and also eat the food they have prepared. An example is the Cookshop Program, in which students were actively involved in cooking in classrooms—and eating what they cooked (Liquori et al. 1998). Classes in which students cooked were compared with classes that involved active hands-on activities but did not include preparing and eating the foods cooked. Although both groups increased in knowledge, only the group that cooked changed its behavior to eat more of the whole grains and vegetables that were offered in the school lunch.

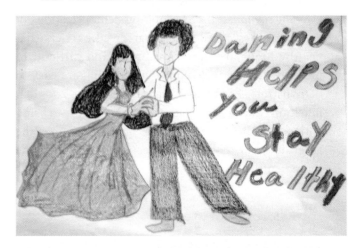

Drawing personal beliefs is a vivid example of personal motivators.

Courtesy of Linking Food and the Environment, Teachers College Columbia University.

BEHAVIOR CHANGE STRATEGIES AND PRACTICAL EDUCATIONAL ACTIVITIES FOR THE THEORY DETERMINANTS OF SOCIAL NORMS AND DESCRIPTIVE NORMS

Behavior Change Strategy: Reframe Perceived Norms

Social norms or social expectations (injunctive norms: what others think you should do) and descriptive norms (experiential norms: what others are thinking or doing) are important determinants of behavior, as you have seen. (See Chapter 4.) We tend to do what others like us are doing. You can design activities in which groups or intended audience members can be made aware of the influence of social norms on their behaviors.

Practical educational activities can include:

- *Analyze television and print ads.* For example, mothers can be provided with activities that analyze TV and print ads about women feeding their children and can be asked to share their feelings about the ads. Discuss their ideas on what they can do to resist negative norms and practices. Schoolchildren can be asked to conduct a survey of Saturday morning food ads, analyze them, and design an ad campaign they think would be effective in making the consumption of fruits and vegetables the norm.
- *Analyze and reflect on social expectations (social norms).* You can assist the groups to identify what important others think they should be doing, such as their spouses', partners', or mothers' approval or disapproval of breastfeeding (injunctive norms), or their doctors' approval that they are eating foods lower in salt for their hypertension.
- *Analyze and reflect on perceptions of the attitudes and behaviors of others (descriptive norms).* Group members can analyze the many other social sources of influences on food choice, such as when eating at work, in the cafeteria, and at home, or eating out with friends. That is, what do they think members of their social networks feel and do about the intervention or program's targeted behaviors?
- *Use positive social models.* Materials, films, and statistics can be used to indicate how individuals similar to the target group are engaging in the healthful behaviors, such as other WIC women breastfeeding, other teenagers drinking water instead of sweetened beverages, and so forth (descriptive norms). You can

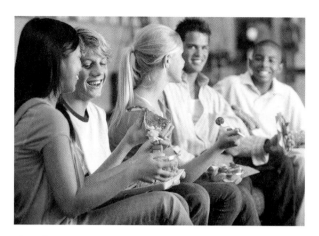

The influence of peers affects the eating patterns of adolescents.
© Monkey Business Images/Dreamstime.com

use sports figures for adolescents, either in person or through other channels such as videos or brochures. You can discuss your own experiences or that of other credible social models. When designing mass media communications, whether visual or print, you can use messages from important people with whom audience members identify. Posters can be designed that show attractive people like themselves (e.g., other schoolchildren or other WIC mothers) enjoying eating the particular foods being emphasized in the intervention.

- *Model resistance.* Show videos, or discuss ways in social situations to politely refuse to participate in the norm (e.g., how much to eat, how to order a dessert in a restaurant, and so forth).
- *Use peer educators.* You can use peer educators to deliver the nutrition education, as has been done effectively in interventions with adolescents, families, and older adults.

BEHAVIOR CHANGE STRATEGIES AND PRACTICAL EDUCATIONAL ACTIVITIES FOR THE THEORY DETERMINANT OF BELIEFS ABOUT THE SELF

Behavior Change Strategy: Stimulate Reflection on Self-Identity and Self-Evaluative Beliefs

Self-representations such as self-identity or social identity often have an important influence on motivation for healthful eating and active living and can be used in your intervention.

Practical educational activities can include:

- *Self-evaluative activities.* You can use written reflection activities for individuals to explore such issues as

"I think of myself as a health-conscious consumer," "I think of myself as someone who is concerned about environmental issues," "I think of myself as a good mother," and so forth. In a group where conditions are safe, these activities can be done as a group. (See Chapters 15 and 17.) You can also use the strategy of self-reevaluation from the transtheoretical model (TTM) to help individuals assess their images of themselves and rethink these images in positive terms.

- *Personal responsibilities and moral obligations.* Develop discussion questions or activities to explore individuals' perceptions about their responsibilities and moral obligations, both personal and social (e.g., as a mother, a spouse, a citizen), in relation to the behavior change goals of your nutrition education session or intervention.

- *Personal ideals.* Help individuals explore ideal-self versus actual-self discrepancies by devising messages or activities to help individuals become aware of their ideals, where they come from, and how realistic or healthful they are. Individuals can then make decisions about how to handle this awareness. In similar fashion, ought-to-be-self versus actual-self discrepancies can be explored through activities that bring to awareness sources of the "oughts," such as being a good mother or being thin, and how to handle them. Active methods of self-exploration and understanding, debates of pros and cons, and discussions are likely to be the most effective strategies, although films and written materials can also be helpful if used appropriately.

Behavior Change Strategy: Prompt Reflection on Personal and Moral Norms

People's sense of personal responsibility for the health and well-being of themselves and their families can be a major motivator of eating behaviors. For example, mothers usually feel a sense of responsibility to feed their families healthy foods. They may also feel a moral obligation to maintain cultural traditions in relation to food.

Practical educational activities can include:

- *Personal responsibilities and moral obligations.* Develop discussion questions or activities to explore individuals' perceptions about their responsibilities and moral obligations, both personal and social (e.g., as a mother, a spouse, a citizen), in relation to the behavior change goals of your nutrition education session or intervention.

BEHAVIOR CHANGE STRATEGIES AND PRACTICAL EDUCATIONAL ACTIVITIES FOR THE THEORY DETERMINANT OF HABITS AND ROUTINES

Behavior Change Strategy: Provide Confrontation with Automatic Behaviors

Many of people's behaviors appear to occur without much thought. Indeed, habit or routines are important motivators of behavior. As we have seen, this results from the frequent pairing of foods and situations in which they are consumed. Nutrition education activities can bring to awareness such attitude–situation cues so that individuals can choose to change behaviors if they wish.

Practical educational activities can include:

- *Awareness of current routines and habits.* You can devise activities to assist individuals to identify cues that seem to trigger behavior directly and unknowingly (such as the smell of baked products or the sight of ice cream) or to identify the chain of events leading to eating a second helping, so that individuals will be conscious of what they are doing.

- *Replacing routines.* Nutrition education activities can be designed to bring the less positive routines (e.g., eating high-calorie snacks) to consciousness so that they can be considered and replaced by more positive routines or habits. Because these more positive behaviors may require more effort (e.g., cutting up fruits and vegetables), tip sheets, checklists, or activities can be designed to assist individuals to develop the new routines.

Behavior Change Strategy: Provide Cues to Action

In many instances, individuals are motivated to some degree but need reminders to take action.

Practical educational activities can include:

- Refrigerator magnets, bookmarks, grocery bags, and pencils with messages on them can provide cues to action. Mass media messages can also be very useful. Billboard messages can serve this role. You can also use more intensive methods, such as telephone calls, email messages, mobile technology apps, or mailed reminders.

BEHAVIOR CHANGE STRATEGIES AND PRACTICAL EDUCATIONAL ACTIVITIES FOR THE THEORY DETERMINANT OF BEHAVIORAL INTENTIONS

After the nutrition education activities have stimulated interest and provoked thought by providing individuals with the opportunity to become more aware of their personal wants, feelings, and behaviors; to understand their own motivations and the factors that seem to control their behaviors; and to deliberate on the issues, you can now provide them with the opportunity to resolve any ambivalences that they have and to make a decision to take action, or not to do so, given their life circumstances.

Individuals' attitudes and their beliefs about the outcomes of a behavior are numerous and may often conflict and compete. Ambivalence reflects the coexistence within individuals of both positive and negative beliefs about outcomes for the same behavior (e.g., eating chocolate is both delicious and fattening), as well as numerous conflicting feelings or attitudes. Individuals can pursue many alternative wishes or actions, and they will have to select among them. This is especially true for food choices, dietary behaviors, and physical activity habits.

The following sections describe several strategies that you may find useful to activate decision making, assist individuals to resolve ambivalences, and facilitate the formation of a behavioral intention or a goal intention. These strategies involve both cognitive and affective domains. In general, they involve individuals' evaluations of the feasibility and desirability of the action or practice. Several of these strategies are similar to the transtheoretical model's processes of self-reevaluation and self-liberation.

Behavior Change Strategy: Initiate Analysis of Decisional Balance/Pros and Cons of Action or Change

Practical educational activities can include:

- *Evaluating costs and benefits of taking action.* Nutrition educators can provide opportunities for individuals to analyze all the benefits or pros of taking action or changing a behavior and the costs or cons of taking action through worksheets or discussions. Individuals should also examine the reverse—that is, what they

will lose by not taking action. This can be done using a pros and cons grid similar to the following:

	Pros	Cons
If I don't take given action		
If I do take given action		

Participants can then make a decision as to whether or not to take action.

- *Choices among several alternatives*: Individuals do not make decisions about making behavior changes or taking action in a vacuum. Any given action is an alternative among several potential actions: for example, eating fruit for dessert or eating cheesecake, breastfeeding or bottle feeding, and going running or working out or watching television. Worksheets thus should help individuals evaluate and make choices among alternative behaviors competing for their time and attention.

Behavior Change Strategy: Promote Values Clarification

Values are an important basis for action. As you have seen, individuals are motivated to take action if the action will lead to outcomes or goals they value. Short-term goals are instrumental values, such as taste, losing weight, looking attractive, or being liked by friends. These are the outcome expectations discussed earlier.

However, people also make choices based on larger, end-state values, such as self-respect, sense of accomplishment, equality, social recognition, pleasure, true friendship, an exciting life, a world of beauty, inner harmony, freedom, happiness, mature love, wisdom, a worthwhile life, and so forth (Rokeach 1973; Buchanan 2000). For some individuals, these values are much more important than short-term, instrumental values. Again, individuals need to clarify for themselves how their current behaviors relate to these larger values and what changing these behaviors would mean to them in terms of these values.

Practical educational activities can be used to assist people to clarify their values:

- *Value statements.* You can present some value statements and ask participants to discuss or explore them in pairs and triads.

- *Visual imagery.* One powerful activity that will help participants understand and process their feelings is to assemble pictures from magazines, the Internet, photographs taken in the community, or drawings showing people engaging in different food- or health-related activities such as shopping for food, going to a farmers' market, preparing food, breastfeeding, eating at fast food restaurants, weighing themselves, or running. Show these pictures to participants and have them either write down or verbally report the feelings evoked by each picture. The answers can be coded, tallied, and reported back to the group as a whole to discuss. Participants may be surprised at their own feelings in response to the pictures as well as those of others. The next phase is to explore why particular emotions or feelings came up and to develop some understanding of these feelings, especially the problematic ones. The group can then come up with some ways to explain the problems depicted or implied by the pictures and to solve them. The Freiere conscientization procedure involves this process (Freiere 1970, 1973).

Behavior Change Strategy: Encourage Resolving Resistance and Ambivalence

To be effective for recipients, nutrition education strategies and messages need to enhance positive thoughts, feelings, and a sense of empowerment to take action. Inevitably, however, group participants or message recipients may resist what is being said. Resistance to change can be useful because it contributes to human consistency and prevents people from constantly swinging from one opinion or behavior to another. Manoff (1985) and other social marketers point out that potential cognitive and emotional "resistance points" of the audience, or their barriers to taking action, must be known and understood by nutrition educators.

Practical educational activities to assist people to understand and resolve their resistance and ambivalence can include:

- *Acknowledge ambivalence and resistance.* Nutrition educators should not try to talk people out of their resistance (it will not work), but instead should respect their position, express understanding, point out contradictions, suggest alternative ways to think

about the issue, and help them make choices. This is also the basis of motivational interviewing (Rollnick, Miller, and Butler 2008). Our task is to assist individuals to resolve their ambivalences and objections, but not in a defensive way. The task is to present the other side in a professional tone. We can talk about the issues and resolve them in a presentation, or provide opportunities for group members to discuss them openly and resolve them in the group discussion.

- *Address internal dialogues.* The effectiveness of nutrition education is improved if the potential internal dialogues of the audience disagreeing with the message are acknowledged, empathy with them is expressed, counterarguments are provided where appropriate or reassurance is given that the doubts do not interfere with taking action, and a way is provided for people to be able to comfortably give up the resistance or to state they are not ready to take action or do not wish to take action. Here are some examples of potential internal dialogues of group participants and how they could be handled:

  - *Internal dialogue of group participant or message recipient.* "My grandfather ate a high-fat diet and smoked all his life and didn't get heart disease, so why should I worry?"
  - *Nutrition educator.* "Some of you may have had a grandparent who ate an unhealthy diet and smoked and yet lived to a ripe old age. However, that grandparent was lucky. You may or may not be so lucky. If that grandparent had 50 friends and half of them practiced poor health habits (as your grandparent did) and the other half ate healthful foods, exercised, and did not smoke, on the average the latter group would live longer, healthier lives. Taking care of yourself lowers your risk of developing chronic diseases such as cancer, heart disease, and stroke."
  - *Internal dialogue of some teenagers with diabetes.* "My mother is always bugging me about doing the right thing to control my diabetes. I hate being told what to do—I'm just not going to do it!"
  - *Nutrition educator.* "I am sure that for many of you, your mothers tend to nag you about taking care of your diabetes. But controlling your diabetes is not your mother's job—it's yours. Consider following your doctor's instructions, but

not for your mother's sake. Do it for yourself. You are worth it. Your mother means well; you need only to reassure her that you've got it under control, and that her way of showing concern is not helpful."

Behavior Change Strategy: Assist Intention Formation

Nutrition educators can assist individuals to evaluate the desirability and feasibility of taking the action or making the behavior change(s) targeted by your sessions or intervention and then making a decision. If they decide to take action, their decision is then their behavioral intention or goal intention.

Practical educational activity can be:

- *Clear statement of intention of goal.* It is best to assist individuals to clearly state their behavioral intention, preferably in writing (e.g., through a commitment form, action plan, contract, or pledge). Alternatively, they can make the commitment orally in the group. When group participants make public commitments, they hold each other accountable and also provide social support to each other to fulfill their commitments.

  In the context of a nutrition education intervention, this intention is usually the intervention's behavior change goal. If your intervention's behavior change goal is quite specific, such as for intervention participants to eat four or more cups of fruits and vegetables daily, the behavioral intention can be stated as "I intend to eat four or more cups of fruits and vegetables daily." How to assist individuals to translate these intentions into action is the subject of the next chapter.

Behavior Change Strategy: Create a Forum for Group Decision Making and Public Commitment

Individuals are more likely to follow through with a specific action or behavior pattern if their attitudes and commitments are made public than if they are kept private, particularly if their peers hold them accountable for fulfilling their commitments. To the extent that individuals, acting in the absence of coercion, make a commitment in front of others to take action, they come to see themselves as believers in that kind of activity.

Lewin's Group Decision Studies

As a result of his research on such issues as group dynamics and social influence, social psychologist Kurt Lewin concluded that commitment to an action is greater when social influence or the social support of the group is involved. During World War II, when food rationing and conservation were important concerns, Lewin conducted a series of experiments to change food habits (Lewin 1943; Radke and Caso 1948). He compared several methods with a "group decision" method in which group discussion was followed by the group setting definite goals for action. These goals could be set up by the group for the group as a whole or by each individual in the group setting. Either way, the message was first presented in a very motivating way, and a public decision was made to try the targeted behavior, through a show of hands or verbal statements. No attempt was made to force a decision.

- *Study with stay-at-home women.* In one study with homemakers, the target behavior was using organ meats such as hearts, lungs, liver, and kidneys instead of the more common cuts of meat. In the control group (or lecture condition), a nutritionist discussed the advantages of using organ meats—low cost, nutritional value, and importance to the war effort. The information was provided in an enthusiastic but formal lecture format, with no group interaction. Recipes for "delicious dishes" were handed out. In the group decision situation, the nutritionist briefly and enthusiastically discussed similar information as for the lecture situation. The group then exchanged views on potential barriers to using organ meats (e.g., their families might not like kidneys, kidneys smell bad during cooking). The nutritionist made suggestions from time to time for dealing with these barriers, but only after group members themselves had expressed their concerns and discussed with each other ways to overcome the barriers. Group members then publicly voted on their decision to serve organ meats during the following week. In follow-up interviews in the women's homes 7 days later, it was found that only 10% of the women in the lecture condition reported serving one of the three targeted organ meats, whereas 52% of the women in the group decision method condition reported trying one of these meats.

- *Study with college students.* In the second study, a request for change (via an announcement) was compared with group decision for increasing the intake of whole wheat bread by male college students in dormitory settings. Similar positive results were obtained.

These studies indicate that a process wherein groups of peers mutually share concerns and make public commitments to each other can exert a powerful effect on individuals' self-image, commitment, and action taking. Nutrition educators can encourage such group decision and public commitment to assist individuals to bridge the intention–behavior gap.

USING DETERMINANTS AND BEHAVIOR CHANGE STRATEGIES TO GUIDE DEVELOPMENT OF PRACTICAL EDUCATIONAL ACTIVITIES: THE FOOD, HEALTH & CHOICES CURRICULUM

The development of the Food, Health & Choices curriculum illustrates how determinants from theory can be used to guide the development of specific objectives, strategies, and practical educational activities to achieve the behavior change goals of the curriculum. This is shown in **NUTRITION EDUCATION IN ACTION 11-3**.

NUTRITION EDUCATION IN ACTION 11-3   Food, Health & Choices Curriculum: Linking Theory, Specific Objectives, and Educational Activities

Food, Health & Choices (FHC) is an obesity prevention curriculum for elementary school children. In Nutrition Education in Action 10-1 in Chapter 10 we describe the curriculum intervention and focus on linking determinants of change with general objectives. Here we describe how the specific objectives of the classroom curriculum are used to design strategies and practical educational activities. There are numerous activities because this list is for the entire 23-lesson curriculum

Behavior Change Goals

The FHC curriculum focuses on the "choose more" behaviors of fruits and vegetables and physical activity, and the "choose less" behaviors of sweetened beverages, processed packaged snacks, fast food, and recreational screen time.

Theory Model

The theory model is based on a combination of determinants of behavior change from social cognitive and self-determination theories.

General Educational Objectives

- Demonstrate understanding and appreciation of the importance of the choose more and choose less behaviors (outcome expectations)
- Identify barriers to doing the choose more and choose less behaviors (perceived barriers)
- Demonstrate increased self-efficacy doing the choose more and choose less behaviors (self-efficacy)
- State intention to do the choose more and choose less behaviors (behavioral intention)
- Analyze their current dietary and physical activity behaviors and choose individual goals for each target behavior (goal setting)
- Express an increased sense of confidence in their skills for choosing more healthful foods and engaging in more physical activity (competence)
- State an increased sense of autonomy in choosing more healthful foods and engaging in more physical activity (autonomy)

Determinant	Behavior Change Strategies	Specific Educational Objectives	Educational Activities, Experiences, and/or Content
Outcome expectations (perceived benefits)	Provide information about positive outcomes	State benefits of eating F&V.	■ "Eat the Rainbow" and "No Connections" puzzles
		State the reasons for eating a "rainbow of colors."	■ Group discusses scientific evidence for how eating F&V benefits our bodies and minds ■ Cards with specific benefits of different colors
		State benefits of doing PA.	■ Squat Jump experiment and how body responds to PA ■ Complete benefits of PA worksheet

Determinant	Behavior Change Strategies	Specific Educational Objectives	Educational Activities, Experiences, and/or Content
Outcome expectations (perceived risk)	Provide information about negative outcomes of behavior/risks	Describe risks to health from eating too few F&V and not engaging in enough PA. Describe risks to eating too many SB, PPS, and FF, and engaging in too much RST.	■ Compare teaspoons of sugar in beverages and fat in fast food to maximum daily recommendation ■ Group activity: blood sugar simulation, clogged blood vessel simulation
Outcome expectations (perceived risk)	Self-assessment to personalize risk	Evaluate personal risk for above behaviors.	■ Recall of own F&V intake and compare to recommendation ■ Recall of own PA levels and compare to recommendation
Perceived barriers	Reframe perception of barriers	Identify barriers to eating F&V and doing PA.	■ Group brainstorms barriers to eating F&V and doing PA
		Propose ways to overcome barriers of above behaviors.	■ Group brainstorms ways to overcome barriers
Behavioral intention	Prompt decisional balance	Evaluate pros and cons of eating more F&V and doing more PA; eating fewer SB, PPS, and FF; and engaging in less RST.	■ Review benefits of eating F&V and doing PA, and cons of eating SB, PPS, and FF and engaging in RST
		State an intention to choose one *eat more* and one *eat less* behavior.	■ Individual worksheet to choose goal(s)
Behavioral capability	Provide factual knowledge	Demonstrate understanding of nutrition and PA concepts related to goal behaviors.	■ Class discussion to review what has been learned
Goal setting skills	Stimulate action goal setting	State action plan to reach behavior goal(s) and monitoring.	■ Student worksheet of individual action plans and write value statements of what they want to be better at and why
Self-regulation	Facilitate self-monitoring and feedback	Appreciate that meeting goal(s) helps them be better at what they enjoy doing.	■ Student worksheet to record successes and challenges of meeting goal(s) and share with peers why it's important
Competence	Facilitate self-monitoring and feedback	Evaluate ability to reach behavior change goal(s).	■ Students share ways they have overcome barriers and successfully met goal(s)
Autonomy	Provide autonomy support	Demonstrate ability to make autonomous choice.	■ Provide support to students for attempts to enact their chosen goals. Students express why their goals are important and how they feel since following goals

F&V = fruits and vegetables; PA = physical activity; SB = sweetened beverages; PPS = processed packaged snacks; FF = fast food; RST = recreational screen time

Source: Abrams, E., M. Burgermaster, P. A. Koch, I. R. Contento, and H. L. Gray. 2014. Food, Health & Choices: Importance of formative evaluation to create a well-delivered and well-received intervention. *Journal of Nutrition Education and Behavior* 44(4S):S137.

Organizing and Sequencing Educational Activities for Delivery with the 4 Es: The Educational or Lesson Plan

As you are creating your educational activities you can also start thinking about how you will arrange them in a way that best promotes learning. Educators use the term *instruction* to mean the deliberate arrangement of educational activities in such a way as to facilitate learning (Gagne et al. 2004; Merrill 2009). The term does not mean just lectures or direct instructions; it includes hands-on interactive and self-directed learning activities as well. A *theory of instruction* is thus about how to select and arrange educational activities (referred to as *events of instruction*) to provide support for people's internal processes of learning. As nutrition educators we can use instructional theory to provide us with practical guidance on how to arrange educational strategies within a session or over several sessions into an instructional sequence, resulting in a plan for instruction, usually referred to as a *lesson plan* or *educational plan*.

SEQUENCING YOUR SESSION OR OTHER COMMUNICATION VENUE WITH THE 4 ES

TABLE 11-2 presents a way to organize and sequence these events of instruction—that is, how you will sequence the various activities you will carry out during sessions. It is based on a theory of instruction proposed by Gagne (Gagne 1965, 1985; Gagne et al. 2004) that has been widely used to design instruction using a variety of media (e.g., oral, written, computer-based, Web-based) for a variety of audiences (e.g., children, adults) and has been modified for health education design (Kinzie 2005). The sequence is similar to the "principles of good instruction or teaching" widely used in the field of education (Merrill 2009; Reigeluth and Carr-Chellman 2009). It also takes into consideration different learning styles. (These are discussed in detail in Chapter 15.) We call the sequence the 4 Es. (Naming the sequence as the "4 Es" was suggested by Koch 2013.) One such educational plan is provided in the case study at the end of this chapter, and another educational plan for the case study is shown in Chapter 12. Do not attempt to accomplish too much in your sessions. People can usually process only small amounts of information at a time, so provide only what is relevant and needed to achieve your behavioral goal. The rule of thumb

TABLE 11-2 Sequencing Nutrition Education Strategies Within Session: The 4 Es	
Sequence of Events of Instruction	**Theory-Based Nutrition Education Strategies**
Excite: Gain attention	■ *Use attention-getter* that is personally relevant for audience about behavior change goal, for example. ■ Increase awareness of *risk* or of *benefits* to taking action, perhaps using self-assessment compared to recommendations. ■ *For ongoing sessions*: Review and reflect.
Explain: Present new material and focus on why-to take action	■ *Tailor messages to audience's prior knowledge and values*: Make message personally meaningful. ■ *Outcome expectations or perceived benefits*: Demonstrate observable effectiveness of the desired behavior to enhance motivation. ■ *Affective attitudes*: Increase reflection on affect/feelings about taking action. ■ *Barriers/self-efficacy*: Make desired action easy to understand and do.
Expand: Provide guidance and practice and focus on how-to take action	■ Provide food- and nutrition-related knowledge and cognitive skills to engage in actions. ■ Provide authentic practice and feedback/coaching and peer collaboration to develop competence and self-efficacy. ■ Use credible social models to demonstrate behavior through media appropriate to the content. ■ Enhance affective skills.
Exit: Apply and close	■ Enhance application. ■ Enhance goal setting skills and action planning. ■ Provide social supports and behavioral cues.

is, plan to cover half as much in twice the time as you think it will take!

The 4 Es sequence is as follows:

■ *Excite—gain attention.* Devise activities that pique interest, excite, provoke thought, and increase awareness. This usually involves focusing on perception of risk through risk information or self-assessment compared to recommendations, or on health benefits of taking action. Visuals, striking statistics, or personal stories that increase awareness of *risk* or of *benefits* to taking action or concrete experiences such as self-assessments are helpful here. In ongoing interventions, review, reflection, and sharing are appropriate.

- ***Explain***—*present stimulus and new material.* The focus is primarily on information that serves a motivational purpose: why-to take action. Tailor the activities and messages to take into consideration the audience's prior knowledge, experience, cultural background, and values. Here, focus on motivation by demonstrating the effectiveness of the targeted behaviors of the intervention to achieve health or food-system–related outcomes, personal benefits, social norms, values, self-efficacy, and so forth. Then, in addition, provide information to make the desired action easy to understand and do. Use mini-lectures, learning activities, and visual presentations.

- ***Expand***—*provide guidance and practice for how-to take action.* Provide the knowledge and skills participants will need for the desired action. To take into account learning styles, use role models to demonstrate action, and hands-on activities, such as food preparation, to help individuals gain practice and mastery and hence increase self-efficacy.

- ***Exit***—*apply and close.* Help participants consider how they will apply what has been learned through goal setting and writing a personal action plan (or implementation intention). For ongoing sessions or an intervention, strengthen self-regulation (self-direction skills and personal agency). Provide social support for participants' action plans. Summarize, wrap up, and bring the session to closure. Participants should be clear about the central action(s) they will take as a result of the session or communication.

Motivational or promotional activities are usually conducted first, whether within a session, over a series of sessions, or in a multicomponent nutrition education intervention. The nutrition science information you present in this phase is of a why-to nature (such as the scientific evidence for the benefits of the behavior change for health). However, motivational activities are still needed throughout the intervention to promote active deliberation and to reinforce motivation.

Strategies to facilitate the ability to take action usually follow motivational activities. The food and nutrition information you present and self-regulation (taking charge) skills participants practice in this phase are of a how-to nature.

This general sequence is useful for all types of sessions and whether they are 20 minutes or 2 hours. If you do not have much time, you can select one or two strategies and activities within each of the 4 Es to focus on, but still address both motivational and skills objectives within the same session and sequence them appropriately. If you have the opportunity to conduct several sessions, you may want to start with the motivational-phase activities and continue with action-phase activities in the second and later sessions. This has a downside—the same participants may not come to all sessions. Or, you may be working with an already motivated group—mothers who keenly want to know how to feed their children, for example, or those at risk of diabetes who want guidance on what to eat. For them, action phase activities are very appropriate. Even in this instance, however, it is helpful to start each session with an attention-getter, and then provide short motivational activities to strengthen the group's attitudes, reinvigorate their motivation, and renew their commitment to act before moving into skill building in the food and nutrition area and in self-regulation.

SEQUENCING BY THE TRANSTHEORETICAL MODEL'S STAGES OF CHANGE

You can also sequence educational activities and learning by individuals' stage of readiness to make dietary changes proposed by the transtheoretical model. **TABLE 11-3** describes the 10 processes of change of the transtheoretical model. Although all of the processes of change are used in all stages, in general, *experiential processes* are used more often during the early stages of motivational readiness, and *behavioral processes* are used more often during the later stages of change. In the early stages, the experiential processes of change emphasized are consciousness-raising, dramatic relief, environmental reevaluation, and self-reevaluation. Educational activities that facilitate the movement through the stages of motivational readiness thus form a sequence rather similar to the 4 Es and steps of health communication just described.

In the later stages, the processes often used for behavior change are the relapse prevention strategies of counterconditioning, management of reinforcements, control of environmental stimuli, and social liberation. (See Chapter 5 for details.) Consequently, if you wish to design educational activities and learning experiences by stages of change, you can use intervention activities that are appropriate for each stage.

TABLE 11-3 Transtheoretical Model: Processes Associated with Stages of Change and Implications for Intervention Strategies

Processes of Change	Stages When More Often Used	Change Process Within the Individual	Intervention Strategies
Consciousness-raising	PC to C	Increasing one's awareness about causes and consequences, seeking new information about healthy behavior	Increase awareness of individuals' eating patterns (e.g., F&V intake) through self-assessment and feedback, confrontations, media campaigns
Dramatic relief/ emotional arousal	PC to C	Emotional experience of threat followed by relief if action is taken	Personalizing risk, personal testimonies, role playing, trigger films, media campaigns to address feelings
Environmental reevaluation	PC to C	Assessing how one's behaviors affect others and the physical environment	Empathy training, documentaries
Self-reevaluation	C to Prep to A	Appraisal of one's image of oneself	Assisting individuals to clarify their values; imagining themselves as active and healthy; believing that behavior change is part of their identity
Self-liberation	C to Prep to A	Believing in ability to change; consciously making a firm commitment to act	Commitment-enhancing techniques such as contracting and public group decisions
Helping relationships	A to M	Enlisting social support for the healthy behavior change	Build rapport; create a supportive environment through groups, buddy systems, and calls
Counterconditioning	A to M	Substituting alternative thoughts and behaviors for less healthful eating behaviors	Teach new ways of thinking (self-talk) about behavior; new food- and nutrition-related skills
Reinforcement and rewards management	M	Increasing rewards for healthful eating and decreasing rewards for unhealthful eating practices	Overt rewards such as tee-shirts, incentives, and verbal reinforcement; teaching individuals to reward themselves
Stimulus or environmental control	M	Removing cues to less healthful eating and adding cues for more healthful eating	Provide instruction on how to restructure environment: refrigerator magnets with reminders, tip sheets
Social liberation	All	Selecting and advocating for environments that support healthful food practices	Provide environmental supports such as more F&V in schools or worksites; advocacy; policy

Note: PC = precontemplation; C = contemplation; Prep = preparation; A = action; M = maintenance; F&V = fruits and vegetables

Exploring Other Audience Characteristics and Intervention Resource Considerations

Before you proceed to creating exciting, motivational activities and writing out your plan for the session, it is important to be clear about some practical considerations in relation to your audience.

IDENTIFYING RELEVANT AUDIENCE CHARACTERISTICS

This is the time to find out some other relevant specifics about the audience or primary group: educational level; the physical and cognitive developmental level of children; literacy and numeracy skills; preferred learning styles and instructional formats; and emotional, social, and special needs. These are explained in more detail in the instructions for the Generate Educational Plans Worksheet shown for the case study at the end of this chapter.

PRACTICAL AND INTERVENTION RESOURCE CONSIDERATIONS

Practical and resource considerations may dictate the duration and intensity of the intervention that are possible, whatever the merits of nutrition education identified in the previous assessments.

- *What resources* will be available for the nutrition education intervention in monetary terms?
- *How long* an intervention is possible or considered desirable? One session or many?
- *What channels are possible given resource constraints?* Will the intervention involve group sessions, audiovisual or print media, health fairs, media campaigns, all of them, or other channels?

- *Time.* How much time do you have for your sessions? How much time will you have for setup and cleanup?
- *Space available and its arrangement.* What is the physical space like? How can you change the space to meet your needs? What space restrictions are you working within? If possible, visit your site ahead of time, or at least discuss with site personnel what the space is like.
- *Equipment available.* What equipment (audiovisual, cooking, etc.) is available to you? What could you bring if you needed to?
- *General administrative/facilities support.* How helpful are your key contact persons in terms of troubleshooting, providing supplies, helping with promotion, and providing technical assistance during your sessions?

Generating the Educational Plan: The Nuts and Bolts

We have now arrived at the ultimate reason for conducting all the activities of Steps 1 through 4: to generate enjoyable and meaningful educational activities, learning experiences, or communication messages to achieve the behavior change goals of your session(s) or intervention. This is an exciting event! These activities should be sequenced into an instructional plan for how to proceed, showing the *events of instruction*, the 4 Es. The resulting plan goes by many names, such as the lesson plan or education plan for a single session, a curriculum for several sequenced sessions, a media message plan, or the intervention guide (for an intervention with many components). And yes, you need educational plans with all audiences, whether they are children in schools, outpatients in a clinic, college athletes, older adults at a congregate meal site, or mothers in a WIC clinic. And yes, you need educational plans whether you will be delivering one 30-minute session or a series of 20 one-hour sessions. You will use these plans to deliver your session(s) with your audience, one educational plan per session. Note that these planning procedures also apply if you are planning indirect educational activities such as newsletters or materials for a website.

The Outline for a Single Session

- *Title* of your session (make it catchy!)
- *The behavior change goal*(s) of this particular educational session. It may be the same as, or a subset of, the behavior change goal(s) you decided on in Step 1.

- *Several general educational objectives* for the session, which may be all those you wrote in Step 4 or only some of them (with others to be used in other sessions in your series). These objectives convert the theory determinants or precursors of behavior change into a format that the nutrition educator can use to create relevant educational activities. Thus, for each general objective, indicate the determinant(s) that the objective seeks to address.
- *An educational plan* describing how you will proceed

START WITH THE PLANNING MATRIX TOOL TO CREATE AN OUTLINE FOR EACH SESSION

You may already have lots of ideas about the activities you want to do with your audience in each session to reach the behavior change goal(s) you have chosen. However, before you actually write up these activities, it is well worth the time it takes to first develop an outline. We provide a planning tool in the form of a matrix for this purpose. The matrix helps you to link the determinants you have selected for the session to your activities through the means of specific educational objectives. After you have planned out the session using this matrix, then you will turn it into a format that you will take with you to use with the group; we call this teaching format the educational plan (or lesson plan). And as we noted, you need an educational plan with all audiences, no matter how informal the session may seem, and whether they are children or adults.

A Planning Tool in the Form of a Matrix

This tool shows you how to use the determinants and behavior change strategies for the determinants to write specific educational objectives; you then create engaging and effective practical educational activities to achieve these specific objectives. The planning tool also helps you to arrange all the activities in a logical sequence. To show you how you can use this planning tool, a completed tool is shown for the case study at the end of the chapter as part of the Step 5 Generate Educational Plans Worksheet.

Start with key determinants from your theory model that you plan to address in this session. Then select one or more behavior change strategies from Table 11-1 and Table 12-1 that you can use to change the determinant(s) and hence the behavior change goals of you session (or intervention). These behavior change strategies will guide the choice of specific educational objectives of the session.

These objectives, in turn, guide your development of activities or learning experiences for the session.

Using the notion of "backwards planning" (i.e., starting with the end you have in mind), the planning outline can be flipped to show the desired end first:

Behavior change goal(s) ← Determinants of change ← Behavior change strategies ← Specific objectives ← Educational activities

Back and Forth Between Objectives and Activities

In working on the outline, go back and forth between objectives and activities. Think of interesting and relevant activities that you can create to help your audience to make changes in their behavior or take action. Then, carefully review the extent to which these activities address the objectives set forth. Use this back-and-forth approach to refine the objectives and create more meaningful and effective activities. Also, make sure that the objectives will engage audience participants in all three domains of the educational experience—head, heart, and hands—and that within each of these domains the activities involve a progression in terms of levels of cognitive difficulty and of affective engagement and internalization, and where needed, the appropriate level of psychomotor skills.

Sequencing Activities Is Important: The 4 Es

As we described earlier, evidence and instructional theory propose that the activities or "events of instruction" in educational sessions need to follow a certain sequence, labeled in this chapter, to be conducive to learning: excite, explain, expand, and exit. Other education developers may use other terms.

In most instances you want to begin each session with activities to gain the attention of the group (*excite*), and then move to activities to enhance motivation and promote contemplation by presenting new material that is motivational and builds on what they already know and can do (*explain*). Next, focus on activities to build skills and strengthen self-efficacy or collective efficacy (*expand*). Finally, some kind of closure or take-home message is crucial (*exit*). At this stage of the session, help the group to consider how to apply the message: usually some kind of individual or group action plan is the most effective. The same systematic process is needed for the design of all nutrition education messages and activities, such as brochures, newsletters, posters, media messages, or campaigns.

Sequencing activities is a very fluid process in which you go back and forth between designing activities and sequencing them appropriately. If you have the opportunity to rehearse (highly recommended) or to pilot test, you may want to change or rearrange activities.

GENERATE THE FINAL EDUCATIONAL PLAN(S): TEACHING FORMAT READY FOR DELIVERING TO YOUR AUDIENCE

In order to actually deliver the educational plan to your audience, the information in the planning tool must be converted into a narrative or teaching format. This is the format you will actually use to teach the session. This teaching format for one session is also shown in detail for the case study at the end of this chapter. It cannot be just a linear outline of activities; that would be too brief. It should have enough detail so that you will have all the food and nutrition information you need as well as the procedures you will follow, but not too long because you will have to be looking at it as you proceed. You do not want to lose eye contact with you audience, so you cannot be reading from a lengthy document. Various communication principles for delivering the lesson to your audience are described in detail in Chapter 15.

Case Study: The DESIGN Procedure in Practice

We now apply the information in this chapter specifically to the ongoing case study. Most educational plans will address both motivational determinants and facilitators of action. The sequence usually is for motivational activities to be conducted first, followed by skills building and application activities. Because there are so many determinants, strategies, and activities that could be used, for illustration purposes the case study presents the educational plan or lesson plan outlines for two hypothetical sessions on increasing intake of fruits and vegetables. One is presented here, focusing on enhancing motivation, and one in Chapter 12, focusing on facilitating change.

SESSION TITLE, BEHAVIOR CHANGE GOAL, AND GENERAL EDUCATIONAL OBJECTIVES

You will recall that in the case study, the nutrition education sessions are being designed for middle school students by a university-affiliated nonprofit health services organization.

The nutrition educator and her colleagues created a catchy title that would pique the interest of the students based on the behavior change goal of the two sessions to increase intake of fruits and vegetables. For this first of two sessions, the title was "In Living Color." They selected several of the general educational objectives from Step 4 and used these to select the strategy and guide the overall development of practical educational activities.

THE EDUCATIONAL PLAN: USING THE PLANNING MATRIX TOOL TO OUTLINE THE SESSION

The nutrition educator and the team used the planning tool to create a matrix showing how the determinants of change from their theory model in Step 3 would be converted to specific objectives for that session. They then brainstormed practical educational activities that they believed would lead to the achievement of these objectives with a primary focus on motivational determinants, and secondarily, on facilitating determinants. These activities were based on the literature and on their assessment in Step 2 of what the middle school students would find engaging, motivating, and meaningful as a learning experience.

Objectives and Activities in All Three Domains of Learning

In designing the educational plan for the case study, the nutrition education planners went back and forth between objectives and activities to ensure that they were in alignment. They also made sure that the objectives would engage students in all three domains of the educational experience—the cognitive, affective, and psychomotor or head, heart, and hands.

Sequencing the Activities

As the nutrition educators were designing the session, they made sure they created activities for each of the components of effective lesson plans and sequenced them appropriately. The final, carefully arranged planning matrix is shown in the case study at the end of this chapter.

THE EDUCATIONAL PLAN: DEVELOPING A TEACHING FORMAT FOR DELIVERING THE SESSION

For use in actually delivering the educational plan to the middle schoolers, the planning matrix was converted into a narrative or teaching format. This is the format the health educator would actually use to teach the session. This teaching format for the session is also shown for the case study in the Step 5 Generate Educational Plans Worksheet at the end of the chapter. For reasons of space the materials, handouts, and worksheets for the session are not shown.

Your Turn to Design Nutrition Education: Completing the Step 5 Generate Educational Plans Worksheet

You can now apply the information in this chapter to state the specific educational objectives for a session and design educational activities, learning experiences, or communication messages to achieve these educational objectives.

SESSION TITLE, BEHAVIOR CHANGE GOAL, AND GENERAL EDUCATIONAL OBJECTIVES

First, create a catchy title for the behavior change goal of your session that will pique the interest of your audience. Then state the general educational objectives from Step 4 that are based on the determinants from your theory model and use these to guide the overall development of practical educational activities. If you plan on devoting more than one session to the same behavior change goal, then select those general educational objectives from Step 4 that you will use to guide a particular session. The same determinants and general educational objectives may be used in more than one session, but typically there will also be some that are unique to each session of your series directed at the same behavior change goal.

USING THE PLANNING TOOL TO OUTLINE EACH EDUCATION PLAN

It is useful to first develop a lesson or educational plan outline using the planning tool in the Step 5 Generate Educational Plans Worksheet. See the Workbook at the end of Chapter 13 for a blank worksheet that you can use. Use the case study as a guide for completing the worksheet. Here, you first state the behavior goal of the session, and then list the general educational objectives to achieve the behavior change goal(s) that you stated in Step 4. These objectives should be directed at the key determinants or precursors of change.

You then complete the planning matrix as follows:

- *In the first column, list each of the four events in the sequence of instruction*: Excite, Explain, Expand, and Exit.
- In the second column, list each of the *potential determinants of behavior change*—which are also the theory constructs—from the theory model you created in Step 3 that *this particular session* will address.
- In the third column, indicate the *behavior change strategies* that you will use to operationalize the potential determinants. The behavior change strategies for each of the determinants are described in this chapter and shown in Table 11-1. Use them as a guide to create

learning experiences, activities, and content that will achieve the specific objectives.

- In the fourth column, state the *specific educational objectives* for each determinant and behavior change strategy. You should check whether the objectives cover all three domains of learning—head, heart, and hands—and include a range of complexity of objectives. These are usually arranged from most simple to most complex within a session or intervention.
- In the fifth column, describe (briefly) all the *practical educational activities*, learning experiences, or messages that will help participants achieve the specific educational objective(s) for the theory determinant listed. The information in Chapters 15 and 17 about practical tips for working with a wide range of groups is very helpful here as you create your practical educational activities.

Event of Instruction	Determinant	Behavior Change Strategy(ies)	Specific Objective(s) for Session	Practical Educational Activities, Learning Experiences, or Messages
Excite				
Explain				
Expand				
Exit				

THE EDUCATIONAL OR LESSON PLAN: DEVELOPING A TEACHING FORMAT FOR DELIVERING THE SESSION

You then convert the planning tool into a more detailed narrative lesson plan that you will actually use when you are with a group. Use the Step 5 Generate Educational Plans Worksheet located at the end of Chapter 13 to develop your educational plan for your real or hypothetical educational session.

- Think of a catchy title that will be meaningful to your audience. It should motivate people to come to your session or pique their interest if they are required to attend.
- State the behavior change goal for the session.
- Restate your general objectives; this can be very helpful here.
- Place an overview or outline of activities and a materials list at the beginning of the teaching plan. That way you will have the entire session in mind and all of the materials ready.
- For each educational activity, create a heading with a title and indicate the determinant(s) addressed as well as the general behavior change strategy. This heading will provide you with a quick visual cue when you are delivering the session with a group. It also indicates the purpose of the activity in terms of which determinant you are attempting to change.
- Convert each of the activities in the matrix into a fuller description or narrative. Include all of the specific content information you will need when you are with the group and a brief statement of the instructions for conducting the activity.
- Write the educational plan in such a way that another nutrition professional could deliver it.
- Be prepared. If the session involves a demonstration, make sure you have all the materials you need. If you plan on a food preparation activity (highly recommended), make sure you have tested the recipes and that you have prepped the foods so they are ready for the participants (such as fruits and vegetables washed, stems cut off, etc.).
- Include essential background information you will need (e.g., teaspoons of fat in the various snacks you will discuss). Lengthy information can be placed in an additional "background" section.
- Sequence the activities based on the order of instruction described in this chapter derived from the work of education instruction specialists: *Excite, Explain, Expand,* and *Exit.* If the session involves hands-on activities, think through the flow—will it work with the size of group that you are addressing?
- A sense of closure is especially important. This is a good time to provide an opportunity to apply what the audience has learned. A clear take-home message or setting action goals and a simple action plan is crucial.
- Make the educational plan several pages long, depending on the length of the session and the complexity of the behavior. You will also have several pages of handouts and other materials.

The case study provides a sample lesson plan showing exactly how the planning matrix is converted to the narrative or teaching format used for delivery.

PILOT TESTING THE EDUCATIONAL PLAN

If your intervention is planned to be more than a one-time event, pilot testing the learning experiences with a similar audience will be very helpful. If food is used, test the recipes and preparation procedures for taste acceptance and feasibility. Using focus groups, direct observation, and interviews, assess whether activities are acceptable and effective with the intended audience.

EDUCATIONAL PLANS IN PRACTICE

It is important to have an educational plan or lesson plan, but it is understood that you will implement the education lesson plans fluidly and naturally in the actual setting. You may find yourself needing to adapt the lessons to the situation on the ground. At the same time, even approaches that seem very informal with a strong focus on learner-centered education require that you develop strong, theory-based educational plans. Ideally, these plans would be developed in collaboration with the intended audience. You will always interact with the group and adjust the content and activities as needed. Tips about how to deliver the educational plans in practice in a group setting and how to develop accompanying materials, such as handouts, posters, or newsletters, are described in Part III of this book, which is about methods of implementing and delivering nutrition education with a variety of audiences.

© Africa Studio/Shutterstock

Questions and Activities

1. In the context of this book, what does learning mean? Describe how learning is related to education and behavior change?

2. Describe carefully the relationship among determinants of behavior change, behavior change strategies, and practical educational activities. Why is it important for a nutrition educator to select activities based on behavior change strategies, and strategies based on determinants?

3. What is a lesson plan or educational plan?

4. Describe the differences among the 4 Es. Describe when and why a nutrition educator would use each during a session. How do you see the sequence as useful for you? If not useful, explain why not.

5. For practice, use the example of increasing intake of calcium-rich foods among teenage girls shown in the accompanying table. For each motivational determinant, describe at least one strategy and one corresponding educational activity.

Potential Motivational Determinant	Behavior Change Strategy	Specific Educational Activity or Learning Experience
Perceived risk		
Outcome expectations/ perceived benefits		
Perceived barriers		
Affect/feelings		
Behavioral intention		

References

Abrams, E., P. Koch, I. R. Contento, L. Mull, H. Lee, J. DiNoia, and M. Burgermaster 2013, July. Food, Health & Choices: Using the DESIGN Stepwise Procedure to Develop a Childhood Obesity Prevention Program. *Journal of Nutrition Education and Behavior* 45(Suppl. 4):S13–S14.

Baranowski, T., E. Cerin, and J. Baranowski. 2009. Steps in the design, development, and formative evaluation of obesity prevention-related behavior change trials. *International Journal of Behavioral Nutrition and Physical Activity* 6: Article 6.

Baranowski, T., T. O'Connor, and J. Baranowski. 2010. Initiating change in children's eating behaviors. *International handbook of behavior, diet, and nutrition*, edited by V. R. Preedy, R. R. Watston, and C. R. Martin. New York:Springer.

Bartholomew, K., S. Parcel, G. Kok, N. H. Gottlieb, and M. E. Fernandez. 2011. *Planning health promotion programs: An intervention mapping approach.* 3rd ed. Hoboken, NJ: Wiley.

Blake C. E., E. Wethington, T. J. Farrell, C. A. Bisogni, and C. M. Devine. 2011. Behavioral contexts, food-choice coping strategies, and dietary quality of a multiethnic sample of employed parents. *Journal of the American Dietetic Association* 111(3):401–407.

Buchanan, D. R. 2000. *An ethic for health promotion: Rethinking the sources of human well-being.* New York: Oxford University Press.

Cohen, M. 1991. A comprehensive approach to effective staff development: Essential components. Presented at Education Development Center, meeting for Comprehensive School Health Education Training Centers. Cambridge, MA.

Contento, I., G. I. Balch, Y. L. Bronner, L. A. Lytle, S. K. Maloney, C. M. Olson, and S. S. Swadener. 1995. The effectiveness of nutrition education and implications for nutrition education policy, programs, and research: A review of research. *Journal of Nutrition Education* 27(6): 277–422.

Dewey, J. 1929. *The sources of a science of education.* New York: Liveright.

Diep, C. S., T. A. Chen, V. F. Davies, J. C. Baranowski, and T. Baranowski. 2014. Influence of behavioral theory on fruit and vegetable intervention effectiveness among children: A meta-analysis. *Journal of Nutrition Education and Behavior* 46(6):506–546.

Freiere, P. 1970. *Pedagogy of the oppressed.* New York: Continuum.

———. 1973. *Education for critical consciousness.* New York: Continuum.

Gagne, R. 1965. *The conditions of learning.* New York: Holt, Rinehart & Winston.

———. 1985. *The conditions of learning and theory of instruction.* 4th ed. New York: Holt, Rinehart & Winston.

Gagne, R., W. W. Wager, J. M. Keller, and K. Golas. 2004. *Principles of instructional design*. Boston: Cengage.

Haidt, J. 2006. *The happiness hypothesis: Finding modern truth in ancient wisdom*. New York: Basic Books.

Heath, C., and D. Heath. 2010. *Switch: How to change when change is hard*. New York: Random House.

Iowa Department of Public Health. 2014. Pick a better snack. http://www.idph.state.ia.us/inn/PickABetterSnack.aspx?pg=Educators Accessed 7/1/15.

Johnson, D. W., and R. T. Johnson. 1987. Using cooperative learning strategies to teach nutrition. *Journal of the American Dietetic Association* 87(9 Suppl.):S55–S61.

Katz, D. L., M. O'Connell, V. Y. Njike, M. C. Yeh, and H. Nawaz. 2008. Strategies for the prevention and control of obesity in the school setting: Systematic review and meta-analysis. *International Journal of Obesity (London)* 32(12):1780–1789.

Kinzie, M. B. 2005. Instructional design strategies for health behavior change. *Patient Education and Counseling* 56:3–15.

Koch, P. A. 2013. The 4Es. Personal communication.

Lewin, K. 1943. Forces behind food habits and methods of change. In *The problem of changing food habits*. Bulletin of the National Research Council. Washington, DC: National Research Council and National Academy of Sciences.

Liquori, T., P. D. Koch, I. R. Contento, and J. Castle. 1998. The Cookshop Program: Outcome evaluation of a nutrition education program linking lunchroom food experiences with classroom cooking experiences. *Journal of Nutrition Education* 30(5):302.

Manoff, R. K. 1985. *Social marketing: New imperatives for public health*. New York: Praeger.

Merrill, M.D. 2009. First principles of instruction. In *Instructional-design theories and models. Volume III. Building a common knowledge base*, edited by C. M. Reigeluth and A. A. Carr-Chellman. New York: Routledge.

Michie, S., S. Ashford, F. F. Sniehotta, S. U. Dombrowski, A. Bishop, and D. P. French. 2011. A refined taxonomy of behavior change techniques to help people change their physical activity and healthy eating behaviors: The CALO-RE taxonomy. *Physiology and Health* 26(11):1479–1498.

Michie, S., M. Richardson, M. Johnston, C. Abraham, J. Francis, W. Hardeman, et al. 2013. The Behavior Change Technique taxonomy (v1) of 93 hierarchically clustered techniques: Building an international consensus for the reporting of behavior change techniques. *Annals of Behavioral Medicine* 46(1):81–95.

Petty, R. E., J. Barden, and S. C. Wheeler. 2009. The elaboration likelihood model of persuasion: Developing health promotions for sustained behavioral change. In *Emerging theories in health promotion practice and research*, R. J. DiClemente, R. A. Crosby & M. C. Kegler, editors (2nd ed., pp. 185–214), San Francisco: Jossey-Bass.

Petty, R. E., and J. T. Cacioppo. 1986. *Communication and persuasion: Central and peripheral routes to attitude change*. New York: Springer-Verlag.

Radke, M., and E. Caso. 1948. Lecture and discussion-decision as methods of influencing food habits. *Journal of the American Dietetic Association* 24:23–41.

Reicks, M., A. C. Trofholz, J. S. Stang, and M. N. Laska. 2014. Impact of cooking and home preparation interventions among adults: Outcomes and implications for future programs. *Journal of Nutrition Education and Behavior* 46:259–276.

Reigeluth, C. M., and A. A. Carr-Chellman. 2009. Understanding instructional-design theory. In *Instructional-design theories and models. Volume III. Building a common knowledge base*, C. M. Reigeluth and A. A. Carr-Chellman, editors. New York: Routledge.

Rokeach, M. 1973. *The nature of human values*. New York: Free Press.

Rollnick, S., W. R. Miller, and C. C. Butler. 2008. *Motivational interviewing in health care: Helping patients change behavior*. New York: Guilford Press.

Sobal, J., and C. A. Bisogni. 2009. Constructing food choice decisions. *Annals of Behavioral Medicine* 38(Suppl 1):LS37–46.

Sobal, J., C. Blake, M. Jastran, A. Lynch, C. A. Bisogni, and C. M. Devine. 2012. Eating maps: places, times, and people in eating episodes. *Ecology of Food and Nutrition* 51(3):247–264.

Thompson, C. A., and J. Ravia. 2011. A systematic review of behavioral interventions to promote intake of fruit and vegetables. *Journal of the American Dietetic Association* 111(10):1523–1535.

Tyler, R. W. 1949. *Basic principles of curriculum and instruction*. Chicago: University of Chicago Press.

Waters, E., A. de Silva-Sanigorski, B. J. Hall, T. Brown, K. J. Campbell, Y. Gao, et al. 2011. Interventions for preventing obesity in children. *Cochrane Database of Systematic Reviews* 7(12):CD001871.

Wong, D., and D. Stewart. 2013. The implementation and effectiveness of school-based nutrition promotion programmes using a health-promoting schools approach: A systematic review. *Public Health Nutrition* 16(6):1082–1100.

Nutrition Education DESIGN Procedure

Decide behavior(s)	**E**xplore determinants of change	**S**elect theory & clarify philosophy	**I**ndicate general objectives	**G**enerate plans	**N**ail down evaluation plan
Step 1	Step 2	Step 3	Step 4	Step 5	Step 6

Step 5: Generate educational plans.

In this step, you use everything you have learned about your audience to generate educational plans for sessions that will help your audience attain your behavior change goal(s). Generate one educational plan for each of your sessions. You use your theory model and general educational objectives to create activities that are engaging, interesting, and meaningful for your audience. This is also the time to take stock of the practical aspects of working with your specific audience.

Use the Step 5 Generate Educational Plans worksheet as an organizational guide to help you design each of your educational sessions and translate theory into practice. You first use the planning matrix tool to outline your session. Then you convert the matrix outline into a narrative teaching format to use with your audience.

What are the practical considerations? Think about the practical considerations that will play a role in how you operationalize your objectives when you begin planning your session(s). When possible, use information from the audience itself; however, the research literature may also be helpful in completing this step.

Audience Trait	Description
Educational level or schooling	7th/8th grade
Physical/cognitive level	Most middle school students are able to integrate motivations and cognitions in a self-regulatory process.
Literacy and numeracy skills	City test scores indicate that the average student is at grade level for math and reading. Seventh grade reading level, operations with whole numbers and fractions, and basic algebra.
Preferred learning style	The school stresses group and hands-on work, and teachers report that students like interactive learning.
Special needs	Each grade has one inclusion class. Students may have difficulty with fine motor skills, comprehension, and behaviors. These classes have aides to help individual students.
Emotional needs	Many middle school students are sensitive about developing their own identity.
Social needs	Many middle school students are preoccupied by peer perceptions. It is important that they receive support and positive reinforcement.
Resources Needed	**Resources Available**
Time	Two 50-minute periods each week for 5 weeks
Space	Regular school classrooms with desks arranged in tables of four
Equipment	Standard classroom equipment: markers, dry erase board, flip charts, and TV/DVDs. Some classrooms have Smart Boards. Most copying will need to occur off premises.
Administrative support	The school is paying the nutrition educator to design and present the lessons.
Other	n/a

Nutrition Education DESIGN Procedure

Decide behavior(s) · Step 1   **E**xplore determinants of change · Step 2   **S**elect theory & clarify philosophy · Step 3   **I**ndicate general objectives · Step 4   **G**enerate plans · Step 5   **N**ail down evaluation plan · Step 6

What is the behavior change goal from Step 1 for this session?

Students will increase fruit and vegetable consumption.

What general educational objectives will you address in this session? Which motivational and/or facilitating objectives from Step 4 will guide your session?

- Participants will be able to recognize how far their fruit and vegetable intake is from recommendations.
- Participants will be able to describe the importance of eating a variety of fruits and vegetables.
- Participants will be able to appreciate the taste of various fruits and vegetables.
- Participants will be able to identify strategies to overcome perceived barriers to fruit and vegetable consumption.
- Participants will be able to have increased confidence in their ability to eat more and/or a greater variety of fruits and vegetables.

Planning matrix to outline your session: What activities will you do to guide your audience to your educational objectives?

Use the determinants and general objectives you have selected to achieve the behavior change goal of this particular session to think about the specific objectives you will need to guide the creation of activities. As you think about your specific objectives and start planning activities, sequence the activities according to the four Es: Excite, Explain, Expand, and Exit. Place the determinants where you think they would best fit into the sequence. Enter this information into columns 1 and 2. Next, refer to Tables 11-1 and 12-1 in the text and choose the behavior change strategy that is best suited to leveraging the motivating and facilitating determinants for your audience and the flow of your lesson. Enter the strategy into the third column. Then, write the specific educational objective for this chosen strategy in column 4. Finally, in column 5, briefly describe the activities you will use with your audience to achieve the specific objective.

Sequencing: 4Es	Determinant(s)	Strategy*	Specific Objective	Activity/Activities
Excite	Provide opportunity for self-assessments to personalize risk	Self-assessments to personalize risk	Students will describe their recent diet.	• Draw most recent meal on blank MyPlate template • Tally different colors of F&V
Explain	Perceived benefits/positive outcome expectations	Provide information about positive outcomes	Students will list benefits of F&V consumption.	Brainstorm benefits of F&V
Explain	Perceived benefits/positive outcome expectations	Provide information about positive outcomes	Students will summarize different benefits of different colored F&V.	• Read F&V superpowers comic • Discussion of benefits of a diet of different colored F&V
Expand	Food preferences	Provide direct experience with healthful food	Students will taste F&V of a variety of colors.	F&V color tasting
Expand	Perceived barriers (self-efficacy)	Reframe perception of barriers	Students will describe a variety of F&V using sophisticated vocabulary.	• Choose vocabulary Post-Its for each F&V dish • Discussion of flavors in F&V dishes and how to describe them

*Behavior change strategies are similar to **behavior change techniques** used in health psychology (e.g., Michie et al., 2011), and **procedures** described by Baranowski (2009).

Planning matrix to outline your session (Continued)

Sequencing: 4Es	Determinant(s)	Strategy	Specific Objective	Activity/Activities
Exit	Perceived risk/ negative outcome expectations	Provide opportunity for self-assessments to personalize risk	Students will evaluate current diet against recommendations.	• Compare recent meal to MyPlate template • Share reactions
Exit	Behavioral intention/goal intention	Promote values clarification	Students will state pros of and strategies for adding a variety of F&V to diet.	Goal intention worksheet with personal pros of eating F&V, strategies, and a goal intention statement

Educational plan in narrative teaching format for delivery to your audience. What is your detailed procedure for delivering the session?

Use the planning matrix outline to design the session in detail. Describe the procedure for each activity in the order in which it will occur during the session. Often motivational determinants correspond with the Excite and Exit part of the session, while facilitating determinants correspond to the Explain and Expand parts of the session. However, each audience and session is different; it is often important to include motivational determinants within the Explain and Expand parts of the session. Don't forget to include how long you expect each activity to take! You should provide a brief overview of the entire session and the necessary materials at the beginning of the session plan. Use the case study as an example.

Write out your narrative teaching plan for your educational session on the following page.

Nutrition Education DESIGN Procedure

Decide behavior(s) — Step 1
Explore determinants of change — Step 2
Select theory & clarify philosophy — Step 3
Indicate general objectives — Step 4
Generate plans — Step 5
Nail down evaluation plan — Step 6

Catchy title: In Living Color!

Behavioral goal: Students will increase fruit and vegetable consumption.

Overview (teaching point):

We get the greatest benefit from eating a variety of fruits and vegetables, so more of our meals should include more, different fruits and vegetables.

General educational objectives:

Participants will be able to:

- Recognize how far their fruit and vegetable intake is from recommendations.
- Describe the importance of eating a variety of fruits and vegetables.
- Appreciate the taste of various fruits and vegetables.
- Identify strategies to overcome perceived barriers to fruit and vegetable consumption.
- Demonstrate increased confidence in their ability to eat more and/or a greater variety of fruits and vegetables.

Materials:

Blank MyPlate worksheet, colored pencils, chart paper, fruit and vegetable superpowers comic, fruit and vegetable dishes highlighting different colored fruits and vegetables (e.g. rice with over-wintered greens, roasted root vegetables, blueberries), small plates, forks, napkins, sophisticated foodie vocabulary cards or Post-It notes (e.g., crisp, tangy, earthy, juicy, umami, hot), recipe newsletter, MyPlate comparison worksheet

Procedure*:

Excite
Self-assessment: Draw your most recent meal (perceived risk).
Distribute the blank MyPlate worksheet to students and ask them to draw their most recent meal. Encourage them to use colored pencils. Once finished, ask the students to tally which colors of fruits and vegetables they ate during that meal (or during the past 24 hours, if they didn't have fruits or vegetables at their most recent meal). (5 minutes)

Explain
Information on positive outcomes: Brainstorm benefits of fruits and vegetables (perceived benefits).
"Adults are always saying, 'Eat your veggies!' Do you think there's something to that statement? What are the benefits of eating fruits and vegetables?" List benefits on chart paper as students raise hands to share. Be sure the following benefits are included: they provide vitamins, minerals, fiber, nutrients; they can increase energy; they help make skin and hair look healthy; they help build strong bones and muscles; they decrease the risk for certain diseases. Also be sure students consider other relevant benefits, such as less packaging, fewer fossil fuels go into their production, and that buying fruits and vegetables at farmers' markets supports local farmers. (5 minutes)

Expand
Provide direct experience with food: "In Living Color" fruit and vegetable tasting (food preferences).
First students must wash hands, and have a quick reminder of how to safely (and politely) serve their own food. Set the ground rule, "Don't yuck my yum." Have students serve themselves a taste of each of the different colored fruit and vegetable dishes. Label each dish with a descriptive and catchy name. (10 minutes)
Reframe perceptions: Use sophisticated vocabulary to describe food (self-efficacy).
Hang sheets of chart paper with the name of each dish around the room. Distribute a set of sophisticated food vocabulary Post-Its to each student. Students do not need to have all of the words, but they should have a few that could apply to each dish. Once students have tasted each of the dishes, have them silently go around the room and stick at least one sophisticated food vocabulary Post-It beneath the name of each dish they tried. After all students have had a chance to participate, discuss the flavors in each dish and the meanings of the different adjectives. Provide positive reinforcement for learning to describe foods in more mature, adult language, instead of childish yuck and yum. (15 minutes)

Exit
Personalize risk: Compare recent intake to MyPlate recommendations (perceived risk).
Have students return to their drawing of a recent meal. Distribute the MyPlate comparison worksheet, with the official MyPlate illustration and recommendation that half your plate be fruits and vegetables. Have students compare their own drawing to the recommendations and evaluate the number of each color of fruits and vegetables they tallied. Have volunteers share their reactions and self-evaluations. (5 minutes)
Promote values clarification: State intention to add a variety of fruits and vegetables to diet (goal intention).
Ask participants to write at least three personal pros about eating more fruits and vegetables, and three strategies that will help them increase fruit and vegetable intake and/or variety. Have a few volunteers share the benefits and strategies they jotted on the worksheet. Encourage participants to make a clear statement that they will take action to include more colors of more fruits and vegetables in their diets in the next week. Provide students with recipes for all of the dishes they tasted during the session. (5 minutes)

*In the headings for each activity, the first phrase is the behavior change strategy; the second is a brief description of your activity; and the words in parenthesis refer to the determinant targeted by the activity.

CHAPTER 12

Step 5: Generating Educational Plans: A Focus on Facilitating the Ability to Change Behavior and Take Action

OVERVIEW

This chapter provides guidance for creating engaging and practical educational activities based on the determinants and strategies of behavior change, and on sequencing these activities to generate educational plans to facilitate the ability of participants to take action on the behavior change goals of your sessions or intervention. The information in Chapters 5, 15, and 17 will help you with this step in the design process.

CHAPTER OUTLINE

- Facilitating the ability to change behavior and take action: an overview
- Translating behavioral theory into educational practice: determinants, behavior change strategies, and educational activities
- Building food- and nutrition-related skills: enhancing behavioral capability
- Strengthening self-regulation (self-directed change) processes and personal agency
- Case study: the DESIGN Procedure in action—Step 5
- Your turn to design nutrition education: completing the Step 5 Generate Educational Plans Worksheet

LEARNING OBJECTIVES

At the end of the chapter, you should be able to:

- Describe the kinds of theory-based behavior change strategies to address determinants that are particularly important in facilitating the ability to take action
- Design specific educational activities or learning experiences to make practical the theory-based educational strategies
- Sequence the behavior change objectives and strategies to create an educational plan

Facilitating the Ability to Change Behavior and Take Action: An Overview

We have seen that motivation is vital for initiating the behavior-change pathway. Chapter 11 describes many behavior change strategies and practical activities nutrition educators can use for communicating food and nutrition content in a way that enhances audience motivation. Once audience members have contemplated their options and decided to make a change or take action given their considerations of family situations, community, and culture, progress towards achieving the behavior change goal(s) of your sessions or intervention still requires that people take the additional step of converting motivations and intention into action. In order to do so, they need to feel empowered and able to make the change or take the action. Our role is to facilitate their movement toward action and provide the conditions to foster their sense of empowerment. At this stage, intervention participants need food- and nutrition-related knowledge and skills in order to carry out the behavior, and self-regulation (that is, skills in self-directed change) in order to be able to follow through with their intentions.

Consequently, this chapter describes behavior change strategies and practical educational activities to:

- Build food- and nutrition-related skills.
- Strengthen self-regulation or skills in self-directed change.

FIGURE 12-1 highlights what we are doing in Step 5 of the DESIGN Procedure; an overview of the action and maintenance component of nutrition education is shown in **FIGURE 12-2**. Note that when individuals are first *initiating action*, the aim of nutrition education is to facilitate the ability to initiate action, and the major nutrition

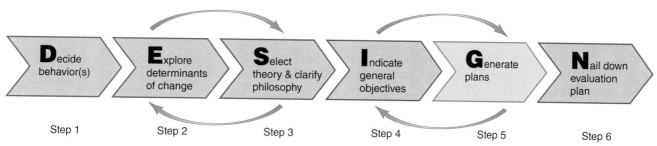

Inputs: Collecting the Assessment Data		Outputs: Designing the Theory-Based Intervention			Outcomes: Evaluation Plan
Tasks: • **Decide** behavior change goal(s) of the intervention, based on: • analyzing issues and behaviors of concern for audience	*Tasks:* • **Explore** determinants of behavior change based on a variety of data sources	*Tasks:* • **Select** theory and draw intervention-specific theory model • Clarify educational philosophy • Articulate perspectives on content	*Tasks:* • **Indicate** general objectives for each determinant in your theory model	*Tasks:* • **Generate** educational plans: • Educational activities to address all determinants in theory model • Sequence for implementation using the 4 Es	*Tasks:* • **Nail down** evaluation plan • Select methods and questions to evaluate outcomes • Plan process evaluation • Create questions to measure how implementation went
Products: *Statement of intervention behavior change goal(s)*	*Products:* *List of determinants to address in the intervention*	*Products:* *Theory model for intervention* *Statement of educational philosophy* *Statement of content perspectives*	*Products:* *A general objective for each determinant in the theory model*	*Products:* *Educational plans that link determinants and educational activities to achieve behavior change or action goal(s)*	*Products:* *List of evaluation methods and questions* *Procedures and measures for process evaluation*

FIGURE 12-1 Nutrition Education DESIGN Procedure: Generate plans—Step 5: Facilitating.

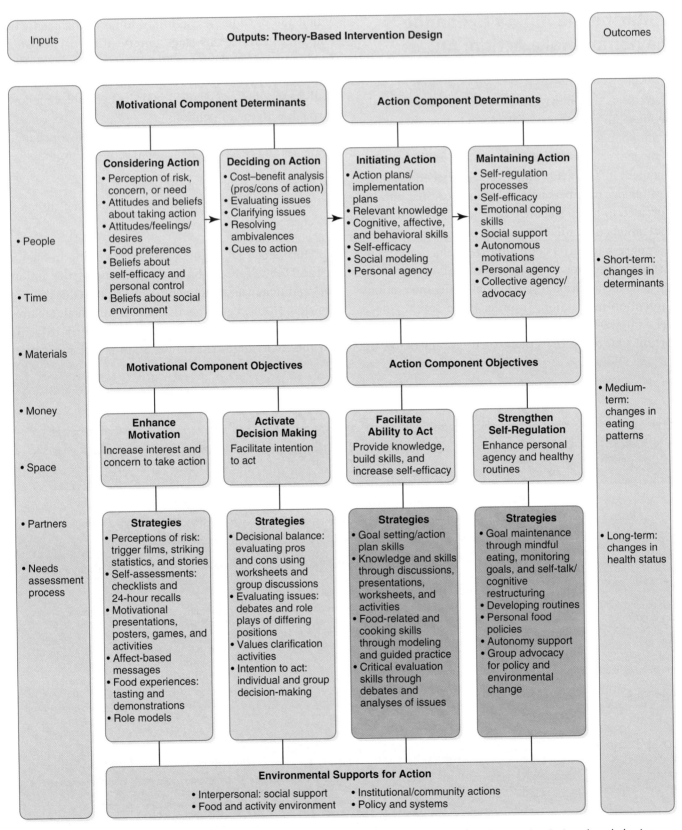

FIGURE 12-2 Conceptual framework for translating behavioral theory into effective nutrition education practice: Action phase behavior change strategies.

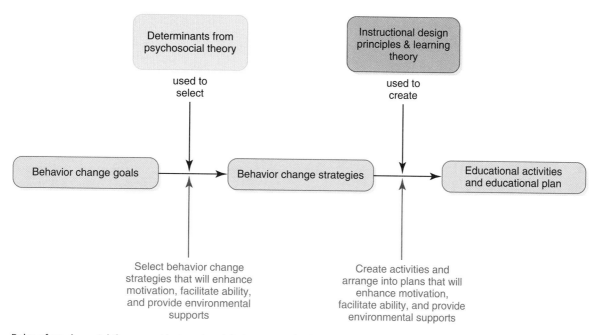

Roles of psychosocial theory and instructional design principles for developing educational activities and an educational plan.

education strategies are to assist people in setting action plans and help them to acquire the relevant knowledge and **cognitive**, **affective**, and **behavioral skills** related to the food and nutrition (or physical activity) behavior change goals set by your sessions or intervention. When individuals are seeking to *maintain the changes* they have made, the aim of nutrition education is to strengthen participants' skills in self-regulation, assist them in developing personal policies, and work with others collectively to advocate for changes in the environment.

Translating Behavioral Theory into Educational Practice: Determinants, Behavior Change Strategies, and Educational Activities

Your selection of behavior change strategies and educational activities depends on the theory or model for the intervention that you created in Step 3 and your educational philosophy. Increasing evidence suggests, however, that for this component or phase of nutrition education, self-regulation models, social cognitive theory, health action process approach, and grounded theory from extensive interviews are the most helpful (Bandura 1997; Pelican et al. 2005; Bisogni et al. 2012; Blake et al. 2011). The strategies appropriate for this component of nutrition education are highlighted in Figure 12-2.

Remember, behavior change strategies are ways to operationalize each of the determinants of behavior change for educational and instructional purposes, and hence the determinants and strategies often have some similarities.

Also remember that behavior change strategies are converted into practical educational activities and learning experiences by using learning theory and the principles of good instruction from the field of education (Gagne et al. 2004; Kinzie 2004; Merrill 2009). (Please read Chapter 15 for more details.) That is, the process of delivering our nutrition education sessions in practice can be summarized as follows:

Choose behavioral change goal → Identify psychosocial theory-based determinants of behavior change → Select determinant-based behavior change strategies → Create educational objectives and activities based on learning theory and instructional design theory from education, as shown in the diagram at the top of the page.

TABLE 12-1 shows the connections among theory determinants of change, behavior change strategies, and practical educational strategies or learning experiences. These strategies and activities are described in more detail later in this chapter. It is important to design educational activities that are engaging and fun, involve the affective as well as the cognitive domain, and include

TABLE 12-1 Linking Theory Determinants, Behavior Change Strategies, and Educational Activities

Determinant of Behavior Change (Theory Construct)	Behavior Change Strategies	Practical Educational Activities, Learning Experiences, Content, or Messages
Behavioral capability/competence: Knowledge and cognitive skills SCT SDT SR	■ Provide factual knowledge related to behavior	Provide factual information related to the behavior change involving *remembering* and *understanding*, using lectures, visuals, slides, and hand-outs
	■ Provide instruction on how to perform the behavior (procedural knowledge)	Provide instruction and create learning experiences on how to perform the behavior, involving *applying* what is learned (such as breastfeeding, safe food handling)
	■ Stimulate cognitive thinking skills related to behavior	Active methods for higher order learning, involving *analysis*, *evaluation*, and *synthesis*: discussions, role plays, debates, games, and interactive learning experiences to teach needed food- and nutrition-related skills to engage in behavior
Behavioral capability/competence: Affective skills SCT SDT SR	■ Build effective communication skills	Discussions, scenarios, role plays, videos, and worksheets to develop affective skills such as communicating needs
	■ Promote delayed gratification	Mindful eating and visualization exercises
	■ Prompt plans for coping responses (to build affective skills; also part of self-regulation skills)	Discussion, videos, and examples of ways to cope with difficulties that arise
	■ Conduct facilitated discussion or dialogue	Group members share feelings and experiences based on questions posed to stimulate reflection and feelings
	■ Build resistance skills to unhealthy norms	Model and provide practice for skills in resistance to unhealthy norms
Behavioral capability/competence: Behavioral skills SCT SDT SR	■ Provide active mastery experiences/guided practice (Also enhances self-efficacy—see below)	Demonstration of food preparation/cooking skills, parenting practices, followed by guided practice with feedback through hands-on activities to develop skills such as cooking, breastfeeding, and safe food handling
Self-efficacy SCT SDT TRA HAPA SR	■ Model/demonstrate the behavior (Separately or as part of guided practice)	Make the desired actions easy to understand and do: Demonstration of the behavior by credible, respected, or relatable social model, such as making a low-fat, whole-grain recipe
	■ Provide guided practice	Assist individuals to achieve success by ■ Providing clear instructions ■ Demonstrating the behavior ■ Providing practice or direct experience (e.g., food preparation or cooking; blood glucose monitoring)
	■ Provide feedback on performance to overcome self-doubt	Give feedback and encouragement on performance, emphasizing achievements and difficulties already overcome. Alleviate concern about responses to the new food or behavior.

Determinant	Behavior Change Strategy	Educational Activity
Self-Regulation: Goal setting SCT SDT HAPA SR	■ Stimulate action goal setting (or action planning/implementation intentions)	Teach goal setting skills for specific behaviors or actions, provide contracts/pledges or action planning forms
Self-regulation: Skills SCT SDT HAPA SR	■ Facilitate self-monitoring and feedback (TTM: Counterconditioning, rewards management, stimulus control)	After setting action goals (or action planning/implementation intentions), provide self-monitoring forms, feedback on progress toward action goals, and action tips
	■ Encourage goal maintenance	Assist participants to identify and prioritize competing goals; reminder to protect action goals from distractions: mindful eating, conscious attention, focus on the big picture, link the action goal to self-identity
	■ Prompt reframing perceptions and attributions/cognitive restructuring	Help participants reinterpret information or reframe how certain foods or situations are perceived; how they interpret their successes and failures
	■ Build skills for planning coping responses (also called coping self-efficacy)	Assist participants to develop ways to cope with difficulties that arise
	■ Build skills for managing cues from environment	Assist participants to develop the mindset of planning ahead for tempting locations or situations
	■ Promote personal food policies and routines	Tip sheets on creating personal policies for purchasing foods, meal patterns (e.g., always eat breakfast, bring lunch to work), and eating out
	■ Encourage repeated consumption of healthful food	Assure participants that with repeated experience with healthful foods, they will come to like them. Flavor substitutes do not change preferences.
Autonomy SDT	■ Provide autonomy support	Provide choice in terms of behavior change and support of choice
Social support SCT SDT SR	■ Enhance skills in management of social context and plan for social support (TTM: Helping relationships)	Facilitate skills in making trade-offs about difficult choices; create supportive group environment; encourage buddy system
Reinforcements SCT SR	■ Provide reinforcements and rewards	Verbal praise, tee-shirts, drawing for prizes, or awards
Cues to action HBM SCT SR	■ Plan cues to action	Billboards, grocery bags, media messages, news articles, refrigerator magnets, and keychains with messages
Collective efficacy/empowerment SCT	■ Enhance skills in advocacy	Working with group to identify and prioritize needs or concerns; develop recommendations or action plans to present to policymakers for desired actions; monitor progress and incorporate feedback for further actions

Note: HBM = health belief model; TRA = the reasoned action approach/theory of planned behavior and extensions; SCT = social cognitive theory; SDT = self-determination theory; HAPA = health action process approach model; Goal = goal model of goal-directed behavior; SR = self-regulation models; TTM = transtheoretical model the psychomotor domain where appropriate. Remember that people generally remember 10% of what they read, 20% of what they hear, 30% of what they see, 50% of what they hear and see, 70% of what they say and write, and 90% of what they say as they do a thing (Wiman and Mierhenry 1969).

Building Food- and Nutrition-Related Knowledge and Skills: Enhancing Behavioral Capability

Although how-to knowledge, or food and nutritional literacy, is not enough to motivate individuals to take food- and health-related actions or to make changes in their diets, it is necessary in order for individuals to act on their motivations and achieve their behavior change goals and action plans. For example, individuals may need help in selecting the appropriate foods from the 40,000-item supermarket; reading food labels; evaluating the nutrition information that bombards them from magazines, newspapers, television news, advertising, and friends; or interpreting medical information provided by their physicians. Food and nutrition education activities must therefore be directed at increasing basic knowledge as well as complex cognitive skills that will enhance people's power to take thoughtful action.

This section describes ways to increase participants' ability to carry out the behavior (labeled as *behavioral capability* in many psychosocial theories) through skill-building in terms of food- and nutrition-related knowledge and cognitive, affective (emotional), and behavioral skills. To increase the ability to carry out the behavior, it is necessary to identify your audience's current level of knowledge and skills (which you did in Step 2) and to design activities that will assist participants to achieve appropriate levels of thinking (cognitive domain), affective or emotional engagement (affective domain), and psychomotor skills in order to fulfill the behavior change goal(s) of your sessions or intervention (Anderson et al. 2000). These levels of understanding and engagement are described in detail in Chapter 10 and Table 10-1 and Table 10-2 and are summarized below. Thus, in designing your educational plans, carefully think through the level of thinking and affective engagement that each activity aims for participants to achieve.

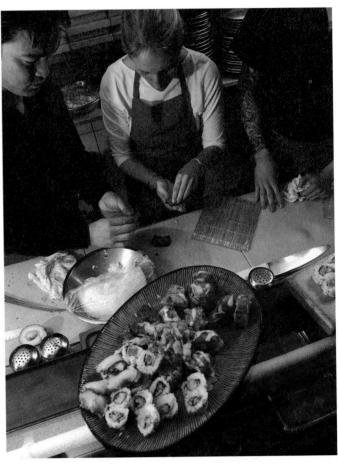

Learning cooking skills can boost confidence.

© Aaron Flaum/Alamy

BEHAVIOR CHANGE STRATEGIES AND EDUCATIONAL ACTIVITIES FOR THE THEORY DETERMINANT OF KNOWLEDGE AND COGNITIVE SKILLS

As you design your activities, consider carefully the levels of knowledge or complexity of understanding and skills you are aiming for the participants to achieve through each activity. In summary, these levels are: (1) *remembering* factual information pretty much as it was learned, (2) *understanding* the information, (3) *applying* or using the learned information in a new and concrete situation or to solve a problem, (4) *analyzing* or taking apart the information into component parts, (5) *evaluating* or judging the value of the information for a particular purpose, and (6) *synthesizing* or putting information together in a new way.

We describe some examples of the kinds of activities that you can use in your sessions or intervention to achieve each of these levels of knowledge and understanding.

Do not focus only on basic factual knowledge. All age groups are capable of all levels of learning; it is only the sophistication of the language and concepts that may differ. For example, do not assume that for young children or low-literacy audiences, educational activities should be set at low levels of cognitive learning such as recall of information or comprehension only. Even second graders can evaluate and low-literacy audiences often bring with them a wealth of practical evaluative and synthesizing skills based on their life experiences. It is good practice to include information about the cognitive level of each activity in your educational plan to ensure that activities are well distributed across levels.

Behavior Change Strategy: Provide Factual Knowledge Related to Behavior

Factual knowledge has been defined for the purposes of developing educational programs as *remembering* factual information (Anderson et al. 2000). In the area of food and nutrition, knowledge might include the ability to recall such facts as the recommended guidelines for healthful diets appropriate for an individual's age, sex, and stage of life; which foods to select to meet the guidelines; or serving sizes and how many servings one should eat of each food group in the MyPlate system or other dietary guidance system. *Understanding*, on the other hand, involves understanding the meaning and interpretation of information (Anderson et al. 2000), such as being able to describe the ecological impact of different food processing techniques and packaging materials. Strategies to both provide factual knowledge and increase understanding are more likely to be effective when they involve the following:

Practical educational activities might include:

- *Presentations and materials made interesting.* Basic information can be provided through lectures, handouts, and slides. How-to nutrition information or nutrition literacy, especially for the general public, is more likely to be remembered if it is vivid and understandable in everyday terms. Personal stories and everyday examples are also effective.
- *Visuals.* Graphs can be made using "foods" visually as units instead of abstract numbers (e.g., a stack of 5 teaspoons on top of each other instead of a plain bar graph to display the number of teaspoons of fat in foods). Show photographs or models of foods to help the audience estimate portion sizes, or bring in boxes or containers

of foods to show nutrient composition. (Tip: Containers should be empty so that audience members don't ask to take the foods home! This has the added advantage that you can use the containers again.)
- *Demonstrations.* These can be very effective, such as spooning out onto a plate the number of teaspoons of fat in a hamburger or burning a cracker to show that it has "calories" in it. (Tip: Use a cracker that has a lot of fat and a loose weave for oxygen to get in.)
- *Other channels.* Other methods involve newsletters, flyers, and Web-based programs, depending on the behavior or practice and the channel chosen (e.g., mass media, in-person).

Provide Instruction on How to Perform the Behavior

Procedural knowledge is the knowledge about how to do something, or decision rules for solving given cognitive tasks. Included are relatively simple skills such as how to read a recipe, or more complex tasks such as how to breastfeed.

Practical educational activities might include:

- *Demonstrations.* These are effective in showing how to perform a behavior, such as how to read a recipe or how to cut up or store foods using safe food handling practices.
- *Visuals.* Visuals such as videos, posters, or handouts can show how to breastfeed.

Behavior Change Strategy: Stimulate Cognitive Thinking Skills

Food and nutrition issues often are complex. To take action and maintain behavior change requires not only knowledge of facts, but also development of conceptual frameworks on which to hang isolated messages, called knowledge structures or schemas. Skills in analysis, evaluation, and synthesis are important here. Building such skills is more difficult than providing factual or procedural information. Active methods are usually more effective with most audiences: worksheets and hands-on, minds-on activities are appropriate to help people see connections between concepts and develop their conceptual frameworks for the given issue.

Higher order learning includes the following cognitive skills:

- *Analysis* may involve examining the sugar content of different beverages or the fat content of different fast foods, or examining the carbon footprint of foods produced by different methods.

- *Evaluation* may involve rating several different food sources of calcium to select the best source based on some criterion such as price or impact on the body, or judging whether different types of food packaging are more environmentally friendly based on some criterion such as amount of energy used to make the package.

- *Synthesis* may be creating a day's menu to incorporate four and a half or more cups of fruits and vegetables (or just a plan for when individuals will incorporate more fruits and vegetables in a day).

Integrating These Skills to Enhance Critical Thinking and Decision Making

You may wish for your nutrition education sessions to include activities directed at enhancing critical reasoning skills. You can do this by integrating the higher-order thinking skills as described above.

You can help your audience to develop such skills by providing them with opportunities to examine the arguments on both sides of an issue related to your target behaviors—for example, whether to reduce dietary fat or carbohydrates to lose weight, eat organic versus "regular" fruits and vegetables, or breastfeed or bottle feed their infant. You can help them analyze and resolve contradictions and create personal policies through synthesis that will guide their food-related activities on an ongoing basis. A cognitive understanding of the food system and its impacts provides a context for action. Food- and nutrition-related behaviors are also embedded in larger social, economic, and political contexts that need to be understood for the continued maintenance of change.

Practical educational activities might include:

- *Trigger films or clips from the Web followed by discussion.* You can use trigger films and discussion to enhance critical thinking skills so participants can learn to evaluate controversial issues or develop complex understandings. The arguments for and against certain practices can be volunteered by the group and recorded on newsprint in a brainstorming format and then discussed and perhaps voted upon.

- *Active methods* such as worksheets and hands-on, minds-on activities are appropriate to help people understand both sides of issues, see connections

between concepts, and develop their conceptual frameworks for specific issues.

- *Debates.* Carefully designed activities such as written or oral critiques or debates can also be used to encourage analysis of issues. Here, participants should focus on the claims of the position, the evidence for and against the position along with the strength of such evidence, and conclusions based on evaluation of the evidence. When selecting opposing groups for a debate, to the extent possible, assign group members to argue for the position that is contrary to their own personal position: this will greatly facilitate discussion and debate based on evidence rather than personal conviction. Use of these activities will depend on the learning style preferences of the audience as well as their comfort level with them. However, debates—oral or written—are interesting for all and should be considered. Low literacy does not preclude oral debates.

BEHAVIOR CHANGE STRATEGIES AND EDUCATIONAL ACTIVITIES FOR THE THEORY DETERMINANT OF AFFECTIVE SKILLS

Even when individuals recognize that they may need to change some of their food practices for health reasons, their current practices are most often psychologically or culturally beneficial. Most people like the way they are eating or it fits family and cultural norms and expectations; that is why they do so. Or, they may want to take action on food system issues to support broader goals and values (such as supporting local agriculture), but doing so is personally inconvenient and more expensive. Consequently, any dietary change is undertaken with some ambivalence. Thus, the nutrition education intervention you are designing needs to create activities that will enhance participants' affective or emotional skills.

Designing Educational Activities at Different Levels of Affective Engagement

Feelings are important, especially for behavior change. As you are designing your sessions or intervention, think about the degree to which your activities will engage your participants emotionally. Maybe you wish only for groups or audiences to: (1) *receive* your message and become aware of the recommended action or behavior change (mass media campaigns may seek this level); or you may seek for your audience to (2) actively *respond* during your sessions or intervention, participating instead of just listening or observing, and beginning to respond with satisfaction to the educational activities and to form their own opinions. However, most educational programs aim for a greater degree of affective engagement resulting in participants (3) *valuing* the recommended action; here, individuals make a commitment to the action recommended by the intervention, perhaps at first tentatively, but later with conviction. At that level of commitment, individuals are ready and willing to take action, moving from intention to action. Or, perhaps you wish for the intervention to have an even more far-reaching impact: (4) the *organizational level* impact, where participants will be able to make the behavior change a priority in their lives and feel self-efficacious to organize their lives and emotions to make the change possible. Finally, you may wish for the intervention to result in people (5) *internalizing* the value of the recommended actions to the extent that they are making the changes consistently and the actions become part of their overall values and worldview.

Because it is appropriate for most nutrition education programs to aim for active commitment to take action and make the change a priority, it would be best for you to design activities to achieve *valuing-* and *organizational*-level objectives. Create activities that will encourage participant engagement and will help individuals address their feelings and emotional concerns as they attempt to convert commitment to action (*valuing* level of engagement) or make the new behavior a priority (*organizational* level).

Behavior Change Strategy: Build Effective Communication Skills

Most individuals live with others and will need to hone their skills in stating their needs in terms of healthy eating (and active living), asking for what they desire and at the same time negotiating with others so that all parties feel heard and have their needs met. For example, different members of the household may have different food likes and habits, and for your participants to ask for more fruits and vegetables to be available or fewer cookies or chips to be lying around may be quite difficult. Additionally, many individuals find it very difficult to refuse foods offered in social situations such as at meals in friends' homes or on special occasions, for fear of offending people. This may mean learning to be assertive but cooperative at the same time. Role playing or discussions may be useful here.

Behavior Change Strategy: Promote Delayed Gratification

There is evidence that when people add healthy items to their diet they do not eat fewer of the less healthy items (Verplankton and Faes 1999). Participants may need help in delaying their gratification in terms of eating the less healthy but tasty food items, with a focus on **mindful eating**. Participants can be led through visualizations about what happens to the less healthy tasty food in our bodies in the short term and over the long term. They can then visualize the health impact of the healthy foods on the body. Or, they can visualize what the areas around their town might look like if all the local farms were gone. This may help them be willing to delay their short-term gratification for long-term positive personal and societal gains.

Behavior Change Strategy: Prompt Plans for Coping Responses

Participants may also need assistance in coping with stressful eating situations: when bored, angry, at parties, and so forth. Have participants acknowledge and explore these stressful situations, brainstorm solutions, and then make plans for how they will handle these situations.

Behavior Change Strategy: Conduct Facilitated Discussion or Dialogue

In small groups, using facilitated discussion or dialogue is one way nutrition educators can help participants deal with feelings and emotional issues. In facilitated discussion, group members share feelings and experiences. The process is described more fully in Chapter 15. Participants can also be divided into groups of three or four where they can talk over questions such as the following: What is the hardest thing about trying to change the way we eat? What are some successful ways we have changed other habits that could be applied to this particular dietary behavior? How will we deal with the desires of various family members when the whole family needs to make changes?

BEHAVIOR CHANGE STRATEGIES AND EDUCATIONAL ACTIVITIES FOR THE THEORY DETERMINANT OF BEHAVIORAL SKILLS

Making dietary changes requires attention to a specific recurring array of sub-behaviors and specific actions that constitute the behavior, such as shopping for food, storing it, and preparing it. The environment in which dietary choices have to be made is often quite challenging. One study found, for example, that to eat more fruits and vegetables, individuals said that they had to make more visits to stores, eating at friends' houses became more difficult, and buying takeout meals became more problematic (Anderson et al. 1998; Cox et al. 1998). Eating behaviors are also very culture bound and hence must be investigated for each intended audience.

Behavioral capability includes a variety of practical skills such as food shopping, household food management skills, or time management skills. Shopping skills include ability to navigate grocery stores, to identify and select the appropriate foods to achieve the targeted behavior change goal(s), knowing which food items can substitute for others, and so forth. Physical skills include such skills as preparing foods, cooking, breastfeeding, growing a vegetable garden, and participating in sports.

Self-efficacy is an important determinant of behavior change. Self-efficacy may increase with increased level of skills, but self-efficacy is not the same thing as skills. Self-efficacy involves both skills and the confidence that individuals can consistently use their skills even in the face of impediments or barriers. Social cognitive theory argues that a person's feeling of self-efficacy or competence in being able to carry out a behavior is crucial to whether that person will perform the target behavior (Bandura 1986). Furthermore, an increased perception of control or feeling of success comes from becoming more skillful in performing the desired behavior. Skill acquisition is thus an essential step leading from intention to behavior.

Behavior Change Strategy: Provide Active Mastery Experiences/Guided Practice

A review of the many strategies for facilitating mastery of skills and enhancing self-efficacy suggests the following specific practical educational activities (Bandura 1997) that can be applied to the acquisition of food preparation, cooking, breastfeeding, safe food handling, or other food- and nutrition-related skills required for participants in your intervention to engage in the intervention's targeted behaviors or practices.

Practical educational activities:

■ *Clear instructions to individuals on how to perform the desired behavior.* You can enhance individuals' sense of confidence in their own abilities to carry out the goal behaviors when you provide them with clear and

realistic instruction on how to perform the behavior. Examples include teaching participants how to make tasty low-fat meals, store fruits and vegetables correctly so that they do not spoil quickly, plant a vegetable garden, breastfeed, or handle foods safely in the home kitchen. Such teaching can be done by direct verbal instruction, using audiovisual media, role playing, or written instructions.

■ *Modeling/demonstration of behavior.* Food demonstrations are a notable example. Such demonstrations can be live, on videotape, through visual mass media such as television, via the Internet, or in printed materials. Note the popularity of food shows and cooking demonstrations on television. Modeling is a powerful factor in motivating behaviors as well as an important instructional tool.

■ *Guided practice with feedback.* This method is highly effective in both teaching skills and increasing self-efficacy. Cooking has been shown to improve cooking-related knowledge, attitudes, and behaviors more than food demonstrations (Levy and Auld 2004). Here, you create opportunities for individuals to practice the behavior (e.g., cooking a particular food) and provide them with specific feedback immediately after they have performed the desired behavior. Encouragement is useful because it can overcome participants' self-doubts. This, of course, requires the availability of food preparation or cooking facilities. However, many nutrition educators have developed ways to

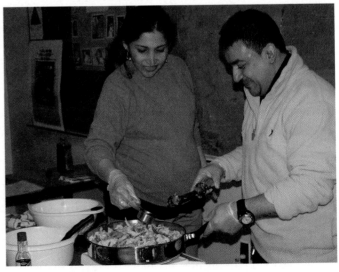

Learning to cook and eat healthfully at the WIC clinic.
Courtesy of USDA.

make cooking demonstrations, and even cooking by participants, possible by bringing with them all the needed food and equipment, including portable butane stoves or electric hot plates. Supermarket tours can enhance skills in shopping practices that are nutritionally healthy and ecologically sound.

Taken together, these three procedures result in a strategy referred to as *guided practice, behavioral rehearsal,* or *skills mastery*. You provide a demonstration of the desired behavior or skills, create opportunities for participants to practice what they observed with guidance on the performance of the task, make suggestions for improvement where necessary, and encourage them in their actions.

These behaviors are, of course, very culture bound and hence must be investigated for each intended audience. In addition, dietary behaviors are complex and the psychological motivations and skills needed are different depending on the food; you need to consider these factors when planning nutrition education.

> The information in Chapters 15 and 17 about practical tips for working with diverse groups is very helpful as you design your educational sessions.

Strengthening Self-Regulation (Self-Directed Change) Processes and Personal Agency

Self-directed change comes about when individuals are not only motivated and have the needed food- and nutrition-related cognitive, affective, and behavioral skills, but also have skills in self-regulation. Self-regulation is the process through which individuals develop the ability to influence and direct their own actions or behaviors though their own efforts: this is often referred to as self-control. However, what is meant by the term is ability to take control or to feel empowered to make voluntary decisions about one's actions. Hence, the action phase of health behavior change is also referred to as the volitional, conscious-choice, or action-control phase. Several models describe the process (Bandura 1997; Gollwitzer 1999; Schwarzer and Renner 2000). These models are discussed in detail in Chapter 5. Self-regulation is not achieved through willpower but

through the development of specific skills in self-directed change. Such skills are needed for both initiating action and maintaining action. As nutrition educators, we can therefore create opportunities for individuals to enhance these skills and, through this, to increase their sense of empowerment or personal agency.

NUTRITION EDUCATION IN ACTION 12-1 describes the Choice, Control & Change program, where the development of a sense of personal agency or self-directed change is the central focus of the intervention. **NUTRITION EDUCATION IN ACTION 12-2** describes the online educational game, Creature 101, based on Choice Control & Change.

Chief among the strategies to achieve self-regulation/self-direction skills is the process known to professionals as goal setting (Locke and Latham 1990; Cullen, Baranowski, and Smith 2001; Shilts, Horowitz, and Townsend 2004, 2009). This process is discussed in detail in Chapter 5. The term *goal setting* refers to a systematic behavior change process that involves many of the educational or behavior change strategies described earlier.

Note: The strategies described here use the language of nutrition education professionals. You would not necessarily use the same terms with the public. Examples are given of terms to use with the intended audience for each strategy.

Behavior Change Strategy: Stimulate Goal Setting/Action Planning

Goals can refer to a variety of levels of states to be achieved: long-term value goals, general behavior change goals, and specific action goals (Bandura 1986; Locke and Latham 1990; Shilts et al. 2004). Because in this text we use the term *goal* to refer to the overall *behavior change goals* you select to be the focus of your entire session(s) or intervention, we will use the specific term *action goals*, and for the process of setting them, *action goal setting* or *action planning*, to avoid confusion. These *action plans* help your audience to achieve the behavior change goals you selected to be the focus of your session(s) or intervention in Step 1. Some audiences actually prefer the term *action plans* because the word goals seems too lofty and unachievable. Consequently, whenever the term *goal setting* is used, it is important to remember we are referring to *action* goal setting—that is, small actionable steps that will help audience members achieve the overall behavior change goals of your intervention. These action plans are also referred to as *implementation intentions* (Gollwitzer 1999).

NUTRITION EDUCATION IN ACTION 12-1 Choice, Control & Change

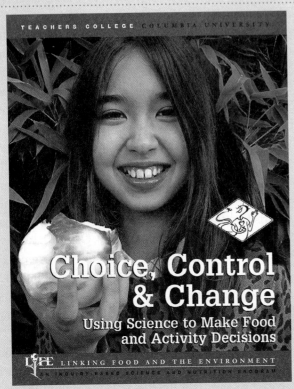

Courtesy of the National Gardening Association and Teachers College Press, Columbia University.

The Choice, Control & Change (C3) program is an inquiry-based science education and health program for preventing overweight among middle school students. Given an environment that encourages overeating and sedentary behavior, the aim of C3 is for youth to become competent eaters who have a sense of personal agency and are able to navigate this environment. It is based on social cognitive and self-determination theories. The *why-to change* information, with a focus on outcome expectations, explores the interplay of biology, personal behavior, and the food system and meets various national standards for science education. Students collect scientific evidence to enable them to understand why healthful eating and ample physical activity are important. The *how-to change* information focuses on teaching cognitive self-regulation skills and enhancing competence and personal agency. It is thus both a science education curriculum and a behavior-focused, theory-based nutrition education intervention. It addresses both why-to and how-to eat healthfully.

THE PROGRAM

The program consists of 19 lessons, broken into five units. The lessons consist of exciting hands-on and minds-on nutrition and science activities:

- *Unit 1 Investigating Our Choices*: Students explore how the environment around us interacts with our biological predispositions to influence what we choose to eat and what activities we do.

- *Unit 2 Dynamic Equilibrium*: Students learn about energy balance in the human body and why and how the body functions better when it is in balance.

- *Unit 3 From Data to Health Goals*: Students collect and analyze their own food and activity data. They compare their data to the C3 goals, create action plans for change, and monitor their change process—through to the end of the curriculum. This gives students opportunities to discuss, debate, and defend the personal changes they are making, both with each other and with significant others in their lives.

- *Unit 4 Effects of Our Choices*: As the students continue to work on their action plans for change they go deeper into why these changes are important to maintain long-term health and decrease risk for cardiovascular disease and type 2 diabetes.

- *Unit 5 Maintaining Competence*: Students integrate their understanding of science, connecting food and activity choices to health, and confirm their personal health commitments.

EVALUATION

In a cluster-randomized controlled study involving 1,146 students in 10 middle schools, students in the program reported consumption of considerably fewer sweetened drinks and processed packaged snacks, as well as smaller sizes at fast food restaurants. There were no reported changes in fruit, vegetable, and water intakes. They also reported intentionally walking more for exercise. Their outcome expectations about the behavior, self-efficacy, goal intentions, sense of competence, and autonomy became significantly more positive.

Sources: Contento, I. R., P. A. Koch, H. Lee, and A. Calabrese-Barton. 2010. Adolescents demonstrate improvement in obesity risk behaviors following completion of Choice, Control & Change, a curriculum addressing personal agency and autonomous motivation. *Journal of the American Dietetic Association* 110:1830–1839.; Choice, Control & Change is a curriculum module of the Linking Food and the Environment (LiFE) curriculum series from Teachers College Columbia University and is available from the National Gardening Association (http://shop.kidsgardening.org/products/choice-control-change-life-3). The book cover is used with permission.

NUTRITION EDUCATION IN ACTION 12-2 **Creature 101: An Online Video Game**

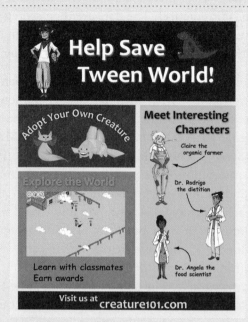

Courtesy of Teachers College Columbia University.

Video games to promote behavior change capitalize on children's pre-existing attention to and enjoyment of them to motivate and help them make behavior changes by embedding behavior change strategies such as goal setting, modeling, and skill development activities into a personally meaningful, entertaining, and immersive game environment. These games are known as "serious video games" and are specially designed to entertain players as they educate, train, or change behavior. Research shows that serious video games may serve as effective behavior change channels for diet and physical activity among children and adolescents as well.

Creature 101 (C101) is a serious game that aims to motivate and help middle school students to engage in energy balances–related behaviors.

THE PROGRAM

C101 is a free, seven session online game based on the inquiry-based nutrition science curriculum of Choice, Control & Change (C3), which aims to promote six healthy eating and physical activity behaviors:

1. Increasing fruit and vegetable intake
2. Increasing consumption of water
3. Increasing physical activity
4. Decreasing consumption of processed packaged snacks (e.g., chips, candy)
5. Decreasing intake of sweetened beverages
6. Decreasing recreational screen time

The storyline features a teen inventor named Murphy who accidentally created a wormhole and found himself in Tween. To befriend the creatures living there, Murphy brought sweetened beverages, processed packaged snacks, video games, and TV sets from Earth. The creatures soon became addicted to these foods and sedentary activities and became sick. Murphy, realizing what he had done, decided to save the creatures. Thus, he brought with him a few experts from Earth who might be able to help. They are a dietitian, a food scientist, and an organic farmer. In the storyline, Murphy recruits helpers (students playing the game) to help. C101 uses social cognitive and self-determination theories as a framework and incorporates the game motif of "virtual companion care" in which students playing the game create an avatar that depicts them in the virtual world of Tween and choose a creature—a virtual companion—to take care of and perform various activities and missions within the virtual world. The students' ultimate mission in the game is to bring their creature back to health, thus achieving the status of "Master Care Taker." Students learn scientific evidence that promotes energy balance by playing mini-games, short educational videos, slideshows, and interactive dialogues with game characters. Students also assess their own behaviors, create their own "real life" food and activity goals, and report their progress.

EVALUATION

The game efficacy was assessed in a pre–post intervention-control study ($n = 531$) with low-income public middle schools (Grades 6–8, 50% male, 63% Hispanic). The students in the intervention group ($n = 359$) played C101 online in science/health education classes (seven sessions, 30 minutes each over the course of 1 month). Students in the control group ($n = 172$) played another game. The intervention students reported significant decreases in the frequency and amount of consumption of sweetened beverages and processed packaged snacks when compared to controls. A dose-response analysis of the levels of game play with behavioral and knowledge outcomes of 224 students in the intervention group indicated that more levels of game play significantly predicted *frequency* ($p = 0.007$, $R^2 = 0.20$) and *amount* ($p = 0.049$, $R^2 = 0.25$) of sweetened beverage consumption among the players. It also predicted increased knowledge of nutrition and physical activity ($p = 0.002$, $R^2 = 0.04$).

These results suggest that behaviorally focused and theory-driven video games can be effective in changing individual energy balance behaviors. The game can be accessed at www.tc.columbia.edu.

Why Action Plans Are Effective

Action goal setting works to motivate, bridge the intention–action gap, and maintain action in nutrition education program participants for a variety of reasons. It engenders a sense of commitment to the action goal. By planning ahead, participants do not have to make a new decision every time a food choice situation arises, thus leading to less mental burden and to development of a routine. The statement of an action goal sensitizes individuals so that they are more conscious or mindful as they make food choices. It gives them a sense of control over their own behavior. It builds their perceptions of self-efficacy and mastery. It creates self-satisfaction and a sense of fulfillment from having achieved their goals and contributes to the cultivation of intrinsic interest through active involvement in the process. Action goal setting is similar to the process of self-liberation in the transtheoretical model. Several reviews have shown that the action goal setting process can be very useful in the dietary arena (Armitage 2004; Cullen et al. 2001; Shilts et al. 2004).

Practical educational activities for action goal setting involve the following:

First, clearly restate the *behavior change goal(s)* of the intervention you are designing. This may be for participants to increase their intake of fruits and vegetables or to decrease their intake of high-fat, high-sugar foods, cook more family meals, buy food with a lower carbon footprint, practice food safety behaviors, and so forth.

Then, help participants set action goals using the following steps:

1. *Select or develop a self-assessment tool for participants.* Self-assessment involves identification of specific actions that participants are currently engaging in that relate to the behavior change goals of the intervention program.

    For example, if the intervention or program's behavior change goal is to reduce fat in the diet, then participants need to identify the foods in their diet that contribute to their fat intake. Is it the amount of meat they are eating or the number of rich desserts? If the intervention's behavior change goal is to encourage eating locally produced foods, then how often do the participants visit farmers' markets or look for foods in the supermarket that are labeled as being local? This may further the recognition of the need for change. The self-assessment usually involves

some kind of recording method, such as food records, 24-hour dietary recalls, or checklists of the targeted foods or practices. The data are then scored in some way. It could be as simple as adding up the frequencies of the behaviors assessed in the self-assessment tool.

2. *Provide instruction for setting effective action goals or action plans: SMART action goals.* A common method for setting specific action goals to achieve the behavior change goals is for the action goals to be SMART:

   - *Specific.* The action goal should be specific. Specific action goals provide clear targets for action, indicating the type and amount of effort needed to achieve the goal. An example might be "I will drink orange juice for breakfast and add a vegetable to lunch" (to increase intake of fruits and vegetables from 1 to 2 cups daily).

   - *Measurable.* The action goal should be stated in such a way that you can measure whether it has been achieved. In the above example, the actions are measurable.

   - *Achievable.* The action goal should stretch and challenge individuals within their ability to achieve the outcome.

   - *Relevant and realistic.* Set action goals that are most important or most likely to result in achieving the overall behavior change goal and that are also realistic for participants, given their life situations.

   - *Time-bound.* Action goals to be accomplished in the immediate future are more likely to be effective than those set for a longer time frame because, in the latter case, it is easy to postpone action. For example, "I will eat 2 and a half cups of fruits and vegetables today by having orange juice at breakfast, eating a fruit for a mid-morning snack, adding a salad to lunch, and eating two vegetables for dinner" is likely to be more effective than stating, "I will eat more fruits and vegetables this month."

In general, action goals should be difficult yet reachable. Those that are challenging but clearly attainable through extra effort are more likely to be motivating and satisfying. It is the discrepancy between where individuals are and where they want to be that is motivating (Bandura 1986, 1997). Motivation can be sustained by setting progressively more difficult action goals, assuming that they are seen as reasonable and within reach. Very difficult or complex changes should be broken down into smaller units, and goals set for each of the units. Heath and Heath (2010) note that when making changes, it is very important not to "spook the elephant." The elephant in us is our emotional side, which is often understandably cautious, reluctant to make drastic changes, and needs to be reassured. The maxim is that the action goal should be small enough to achieve but large enough to matter. For example, rather than set one large goal, such as "to eat less fat and sugar and to eat more fruits and vegetables," individuals should set separate action goals and make them specific, such as "to add one dark green vegetable to my diet each day this week" or "to eat ice cream only twice this week."

3. *Create an action plan form for the SMART action goals.* Commitment to an action goal is the personal resolve to pursue the goal. Personal commitment is strengthened by pledges that bind the individual to future action. The motivational effect of binding themselves to future action is largely the result of not wanting to renege on an agreement they have made.

It is helpful to provide some kind of action plan form or worksheet on which group participants can state their SMART action goals or pledge. See the example in **FIGURE 12-3**. Each participant should create and sign one. Given that public commitment enhances

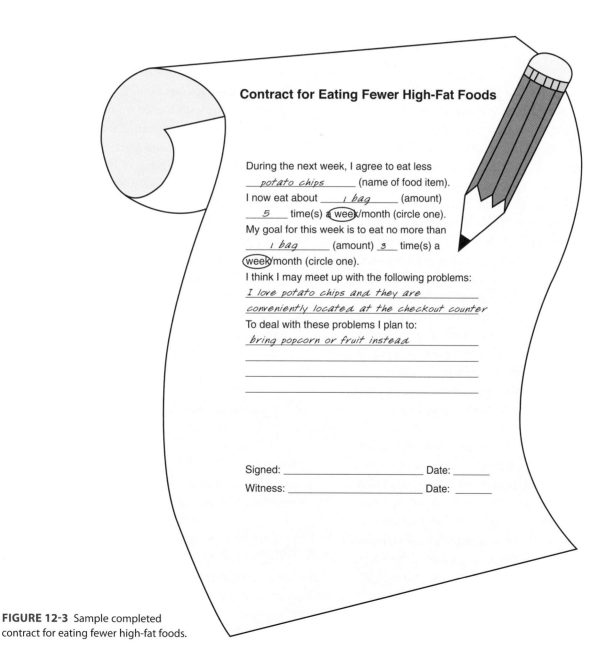

FIGURE 12-3 Sample completed contract for eating fewer high-fat foods.

TABLE 12-2 What Works and Doesn't Work in Making Changes

What Works	What Doesn't Work
Setting realistic goals and breaking your goal into small steps you can achieve	Setting unrealistic goals
Allowing for your food dislikes	Trying to include foods you don't like
Making small changes	Making drastic changes
Choosing foods you can get easily	Choosing foods you have to search for
Getting support from your family and friends	Trying to make changes all by yourself
Being flexible: compromising in some situations	Being rigid: trying to live up to your changes with absolutely no exceptions

the likelihood of following through on a pledge, it is best to have another member of the group, a friend, or a family member also sign as a witness. A couple of really simple formats are shown in Chapter 5, Figures 5-2a and 5-2b. **TABLE 12-2** contains some tips to go with the contract form, which can be made into a handout for the group. Some nutrition educators who work in classroom settings with younger children have students voluntarily sign a class book instead. The children then check off when they have attained the goal. This often is called a *challenge sheet*. Or a *collective contract* can be hung up in the room as a reminder, such as in a classroom or community center in which the group meets. Or, in a group setting with adults, particularly a low-literacy audience, a *public verbal commitment* may be appropriate. If you are providing only one session, this is probably as far as you can go. This activity will provide a good closure to your session.

4. *Develop a tracking and feedback form (self-observation and self-evaluation).* If you plan on a series of sessions, the next step is for individuals and groups to track their progress to see how well they are doing compared with their action goals. Self-observation and self-evaluation are considered extremely important for maintaining behavior change. Such feedback can be provided through a tracking system that you develop for use by intervention participants. This may be easy for behaviors that are clearly visible or identifiable, such as eating fruits and vegetables; however, other

behaviors may not be so easy, such as reducing fat in foods. In the latter case, you could come up with some clear definitions of higher-fat and lower-fat foods to make tracking possible.

This tracking is mostly for the participants' own use. However, you can review the completed tracking forms and give individual feedback as well. Or, the participants can give oral reports in group settings and get feedback from the group if the action goals have been made public and it is appropriate to do so. The focus should be on positive accomplishments rather than failures.

5. *Create rewards and encouragement.* Achievement of the action goals can be rewarded by you, by collective action on the part of the participants, or by the individuals themselves, depending on the situation. **Reinforcement** may include verbal encouragement, smiles, and an approving, nonjudgmental tone of voice in all interactions with the group or it could be material rewards such as key chains, magnets, tee-shirts, or sweatshirts to those who participate or complete the program. You can also give out raffle tickets to be drawn for prizes upon completion of the contract. The hidden messages in these reinforcements should be consistent and support the spoken, overt message. For example, rewarding children for being physically active with high-fat, high-sugar food products would not be supportive of the message. Present participants with certificates of achievement when they achieve their goals.

Individuals can also be encouraged to reinforce themselves in tangible ways, such as buying a new piece of clothing or a new piece of exercise equipment, or through their affective reactions, such as praising themselves when they meet their goals and problem solving when they fall short. Physiological and external reinforcements also influence goal achievement. Thus, knowledge that one's serum cholesterol level has declined can enhance an individual's commitment to eating a low-fat diet.

Behavior Change Strategy: Encourage Goal Maintenance (Relapse Prevention)

If you have the opportunity to work with participants over time or the group is already taking action on the behavior change goals of your intervention, assisting them to maintain the behavior change becomes a possibility, and a priority. In the area of food and dietary behavior, goal maintenance is a more appropriate concept than relapse prevention. Eating requires daily food choices and constant trade-offs among numerous alternative actions. Healthy food practices need to be maintained for the long term—indeed, permanently. Studies have found that no magic food changes are involved in making dietary changes. Adding foods to the diet, such as fruits and vegetables, appears easier to do and maintain than removing a food or a food constituent such as fat or sugar.

Practical activities can involve the following:

- *Provide a general dietary framework.* An effective approach is to use a general dietary framework, not a specific prescriptive diet (Bowen et al. 1993; Urban et al. 1992). This gives individuals control over their diets. You can provide them with more than one way to change their diets and give alternative menu suggestions to enhance their ability to make their own trade-offs.

- *Self-monitoring protocols.* Another effective approach is to devise and provide program participants with some sort of self-monitoring system that is feasible and easy to use. For foods that are easily identifiable, such as fruits and vegetables, such a system is relatively simple—counting items and estimating the amounts in foods. See **FIGURE 12-4** for examples. In the dietary fat arena, visible fats are easily identified (such as butter and oils), and changes can be monitored. However, many nutrients, such as fat, salt, or fiber, are not visible. Here, some kind of point system needs to be devised for self-monitoring purposes, and label-reading skills become important.

    In general, whereas the initial motivation for change is driven by *anticipated* positive consequences of making the change, maintenance of change is motivated by *actual* positive consequences from the change, such as finding that eating healthful food is satisfying and pleasurable.

- *Prioritizing competing goals.* For many program participants (as for most of us), a major ongoing challenge in maintaining healthful practices is setting priorities between conflicting goals or desires, such as between the goal to eat more healthfully and a personal agenda that may involve work-related aspirations or family obligations that do not leave much mental and physical time for planning and eating healthfully. In this situation, help participants to evaluate their chosen

action goal, such as to eat healthful lunches at work, in relation to competing goals, such as the desire to be a productive worker and hence not be gone too long from one's desk. They can then think of ways to protect the chosen behavior change goal from these competing goals if it is determined to be more important. Encourage participants to review each goal they are trying to achieve (e.g., eating fruits and vegetables, breastfeeding) in terms of its positive value to them, how important or desirable it is to them, how it relates to their larger life goals, how they will feel about achieving or not achieving the action goal, and how much they have already invested, and then to reaffirm their commitment to their chosen goal. Your role is that of a collaborator and coach.

- *Protecting action goals from distractions: practice mindful eating.* Maintaining action goals relies on conscious control and attention. It is important to assist program participants to protect their action goals from being interrupted and given up prematurely because of competing distractions. For example, a table that is full of tasty, high-fat foods presents a distraction to someone who has chosen the goal of eating lower-fat foods. The eating setting—ambiance, lighting, eating with others, or look of the menu—influences the amount of food eaten (Wansink 2006). Ask individuals to identify potential distracting situations and to make plans ahead of time to ignore these anticipated distractions. This can be done when participants verbally describe or imagine the situation and rehearse exactly what they will do and the positive outcomes they can expect from staying with their goals. You also can remind individuals just to be mindful about what they eat—to think before they eat.

- *Focusing on overall behavior change goals in the achievement of specific action goals.* When program participants find themselves in difficult situations for fulfilling their specific action goals, help them to remember the big picture—the overall behavior change goal they are aiming to achieve. This can provide stability and facilitate choices among specific action goals. For example, individuals may find themselves unable to eat the vegetables at lunch like they had planned because of a birthday party for a coworker. They can fulfill their personal social goal at lunch and "reschedule" an extra vegetable serving at dinner to achieve their major health goal of eating more fruits and vegetables.

Bite and Write Food Log (sample)

Use this sample to help you fill out your food log completely and accurately

Date: _25 October_   Day of the Week: _Tuesday_

Time	Place	What I Ate	How Much?
3:30 p.m.	On the way home from school	1 can of root-beer eats and potato chips	12-oz. can and small bag
5:30 p.m.	Sitting in front of the TV	1 green apple	Medium sized, about the size of a baseball
7:30 p.m.	Double-Quick-Eats fast food place	Cheese burger with lattuce and tomatos and bun, French fries, cola	Small, I think, they were from the dollar menu
10 p.m.	My kitchen	Glass of water	Not sure exactly how much, but it filled the blue cup we have in our kitchen
11 p.m.	My kitchen	Glass of cola	Not sure exactly how much, but it filled the blue cup we have in our kitchen
7:30 a.m.	My kitchen	Banana, packaged cinnamon bun, water	Large, medium sized bun 1 cup
11:30 a.m.	cafeteria	Chicken nuggets, green beans, bread roll, grape soda	6 nuggets, 1/2 cups 1 small roll, 20-oz. bottle

Assessment of current intake.

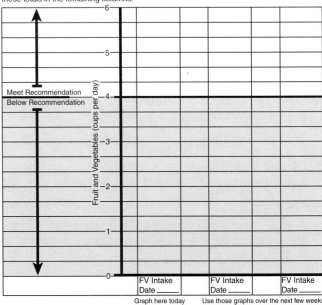

Comparison of Fruit and vegarable (FV) Intake to the Recommendation

In the FIRST "FV intake" column, make a bar graph of your total cups of fruits and vegetables, as recorded on the previous page.

Over the next few weeks, choose two days to tract your fruit and vegetable intake, and graph these totals in the remaining columns.

Graph here today   Use those graphs over the next few weeks

Comparing current intake to recommendations.

My Plan

Add a fruit or vegetable at (circle one): **Breakfast**   **Lunch**   **Dinner**   **Snacks**

On these days: **Monday   Tuesday   Wednesday   Thursday   Friday   Saturday   Sunday**

Tracker

Date	Day of Week	Did you do it?	What did you eat?	Notes*
		YES NO		
		YES NO		
		YES NO		
		YES NO		
		YES NO		
		YES NO		
		YES NO		
		YES NO		
		YES NO		
		YES NO		
		YES NO		
		YES NO		
		YES NO		
		YES NO		

*In the notice section write about how you did, If you ate a fruit or vegetable – How did you do it? How did it feel? If you did not eat a fruit or vegetable – What were the challenges? What could you do differently next time?

Making an action plan and monitoring progress.

FIGURE 12-4 Tools for self-assessment and comparison to recommendations for fruit and vegetable intake, setting action goals, and self-monitoring in the Food, Health & Choices curriculum program for upper elementary school students.

Reprinted from *Journal of Nutrition Education and Behavior* 44(4S), I.R. Contento, P.A. Koch, and H. Lee Gray, Reducing childhood obesity: An innovative curriculum with wellness policy support, Page S190; and Abrams, E., M. Burgermaster, P.A. Koch, I.R. Contento, & H. Lee Gray, Food, Health & Choices: Importance of formative evaluation to create a well-delivered and well-received intervention, Page S137. Copyright 2014 with permission from Elsevier.

- *Linking action goals to self-identity.* If the chosen goals can be seen as part of the identity of intervention participants, they are less likely to be devalued or postponed when competing goals emerge (such as deadlines at work). For example, the nutrition educator can help individuals reflect on how they think of themselves. If they come to think of themselves as health-conscious or ecologically responsible eaters, they will be more likely to stay with their action goals to eat more fruits and vegetables.

Behavior Change Strategy: Prompt Reframing of Perceptions and Attributions/Cognitive Restructuring

When individuals attempt to make changes in their eating patterns, they will likely experience both successes and failures. Their attributions of why they were successful or not will influence their sense of self-efficacy and future behavior.

Practical activities can include the following:

- *Help participants reinterpret information or reframe* how certain foods or situations are perceived. They may think of the situation as insurmountable. Helping them to reframe the barriers and think of small steps they can take can be very effective.
- *Attributions of success and failure.* If they think their success (for example, in cooking) was because of a stable cause, such as their ability, they will have a higher expectation of success the next time compared with individuals who attribute their success to something unstable, such as luck. After failure, these effects are reversed. These attributions are sometimes called self-talk. You can assist individuals to develop more accurate attributions and new ways of thinking or self-talk. For example, encourage individuals to tell themselves they are not clumsy, but skillful, and to recognize that the great dish they have prepared results from the skills they have acquired, not luck, and to tell themselves they can do it again. This process is called counterconditioning in the transtheoretical model.

Behavior Change Strategy: Build Skills for Planning Coping Responses

Goal maintenance also relies on emotion-coping strategies, such as the ability to ignore feelings of worry or of disappointment in not meeting the goals that were set. These strategies are important because many desirable food- and nutrition-related practices require effort—for example, seeking out farmers' markets to eat locally or learning to cook in order to gain control over what is eaten personally or by the family. Individuals' optimistic beliefs about their ability to deal with barriers, though a major hindrance in getting them motivated, may be helpful here because a new behavior may turn out to be much more difficult to adhere to than they had anticipated. These beliefs are referred to as coping self-efficacy.

Practical activities can include the following:

- *Help participants plan ways to cope with these emotions.* Examples are "I can stick with a healthful diet even if I have to try several times until it works," or "I can stick with a healthful diet even if I need a long time to develop the necessary routines" (Schwarzer and Renner 2000). Or, "I can stick with a healthful diet even when others in the family do not wish to do so." Thus, the nutrition educator should help program participants become aware that they have coping resources. Again, having program participants practice positive, action-oriented self-talk (or cognitive restructuring) can be useful in order to remind themselves that they are capable of taking action.

Behavior Change Strategy: Build Skills for Managing Environmental Cues

Cue management is the process in which individuals remove cues to less healthful eating and add cues for more healthful eating.

Practical activities can include the following:

- *Provide instruction to program participants on how to restructure their personal or family environments.* For example, they can reduce the number of less healthful foods in the household and keep them out of sight or make them less accessible and convenient. Such foods can be purchased and eaten occasionally or as treats. On the other hand, fruit can be washed, ready to eat, and left on the counter or in the refrigerator. Likewise, vegetables can be washed, cut up, and ready to eat, and conveniently placed in the refrigerator. If a goal is to reduce the number of plastic bags used for groceries, then canvas bags can be placed on the front doorknob or in the car, ready for use in the grocery store.

■ *Help participants to be aware of environmental cues,* even in situations where they cannot control them, and to develop coping strategies. Two-thirds of food purchases are unplanned and influenced by store displays and other marketing strategies. Participants should write out shopping lists.

Behavior Change Strategy: Promote Developing Personal Food Policies and Routines

A major aim during the maintenance phase of dietary change is for the new behaviors to become automatic or habitual (Bargh and Barndollar 1996).

Practical activities can include the following:

■ *Remind people that repeating the behavior makes it easier.* Help participants recognize that when people repeatedly perform a behavior in a specific context (such as drinking orange juice at breakfast), the motivation (to eat more fruit) and its implementation instructions (drink orange juice at breakfast) become so integrated that as soon as they experience the situation (breakfast) the specific action is triggered in memory without the need for conscious decision making. Thus, repeated context-specific action leads to increasingly effortless enactment of the behavior.

■ *Create worksheets or discussion guides* that lead individuals through a process of developing personal food policies to guide their dietary choices and food-related actions. They can decide, for example, that they will always eat breakfast, always have a vegetable at lunch, only eat desserts once a week, buy organic or local foods whenever there is a choice, shop at farmers' markets in season, eat at a fast food chain restaurant only once a week (or whatever frequency), and so forth. These food policies help guide decisions on an ongoing basis.

Behavior Change Strategy: Encourage Repeated Consumption of Healthful Food

Program participants are more likely to maintain behavior change if they come to enjoy eating the healthful foods that are the target of the interventions. As you saw earlier, there is considerable evidence that repeated experience with a food can increase liking and preference for it.

Practical activities can include the following:

■ *Remind participants that studies have found that those who decide to change their eating patterns usually come to like them.* For example, studies have found that people who decide to eat less salt (or fat) come to like foods with less salt (or fat). The same applies for fruits and vegetables and other healthy foods.

■ *Point out that using sugar and fat substitutes is easily adopted but does not change their preferences* for their flavor or change their behavior (Bowen et al. 1993). For example, individuals who eat foods with fat substitutes will still like the taste of fat, but when they switch to naturally low-fat foods, they decrease their liking for the fatty taste (Mattes 1993; Grieve and Vander Weg 2003).

■ *Reassure participants* that at first they may feel deprived, but studies have found that over time this will change. It is clear that people eat what they like, but they also come to like what they eat (Bowen et al. 1993). Hence, remind program participants to stay with their chosen dietary change long enough for them to come to like the new foods and, indeed, to find them pleasurable to eat.

Behavior Change Strategy: Enhance Skills in Management of Social Context and Plan for Social Support

Most eating occurs in a social context, even if some meals are eaten alone, involving others in the household and extended family and friends.

Practical activities can include the following:

■ *Help participants to consider and make trade-offs.* For most people, dietary change requires consideration of household needs as well as personal needs. For example, the mother of the household may decide to eat more plant-based, whole grain meals to reduce her weight and risk of hypertension, whereas the other family members want to eat hamburgers and French fries. Will she make two meals? She will have to make trade-offs and negotiations between her desire for health for herself and her desire to maintain good family relationships. And of course, mothers of young children constantly need to make trade-offs in terms of when to insist that they eat their vegetables.

■ *Facilitated group discussions* can be invaluable as individuals meet with others like themselves to share ideas and challenges and how to overcome them. Such a group can provide welcomed social support. The

NUTRITION EDUCATION IN ACTION 12-3 Sisters in Health: An Experiential Program Emphasizing Social Interaction to Increase Fruit and Vegetable Intake Among Low-Income Adults

Sisters in Health was a community-based program to increase fruit and vegetable intake among low-income women that was designed to be implemented in small groups in real-life community settings, to be flexible, and to be easy to implement by community nutrition educators. It was based on facilitated group discussion and experiential learning, in which group members were interactively involved in discussing their knowledge, experiences, problems, and solutions with other group members.

THE PROGRAM

The program consisted of six 90-minute weekly meetings for groups of approximately 10 women, facilitated by community nutrition paraprofessionals trained through the Cooperative Extension Service. The program was based on extensive formative research or needs assessment.

Each session included the following:

- A welcome or warm-up activity, such as how the family liked the new dish tried at home

- A food preparation and tasting experience, such as creating and tasting a salad bar

- A group learning activity, such as adding or subtracting ingredients from a salad to boost nutrient density

- A take-home challenge, such as making at least one "enhanced salad" at home

- Feedback on the meeting used for planning the next one

- Low-cost incentives, such as cooking utensils and notebooks for recipes

All groups received the sessions "Getting Started," which focused on participants' familiarity with and preferences regarding fruits and vegetables, and "All About Me," which focused on recommendations and portion sizes. Four other sessions were chosen (from eight) by the group on topics such as "Scoring with Salads," "Kids and Vegetables," "Easier Than Pie: Fruit Anytime," and "Beat the Clock with Meals in Minutes." Such an approach combined flexibility and the needs and interests of the group with the need for pre-prepared education plans for effective education.

EVALUATION

The program's impact was evaluated in a nonrandom sample of 269 low-income adults in 32 intervention and 10 control groups using a quasi-experimental, pre- and post-program evaluation design in which a control group received a budgeting or parenting program of the same duration and intensity. Intervention groups reported an increase in fruit and vegetable consumption, measured by a brief screener, of 1.6 times a day (compared to 0.8 in the control groups). Knowledge of the number of servings people should eat and self-efficacy did not increase (they may have already been high), but attitudes, knowledge of preparation methods, and satisfaction with how vegetables turned out did increase significantly. Group support, active learning experiences, food tastings, and food skill development were thus effective in increasing fruit and vegetable intake in these low-income adults.

Source: Devine, C. M., T. J. Farrell, and R. Hartman. 2005. Sisters in Health: Experiential program emphasizing social interaction increases fruit and vegetable intake among low-income adults. *Journal of Nutrition Education and Behavior* 37:265–270.

nutrition educator can provide valuable assistance in the process. An example of such an intervention is discussed in **NUTRITION EDUCATION IN ACTION 12-3.**

Behavior Change Strategy: Enhance Skills in Advocacy

Collective efficacy is the belief of groups and community members that they have the capacity to take collective action to create change in their environment. It is enhanced by a process that is somewhat like goal setting where group members identify the issue of concern, set small goals to address the concern, and, when these produce tangible results, come to believe that they have the capability to change the social and political environments in which they live. A major way to convert goals to action on the environment is through advocacy.

Practical activities to enhance advocacy skills can include the following:

- *Work in collaboration with group members to develop a group procedure* whereby they identify issues of concern to them, participate in authentic dialogue about the issues, drawing on their prior knowledge and experience, come to an understanding about the root causes of the issues, and set action goals to address the concern. These outcomes may be recommendations or requests to local businesses, government agencies, decision-makers, and policymakers to act on their concerns. The group then monitors progress towards the status of the recommendations and takes further advocacy actions as appropriate.
- *Share tips or other commonly used practices,* if needed, on how to contact and lobby their representatives through a variety of media such as letters, telephone, and electronic media.
- *Provide technical assistance* such as computer access, website development, letter writing, and contacts with other like-minded groups for collaboration or with policy-makers.

Case Study: The DESIGN Procedure in Action—Step 5

We now apply the information in this chapter specifically to the ongoing case study to illustrate the process of selecting appropriate behavior change strategies for each of the determinants of the theory model of Step 3 and of designing fun, enjoyable educational activities and needed food and nutrition content for group participants to achieve the educational objectives. In the case study, the sessions are provided to middle school students by a university-affiliated nonprofit health services organization. This lesson is a follow-up to the one described in Chapter 11. The behavior change goal of the two hypothetical sessions is to increase intake of fruits and vegetables.

SESSION TITLE, BEHAVIOR CHANGE GOAL, AND GENERAL EDUCATIONAL OBJECTIVES

The nutrition educator and her colleagues created a catchy title that would pique the interest of the students. For this, the second of two sessions, the title was "SMART

Goals for Smart Snacking." They then selected the general educational objectives from Step 4 that were relevant to this session. From these they selected strategies they would use to guide the overall development of practical educational activities.

EDUCATIONAL PLAN: THE PLANNING MATRIX FOR DESIGNING THE SESSION

The team then used the matrix planning tool to create a matrix showing how the determinants of change from their theory model in Step 3 would be converted to specific objectives for that session. They then brainstormed engaging, motivating, and meaningful practical educational activities to increase fruit and vegetable intake, focusing on both motivational and facilitating determinants. They especially wanted to provide students with some food preparation activities.

THE EDUCATIONAL PLAN: TEACHING FORMAT FOR DELIVERING THE SESSION

The teaching or narrative form for delivering the lesson is also shown for the case study. This is what the nutrition educator in this school will take with him or her to implement the session. The numerous handouts, worksheets, and other materials are not shown due to space constraints.

Your Turn to Design Nutrition Education: Completing the Step 5 Generate Educational Plans Worksheet, with a Focus on Taking Action

You can now apply the information in this chapter to the process of selecting appropriate behavior change strategies and designing interesting and relevant learning experiences for your audience to achieve the behavior change goals of the intervention. You will need one educational plan per session.

SESSION TITLE, BEHAVIOR CHANGE GOAL, AND GENERAL EDUCATIONAL OBJECTIVES

First, create a catchy title for the behavior change goal of your session that will pique the interest of your audience. Then, state the general educational objectives from

Step 4 that are based on the determinants from your theory model and use these to guide the overall development of practical educational activities. The same determinants and general educational objectives may be used in more than one session devoted to the same behavior change goal, but typically there will also be some that are unique to each session of your series. By now you probably realize that designing educational activities or learning experiences is a very fluid process and that you will be going back and forth between designing activities, sequencing them, and writing educational objectives.

SEQUENCING ACTIVITIES IS IMPORTANT: THE 4 ES

How exactly you arrange your sequence of educational strategies depends on many factors that are specific to the needs of your audience and the theory guiding your intervention. In general, though, sequencing activities is extremely important, using the "4 Es" or some similar format. (Sequencing of activities is discussed in detail in Chapter 11.)

- *Excite—gain attention.* You want to begin each session or series of sessions with activities to gain the attention of the group. Even if they appear motivated, booster shots of motivation are always useful.
- *Explain—present stimulus and new material.* You then move to activities to promote motivation, action, or maintenance of the behavior change (depending on the stage of change of participants and aim of your session) by presenting new explanatory material that builds on what they already know and can do.
- *Expand—provide guidance and practice for how-to take action.* You then focus on activities to build skills and strengthen self-efficacy or collective efficacy.
- *Exit—apply and close.* Some kind of closure or take-home message or action goals setting is important (Gagne et al. 2004).

Completing an action goal setting or action planning process is especially powerful as an Exit apply and close activity. Provide a worksheet, if possible. This can be quite simple for low-literacy audiences, or you can discuss the process orally. The activity can help program participants plan how they will monitor their progress toward their action goal. If you see them in another session or sessions, be sure to provide opportunities for feedback and rewards and setting new action plans. The same systematic process is needed for the design of all nutrition education messages and activities, such as brochures, newsletters, posters, media messages, or campaigns.

THE EDUCATIONAL PLAN: USING THE MATRIX TOOL TO OUTLINE SESSIONS

It is extremely useful to first develop a lesson or educational plan outline using a matrix format. The Generate Educational Plans Worksheet is located in the workbook at the end of Chapter 13. The first column in the worksheet lists the *4 Es* so that you can be aware at all times of the sequence of activities. The second column lists each of the *potential determinants* of behavior change from the intervention's theory model that you plan to address in this session. The third column shows *the behavior change strategy or strategies* that you will use to operationalize the potential determinants. The behavior change strategies for each of the determinants are described in this chapter and shown in Table 12-1. The fourth column indicates the *specific educational objectives* for the determinant of behavior change. The final column briefly describes all of the *practical educational activities*, learning experiences, or messages that are used to carry out the educational strategies.

The matrix format enables you to easily see whether you have addressed all the determinants of behavior change needed to accomplish the behavior change goals of your session. This is also the time to check that the specific educational objectives that you set and the activities are appropriate for your audience in terms of domain of learning—cognitive, affective, or psychomotor—and level of complexity within domains. The information in Chapters 15 and 17 about practical tips for working with groups is also very helpful as you design your educational sessions.

THE EDUCATIONAL PLAN: DEVELOPING A TEACHING FORMAT FOR DELIVERING THE SESSION

Next, convert the matrix into a more detailed narrative or teaching format that you will actually use when you are with a group. The case study provides a sample lesson plan showing how the planning matrix is used to design the session and how the narrative teaching format is used for delivery. Completing the Generate Educational Plans Worksheet will help you develop your educational plan for a real or hypothetical educational session.

- Think of a catchy title that will be meaningful to your audience. It should motivate people to come to your session or pique their interest if they are required to attend.
- Restate your general objectives, which can be very helpful here.
- Place an overview or outline of activities and a materials list at the beginning of the teaching plan. That way you will have the entire session in mind and all of the materials ready.
- Convert each of the activities in the matrix into a fuller description or narrative. Include all the specific information you will need. Don't count on remembering everything.
- Arrange the activities according to the 4 Es: Excite, Explain, Expand, and Exit.
- Create a heading with a title for each educational activity. This heading will provide you with a quick visual cue when you are delivering the session with a group. In this heading list three items: the first item in the heading is the *behavior change strategy* being used, indicating the purpose of the activity. Then comes a *brief description of the activity*. Finally, indicate the *determinant(s)* from your theory model being addressed in parentheses at the end of the title.
- Describe the activities within the educational plan with sufficient detail that some other nutrition professional could deliver it.
- Include essential background information you will need (e.g., teaspoons of sugar in the various beverages you will discuss). Lengthy information can be placed in an additional "background" section.
- Be prepared and organized. If the session involves demonstration, make sure you have all the materials you need. If you plan on a food preparation activity (highly recommended), make sure you have tested the recipes and that you have prepped the foods so they are ready for the participants to use (such as fruits and vegetables washed, stems cut off, etc.).

- Think through the flow if the session involves hands-on activities. Once the group starts to do food preparation, for example, it may be hard to get them back into a group listening mode, so you may want to do that at the end. Can some of the instruction be provided concurrently with the activity?
- Provide a sense of closure; this is especially important. This is a good time to offer an opportunity to apply what the audience has learned. A clear set of action steps or a goal setting worksheet for setting SMART action goals is highly recommended.
- Make the educational plan several pages long, depending on the length of the session and the complexity of the behavior. You will also have many pages of handouts, worksheets, or other materials.

PILOT TESTING THE EDUCATIONAL PLAN

If your intervention is planned to be more than a one-time event, pilot testing the learning experiences with a similar audience will be helpful. If food is used, test the recipes and preparation procedures for taste acceptance and feasibility. Use focus groups, direct observation, and interviews to assess whether activities are acceptable and effective with the intended audience.

EDUCATIONAL PLANS IN PRACTICE

It is very important to have an educational plan or lesson plan. (See Chapter 11.) Otherwise, the sessions will not have a clear focus that serves the cause of helping program participants to achieve the behavior change goals that your program has set out. You may find yourself needing to adapt the education plans to the situation on the ground and to the backgrounds and interests of the specific group with whom you are working. Note that even approaches that seem very informal with a strong focus on learner-centered education require that you develop strong, theory-based educational plans. Ideally, these plans would be developed in collaboration with the intended audience. Practical delivery methods and tips for developing accompanying materials, such as handouts, posters, or newsletters, are described in more detail in Part III of this book.

Questions and Activities

1. Why is action planning important for the effectiveness of nutrition education interventions? Discuss.
   a. What are characteristics of effective action goals?
   b. Describe some practical ways that goal setting can be taught.
2. Describe three kinds of specific educational activities or learning experiences that you could conduct to strengthen self-regulation skills.
3. For practice, think of a session on increasing the intake of calcium-rich foods among teenage girls. For each facilitating behavior change–related determinant,

describe at least one behavior change strategy and one corresponding educational activity.

Potential Determinant of the Ability to Take Action	Behavior Change Strategy	Educational Activities or Learning Experiences
Coping self-efficacy		
Social support		
Cues to action		

References

Anderson, A. S., D. N. Cox, S. McKellar, J. Reynolds, M. E. Lean, and D. J. Mela. 1998. Take Five, a nutrition education intervention to increase fruit and vegetable intakes: Impact on attitudes towards dietary change. *British Journal of Nutrition* 80(2):133–140.

Anderson, L. W., D. R. Krathwohl, P. W. Airasian, K. A. Cruikshank, R. E. Mayer, P. R. Pintrich, et al. 2000. *A taxonomy for learning, teaching, and assessing: A revision of Bloom's Taxonomy of Educational Objectives.* New York: Pearson, Allyn & Bacon.

Armitage, C. 2004. Evidence that implementation intentions reduce dietary fat intake: A randomized trial. *Health Psychology* 23:319–323.

Bandura, A. 1986. *Foundations of thought and action: A social cognitive theory.* Englewood Cliffs, NJ: Prentice Hall.

———. 1997. *Self-efficacy: The exercise of control.* New York: WH Freeman.

Baranowski, T., E. Cerin, and J. Baranowski. 2009. Steps in the design, development, and formative evaluation of obesity prevention-related behavior change trials. International Journal of Behavioral Nutrition and Physical Activity 6-6.

Bargh, J. A., and K. Barndollar. 1996. Automaticity in action: The unconscious as repository of chronic goals and motives. In *The psychology of action: Linking cognition and motivation to behavior,* P. M. Gollwitzer and J. A. Bargh, editors. New York: Guildford Press.

Bisogni, C. A., M. Jastran, M. Seligson, and A. Thompson. 2012. How people interpret healthy eating: Contributions of qualitative research. *Journal of Nutrition Education and Behavior* 44(4):282–301.

Blake C. E., E. Wethington, T. J. Farrell, C. A. Bisogni, and C. M. Devine. 2011. Behavioral contexts, food-choice coping strategies, and dietary quality of a multiethnic sample of employed parents. *Journal of the American Dietetic Association* 111(3):401–407.

Bowen, D. J., H. Henry, E. Burrows, G. Anderson, and M. H. Henderson. 1993. Influences of eating patterns on change to a low-fat diet. *Journal of the American Dietetic Association* 93:1309–1311.

Contento, I. R., P. A. Koch, H. Lee, and A. Calabrese-Barton. 2010. Adolescents demonstrate improvement in obesity risk behaviors following completion of Choice, Control & Change, a curriculum addressing personal agency and autonomous motivation. *Journal of the American Dietetic Association* 110:1830–1839.

Cox, D. N., A. S. Anderson, J. Reynolds, S. McKellar, M. E. J. Lean, and D. J. Mela. 1998. Take Five, a nutrition education intervention to increase fruit and vegetable intakes: Impact on consumer choice and nutrient intakes. *British Journal of Nutrition* 80(2):123–131.

Cullen, K. W., T. Baranowski, and S. P. Smith. 2001. Using goal setting as a strategy for dietary behavior change. *Journal of the American Dietetic Association* 101:562–566.

Gagne, R., W. W. Wager, J. M. Keller, and K. Golas. 2004. *Principles of instructional design.* Boston: Cengage.

Gollwitzer, P. M. 1999. Implementation intentions: Strong effects of simple plans. *American Psychologist* 54:493–503.

Grieve, F. G., and M. W. Vander Weg. 2003. Desire to eat high- and low-fat foods following a low-fat dietary intervention. *Journal of Nutrition Education and Behavior* 35:93–99.

Heath, C., and D. Heath (2010). *Switch: How to change when change is hard.* New York: Random House.

Kinzie, M. B. 2005. Instructional design strategies for health behavior change. *Patient Education and Counseling* 56:3–15.

Levy, J., and G. Auld. 2004. Cooking classes outperform cooking demonstrations for college sophomores. *Journal of Nutrition Education and Behavior* 36:197–203.

Locke, E. A., and G. P. Latham. 1990. *A theory of goal setting and performance.* Upper Saddle River, NJ: Prentice Hall.

Mattes, R. D. 1993. Fat preference and adherence to a reduced fat diet. *American Journal of Clinical Nutrition* 57: 373–377.

Merrill, M. D. 2009. First principles of instruction. In *Instructional-design theories and models. Volume III. Building a common knowledge base.* C. M. Reigeluth and A. A. Carr-Chellman, editors. New York: Routledge.

Michie, S., S. Ashford, F. F. Sniehottac, S. U. Dombrowskid, A. Bishop, and D. P. French. A refined taxonomy of behaviour change techniques to help people change their physical activity and healthy eating behaviours: The CALO-RE taxonomy. Psychology and Health 26(11): 1479–1498.

Pelican, S., F. Vanden Heede, B. Holmes, S. A. Moore, and D. Buchanan. 2005. The power of others to shape our identity: Body image, physical abilities, and body weight. *Family and Consumer Sciences Research Journal* 34:57–80.

Schwarzer, R., and B. Renner. 2000. Social cognitive predictors of health behavior: Action self-efficacy and coping self-efficacy. *Health Psychology* 19:487–495.

Shilts, M. K., M. Horowitz, and M. Townsend. 2004. An innovative approach to goal setting for adolescents: Guided goal setting. *Journal of Nutrition Education and Behavior* 36:155–156.

———. 2009. Guided goal setting: Effectiveness in a dietary and physical activity intervention with low-income adolescents. *International Journal of Adolescent Medicine and Health* 21(1):111–122.

Urban, N., E. White, G. Anderson, S. Curry, and A. Kristal. 1992. Correlates of maintenance of a low fat diet in the Women's Health Trial. *Preventive Medicine* 21:279–291.

Verplanken, B., and S. Faes. 1999. Good intentions, bad habits, and effects of forming implementation intentions on healthy eating. *European Journal of Social Psychology* 29:591–604.

Wansink, B. 2006. *Mindless eating: Why we eat more than we think.* New York: Bantam Dell.

Wiman, R. V., and W. C. Mierhenry. 1969. *Editors, educational media: Theory into practice.* Columbus, OH: Charles Merrill.

Nutrition Education DESIGN Procedure

| **D**ecide behavior(s) | **E**xplore determinants of change | **S**elect theory & clarify philosophy | **I**ndicate general objectives | **G**enerate plans | **N**ail down evaluation plan |
| Step 1 | Step 2 | Step 3 | Step 4 | Step 5 | Step 6 |

Step 5: Generate educational plans.

What is the behavior change goal from Step 1 for this session?

Students will increase fruit and vegetable consumption.

What general educational objectives will you address in this session? Which motivational and/or facilitating objectives from Step 4 will guide your session?

- Participants will be able to describe the importance of eating a variety of fruits and vegetables.
- Participants will be able to identify strategies to overcome perceived barriers to fruit and vegetable consumption.
- Participants will be able to know how to increase their fruit and vegetable consumption and variety.
- Participants will be able to recognize the influence of peers in their snacking choices.
- Participants will be able to prepare fruit and vegetable snacks.
- Participants will be able to set and monitor goals to eat more and/or a greater variety of fruit and vegetables.
- Participants will be able to have increased confidence in their ability to eat more and/or a greater variety of fruits and vegetables.

Planning matrix to outline your session: What activities will you do to guide your audience to your educational objectives?

Use the determinants and general objectives you have selected to achieve the behavior change goal of this particular session to think about the specific objectives you will need to guide the creation of activities. As you think about your specific objectives and start planning activities, sequence the activities according to the four Es: Excite, Explain, Expand, and Exit. Place the determinants where you think they would best fit into the sequence. Enter this information into columns 1 and 2. Next, refer to Tables 11-1 and 12-1 in the text and choose the behavior change strategy that is best suited to leveraging the motivating and facilitating determinants for your audience and the flow of your lesson. Enter the strategy into the third column. Then, write the specific educational objective for this chosen strategy in column 4. Finally, in column 5, briefly describe the activities you will use with your audience to achieve the specific objective.

Sequencing: 4Es	Determinant(s)	Strategy*	Specific Objective	Activity/Activities
Excite	Perceived benefits/ positive outcome expectations	Provide information about positive outcomes	Students will recall benefits of eating a colorful variety of F&V.	Class review of benefits of F&V
Excite	Perceived barriers (self-efficacy)	Reframe perception of barriers	Students will describe barriers to consuming a colorful variety of F&V.	Class discussion of their experiences with barriers to eating a wider variety of more F&V since the last lesson
Explain	Behavioral capability/ competence: cognitive skills	Provide factual knowledge	Students will identify enjoyable F&V snacks.	Class discussion of possible F&V snacks and tips for making F&V snacks easier
Explain	Perceived social norms	Reframe perceived norms	Students will become aware of positive social norms for F&V snacking.	• Discussion of peer influence on snacking choices • Identification of positive F&V role models
Expand	Behavioral capability/ competence: behavioral skills	Provide guided practice	Students will prepare palatable F&V snacks.	Class snack prep and tasting

*__Behavior change strategies__ are similar to __behavior change techniques__ used in health psychology (Michie et al., 2013), and __behavior change procedures__ described by Baranowski (2009).

*Nutrition Education DESIGN
Procedure*

Decide
behavior(s)
Step 1

Explore
determinants
of change
Step 2

Select
theory & clarify
philosophy
Step 3

Indicate
general
objectives
Step 4

Generate
plans
Step 5

Nail down
evaluation
plan
Step 6

Planning matrix to outline your session (Continued)

Sequencing: 4Es	Determinant(s)	Strategy	Specific Objective	Activity/Activities
Expand	Goal setting	Action goal setting	Students will develop goals and action plans for eating more of a variety of F&V.	SMART goals instruction, modeling, and guided practice
Exit	Social support	Social support	Students will share goals with important others.	Goal sharing or plan for sharing

Educational plan in narrative teaching format for delivery to your audience. What is your detailed procedure for delivering the session?

Use the planning matrix outline to design the session in detail. Describe the procedure for each activity in the order in which it will occur during the session. Often motivational determinants correspond with the Excite and Exit part of the session, while facilitating determinants correspond to the Explain and Expand parts of the session. However, each audience and session is different; it is often important to include motivational determinants within the Explain and Expand parts of the session. Don't forget to include how long you expect each activity to take! You should provide a brief overview of the entire session and the necessary materials at the beginning of the session plan. Use the case study as an example.

Write out your narrative teaching plan for your educational session on the following page.

Nutrition Education DESIGN Procedure

Decide behavior(s)	**E**xplore determinants of change	**S**elect theory & clarify philosophy	**I**ndicate general objectives	**G**enerate plans	**N**ail down evaluation plan
Step 1	Step 2	Step 3	Step 4	Step 5	Step 6

Catchy title: SMART Goals for Smart Snacking

Behavioral goal: Students will increase fruit and vegetable consumption.

Overview (teaching point):

There are many barriers to adopting a healthy lifestyle; one way to overcome them is to set SMART goals for yourself.

General educational objectives:

Participants will be able to:

- Describe the importance of eating a variety of fruits and vegetables.
- Identify strategies to overcome perceived barriers to fruit and vegetable consumption.
- Describe how to increase their fruit and vegetable consumption and variety.
- Recognize the influence of peers in their snacking choices.
- Prepare fruit and vegetable snacks.
- Set and monitor goals to eat more and/or a greater variety of fruits and vegetables.
- Demonstrate increased confidence in their ability to eat more and/or a greater variety of fruits and vegetables.

Materials:

Chart paper, fruit and vegetable superpowers comic, fruit and vegetable snacks highlighting different colored fruits and vegetables, small plates, napkins, snack tips to take home, SMART goal worksheet

Procedure*:

Excite

Provide information about positive outcomes: Review reasons for eating a variety of F&V (perceived benefits).
Begin by reviewing the reasons to eat a colorful range of F&V. Ensure the following are mentioned: provides essential vitamins, minerals, fiber, and other nutrients; can increase energy; helps make hair and skin healthy; builds strong bones and muscles for athletic performance; and decreases risk for certain diseases. F&V can be wonderful snacks. (5 minutes)

Reframe perception: Brainstorm barriers to eating a variety of F&V (perceived barriers).
Ask for volunteers to suggest what made it difficult for them to eat a variety of F&V since the last lesson. Accept all answers and record on chart paper. Ensure that the following topics are mentioned: lack of time, not available, my parents don't buy/cook them, friends think it's uncool, dislike taste, don't know how to make them myself. Briefly discuss possible strategies to overcome the barriers mentioned. (5 minutes)

Explain

Provide factual knowledge: Describe how F&V can be used as snacks (cognitive skills).
Ask participants if they have a favorite fruit and vegetable snack to share. Suggest tips, such as leaving fruit on the kitchen table or cutting up veggies for a grab-and-go snack. (5 minutes)

Reframe perceived norms: Discuss peer influence and provide role models (perceived social norms).
"What might your friends say when you choose to eat F&V or bring them as a snack?" Allow for adequate discussion time. If the participants suggest that it might be seen as "uncool," provide alternate stories or media models that show F&V consumption as "cool." Make sure that the models are appropriate for the specific age, gender, and culture of the group. If possible, get some pictures of students or teachers from the school posing while eating fruits and vegetables. (5 minutes)

Expand

Provide guided practice: Quick and easy F&V snack prep and tasting (behavioral skills).
Snack suggestions: veggies and dips, like hummus, lemon yogurt, nut or seed butters; fruit salad; green salad with dressing. Make sure all of the students are involved in the preparation, and be sure to demonstrate and assist with any measuring skills necessary. Encourage everyone to taste the food. Insist that students follow the rule, "Don't yuck my yum!" and encourage them to use the sophisticated food vocabulary they learned in the previous lesson. Practice good food safety and involve students in cleanup. (15 minutes)

Stimulate action goal setting: SMART goals (goal setting).
Distribute SMART goals worksheets and discuss with students the value of setting goals when you're trying to change a behavior, using a personal anecdote if appropriate. Model how to create a SMART goal for choosing a variety of colored fruits and vegetables as snacks, starting with the barrier you're overcoming (e.g., not sure how to prepare something tasty) and why the goal is important to you (e.g., eating a variety of fruits and vegetables will help keep me from catching a cold, feeling crummy, and missing out on fun stuff). Then explain to students how to formulate a goal that is specific, measurable, achievable, relevant, and time-framed (e.g., In the next week, I will prepare one of the snack recipes we tried in class and eat that instead of my usual snack four out of the seven days). Then have the students develop a SMART goal for themselves; go around the room to help students as they work independently. (10 minutes)

Exit

Provide social support: Share your goal with others (social support).
Have volunteers share their SMART goals with the whole group. Have other students share in small groups. If some students do not feel comfortable sharing with the class, have them name a trusted person they will share their goal with after class. Distribute F&V tips to students to take home. (5 minutes)

*In the headings for each activity, the first phrase is the behavior change strategy; the second is a brief description of your activity; and the words in parenthesis refer to the determinant targeted by the activity.

CHAPTER 13

Step 6: Nail Down the Evaluation Plan

OVERVIEW

Finding out whether and how the sessions or intervention you are designing will be effective is helpful to all involved and can be very satisfying. Thinking about how you will evaluate your activities at the same time as you develop them improves both the intervention and the evaluation. Thus, planning the evaluation is included in the steps of the DESIGN Procedure. This chapter leads you through the process of nailing down the plan for evaluating the behavior change goals of your sessions or intervention. Chapter 14 describes evaluating the environmental support components for your intervention behavior change goals.

CHAPTER OUTLINE

- Introduction: why evaluate?
- What should be evaluated? Types of evaluation
- Planning the outcome evaluation
- Planning the process evaluation

- Case study: the DESIGN Procedure in action—Step 6
- Your turn to conduct nutrition education: completing the Step 6 Nail Down Evaluation Plan Worksheet

LEARNING OBJECTIVES

At the end of the chapter, you should be able to:

- State reasons for conducting evaluations of nutrition education interventions
- Distinguish between the major types of evaluation: formative, outcome, and process
- Explain the relationships among educational objectives, determinants, and measures of outcome

- Describe types of measures for evaluating determinants and behaviors
- Describe key features to consider in creating evaluation measures
- Judge the appropriateness of different evaluation designs for the given intervention and audience
- Demonstrate skills in designing an evaluation for a nutrition education intervention

Introduction: Why Evaluate?

You have designed your intervention activities carefully, basing them on theory and evidence so that the intervention will be effective. Why do you need to evaluate it?

Consider this example: An American Peace Corps volunteer went to Malawi to work in an under-fives clinic. There he saw many malnourished children and started trying to convince mothers to enrich their babies' food. He finally wrote and recorded a song with the following message: put pounded peanut flour in your baby's maize porridge and feed it to the baby three times a day if you want your child to weigh a lot. The song was a success; it became number one on the national radio hit parade. He had decided on a clear behavior, and addressed it with appropriate motivators for the behavior and instructions for how-to take action. Did this very original and apparently successful approach to nutrition education change

the mothers' behavior and improve the nutritional status of children in Malawi? Unfortunately, no one will ever know because no evaluation was conducted. Large amounts of dedication, creativity, and resources have often been invested in programs and no one knows their impact because the programs were not evaluated.

You will want to know whether the sessions or intervention you designed had the effect that you hoped, and if not, why not. Thus, at the same time that you are designing the sessions and other activities, it is important to consider how you will evaluate them and nail down a plan for doing so. As we can see in **FIGURE 13-1**, evaluation is considered an integral component of nutrition education planning. In general, with the word *value* embedded in the term *evaluation*, it is not surprising that a simple definition of the term is the process of determining the value or worth of an enterprise and that it is considered crucial to nutrition education and health promotion (Contento, Randell, and

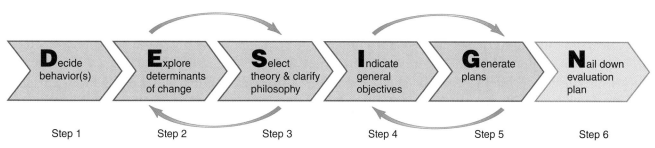

Decide behavior(s)	**E**xplore determinants of change	**S**elect theory & clarify philosophy	**I**ndicate general objectives	**G**enerate plans	**N**ail down evaluation plan	
Step 1	Step 2	Step 3	Step 4	Step 5	Step 6	

Inputs: Collecting the Assessment Data		Outputs: Designing the Theory-Based Intervention			Outcomes: Evaluation Plan

Tasks:
• **Decide** behavior change goal(s) of the intervention, based on:
  • Analyzing issues and behaviors of concern for audience
	Tasks:
	• **Explore** determinants of behavior change based on a variety of data sources
		Tasks:
		• **Select** theory and draw intervention-specific theory model
		• Clarify educational philosophy
		• Articulate perspectives on content
			Tasks:
			• **Indicate** general objectives for each determinant in your theory model
				Tasks:
				• **Generate** educational plans:
				  • Educational activities to address all determinants in theory model
				  • Sequence for implementation using the 4 Es
					Tasks:
					• **Nail down** evaluation plan
					  • Select methods and questions to evaluate outcomes
					  • Plan process evaluation
					  • Create questions to measure how implementation went

Products: Statement of intervention behavior change goal(s)	*Products:* List of determinants to address in the intervention	*Products:* Theory model for intervention Statement of educational philosophy Statement of content perspectives	*Products:* A general objective for each determinant in theory model	*Products:* Educational plans that link determinants and educational activities to achieve behavior change or action goal(s)	*Products:* List of evaluation methods and questions Procedures and measures for process evaluation

FIGURE 13-1 Nutrition Education DESIGN Procedure: Nail down evaluation plan—Step 6.

Basch 2002; Green and Kreuter 2005; Institute of Medicine 2007). Evaluating a program can tell you whether:

- Your intervention had the intended impacts on the intended health outcomes, targeted behavior changes or actions, or determinants of those behaviors and actions
- The message or content was suitable for your audience
- The educational activities (such as format, duration, and frequency) were appropriate for your audience and contributed to the achievement of the behavior change goals and educational objectives of your intervention
- The intervention was implemented as planned, and if not, why not
- The intervention achieved the goals of the funding or sponsoring organization, or the larger goals of society (such as chronic disease reduction, healthy eating for low-income families, or a more sustainable food system)

You can use information such as this to improve the planning and implementation of the nutrition education program the next time around and to judge its overall worth.

Evaluation can also serve sociopolitical functions. For example, evaluation may be used to improve public relations by demonstrating to the public how good the program or intervention is and how worthy it is of further public- or private-sector funding. An evaluation report released to the various media may also be used to increase the visibility of the work of your organization or to apply political pressure for legislative action in some area of nutrition education.

Finally, evaluation may serve psychological functions. Learning that your sessions or other activities have been effective can be very motivating for all involved in the nutrition education intervention, but especially to those actually delivering the programs to the intended audience—such as you and others involved. Even if the behavior change or other goals of your evaluation were not fully achieved, an evaluation can provide guidance on where and how to make changes in the intervention to improve effectiveness.

What Should Be Evaluated? Types of Evaluation

There are three major types of evaluation that you can use to evaluate your intervention, depending on your needs and the duration and intensity of your series of sessions or related activities: formative, outcome, and process. **Formative evaluation** involves pilot testing near the beginning of your program. *Outcome evaluations* are carried out at the end of the program to provide information on the overall effects of the program or intervention, and they are sometimes called *effect* evaluations. In **process evaluation**, you want to know how many people participated in your program and their evaluations of the worth of the sessions or program. You also want to know whether the program was implemented as designed, in order to help shed light on why your intervention worked well or not and to provide rich descriptions of how it worked and with whom.

FORMATIVE EVALUATION OR PILOT TESTING

If you are creating sessions or an intervention and related indirect but individual-level activities (such as newsletters, social media, or other channels) that will be used again or on an ongoing basis, you will want to do some pilot testing or formative evaluation in order to improve it for its final use. The information collected in this type of evaluation is intended to serve decision making about the sessions or program.

Formative research ahead of time with an audience similar to your intended audience can help you learn whether the educational objectives are appropriate and the activities are interesting to the audience, sequenced logically, and can be delivered within the allotted time. You can then use such information to revise the objectives and educational activities of the program. You also will want to test the food-related activities and recipes in your educational plan. It will be very important to test whether the evaluation instruments you have developed are appropriate to your audience and are valid and reliable. If your program is designed for wide-scale use, formative evaluation can involve more systematic field tests of the sessions or intervention materials before the final product is printed for use. For example, you can send your educational plans or manual of activities to a sample of community nutrition educators or teachers and ask them to implement the educational plans with a similar group to find out if: (1) the objectives are clear; (2) the issues included are considered relevant; (3) the educational activities are appropriate, interesting, and feasible to carry out; and (4) the evaluation procedures are useful.

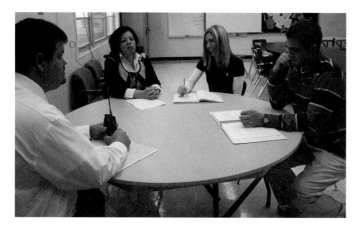

Among the considerations for practitioners as they design programs for a given audience are behavior change goals, educational objectives, and appropriate activities.

© Jones & Bartlett Learning. Photographed by Christine Myaskovsky.

OUTCOME EVALUATION: OUTCOMES IN THE SHORT, MEDIUM, AND LONG TERM

Outcome evaluations are based on the behavior change goals and general educational objectives of your nutrition education sessions or intervention and can represent outcomes that are achievable in the short, medium or long term. See **FIGURE 13-2**.

Outcomes Achievable in the Short Term: Determinants of Behavior Change

Although demonstration of achievement of actual actions or behaviors is most often sought for many nutrition education programs, achievement of *short-term outcomes* may be all that can be expected for some interventions given their short duration, intensity, or scope. These are usually outcomes in terms of the *determinants* of targeted behavior change, such as the participants, perception of risk of current issue or behaviors, perception of benefits of taking action, preferences for healthful foods, self-efficacy, and intentions. Food- and nutrition-related knowledge and skills or goal setting and self-direction skills are sometimes measured as well. These are called short-term outcomes in the logic model not because they will only last for a short while, but because it may be possible to find an effect in the short term. In some cases, movement of participants through the stages of readiness to change may be measured.

If the research evidence indicates that there is a strong relationship between these determinants and the behavior itself, then changes in these determinants can serve as good indications that the impacts may be translated into action under suitable conditions. For example, in some

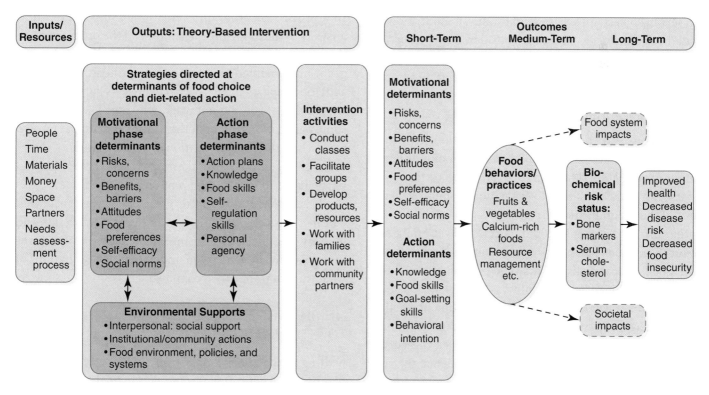

FIGURE 13-2 Designing the evaluation for theory-based nutrition education using a logic model.

studies the relationship between self-efficacy and behavior is strong enough that an increase in self-efficacy in program participants may be meaningful. Information about changes in these determinants of behavior can also help to explain how and why the intervention or its component activities worked or not.

Outcomes Achievable in the Medium Term: Behavior Change

In behavior-focused, theory-based nutrition education interventions or social and behavioral change communications, the primary outcomes to be assessed are usually the behaviors that are targeted by the program and that help to resolve the health- or food-related issue, such as an increase in consumption of fruits and vegetables, breast-feeding, or use of electronic benefit transfer cards to shop at a farmers' market. These behavioral outcomes are considered achievable in the *medium term* in the community nutrition education logic model described in Chapter 14, Figure 14-3 (Chipman 2014).

Outcomes Achievable in the Long Term: Physiological or Health Outcomes

In some educational interventions, physiological parameters are the desired primary end points, such as changes in serum cholesterol levels, weight status, malnutrition, or vitamin deficiencies. These are considered *long-term outcomes* because they may be expected only after educational interventions of considerable intensity and/or duration.

Outcome Evaluation: Clarifying Terms

When you read the intervention evaluation literature, you will come across some distinctions among different kinds of evaluation. The terms **outcome evaluations** and **impact evaluations** refer to evaluations conducted at the end of the program and are statements of the results of the program (Medeiros et al. 2005). That is, did your nutrition education intervention actually accomplish what it was designed to accomplish? This type of evaluation carries the connotation of accountability.

Outcome evaluations address the question of whether anticipated group changes or differences occur in connection with the intervention. By itself, however, measuring outcomes may not provide definitive evidence that the observed outcomes are truly the result of the intervention: maybe they were the result of something else that was going on at the same time, such as a community-wide media campaign or another related program. To definitively conclude that the observed outcomes are a result of the intervention, an impact evaluation must be conducted.

Impact evaluations involve the use of a systematic research design (such as controlled trial) or an evaluation plan to eliminate alternative explanations for the observed differences (U.S. Department of Agriculture [USDA] 2005). The impact evaluation design is described later in this chapter.

Efficacy and effectiveness evaluations are also terms used in the research literature. An *efficacy evaluation* is conducted under optimal conditions (such as when the researchers or program designers themselves deliver the program with outside funding and supports), whereas an *effectiveness evaluation* evaluates a program under real-world circumstances (such as when interventions are conducted by teachers or by practitioner staff as part of their jobs).

Evaluation of nutrition education in practice settings such as community settings, group sessions with families, outpatient education, and so forth will most likely be outcome evaluations focusing on effectiveness. They may also include process evaluation, described next.

PROCESS EVALUATION

In a process or program evaluation, you want to know answers to the following questions: Did the program reach the intended audience? How many attended? Was the program implemented as designed or planned? Were all the activities implemented? To what degree? What worked and what did not? If it did not work, why not? Did it work for some participants but not others? From participants' own words, how did the intervention or sessions work for them? What changes did they make and why and how? How did participants judge the intervention activities?

It is just as important to probe failures as successes. Failures may bring to light flaws in the original design and identify breakdowns in the internal operations of the program. Failures also help you understand the limitations of what the program can accomplish.

LINKING THE EVALUATION PLAN TO INTERVENTION DESIGN

Nailing down the evaluation procedures when you are planning the educational intervention enables the evaluation procedures to be incorporated into activities you design. Even before you have implemented the intervention, you can plan for the kinds of information you will need as you go along and at the end of the intervention, and design appropriate measurement tools.

Planning the Outcome Evaluation

Figure 13-2 provides the framework for designing the outcome evaluation. As you can see, you can measure outcomes that are achievable in the short, medium, and long term. Planning the outcome evaluation generally involves the following steps:

- Clarifying the outcomes that will be evaluated
- Specifying data collection methods and instruments or tools
- Selecting or creating evaluation tools for your intervention
- Constructing an appropriate evaluation plan to measure outcomes and impacts

CLARIFYING THE OUTCOMES THAT WILL BE EVALUATED

Outcome evaluations are based on the behavior change goals and educational objectives of the nutrition education sessions or intervention. Indeed, the way you state these goals and objectives can serve as your statements of desired evaluation outcomes. For example, if your behavior change goal is that "youth will increase their intake of fruits and vegetables," the outcome you evaluate is "youth will increase their intake of fruits and vegetables." Or if your general educational objective is that "participants will have increased confidence in their ability to eat more and/or a greater variety of fruit and vegetables," then that is exactly what you will use to measure self-efficacy at the end in a post-test. Hence, if your objectives are carefully written, all you have to do for an evaluation is to specify the actual methods or instruments you will use to measure these outcomes.

Determinants of Behavior Change

If you are conducting only one or two sessions, statements of behavioral intentions and improvements in determinants of behavior change such as motivations and relevant knowledge and skills that are achievable in the short term may be

all that are possible. These are the substance of your general educational objectives. Thus, will changes in determinants in the desirable direction, or behavioral intentions, be sufficient? Will improvement in the stages of motivational readiness to change be sufficient? Depending on your intervention, demonstration of personal or collective agency or empowerment may be an important outcome.

Behavior Changes Made or Actions Taken

Will the effectiveness of your sessions or intervention activities be judged on achievement of the behavior change goals of the intervention? In behaviorally focused nutrition education, changes in behavior are often a major outcome of interest. You need to clarify what exactly is meant by "behavior" for your intervention. For example, will achievement of the actual behavior change (such as increased intakes of fruits and vegetables) and engagement in the targeted actions by the intended audience (such as buying at farmers' markets) be used as the criterion of outcome effectiveness? For an intervention of short duration, will a small behavior change be acceptable, such as trying new vegetables when offered? For some interventions, perhaps maintenance of an existing healthy behavior is most appropriate.

Physiological or Health Outcomes

Will the effectiveness of your sessions or intervention activities be judged on whether there were changes in the physiological parameters or risk factors for health problems that result from engagement in the targeted actions, such as change in weight or biochemical markers related to diabetes?

Participant Choice

Perhaps the philosophical approach of your intervention is that participants will choose which changes to make or whether to make any changes at all. What criteria will you use to evaluate effectiveness of your program in this case?

SPECIFYING DATA COLLECTION METHODS AND INSTRUMENTS OR TOOLS FOR OUTCOMES

Once you are clear on what outcomes to evaluate, the next step is to think about *methods* of collecting the outcome data and the measures you will use. *Measures* are the specific tools or instruments that you use to collect the outcome data. In the case of group sessions and related nutrition education activities, these are usually questions on a survey instrument, which can be administered via pen and paper, interview, online, or other medium.

Linking Outcomes, Methods, and Instruments/Questions

To evaluate outcomes you will develop tables that have the following columns: "Outcomes," "Methods," and "Instruments or Questions." Examples are shown here:

Outcomes	Method of Data Collection	Instruments/Tools/Questions to Evaluate Outcomes
Outcomes for Determinants (addressed by general educational objectives) increased importance of eating a variety of fruits and vegetables	Survey	How important is eating a variety of fruits and vegetables to you? (not at all important, somewhat important, important, very important)
Behavior Change Outcomes Decreased intake of sweetened drinks	Food frequency questionnaire	How many sugary drinks, such as soda, sweetened iced tea, and fruit drinks, did you drink yesterday? (fill in number _____)
Health Outcomes Improved serum cholesterol levels	Blood test	Finger prick or blood draws and lab analysis for serum cholesterol level

The following subsections discuss some potential methods and instruments/tools/questions in three categories: (1) short-term achievable outcomes: determinants of behavior change goals; (2) medium-term achievable outcomes: behavior change goals; and (3) long-term achievable outcomes: physiological parameters. For each, the methods for collecting the data are described along with the instruments.

EVALUATING EFFECTS ON DETERMINANTS OF CHANGE: OUTCOMES ACHIEVABLE IN THE SHORT TERM

You used determinants of behavior change as the basis of your general educational objectives, and you used them as the basis for selecting strategies and creating your activities. Now, they can also be the basis of your evaluation of outcomes achievable in the short term, which is another reason why you design the evaluation at the same time as behavior change goals, educational objectives, and activities.

To illustrate, excerpts from the ongoing case study of nutrition education with middle school students are shown in **TABLE 13-1**. The full set of outcomes, methods, and instruments is shown in the case study at the end of the chapter.

You may not want to measure impacts on all of the determinants (embodied in your general educational objectives). Some may be more important than others for judging the effectiveness of your sessions or intervention, and some determinants may be useful for guiding the creation of activities but not very useful as an evaluation tool, such as social modeling of a behavior by others (because

Table 13-1 Evaluating Impacts on Potential Psychosocial Determinants of Behavior Change: Examples

Outcomes for Determinants	Methods	Instruments/Tools/Questions
Outcome expectations/perceived benefits	Survey	How important is eating a variety of fruits and vegetables to you? (not at all important, somewhat important, important, very important)
Barriers	Worksheet	What tips sound like they would work to help you, personally, to eat more and a greater variety of fruits and vegetables? (open-ended written response)
Preferences	Group discussion	What specific, sophisticated adjectives can you use to describe this food? (open-ended oral response)
Self-efficacy	Survey	How confident are you that you can eat more fruits and vegetables? (not at all confident, somewhat confident, confident, very confident)
Behavioral capability	Observation	Are the students able to safely cut, mix, and serve fruit and vegetable snacks from the recipe? (checklist observation form)

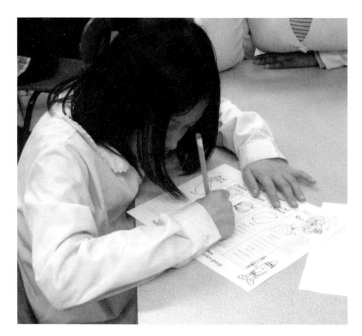

Children like questionnaires if the questions are interesting.

Courtesy of Linking Food and the Environment, Teachers College Columbia University.

this is external to the participants). Now is the time to specify which determinants you will actually measure (usually three to five).

Survey Instruments

- *Survey tool or questionnaire.* You can measure outcomes about determinants in various ways, although the most common method is by asking questions using survey instruments. Theory constructs or determinants are operationalized as a series of questions that participants answer or a series of statements to which participants respond. Many formats can be used. For most determinants, participants are given a series of statements and asked to indicate their opinion on a five-point agreement scale such as whether they strongly disagree (given a score of 1), disagree (given a score of 2), are neutral (given a score of 3), agree (given a score of 4), or strongly agree (given a score of 5). Statements might include "I feel that I am helping my body by eating more fruits and vegetables" (perceived benefits), "I feel that fruit is too expensive" (perceived barriers), or "People in my family think that I should eat more fruits and vegetables" (perceived social norms).

  For determinants, scales may use different anchors. For example, "In your household, how much control do you have in buying/preparing the food you eat?" with a scale ranging from "very little control" to "complete control." Self-efficacy is often measured in terms of how confident individuals are in being able to carry out a given action, such as "How sure are you that you can eat two or more vegetables at dinner?" or "How sure are you that you can add more vegetables to casseroles and stews?" The range of responses might be from "not at all sure" (score of 1) to "very sure" (score of 5). Individuals' readiness to take action can be measured using a series of statements that place them in one of the stages of change: "I am not thinking about eating more fruit" (precontemplation), "I am thinking about eating more fruit" (contemplation), "I am planning to start eating more fruit within 6 months" (contemplation), "I am definitely planning to eat more fruit in the next month" (preparation), "I am trying to eat more fruit now" (action), and "I have been eating two or more servings of fruit a day for at least 6 months" (maintenance).

- *Scoring the survey data.* To evaluate whether there have been improvements in the selected determinants of behavior change, you calculate changes in scores in these variables. You average the score of all participants for each of the questions in the pretest given at the beginning of the intervention, and you average the score of all participants on the same instrument given as a post-test at the end of the program. You then examine whether there has been an improvement in scores and whether this improvement is statistically significant. (If possible, you can also compare this improvement to that of a group that did not participate in the intervention—a control group—to see whether the improvement is truly a result of your intervention.)

Making Survey Instruments Cognitively Appropriate and Motivating

- The questionnaires should look inviting and be motivational to complete, using pictures, drawings, or other visuals to add interest. For low-literacy audiences, use of visuals is crucial to understanding the questions (see section later in this chapter). Use appropriate formatting and white space. The literacy level of the questions is also very important. This also applies to surveys of children. An example of an instrument used with fifth graders in the Food, Health & Choices curriculum

EXPERIMENTING ACTIVITY SHEET

Read each statement and choose the answer that best describes how true it is for you.

Eating lots of packaged snacks such as chips, candy, and cookies...	Not at all true for me	Not true for me	Neutral	Somewhat true for me	Very true for me
20. helps me do well in school.	O	O	O	O	O
21. helps me stay at a healthy weight.	O	O	O	O	O
22. makes me feel good about myself.	O	O	O	O	O

Mark each statement that best describes **how sure** you are that you can do each.

I am sure I can...	Not at all sure	A little sure	Neutral	Sure	Very sure
23. avoid eating processed packaged snacks such as chips, candy, or cookies at home.	O	O	O	O	O
24. avoid bringing processed packaged snacks to lunch at school.	O	O	O	O	O
25. avoid eating processed packaged snacks when I'm with my friends.	O	O	O	O	O

Read each statement and choose the answer that best describes how true it is for you.

I believe that...	Not at all true for me	Not true for me	Neutral	Somewhat true for me	Very true for me
26. I can set a goal for healthy eating	O	O	O	O	O
27. when I have a goal I can follow through with it pretty well	O	O	O	O	O
28. I know how to assess my food intake	O	O	O	O	O
29. I know how to keep track of my eating patterns	O	O	O	O	O

→ Go to the next page

FIGURE 13-3 Instrument for fifth-grade students to measure self-efficacy and goal setting skills for eating fewer packaged processed snacks.

Food, Health & Choices, Contento, Koch & Lee, 2014.

study is shown in **FIGURE 13-3** (Contento, Koch, and Lee 2014). It asks about the determinants related to eating packaged, processed snacks: self-efficacy and goal setting skills. The questions use vocabulary that is understandable by this audience (ages 10–11 years), with a minimum of words. The stems of the questions provide very clear instructions. Such instruments can also be administered through handheld devices in which participants enter the data electronically, such as iPads or an audience response system. Here, the data are transported directly into an associated computer program.

■ Formatting a tool for measuring psychosocial determinants of fruit and vegetable intake to make it appropriate for low-income audiences is shown in **FIGURE 13-4**. The wording for the entire instrument is in Chapter 8, Table 8-2. Note that the items are written at the appropriate reading level for this audience, the text is made up of short sentences with declarative statements, there are visuals on the page, and there is lots of white space. It looks inviting and easy to complete. Such tools can be given using a pencil-and-paper format (most common). For young children or low-literacy audiences, the questions can be read aloud with participants completing the instruments on their own.

Qualitative Methods

■ *Qualitative data.* Information on the outcomes of your sessions on determinants can also be obtained through in-depth interviews, focus groups, and other qualitative methods (Straus and Corbin 1990). In the case of interviews, they are first transcribed and then analyzed for categories and emerging themes through an interpretive approach. The analysis involves an iterative or repeated process in which cases are first reviewed and the data grouped into categories or codes that may be based on prior research or program goals. As new cases are reviewed and added to the coding scheme, the categories and themes may change. This is repeated until there is consensus that the codes have captured all the information. The findings may also be checked with the recipients as validation.

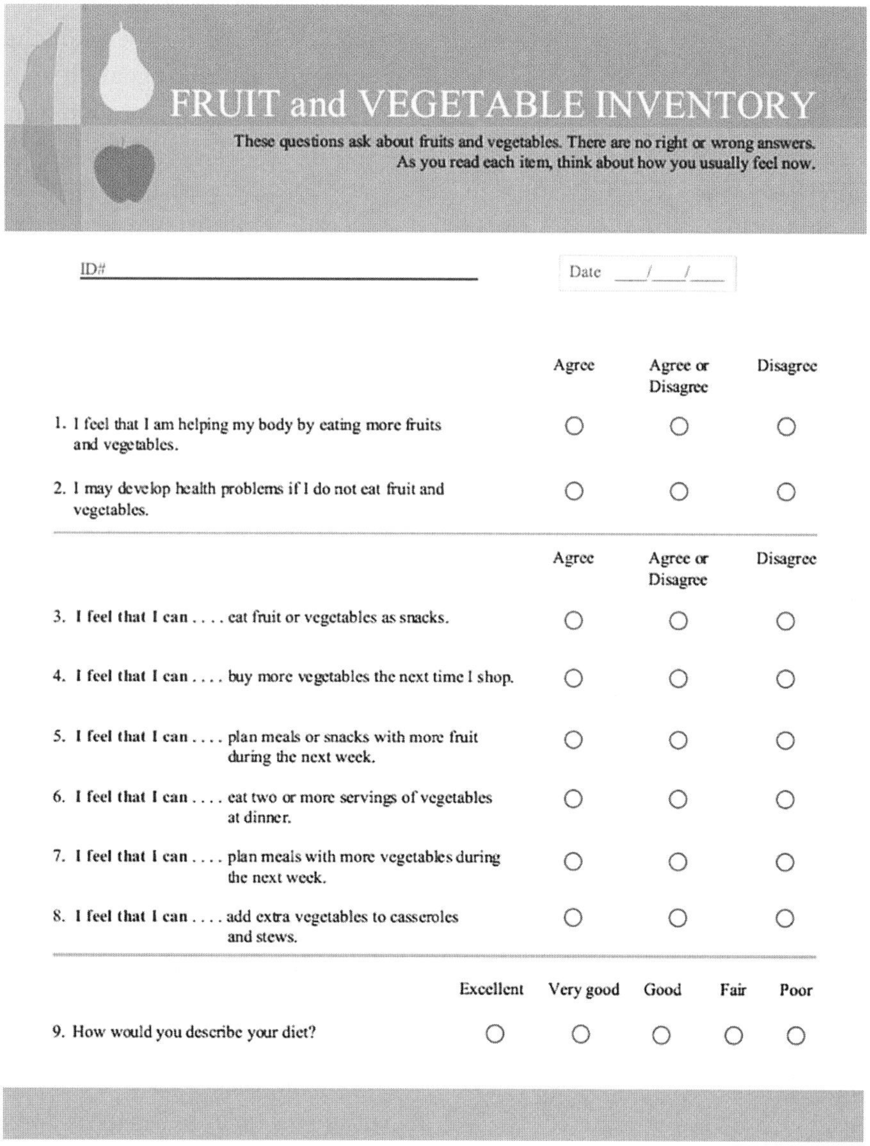

FRUIT and VEGETABLE INVENTORY

These questions ask about fruits and vegetables. There are no right or wrong answers. As you read each item, think about how you usually feel now.

ID# _____   Date ___/___/___

	Agree	Agree or Disagree	Disagree
1. I feel that I am helping my body by eating more fruits and vegetables.	○	○	○
2. I may develop health problems if I do not eat fruit and vegetables.	○	○	○

	Agree	Agree or Disagree	Disagree
3. I feel that I can . . . . eat fruit or vegetables as snacks.	○	○	○
4. I feel that I can . . . . buy more vegetables the next time I shop.	○	○	○
5. I feel that I can . . . . plan meals or snacks with more fruit during the next week.	○	○	○
6. I feel that I can . . . . eat two or more servings of vegetables at dinner.	○	○	○
7. I feel that I can . . . . plan meals with more vegetables during the next week.	○	○	○
8. I feel that I can . . . . add extra vegetables to casseroles and stews.	○	○	○

	Excellent	Very good	Good	Fair	Poor
9. How would you describe your diet?	○	○	○	○	○

FIGURE 13-4 Measuring psychosocial determinants of fruit and vegetable consumption: University of California Fruit and Vegetable Inventory, 2006.

Townsend MS, Kaiser L. Fruit and Vegetable Inventory. University of California, Davis. All rights reserved. From *J Am Diet Assoc.* 2007;107:2120–2124.

Indirect Nutrition Education Activities

For other related communications, materials, and activities, the following are some methods and instruments you can use:

- Recall of having seen the materials, such as posters or flyers
- Short questionnaire to test understanding of material ("Check out what you learned")
- Short survey to ask about perceived benefits of taking action and some actions they can do, or similar questions
- Participation in a quick survey through social media

EVALUATING EFFECTS ON INTERVENTION BEHAVIOR CHANGE GOALS: MEDIUM-TERM OUTCOMES

In nutrition education that is focused on behavior change and based on evidence, increased engagement in the behavior change goal(s) of the intervention is usually the major outcome sought by various stakeholders, including participants themselves. Individuals usually invest their time and effort to participate in nutrition education programs because they desire to lose weight, be good parents, or eat more healthfully or in a way that fosters sustainability of the food system or for other reasons.

Tools for measuring behaviors depend on the level of accuracy desired, the purpose of the evaluation, the size of the group, and the resources available. A detailed discussion of these methods is outside the scope of this book; they are usually described in nutritional assessment books (Willett 2012). Many of the tools commonly used in nutrition education interventions have been reviewed (Hersey et al. 2001; Keenan et al. 2001; Medeiros et al. 2001; Contento et al. 2002; National Collaborative on Childhood Obesity Research [NCCOR] 2013). Some key methods are described briefly below. These are arranged from those that are quick, easy to use, and most useful in practice settings or evaluation studies that do not need rigorously accurate data to the most accurate, which are usually used only when a comprehensive and accurate evaluation tool is needed.

Intake of Targeted Foods

- *Brief food intake checklists or screeners.* These are very short food frequency questionnaires involving a short list of the foods of interest, such as fat intake screeners or fruit and vegetable screeners. Some examples are the Centers for Disease Control and Prevention's Behavioral Risk Factor Surveillance System (BRFSS) (Serdula et al. 1993), the National Cancer Institute's 5 A Day fruit and vegetable screener (National Cancer Institute 2000), or the rapid food screener to assess fat and fruit and vegetable intake (Block et al. 2000). The burden for the participants or respondents is low. This is called *respondent burden.*

- *Food frequency questionnaires.* There are standard food frequency questionnaires that contain fairly long food lists. Individuals indicate how frequently they have eaten foods on this list during the past year or some other time period. The foods on this list can be scored for the individual foods that are your behavioral change goals, manually if you have a small group or using a computer-based diet analysis program. These standardized questionnaires usually use forms that can be optically scanned. These can be self-administered in a group setting. The respondent burden for participants is moderate (Willett et al. 1987; Block et al. 1992).

  A note about short and standard food frequency questionnaires. The food list must consist of an appropriate inventory of foods commonly eaten by the audience with which you are working, and the names of the foods should be clearly understood by the audience. (These often differ by ethnic group, or by country and region within an ethnic group.) Food frequency questionnaires are quick to administer but are often insensitive to change following an intervention, particularly if it is short. They also ask about intake over a time span of a month to a year, and hence may not be suitable for short-term programs.

- *Recalls of foods consumed, usually over the previous 24 hours* (called a 24-hour dietary recall) (Willett 2012). Here, participants in your intervention are individually asked to recall all the foods and beverages that they consumed during the previous 24-hour period. You will need some special training to conduct these interviews (Raper et al. 2004; http://www.ars.usda.gov/Services/docs.htm?docid=7710).

  You then score the recalled foods for the quantity of intakes of the foods targeted by your intervention, such as fruits and vegetables or iron-rich foods, either manually, by using a computer diet-analysis program, or with the U.S. government's Supertracker program (www.supertracker.usda.gov/foodtracker.aspx). The latter can provide information on calories, empty calories, and whether the food group guidelines have been met. The respondent burden for 24-hour recalls is moderately high. Automated online self-administered 24-hour dietary recalls are also available: ASA24 (Subar et al. 2012) and FIRSSt4 (Baranowki et al., 2014).

■ *Food records.* In this instance, participants keep a record of their intakes of foods and drinks over a 1-, 3-, or 7-day period. The records can be analyzed for foods targeted by the program, as for the 24-hour dietary recalls. The respondent burden is high.

■ *Observations of intake.* This usually involves observing how much of meals that were served is eaten or thrown away; thus, the method is often called measurement of estimated plate waste. This can be done by preweighing the average serving size of each item served so that you know how much is in an average serving. Then, individuals or groups, such as students sitting together, are observed or asked to leave their trays, and the amount left on each plate is recorded on a predesigned recording sheet. Or the meal can be photographed

pre- and post-consumption and analyzed later. This analysis can be used for total quantity of food eaten, or for foods in specific food groups, such as fruits and vegetables, grains, or dairy. This is done before and after the intervention, and the difference in quantity of items consumed is calculated. This is a very labor-intensive method and requires trained personnel; consequently it is usually used only in research intervention studies.

Food Behaviors or Patterns

■ *Food behavior checklists and questionnaires.* These instruments or tools measure specific observable food-related behaviors, such as eating fruits and vegetables, buying local or organic foods, shopping practices, food safety behaviors, or food insecurity (Kristal et al. 1990; Yaroch, Resnicow, and Khan 2000). One validated instrument, the Food Behavior Checklist (Townsend et al. 2003; Townsend et al. 2008), is widely used for evaluating nutrition education in U.S. government assistance programs. Excerpts are shown in **FIGURE 13-5**.

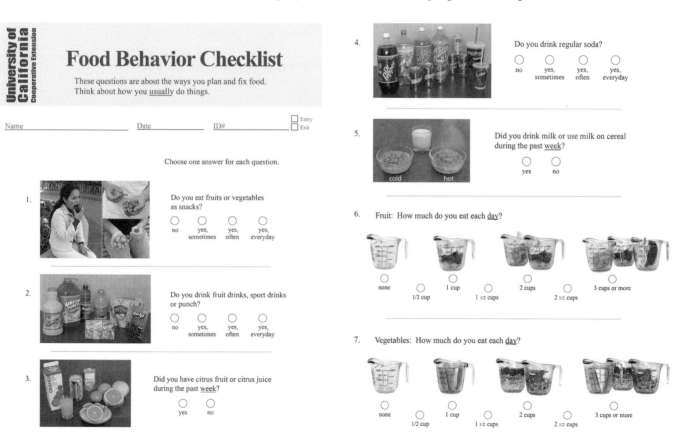

FIGURE 13-5 Excerpts from the 4-page California Food Behavior Checklist.

Townsend, M. S., L. L. Kaiser, L. H. Allen, A. Block Joy, and S. P. Murphy. 2003. Selecting items for a food behavior checklist for a limited-resources audience. *Journal of Nutrition Education and Behavior* 35:69–82. University of California Cooperative Extension; University of California, Davis. http://townsendlab.ucdavis.edu. Reprinted with permission.

The wording for the full instrument is shown in Chapter 7, Table 7-1. The respondent burden is low.

- *Food habits questionnaire.* In this instrument (Shannon et al. 1997), the behaviors related to reducing fat in the diet are categorized as modifying foods to make them lower in fat, avoiding fat as a seasoning or condiment or in cooking, using lower-fat substitutions, or replacing high-fat foods with fruits and vegetables and other lower-fat foods. Those related to fiber are categorized as eating cereals and grains, eating fruits and vegetables, and substituting high-fiber for low-fiber foods.
- *Eating patterns instruments.* You can create tools to provide information on specific eating patterns that are targeted by your program or sessions, such as whether the participants are eating a healthy pattern of foods, judged in terms of health outcomes, carbon footprint, or other criteria. The MyPlate eating pattern can be very useful here.
- *Food-related behaviors such as meal planning and food safety:* These can be measured using instruments such as the EFNEP Checklist (Townsend et al. 2012).

Diet Quality

- *Dietary quality questions or indices.* Sometimes a single question can be used, such as "How would you describe the quality of your diet?" Other instruments provide an assessment of the overall quality

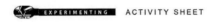

EXPERIMENTING ACTIVITY SHEET

Date	School	Class	Name

My Drinks and Snacks Assessment

Please think about what you ate and drank **during the past week** as you complete this survey. Some questions ask you about how often or how much you ate or drank, and some ask about your opinions about foods and drinks.

Example:

In the past week, I drank...	0 times	About 1-2 times	About 3-4 times	Almost every day	2 or more times every day
Water	O	O	●	O	O

For each question mark **how many times** you had this kind of drink **in the past week.**

In the past week, I drank...	0 times	About 1-2 times	About 3-4 times	Almost every day	2 or more times every day
1. fruit drinks & sweetened iced teas (such as Snapple, Capri Sun, Kool-Aid, or Arizona)	O	O	O	O	O
2. sodas (such as Coke, Pepsi, 7-Up, Sprite, or root beer)	O	O	O	O	O
3. sport drinks (such as Gatorade or PowerAde)	O	O	O	O	O
4. flavored waters (such as Propel or Vitamin Water)	O	O	O	O	O
5. energy drinks (such as Rockstar, Red Bull, Monster, or Full Throttle)	O	O	O	O	O
6. milk (includes white, chocolate, or strawberry)	O	O	O	O	O

FIGURE 13-6 Food frequency instrument for fifth-grade students.

Food, Health & Choices, Contento, I. R., P. A. Koch, and H. Lee Gray. 2014.

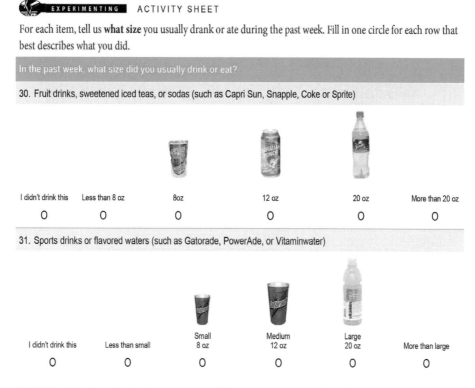

FIGURE 13-7 Food intake instrument for fifth-grade students asking about size of item consumed with photos of different sizes.

Food, Health & Choices. Contento, I. R., P. A. Koch, and H. Lee Gray. 2014.

of the diet. The USDA Healthy Eating Index provides overall diet quality information but is also a research tool.

BEHAVIORAL INSTRUMENT DESIGN: MAKING THEM COGNITIVELY APPROPRIATE AND MOTIVATING

Just as it is important to make the nutrition education or intervention motivating and engaging to your audiences, it is important that the evaluation instruments or tools you design are inviting and motivational to complete. Most pre- and post-assessments are conducted using paper and pencil in practical, real-world settings. Careful design, layout, and formatting are important to make the instrument appealing. In many instances, adding photos is

crucial for the audience to clearly understand what you are asking. These issues are illustrated in the following figures. **FIGURE 13-6** shows the text version of an instrument asking fifth-grade students about their intake of sweetened drinks (Contento et al. 2014). Note the clear instructions and clear about color-coded layout. However, examples to illustrate the question are given in words because there are no photos, given that the questions ask about several food items. **FIGURE 13-7** shows another version of the instrument with photos of different sizes of drinks, so participants are clear about what the question is asking. **FIGURE 13-8** shows a similar instrument placed online for middle school students to complete (Majumdar et al. 2013). By showing numerous examples in the photo, examples are not needed in the wording of the question, and there is no confusion about the intent of the question.

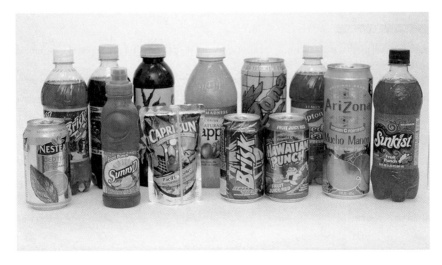

6. How often do you drink fruit drinks or flavored sweetened teas?

○ more than 2 times per day   ○ about 3-4 times per week

○ about once per day   ○ about 1-2 times per week

○ about 5-6 times per week   ○ never drink this

FIGURE 13-8 Food frequency instrument for middle school students completed online showing photos of the kinds of drinks referred to in the question.

Majumdar D, Koch PA, Lee H, Contento IR, Islas-Ramos AD, Fu D, "Creature-101": A Serious Game to Promote Energy Balance-Related Behaviors Among Middle School Adolescents. *Games Health J.* 2013 Oct;2(5):280–290.

EVALUATING EFFECTS ON PHYSIOLOGICAL PARAMETERS: LONG-TERM OUTCOMES

In some nutrition education programs, the expected outcomes are reduced risk for chronic disease or improved health. Indicators are improvements in nutritional status (iron deficiency, bone health) or in physiological disease-risk status.

Measures include the following:

- *Biochemical or physiological measures.* A variety of measures is used. For example, for people with diabetes, maintenance of appropriate blood glucose levels may be the appropriate measure; for weight gain prevention programs, body mass index (BMI) may be the primary outcome measure; and for heart disease prevention programs, serum cholesterol levels may be used as the outcome measure.

Criteria of Effectiveness

For each of the measures you choose to evaluate the program, you also need to decide the level of change that you will consider as necessary to judge effectiveness. Will a statistically significant change be the demonstration of effectiveness, such as a significant increase in intake of fruits and vegetables or rate of breastfeeding? Or will the change have to reach some criterion level (such as 4 or more cups of fruits and vegetables per day or exclusive breastfeeding for 6 months)? For stages of readiness to change, will any movement be considered acceptable, or does the movement have to be from motivation to action (e.g., from precontemplation or contemplation to preparation or action)?

SELECTING OR CREATING EVALUATION TOOLS FOR YOUR INTERVENTION

For an intervention consisting of a single session or several sessions that you may or may not present again and for which there are no requirements by the agency or funding source for evaluation data, the evaluation tool you develop can be quite simple. Because your intervention is directed at changing specific behaviors, you will want to select or create instruments to measure whether there are any improvements in these behaviors as your primary outcome. However, for short interventions, you may only be able to measure improvements in *behavioral intention* and the *psychosocial determinants* of behavior change, with the assumption that if these are strong, they will in time lead to behavior change.

To the extent possible, use an existing validated instrument. However, it is difficult to select one that is perfectly right for you even though there are many published instruments and a registry of over 1000 of them (NCCOR 2013). There are many reasons for this. Rarely are two interventions identical. Tools need to be appropriate to the specific intervention, so it is not easy to find one that is exactly appropriate for the sessions or intervention you are designing. For example, some instruments have been validated with low-resource adult audiences but only in the domains of reducing fat in the diet or increasing fruit and vegetable intake; some have been validated for upper elementary school–aged children, but not for adults, and so forth. When selecting, adapting, or developing a new instrument, you need to consider the issues discussed below (Coaley 2014).

Appropriateness

Maybe the educational activities that participants will complete can also serve as evaluations. For example, in school food and nutrition education, activities in community nutrition education, or WIC clinics, many of the evaluations work best as activities that participants will complete as part of the learning units. In this case, some system must be set up to record the results of these evaluation activities.

In most cases, nutrition educators use specific instruments administered separately from the educational activities. These measures need to be appropriate for the intended audience. If you need to design your own instruments, remember that designing such instruments is not easy, even for a one-time session or for short interventions. How much time and effort you should spend on such instruments depends on the purpose of evaluation and the degree of measurement accuracy needed or desired.

The most commonly used procedure is to identify those instruments that are close to your sessions or intervention in terms of behavioral focus and determinants addressed and to modify or adapt them for use with your specific audience. If you are working with adolescents or a low-income audience, for example, check whether the instrument you have identified as potentially useful has been developed and validated for that group.

Validity

Validity is a generic term that refers to different kinds of accuracy—the degree to which the instrument adequately or correctly measures the variable or concept under study, whether that variable is in the domain of knowledge or of determinants of change or is a behavior. The following is a brief description of the different types of validity. Check for these when you are selecting your instrument or developing your own:

- *Content validity.* Are the items on the checklist, test, or questionnaire reasonably representative of the larger domain or content covered? For dietary intake, are the items on the food frequency questionnaire truly representative of what is typical for this audience? If you are interested in knowledge about fruits and vegetables, are the items representative of that domain?
- *Face validity.* Face validity comes from pilot testing with the intended audience and finding out if the tool is suitable. That is, are the language used to ask the questions, the formats, and the procedures of the instrument understandable and reasonable from the program participants' point of view?
- *Criterion validity.* Does the score generated by the instrument correlate well with data obtained with a criterion measure? For example, does the fruit and vegetable questionnaire correlate well with 7-day food records or serum carotenoid levels (which are considered as standards)?
- *Construct validity.* Does the instrument clearly measure the construct it is supposed to be measuring, such as outcome expectations or self-efficacy?

Reliability

Reliability is a measure of the consistency and dependability of the instrument. There are several kinds of reliability:

- *Reproducibility or test-retest reliability.* Consistency or stability over time. It is the degree to which the instrument, used at different times with the same people, will give the same result. This type of reliability is usually examined by giving the same instrument to the same individuals twice within a short time, such as 2–3 weeks.

■ *Internal consistency.* Consistency within a set of items. Is the instrument internally reliable or consistent? For example, if you have four self-efficacy items, is there consistency among them? For such determinants, the correlations of each item to the total items, or Cronbach's alpha coefficient, where the items are correlated with each other (Cronbach 1951; Coaley 2014), are calculated. For knowledge items, split-half reliability or KR-20 coefficient is usually calculated.

■ *Interrater reliability.* Consistency among data collectors. If two or more people will be collecting the information or coding it, has interrater reliability been established? For example, do two nutritionists code the fruit and vegetable intake data from 24-hour recalls in the same way?

Sensitivity to Change

Sensitivity is the degree to which an instrument can detect changes resulting from an intervention.

Cognitive Testing: Readability and Understandability

■ *Readability* is the ease of comprehension of the evaluation tool by the intended audience, given its vocabulary, sentence length, writing style, or other factors. Reading-level formulas can help make that determination (Nitschke and Voichick 1992). Two commonly used systems are the SMOG Readability Formula (McLaughlin 1969) and the Flesch-Kincaid Grade Level Formula and Flesch Reading Ease Score (Klare 1984). The easiest way to assess readability is to use the Microsoft Office software on most computers that is based on the Flesch-Kincaid Grade Level Formula (Microsoft Office 2010; Stockmeyer 2009).

■ *Understandability* goes beyond readability to assess whether the instrument content is understood by the audience in the way you intend. This can be judged by having participants tell you what they think each question means or is asking about, a process called *cognitive testing* (Alaimo, Olson, and Frongillo 1999). Even if you choose to use an existing instrument, you should still test it for understandability with your particular audience.

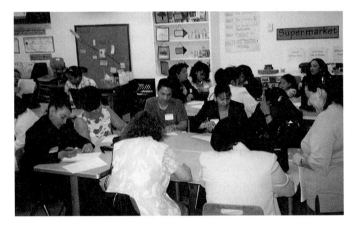

Evaluation instruments need to be tailored to the literacy levels of the audience to ensure accurate data and to be rewarding for participants to complete.

Courtesy of Linking Food and the Environment, Teachers College Columbia University.

Qualitative Data

Qualitative data, such as information from observations, in-depth interviews, focus groups, or open-ended surveys, also are subject to reliability and validity considerations. In this case, the criteria are dependability, credibility, and trustworthiness.

■ *Dependability* is somewhat like reliability in that other people need to be able to follow the procedures and decision trail of the original investigator to understand how the findings were obtained; documentation of all steps is thus crucial.

■ *The credibility or trustworthiness* of the findings is indicative of validity. Credibility is increased through engagement with the individuals over a sufficient length of time to understand the phenomenon being studied, through persistent observation, and through the use of several sources and methods to study the same phenomenon, yielding consistent information. This process is called *triangulation*. Often, the findings are shared with the participants for verification, called *peer debriefing*. In addition, the findings need to ring true to readers, in that they can recognize that an aspect of human experience is being described, even though they have only read the study.

Validating and Pilot Testing Instruments

Pilot testing of instruments and data collection procedures is absolutely essential. Whether borrowed or developed anew, instruments must be tested with your particular audience if you want accurate and meaningful data. When you are conducting a one-time or several-session program, you may not have the opportunity to pilot test the instrument. But even here, if at all possible, check for content validity by asking colleagues to review your instrument. Also, have a few members of the intended audience complete it: check for readability and understanding, and ask them what they think of it. Revise accordingly before using. Readability of the instrument is very important in enhancing validity and reliability—and to be motivating for the audience to complete.

Examples of Validation Studies of Instruments

The general procedure is to compare your instrument to a criterion. One study compared a short food frequency tool for calcium-rich foods (taking about 5 minutes to complete) in an online version and printed version, with 3-day food records as the criterion, and found it to have a good correlation (Hacker-Thompson, Robertson, and Sellmeyer 2009).

The Food Behavior Checklist shown in Figure 13-5 was validated for low-income audiences as follows: items related to fruits and vegetables were compared to serum carotenoid levels. (The checklist is also shown in Table 7-1.) Other food items were compared to nutrient intakes derived from three 1-day dietary recalls (Murphy et al. 2001; Townsend et al. 2003; Townsend and Kaiser 2007). A similar process was used to validate a brief fruit and vegetable tool to measure determinants of behavior change (Townsend and Kaiser 2007).

DESIGNING BEHAVIORAL EVALUATION TOOLS FOR LOW-LITERACY AUDIENCES

According to surveys, about one in seven adults (or about 32 million) in the United States cannot read; another 21% read below a 5th-grade level, and 19% of high school graduates can't read (National Center for Educational Statistics 2003). Many community nutrition education program participants are functioning at a 5th-grade level or below, and recent immigrants may be functioning at even lower levels. Consequently, any evaluation tool we devise must be written so that it is understood by our audiences if we are to obtain valid evaluation information from them. This involves question wording, sentence structure, format, and the cognitive task required to complete the instrument. In addition, the finding that adding visuals to text information enhances learning (Levie and Lintz 1982) suggests that adding visuals to text in a tool will make it easier for low-literacy nutrition education participants to understand evaluation questions.

Townsend and colleagues have conducted research and developed many evaluation tools for the low-literacy audience (Townsend 2006; Townsend and Kaiser 2005, 2007; Townsend et al. 2003; Townsend et al. 2008; Townsend et al. 2012; Townsend et al. 2014). They have based their work on several relevant theories, which they summarize as follows (Johns and Townsend 2010): Sudman's general principle of formatting (Bradburn, Sudman, and Wansink 2004) is that the participants' needs must come first (not the professionals' needs), particularly if it is a self-assessment tool. Realism theory suggests that adding realistic visual cues makes it easier for participants to store and retrieve information (Berry 1991). Cue summation theory (Severin 1967) suggests that learning increases as the number of visual cues increases. In particular, color makes the cues more realistic and thus easier to remember and use.

Townsend and colleagues started with existing tools or created their own text. Then they created the visuals to accompany the text, based on these theories. First they used line drawings and then they took relevant realistic photographs that were specific to the items in the text. The researchers tested photographs in black and white and then in color. They conducted extensive cognitive interviews about the text and visuals with members of the audience at each stage, using think-aloud and paraphrasing techniques (Johns and Townsend 2010; Townsend et al. 2008). In addition, the interviews inquired about the formatting, graphics, layout, and so forth of the instrument. They also assessed the readability of the final evaluation tool.

They found that low-literacy audiences preferred photographs over words or line drawings, color over black and white, and specific recognizable brands of items over generic ones (Townsend et al. 2008). The photographs serve two important functions. First, they explain the question content. Second, they replace text in questions. For example, color food photographs explain the color and shape cues associated with the apple shown

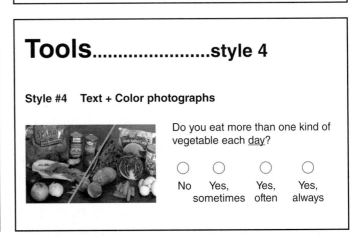

FIGURE 13-9 Progression in formats in the development of the food behavior checklist.

University of California Cooperative Extension; University of California, Davis. [refer to Townsend MS, Sylva K, Martin A, Metz D, Wooten Swanson P. Improving readability of an evaluation tool for low-income clients using visual information processing theories. *J Nutrition Education Behavior* 2008;40:181–186.]

in **FIGURE 13-9**. Limiting the total number of words and words of three or more syllables was also important. Figure 13-9 shows the progression of the development of the instrument. The final instrument is the Food Behavior Checklist, excerpts of which are shown in Figure 13-5. A shortened version of it to measure fruit and vegetable intake only, the Fruit and Vegetable Checklist, is shown in **FIGURE 13-10**. Validity and reliability of this instrument have been established in both the English- (Townsend et al. 2008) and Spanish-language versions (Banna et al. 2010; Banna and Townsend 2011). Participants in group interviews reported that the visually enhanced tools captured their attention, improved their understanding of the questions, and made them more interested in the evaluation process (Johns and Townsend 2010).

Townsend and colleagues also developed instruments to measure other food-related behaviors such as meal planning and food safety, including the EFNEP Checklist (Townsend et al. 2013). After 77 cognitive interviews,

the researchers found that declarative statements, such as "I plan meals," were much more understandable than questions. The instrument is shown in **FIGURE 13-11**.

CONSTRUCTING AN APPROPRIATE EVALUATION PLAN TO MEASURE OUTCOMES AND IMPACTS

When you give out an evaluation instrument at the beginning and end of a one-time session or a series of sessions, you are following an evaluation plan whether you are aware of it or not. In this case it is a *one-group pretest post-test* design. This design provides you with *outcome evaluation* information.

The purpose of an evaluation plan or design is to ensure that evaluation results are caused by the nutrition education program and not by other confounding factors. Thus, evaluation plans are designed to rule out competing explanations for the results that you obtain. This allows you to measure the true *impact* of the program.

The one-group pretest post-test design is highly practical and can be quite useful but is not a very strong design for ruling out competing explanations. Other designs that can be used are outlined in the following sections. Your choice of design depends largely on which plan is most feasible given the type of power, duration, or intensity of your educational intervention; the context in which it takes place; and the financial and time resources and expertise available to you.

Experimental Designs

We have all heard of the *true experimental design* or *randomized control trial* (RCT) from our familiarity with nutrition science and clinical nutrition research studies, where it is routinely used. It is considered ideal for research purposes. In this design, individuals, WIC clinics, schools, or worksites are randomly assigned to two groups, one of which receives the nutrition education program (intervention condition) and the other of which receives the usual education or another unrelated intervention (the control condition) of equal duration and intensity. Both groups are given test instruments before and after the intervention. One major advantage of this design is that the randomization process ensures that significant differences in outcomes are attributable to the program. A major disadvantage is that randomization is very difficult to accomplish in nutrition education practice settings.

Quasi-experimental Designs

Quasi-experimental designs are traditionally viewed as more realistic models for field evaluation studies. The most

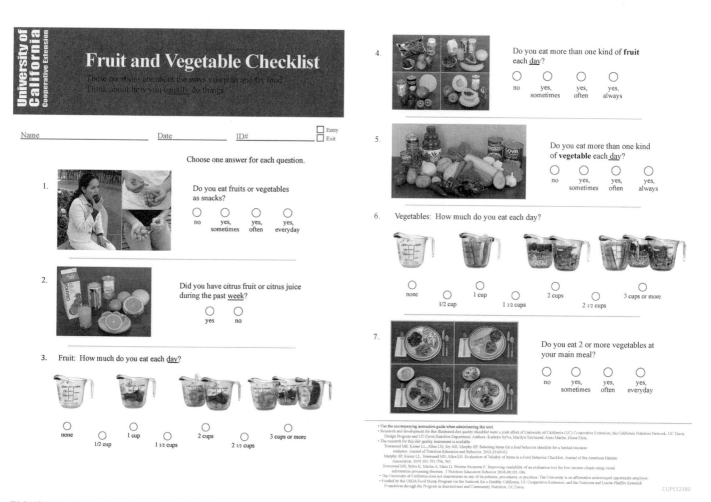

FIGURE 13-10 Fruit and vegetable checklist.

Sylva, K., Townsend, M. S., Martin, A., and Met,z D. 2007. Fruit and Vegetable Checklist. University of California Cooperative Extension; University of California, Davis. http://townsendlab.ucdavis.edu. Reprinted with permission.

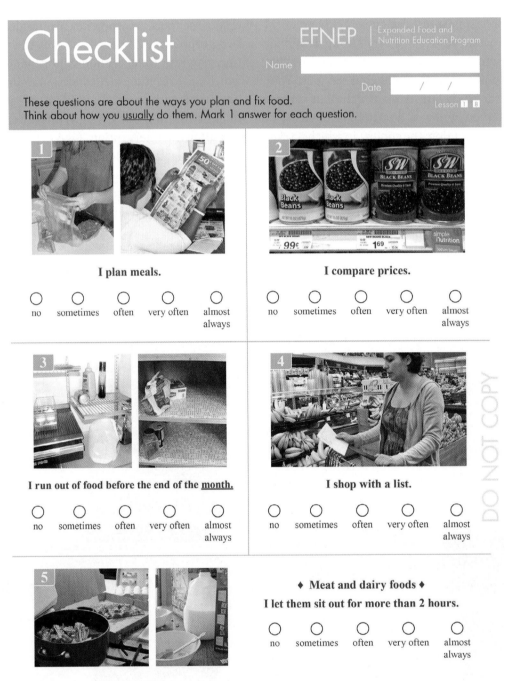

FIGURE 13-11 EFNEP checklist.

Source: Townsend M. S., M. Johns, S. Donohue, et al. Checklist version 3 for 2013–2014. Outcome evaluation tool of selected food behaviors for low-literate EFNEP participants. 4-page booklet using color visuals to replace text to improve readability. Accompanies other data collection tools.

common design within this category is the *comparison-group design with pretest and post-test* in which one group receives the program and is compared with a second matched comparison group that does not receive the program and is selected from a similar population and matched on various characteristics, such as age, gender, ethnicity, or socioeconomic status. Both groups are given pre- and post-tests. Gain scores are compared between the two groups. In school settings, this means that entire classes may be matched with similar classes in the same school, or entire schools matched with other schools. WIC clinic groups receiving an intervention may be matched with groups from WIC clinics with similar characteristics not receiving the intervention. Although these designs do not guard against all competing explanations for the results, they do control for various important sources of error while remaining a fairly workable method for many programs in practice settings.

Nonexperimental Designs

Nonexperimental designs use two common approaches. In the *one-group pretest and post-test design,* described above, scores are compared before and after the program in the same group. There is no comparison group. In the *post-test-only design with nonequivalent comparison groups,* the scores of those who have received the program are compared with a similar group that did not receive the program. There is no pretest. These designs make it difficult to rule out other explanations of results. However, such designs are often the only ones feasible in practice settings and can provide important insights.

Time Series Designs

In *interrupted time series designs,* a number of observations are made over a period of time as a baseline, and then the program is introduced. A series of observations is then made after the program. If the scores remain constant for a time before the program and then increase immediately after the program and remain constant at that higher level for some time after the program, the increase may be attributable to the program. This conclusion is strengthened if the observations are accompanied by time series observations of a no-treatment comparison group. Again, although many sources of error remain, this design can provide some insight into the effectiveness of the program.

Surveillance Studies

Surveillance studies monitor the status of a population or group on outcomes of interest such as dietary intakes or attitudes toward healthful eating. Such studies can document how a group is doing over time but cannot explain what causes the observed status.

Qualitative Evaluation Designs

Qualitative evaluation designs can be used as an alternative to quantitative designs or as a complement to them. The methods used are generally inductive in nature and rely on such strategies as observations, structured and semistructured individual and group interviews, focus groups, historical records, photo voice interviews (where participants take photos of relevant practices and then talk about them), and questionnaires. Qualitative methods can boost the usefulness of quantitative methods by focusing on the dynamics and contexts of change because the quantitative methods tend to focus only on the outcomes of the interventions. Qualitative methods also enlarge the observational field to capture actual, and often unintended, changes. By focusing on the participants' viewpoints, they can also help us understand how the intervention affected participants and with whom and how the program was effective. Qualitative methods can help us identify and understand program elements such as current practices, values, and attitudes of participants; leadership styles; staffing patterns; and relationships among program activities.

CONDUCTING EVALUATIONS ETHICALLY: INFORMED CONSENT

Evaluations should be conducted ethically. This means that you should obtain informed consent from program participants to participate in the evaluation. Participants should not be coerced into completing evaluation activities. Their responses should be anonymous or confidential and should not jeopardize them in any way. Participants should not be denied essential services on the basis of their responses or lack thereof.

Planning the Process Evaluation

The process evaluation, in its simplest form, is the kind of evaluation most familiar to nutrition educators. It tends to be done routinely and it is also easier to design than an outcome evaluation. You are participating in a process evaluation when, as a student, you complete an end-of-semester evaluation of the course and the instructor, or when, as a professional, you complete an evaluation form asking for your opinions about the learning experience at the end of a conference or professional meeting. When you have completed your sessions or intervention you, too, will want to do it to find out how the intervention went. Process evaluation can be much more extensive than just finding out how well participants liked the program. Information about many other aspects of the intervention can be extremely useful in helping to make it more effective and to provide a context for understanding the outcome evaluation as well as how the intervention was received and acted on, or not, by your audience (Baranowski and Stables 2000; Steckler and Linnan 2002; Baranowski and Jago 2005; Lee, Contento, and Koch 2013). This section describes the kinds of questions you might want to ask. How you collect the evaluative data depends on the size of the program and the time and resources available to evaluate the program. Gathering the evaluative data may also involve the development of appropriate instruments or forms for recording the data or for reviewing existing material.

PROCESS EVALUATION TO UNDERSTAND HOW THE INTERVENTION WAS IMPLEMENTED

Process evaluation can help us understand how the intervention was actually implemented. Who was reached? Were the participants satisfied with the intervention? Were the behavioral goals and activities appropriate? These and other questions are listed below with suggestions on how you might collect data to answer them. Answers to these will help you understand and explain your outcome results.

Program Reach

- Did your sessions or program reach the intended target audience? To what extent? For example, you planned the sessions for parents of fifth-grade students, but half of those attending were parents of students in grades 1 and 2. Or you conducted a workshop on prevention of type 2 diabetes in an outpatient clinic that serves about 100 such individuals but only 10 attended. This is called *reach.*

Data Collection Methods

Attendance sheets can provide information on the number of participants and demographics or other information

relevant to your intervention. For Web-based activities, you can devise some sort of tracking system.

Participant Satisfaction

- What were participants' and practitioners' degrees of satisfaction with both the content of materials, learning activities, or media messages and the form in which they were delivered? That is, which aspects of the program did they like or find useful and which did they not?

Data Collection Methods

You can develop an evaluation form for participants to complete in person or online, asking them to rate their satisfaction with the nutrition education experience—whether it was one session or an intervention of several months. More important, the evaluation should ask them to state which parts of the sessions or intervention were most useful and which least useful, what material should have been covered in greater depth or less, and which activities they liked and did not like and why.

Program Implementation and Fidelity

When you conduct an outcome evaluation using some kind of pre- and post-assessment, you are assuming that the sessions were fully and completely delivered as you designed them. But maybe this did not occur; you or the nutrition educator(s) actually delivering the sessions may have been unable to complete the sessions because there were internal factors, such as group management issues, or external factors beyond the educator's control. Or the educator decided to change the lessons as he or she was delivering them. These changes will have an effect on your pre and post-assessment results. Process evaluation can thus be used to help you understand to what extent the sessions or intervention that you designed were delivered fully and completely. You will want to ask:

- To what extent was the material or activities designed for the program fully delivered? This is called *completion of implementation.* Were you or the presenting nutrition educator able to complete all the activities? If not, why not?
- Was the program implemented as designed? This is called *fidelity or faithfulness to the program.* Did you or the presenting nutrition educator add material or

activities in the course of implementing, If so, why? Did you leave out material or activities? If so, why?

- Implementation completion and fidelity together are referred to as *dose delivered*. If the dose was not fully delivered as designed, why not? What were the obstacles?
- Was the program that was delivered fully received? That is, was the audience able to devote attention to the program without competing or distracting physical conditions, such as noise, lighting, poor slides or speaking voice, equipment that did not work, or social conditions such as management issues in school classrooms? This is referred to as *program reception* or *dose received*.

Data Collection Methods

To assess completeness of implementation and fidelity to the program, devise an instrument such as a checklist of activities for each session so that the nutrition educator can check off how much of the session content was delivered and note which parts were omitted and whether other material was added (Lee et al. 2013). If ongoing records are to be obtained from the participants, such as 3-day food records, to see if they are adhering to the program's behavioral goals, you need to design some way to keep track of whether these records were turned in.

Intervention Design Review

- Were the program behavioral goals and educational objectives that you designed directed at, or consistent with, the issues you identified in Step 1?
- Were the behavior change strategies and learning experiences appropriately designed to achieve stated behavioral goals and educational objectives?
- Were the behavior change strategies and learning experiences appropriately based on nutrition behavior theory and research findings?
- Were the behavior change strategies and learning experiences appropriate to the age group, learning styles, and other relevant characteristics of the participants?

Data Collection Methods

The materials that you designed, such as the description of the overall intervention, the lesson or education plans you used, or handouts given to participants, should be maintained and easily accessible (in binders or in physical or computer files). These materials provide the needed information to assess whether the behavioral goals and educational objectives are directed at, or are consistent with, the needs analysis data from Steps 1 and 2, and whether the behavior change strategies and learning activities are consistent with theory and evidence.

Program Management

- If your intervention has several types of activities that may be done by different people, such as group sessions, Web-based materials, or newsletters, was the flow of information to those needing it timely and adequate? If appropriate to your intervention or program, how well was the program managed?

Data Collection Methods

To obtain such management information, if needed, you may want to interview key individuals or conduct a survey, in-person or online, of the individuals involved. A review of existing documents may also shed light on the issue.

PROCESS EVALUATION DATA TO UNDERSTAND THE LINK BETWEEN IMPLEMENTATION AND OUTCOMES

Designing and delivering a group of sessions or an intervention requires a number of steps and components: designing the intervention, providing professional development for those who will deliver the sessions if you are not doing so yourself, ensuring that the intervention is delivered with the intended dose, and ensuring that this intended dose is fully received by the audience. There are barriers at each of these steps that need to be noted and resolved, if possible. There are also external factors and competing programs that influence the implementation process. All of these factors will have an impact on whether and how your sessions will change the determinants and behaviors that are the target of your sessions or intervention. Quantitative data in the form of observational checklists, interviews, or surveys can be used. Qualitative methods can be a rich source to help you understand whether and how the sessions may have impacted audience members differently.

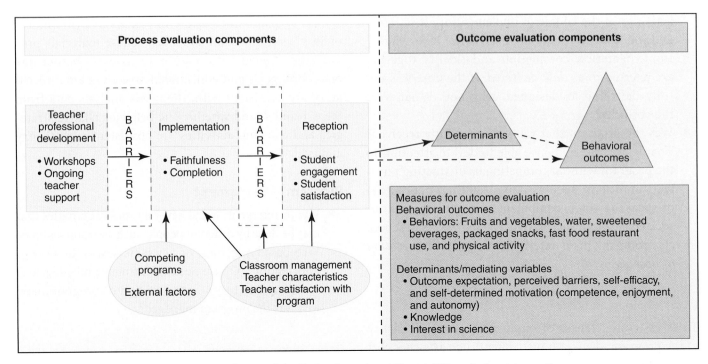

FIGURE 13-12 Conceptual model for the evaluation of the Choice, Control, and Change (C3) curriculum intervention.

Lee, H. W., I. R. Contento, and P. Koch. 2013. Using a systematic conceptual model for process evaluation of a middle-school curriculum intervention: *Choice, Control & Change. Journal of Nutrition Education and Behavior.*45(2):126–36

A conceptual framework for conducting a process evaluation is shown in **FIGURE 13-12**. It is for a middle school obesity prevention intervention that is described in Chapter 12 in Nutrition Education in Action 12-2. The conceptual framework can just as easily be applied to other settings, such as diabetes prevention or management sessions in an out patient setting or workshops for low-income parents. Here, the dose delivered is called *implementation* and consists of *faithfulness* to, and *completion* of, the sessions or intervention as designed. The data for estimating these consisted of specifically designed forms for each session that were completed by observers for a sample of sessions, and interviews with the teachers. Dose received is called *reception* and consists of *student engagement* and *student satisfaction*. Student engagement was measured (for a sample of sessions) using observation forms developed for each session, and student satisfaction was determined from a survey at the end of the intervention.

Contextual factors are also important to capture and describe. In this example, they consisted of classroom management issues, teacher characteristics, and teacher satisfaction with intervention. For this study,

these implementation factors were found to influence the psychosocial and behavioral outcomes (Lee, Contento, and Koch 2013).

USE OF THE PROCESS DATA

You can use the data collected in a formative way to decide how to improve participation rates and degree of satisfaction with your intervention; how to improve the process of delivery, such as better training for personnel, better materials, or more clarity about intervention strategies; or how to improve management. The data collected in an evaluation during or at the end of an intervention can provide rich descriptions of what went on for all stakeholders during the intervention. Process evaluation data can also be used to identify specifically why your intervention was or was not effective in bringing about desired nutritional goals. In other words, information obtained about program functioning can help to interpret the results obtained from the outcome evaluation about the effectiveness of your intervention (or lack of it). For example, an outcome that is negative may be because your intervention was not implemented completely or with full fidelity, or because the distractions were numerous. This tells you that your intervention itself may be sound and that the implementation process needs to be improved.

Case Study: The DESIGN Procedure in Action—Step 6

The ongoing case study with middle school youth addresses several behavior change goals, including increasing their intake of fruits and vegetables. Given the resources available, the case study intervention will measure student outcomes in terms of improvements in the determinants of change, behavioral outcomes (improvements in fruit and vegetable intake), and weight status (health outcome). The nutrition educator plans on collecting the data pre- and post-intervention in these students and in a matched comparison class of middle school students so that they can compare the changes in students who receive the intervention with those who do not. This is a quasi-experimental evaluation design. The completed Step 6 Nail Down Evaluation Plan Worksheet for the case study is shown at the end of the chapter.

OUTCOME EVALUATION

- *Outcomes in terms of psychosocial determinants of change.* The worksheet asks for ways to measure the outcomes for determinants of change first. The nutrition educator and her colleagues restated the general educational objectives that were based on their theory model determinants and then indicated the method they would use to get the information they needed and the actual questions directed at the objective/determinant. You can see that they chose to use a variety of methods: surveys, worksheets, group discussions, and observations. A sampling of their questions is shown.
- *Outcomes in terms of intervention behavior change goals.* The behavior change goals for these adolescents included to increase their intake of a variety of fruits and vegetables. The instrument to be used is a 24-hour food intake recall, where the students' intakes for one day will be analyzed for several behaviors including increases in the consumption of fruits and vegetables. The criterion of effectiveness is a statistically significant increase in the intake of fruits and vegetables compared with baseline and compared with

the intakes in a matched comparison class of middle school students.
- *Outcomes in terms of health issue of concern.* Recall that the major rationale for the intervention was the concern for the high obesity rate in these youth. Consequently, the health outcome is to be measured in terms of pre- and post-intervention weight status for the 10 sessions spread over time, compared to a matched comparison class of middle school students.

The criterion of effectiveness for all three outcomes is set as statistically significant improvements in determinants of change. Behaviors including fruit and vegetable intake and weight status, compared with baseline and compared with the intakes in a matched comparison class of middle school students.

PROCESS EVALUATION

The process evaluation component of the worksheet asks about how the sessions went: Did the health education teacher complete the sessions? Did he or she follow the plans without adding or omitting parts? Were the students satisfied with the sessions? What could be improved according to the students? Surveys and observations are the methods proposed for obtaining this information.

Your Turn to Conduct Nutrition Education: Completing the Step 6 nail down evaluation plan Worksheet

As noted previously, designing nutrition education programs is an iterative process in which you go back and forth between various tasks. Nailing down the evaluation plan goes hand in hand with the design of educational activities. Thus, at the time when you are stating the general educational objectives directed at the determinants of change in Step 4 and creating your educational activities in Step 5, consider how you will evaluate the achievement of the objectives and the impact of the activities. Step 6 is the time to finalize the evaluation methods.

Complete the Step 6 Nail Down Evaluation Plan Worksheet in the DESIGN Workbook at the end of the chapter, using the case study as a guide. There are many ways to evaluate the outcomes. This is an important activity and can be a very satisfying one.

© Africa Studio/Shutterstock

Questions and Activities

1. Give three reasons why it is important to evaluate nutrition education, no matter how briefly.
2. Distinguish between outcome and process evaluation.
3. In terms of evaluation, describe each of the following terms, indicating the relationships among them and to the general educational objectives:
   a. Outcomes
   b. Instruments
   c. Evaluation plan
   d. Data collection methods
4. Describe four ways for measuring each of the following:
   a. Behavioral outcomes
   b. Potential determinants of behavioral change goals
5. Distinguish between validity and reliability in terms of evaluation instruments. What is the relationship between these two features?
6. Describe ways to make evaluation instruments of nutrition education with low-literacy participants more effective.
7. Think of a practice setting in which you will provide six nutrition sessions to low-income women. What would be a good evaluation design to measure the impact of your program? Describe the design and the kinds of outcomes you think would be practical to measure.

References

Alaimo, K., C. Olson, and E. Frongillo. 1999. Importance of cognitive testing for survey items: An example from food security questionnaires. *Journal of Nutrition Education* 31:269–275.

Banna, J., and M. S. Townsend. 2011. Assessing factorial and convergent validity and reliability of a food behavior checklist for Spanish-speaking participants in USDA nutrition education programs. *Public Health Nutrition* 14(7):1156–1176.

Banna J., L. E. Vera-Becerra, L. L. Kaiser, and M. S. Townsend. 2010. Using qualitative methods to improve questionnaires for Spanish speakers: Assessing face validity of a food behavior checklist. *Journal of the American Dietetic Association* 110:80–90.

Baranowski, T., N. Islam, D. Douglass, H. Dadabhoy, A. Beltran, J. Baranowski, et al. 2014. Food Intake Recording Software System, version 4 (FIRSSt4): a self-completed 24-h dietary recall for children. *Journal of Human Nutrition and Dietetics* 27 Suppl 1:66–71.

Baranowski, T., and R. Jago. 2005. Understanding the mechanisms of change in children's physical activity programs. *Exercise and Sport Science Reviews* 33(4): 163–168.

Baranowski, T., and G. Stables. 2000. Process evaluations of the 5-a-day projects. *Health Education and Behavior* 27(2):157–166.

Berry, L. H. 1991. The interaction of color realism and pictorial recall memory. *Proceedings of Selected Research Presentations at the Annual Convention of the Association for Educational Communications and Technology, 1991.*

Block, G., C. Gillespie, E. H. Rosenbaum, and C. Jenson. 2000. A rapid screener to assess fat and fruit and vegetable intake. *American Journal of Preventive Medicine* 18:284–288.

Block, G., F. E. Thompson, A. M. Hartman, F. A. Larkin, and K. E. Guire. 1992. Comparison of two dietary questionnaires validated against multiple dietary records collected during a 1-year period. *Journal of the American Dietetic Association* 92:686–693.

Bradburn, N. M., S. Sudman, and B. Wansink. 2004. *Asking questions: the definitive guide to questionnaire design for market research, political polls, and social and health questionnaires.* Newark, NJ: John Wiley & Sons.

Chipman, H. 2014. *Revision 3 of the CNE Logic Model (February 2014). Aligns with Dietary Guidelines for Americans, 2010.* NIFA/USDA.

Coaley, K. 2014. *An introduction to psychological assessment and psychometrics.* Thousand Oaks, CA: Sage.

Contento, I. R., P. A. Koch, and H. Lee. 2014. Reducing childhood obesity: An innovative curriculum with wellness policy support. *Journal of Nutrition Education and Behavior* 45(Suppl. 4):S80.

Contento, I. R., J. S. Randell, and C. E. Basch. 2002. Review and analysis of evaluation measures used in nutrition education intervention research. *Journal of Nutrition Education and Behavior* 34:2–25.

Cronbach, L. J. 1951. Coefficient alpha and the internal structure of tests. *Psychometrika 16*(3):297–334.

Green L., and M. W. Kreuter, 2005. *Health program planning: An educational and ecological approach.* 4th ed. New York: McGraw-Hill.

Hacker-Thompson, A., T. P. Robertson, and D. E. Sellmeyer. 2009. Validation of two food frequency questionnaires for dietary calcium assessment. *Journal of the American Dietetic Association 109*(7):1237–1240.

Hersey, J., J. Anliker, C. Miller, R. M. Mullis, S. Daugherty, S. Das, et al. 2001. Food shopping practices are associated with dietary quality in low-income households. *Journal of Nutrition Education and Behavior 33*:S16–S26.

Institute of Medicine. 2007. *Progress in preventing childhood obesity: How do we measure up?* Washington, DC: National Academies Press.

Johns, M., and M. S. Townsend. 2010. Client driven tools: Improving evaluation for low-literate adults and teens while capturing better outcomes. *The Forum for Family and Consumer Issues 15*(3):1540–5273. http://ncsu.edu/ffci/publications/2010/v15-n3-2010-winter/johns-townsend.php Accessed 5/29/15.

Keenan, D. P., C. Olson, J. C. Hersey, and S. M. Parmer. 2001. Measures of food insecurity/security. *Journal of Nutrition Education 33*(Suppl. 1):S49–S58.

Klare, G. R. 1984. Readability. In *Handbook of Reading Research*, P. D. Pearson, ed. (pp. 681–744). New York: Longman.

Kristal, A. R., B. F. Abrams, M. D. Thornquist, L. Disogra, R. T. Croyle, A. L. Shattuck, and H. J. Henry. 1990. Development and validation of a food use checklist for evaluation of community nutrition interventions. *American Journal of Public Health 80*:1318–1322.

Lee, H. W., I. R. Contento, and P. Koch. 2013. Using a systematic conceptual model for process evaluation of a middle-school curriculum intervention: Choice, Control & Change. *Journal of Nutrition Education and Behavior 45*(2): 126–136.

———. 2015. Linking implementation process to intervention outcomes in a middle school obesity prevention curriculum: Choice, Control & Change. *Health Education Research.*

Levie, W. H. and R. Lentz. 1982. Effects of text illustrations: a review of research. *Education and Communication Technology Journal 30*(4):195–232.

Majumdar, D., P. A. Koch, H. Lee, I. R. Contento, A. Islas de Lourdes Ramos, and D. Fu. 2013. A serious game to promote energy balance-related behaviors among middle school adolescents. *Games for Health: Research, Development, and Clinical Applications 2*(5):280–290.

McLaughlin, G. H. 1969. SMOG grading: A new readability formula. *Journal of Reading 12*:639–646.

Medeiros, L. C., S. N. Butkus, H. Chipman, R. H. Cox, L. Jones, and D. Little. 2005. A logic model framework for community nutrition education. *Journal of Nutrition Education and Behavior 37*:197–202.

Medeiros, L., V. Hillers, P. Kendall, and A. Mason. 2001. Evaluation of food safety education for consumers. *Journal of Nutrition Education 33*:S27–S34.

Microsoft Office. 2010. Test your document's readability. https://support.office.com/en-us/article/Test-your-documents-readability Accessed 4/26/15.

Murphy S., L. L. Kaiser, M. S. Townsend, and L. Allen. 2001. Evaluation of validity of items in a Food Behavior Check-list. *Journal of the American Dietetic Association 101*:751–756, 761.

National Cancer Institute. 2000. *Eating at America's Table Study: Quick food scan.* Bethesda, MD: National Cancer Institute, National Institutes of Health. http://riskfactor.cancer.gov/diet/screeners/fruitveg/allday.pdf Accessed 1/26/15.

National Center for Educational Statistics. 2003. The 2003 National Assessment of Adult Literacy. Institute of Education Sciences, U.S. Department of Education. http://nces.ed.gov/NAAL/ Accessed 1/26/15.

National Collaborative on Childhood Obesity Research (NCCOR). 2013. Measures registry. http://tools.nccor.org/measures Accessed 2/16/15.

Nitzke, S., and J. Voichick. 1992. Overview of reading and literacy research and applications in nutrition education. *Journal of Nutrition Education 24*:262–266.

Raper, N., B. Perloff, L. Ingwersen, L. Steinfield, and J. Anand. 2004. An overview of USDA's dietary intake data system. *Journal of Food Composition and Analysis 17*:545–555.

Serdula, M., R. Coates, T. Byers, et al. 1993. Evaluation of a brief telephone questionnaire to estimate fruit and vegetable consumption in diverse study populations. *Epidemiology 4*:455–463.

Severin, W. 1967. Another look at cue summation. *AV Communication Reviews 15*:233–245.

Shannon, J., A. R. Kristal, S. J. Curry, and S. A. Beresford. 1997. Application of a behavioral approach to measuring dietary change: The fat and fiber-related diet behavior questionnaire. *Cancer Epidemiology, Biomarkers and Prevention 6*:355–361.

Steckler, A. and L. Linnan. 2002. *Process Evaluation for Public Health Interventions and Research.* San Francisco, CA: Jossey-Bass.

Stockmeyer, N. O. 2009, January. Using Microsoft Word's readability program. *Michigan Bar Journal*: 46–47.

Straus, A. L., and J. Corbin. 1990. *Basics of qualitative research: Grounded theory procedures and research.* Newbury Park, CA: Sage.

Subar, A. F., S. I. Kirkpatrick, B. Mittl, T. P. Zimmerman, F. E. Thompson, C. Bingley C, et al. 2012. The Automated Self-Administered 24-hour dietary recall (ASA24): a resource for researchers, clinicians, and educators from the National Cancer Institute.

Townsend, M. S. 2006. Evaluating Food Stamp nutrition education: Process for development and validation of evaluation measures. *Journal of Nutrition Education and Behavior* 38:18–24.

Townsend, M. S., C. Ganthavorn, M. Neelon, S. Donohue, and M. C. Johns. 2014. Improving the quality of data from EFNEP participants with low literacy skills: A participant-driven model. *Journal of Nutrition Education and Behavior* 46(4):309–314.

Townsend, M. S., and L. L. Kaiser. 2005. Development of a tool to assess psychosocial indicators of fruit and vegetables intake for two federal programs. *Journal of Nutrition Education and Behavior* 37:170–184.

———. 2007. Brief psychosocial fruit and vegetable tool is sensitive for the U.S. Department of Agriculture's Nutrition Education Programs. *Journal of the American Dietetic Association* 107(12):2120–2124.

Townsend, M. S., L. L. Kaiser, L. H. Allen, A. Block Joy, and S. P. Murphy. 2003. Selecting items for a food behavior checklist for a limited-resources audience. *Journal of Nutrition Education and Behavior* 35:69–82.

Townsend, M. S., C. Schneider, C. Ganthavorn, et al. 2012. Enhancing quality of EFNEP data: Designing a diet recall form for a group setting and the low literate participant. *Journal of Nutrition Education and Behavior* 44(Suppl. 4): S16–S17.

Townsend, M. S., K. Sylva, A. Martin, D. Metz, and P. Wooten-Swanson. 2008. Improving readability of an evaluation tool for low-income clients using visual information processing theories. *Journal of Nutrition Education and Behavior* 40(3):181–186.

U.S. Department of Agriculture. 2005, September. Nutrition education: Principles of sound impact evaluation. Office of Analysis, Nutrition, and Evaluation Newsletter. http://www.fns.usda.gov/ora/menu/FSNE/FSNE.htm Accessed 2/10/13.

U.S. Department of Agriculture. USDA Automated Multiple-Pass Method http://www.ars.usda.gov/services/docs.htm?docid=7710.

Willett, W. C. 2012. *Nutritional epidemiology.* 3rd ed. New York: Oxford University Press.

Willett, W. C., R. D. Reynolds, S. Cottrell-Hoehner, L. Sampson, and M. L. Browne. 1987. Validation of a semi-quantitative food frequency questionnaire: Comparison with a 1-year diet record. *Journal of the American Dietetic Association* 87(1): 43–47.

Yaroch, A. L., K. Resnicow, and L. K. Khan. 2000. Validity and reliability of qualitative dietary fat index questionnaires: A review. *Journal of the American Dietetic Association* 100(2):240–244.

Nutrition Education DESIGN Procedure

Decide behavior(s) — Step 1
Explore determinants of change — Step 2
Select theory & clarify philosophy — Step 3
Indicate general objectives — Step 4
Generate plans — Step 5
Nail down evaluation plan — Step 6

Step 6: Nail down evaluation plan.

Of course, you will want (and possibly be required) to show how effective your educational sessions were in achieving your objectives. By planning an evaluation before you begin your sessions, you will ensure success. Don't be afraid to go back and tweak your session plans after you nail down your evaluation plan in order to make sure they are perfectly aligned.

As you work through your evaluation plan, first determine what the outcomes would be if you are successful in achieving your general educational objectives and behavioral goal(s). Then decide how to measure those outcomes.

Use the Nail Down Evaluation Plan worksheet to help you design your evaluation plan.

How will you know if your audience achieved your objectives? Copy your general educational objectives and paste them into column 1. Then complete column 2 with the appropriate methods to help you determine if your objectives have been met. Finally, complete column 3 with questions you might ask your audience as part of your evaluation.

General Educational Objective (Theoretical Determinant)	Method	Sample Question(s) to Evaluate Outcome
Participants will have increased confidence in cooking vegetables at home. (Self-efficacy)	Survey	How confident are you that you can cook a healthy vegetable recipe at home? (not at all confident, somewhat confident, confident, very confident)
Participants will appreciate the importance of eating a variety of fruits and vegetables. (Perceived benefits)	Survey	How important is eating a variety of fruits and vegetables to you? (not at all important, somewhat important, important, very important)
Participants will recognize how far their fruit and vegetable intake is from recommendations. (Perceived risk)	Worksheet	How does the drawing of your recent meal match up with the USDA's MyPlate template? (open-ended written response)
Participants will appreciate various qualities of fruits and vegetables. (Food preferences)	Group discussion	What specific, sophisticated adjectives can you use to describe this food? (open-ended oral response)
Participants will identify strategies to overcome perceived barriers to fruit and vegetable consumption. (Perceived barriers)	Worksheet	What tips sound like they would work to help you, personally, eat more and a greater variety of fruits and vegetables? (open-ended written response)
Participants will recognize the influence of peers in their snacking choices. (Perceived social norms)	Group discussion	In what ways do your friends and peers influence what you eat? (open-ended oral response)
Participants will know how to increase their fruit and vegetable consumption and variety. (Behavioral capability: Cognitive skills)	Survey	What would you tell an audience of 6th graders in order to help them eat more fruits and vegetables? (open-ended written response)
Participants will be able to prepare fruit and vegetable snacks. (Behavioral capability: Behavioral skills)	Observation	Are the students able to safely cut, blend, and serve fruit and vegetable snacks from the recipe? (checklist observation form)
Participants will be able to set and monitor goals to eat more and/or a greater variety of fruits and vegetables. (Goal setting)	Worksheet	What is your fruit and vegetable SMART goal? What steps do you plan to take to reach your SMART goal? (open-ended written response)
Participants will have increased confidence in their ability to eat more and/or a greater variety of fruits and vegetables. (Self-efficacy)	Survey	How confident are you that you can eat more fruits and vegetables? (not at all confident, somewhat confident, confident, very confident)

Nutrition Education DESIGN Procedure

Decide behavior(s)	**E**xplore determinants of change	**S**elect theory & clarify philosophy	**I**ndicate general objectives	**G**enerate plans	**N**ail down evaluation plan
Step 1	Step 2	Step 3	Step 4	Step 5	Step 6

How will you know if your audience achieved your behavior change goal(s)? Copy your behavior change goal(s) and paste them into column 1. Then complete column 2 with the appropriate methods to help you determine if your goal(s) have been met. Finally, complete column 3 with questions you might ask your audience as part of your evaluation.

Behavior Change Goal	Methods	Sample Question(s) to Evaluate Outcome
Participants will drink fewer sweetened beverages.	Food frequency questionnaire	How many sugary drinks, such as soda, sweetened iced tea, and fruit drinks, did you drink yesterday? (fill in number _____)
Participants will increase fruit and vegetable consumption.	24-hour recall	Select fruits and vegetables from overall diet (pre-post)

How will you know if the issue of concern has been improved? This is only applicable for multi-session interventions. Record the issue(s) of concern you identified in step 1 in column 1. Then complete column 2 with the appropriate methods to help you determine if your issues of concern have been improved. Finally, complete column 3 with questions you might ask your audience as part of your evaluation.

Issue of Concern	Methods	Sample Measurement(s) to Evaluate Outcome
Childhood obesity	Anthropometric measurements	Height (pre-post); Weight (pre-post)
Childhood obesity	Anthropometric measurements	Height (pre-post); Weight (pre-post)

Possible Methods
Survey, Interview, Focus group, Dietary recall, Food frequency questionnaire, Food diary, Group discussion, Projects, Worksheets, Group show of hands in response to questions, Participant engagement, Participant responses, Anthropometric measurements, Physiological parameters, Observation

How did your session go? Use the prompts in the table below to think about how you might gather information for the process evaluation of your educational session. Consider your audience and the amount of time you have to gather this information. This step is especially important if you plan to teach a similar lesson or present to a similar audience in the future.

Process Component	Methods	Sample Question(s)
Did you complete your session?	Observational checklist	How much of the lesson did you complete?
Did you follow your plan?	Observational checklist	Which activities were completed? Which activities were not completed?
Was your audience satisfied with the session?	Survey	How much did you like the lesson? (not at all, a little, some, a lot)
What did the audience think could be improved?	Survey	Select fruits and vegetables from overall diet (pre-post)
Other:		

What sources did you use to complete the Nutrition Education DESIGN Procedure?
Include your reference list or bibliography here.

[1] Ogden CL, Carroll MD, Flegal KM. High body mass index for age among US children and adolescents, 2003-2006. JAMA. May 28 2008; 299(20): 2401-2405.

[2] U.S. Department of Health and Human Services. The surgeon general's call to action to prevent and decrease overweight and obesity. Washington, D.C.: Author; 2001.

[3] U.S. Department of Health and Human Services. The surgeon general's call to action to prevent and decrease overweight and obesity. Washington, DC: Author; 2001.

[4] U.S. Department of Health and Human Services. Healthy People 2020: Understanding and improving health. Retrieved from: http://www.healthypeople.gov/2020

[5] Enns CW, Mickle SJ, Goldman JD. Trends in food and nutrient intakes by children in the United States. Family Economics and Nutrition Review. 2002; 14(2): 56-68.

[6] Munoz KA, Krebs-Smith SM, Ballard-Barbash R, Cleveland LE. Food intakes of US children and adolescents compared with recommendations. Pediatrics. Sep 1997; 100(3 Pt 1): 323-329.

[7] Tam CS, Garnett SP, Cowell CT, Campbell K, Cabrera G, Baur LA. Soft drink consumption and excess weight gain in Australian school students: results from the Nepean study. Int J Obes (Lond). Jul 2006;30(7):1091-1093.

[8] Agricultural Research Service U.S. Department of Agriculture. Continuing food intake by individuals 1994-1996 (CSFII 1994-1996). Washington, D.C.: Author; 2000.

[9] Paeratakul S, Ferdinand DP, Champagne CM, Ryan DH, Bray GA. Fast-food consumption among US adults and children: dietary and nutrient intake profile. Journal of the American Dietetic Association. Oct 2003;103(10):1332-1338.

[10] National Center for Chronic Disease Prevention and Health Promotion. Data and statistics: YRBSS: Youth Risk Behavior Surveillance System. http://www.cdc.gov/HealthyYouth/yrbs/index.htm.

[11] Any Town Health Department. Any Town health statistics. Any Town, USA: Author; 2008.

[12] University-Town Partnership. Intervention needs assessment findings: Survey and interview results 2014.

Congratulations!
You've completed the Nutrition Education DESIGN Procedure.
Good luck teaching and evaluating your sessions!

The Nutrition Education DESIGN Procedure

Nutrition Education:

Linking Research, Theory, and Practice

Isobel R. Contento

with contributions from
Pamela Koch and Marissa Burgermaster
Teachers College Columbia University

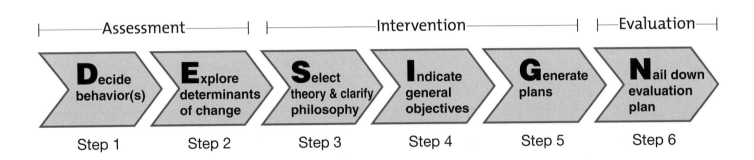

Nutrition education is a valuable part of improving the health and well-being of people everywhere. The Nutrition Education DESIGN Procedure provides a simple and systematic way to link behavioral theory with your creativity as a nutrition educator to generate educational plans that are engaging, evidence-based, and meaningful in promoting healthful eating.

During the course of six easy steps, you will learn a good deal about your audience and use that information to design group sessions, anywhere from one session to multi-session intervention. First, you will examine your audience's issues and behaviors of concern and their assets and decide on the behavior change focus of your session(s) or intervention. Next, you will seek out information about how the audience might effectively be motivated to change their behavior as well as what information and skills they need to learn in order to be empowered to do so. Then, you will use the information you have gathered to choose an appropriate behavior change theory to guide your session or intervention design. At this point you will also reflect on your personal perspectives on nutrition education. Next you will indicate the objectives for your session(s) or intervention, and generate the educational plans you will use to teach your session(s) or intervention. Finally, you will conclude the procedure by developing a plan for evaluating your session(s) or intervention.

Throughout the procedure you should refer to corresponding chapters in *Nutrition Education: Linking Research, Theory, and Practice*. As you learn about your audience through research literature, web sites, and stakeholders themselves, be sure to cite these information sources as appropriate in the bibliography at the end of the workbook.

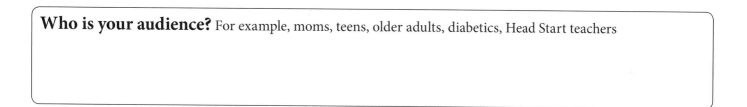
Step 1: Decide behavior change or action goal(s).

Before you design any nutrition education intervention, whether it is a few sessions or a larger intervention with several components, it is important to learn about your primary audience. From this you will be able to determine the behaviors and issues upon which to focus your intervention.

The Decide Behavior Change Worksheet will help you conduct assessments to obtain the information you will need within a framework that allows for your creativity. Use this worksheet as a guide to help you decide behavioral goals for your educational session.

Who is your audience? For example, moms, teens, older adults, diabetics, Head Start teachers

What can you learn about your audience in general? What do general sources, including the research literature and policy documents, tell you about your audience's issues and behaviors of concern? Consider demographics, eating patterns, and health risks. Remember, issues are health problems such as diabetes and obesity, food system problems such as excessive energy use from over processed food, and societal issues such as unfair wages for food workers. Behaviors include not enough fruits and vegetables, too many energy-dense snacks, etc.

Nutrition Education DESIGN Procedure

Decide behavior(s)	**E**xplore determinants of change	**S**elect theory & clarify philosophy	**I**ndicate general objectives	**G**enerate plans	**N**ail down evaluation plan
Step 1	Step 2	Step 3	Step 4	Step 5	Step 6

What can you learn about your specific audience? What do you learn from your specific audience about their issues and behaviors of concern through questionnaires, focus groups, interviews, and visiting the neighborhood?

What could be the behavioral goals for your session? Given the assets and concerns you described on the previous page, list potential behavior change goals for your session(s) or intervention in the left column of the table. Then, in the right column, consider the importance, feasibility, and desirability of each of these potential behavior change goals and think about how modifiable and measurable each would be.

Potential Goal Behaviors	Considerations • How **important** is this behavior in addressing the issues of concern? • How **feasible** is changing this behavior, given the time allotted and resources available? • How **desirable** is changing this behavior from the audience's point of view? • How **modifiable** is this behavior by educational means? • How **measurable** is change in this behavior?

Nutrition Education DESIGN Procedure

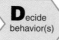

Decide behavior(s)	**E**xplore determinants of change	**S**elect theory & clarify philosophy	**I**ndicate general objectives	**G**enerate plans	**N**ail down evaluation plan
Step 1	Step 2	Step 3	Step 4	Step 5	Step 6

What is your behavior change goal? Evaluate the information in the above table and decide on the behavioral goal(s) for your session(s) or progam. This decision will guide you as you complete the DESIGN Procedure.

How would adopting this behavior benefit your audience? What issues of concern* will be made better if your audience reaches your behavior change goal(s)?

* Note: You may or may not discuss these issues of concern with your audience.

Nutrition Education DESIGN Procedure

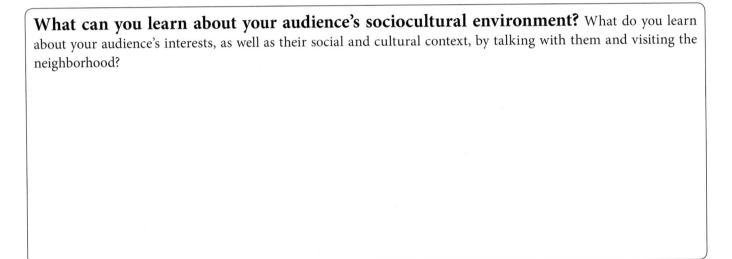

| **D**ecide behavior(s) | **E**xplore determinants of change | **S**elect theory & clarify philosophy | **I**ndicate general objectives | **G**enerate plans | **N**ail down evaluation plan |
| Step 1 | Step 2 | Step 3 | Step 4 | Step 5 | Step 6 |

Step 2: Explore determinants of behavior change or action(s).

After deciding on the behavioral goal for your educational session(s), it is important to figure out what might motivate and facilitate your audience in taking on the goal behavior(s). You should always strive to keep in mind what you have learned about your audience as you proceed through the Nutrition Education DESIGN Procedure. By combining these insights with new information about your audience's beliefs and feelings about the goal behavior and their knowledge and skills related to the goal behavior, you will be able to identify the theoretical determinants that will become the framework for your session(s).

Use the Explore Determinants of Change worksheet as a guide to help you identify and select motivations and skills that relate to the behavioral goals of your educational session or intervention.

What can you learn about your audience's sociocultural environment? What do you learn about your audience's interests, as well as their social and cultural context, by talking with them and visiting the neighborhood?

What can you learn about your audience's assets? What can you learn about individual or community strengths by talking with your audience and visiting the neighborhood?

Nutrition Education DESIGN Procedure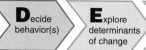

Decide behavior(s)	**E**xplore determinants of change	**S**elect theory & clarify philosophy	**I**ndicate general objectives	**G**enerate plans	**N**ail down evaluation plan
Step 1	Step 2	Step 3	Step 4	Step 5	Step 6

Why would your audience want to engage in the behavior change goal(s)? Being mindful of what you learned about your audience's sociocultural environment and community assets, find out your audience's beliefs and feelings about the goal behavior. What would motivate them to change their behavior or take action? If possible, use information from your audience; however, the research literature may be equally helpful in identifying motivators. After you've listed the motivators in the left column of the table, identify the motivational determinants from psychosocial theories to which they correspond in the right column.

Audience-Identified Motivators	Psychosocial Determinant(s)
Teenage girls say they would eat vegetables if they tasted good.	Outcome expectations
Teenage girls say they would eat fruits and vegetables at school if it were perceived as "cool" by their peers.	Perceived social norms

Nutrition Education DESIGN Procedure

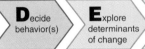

Decide behavior(s)	**E**xplore determinants of change	**S**elect theory & clarify philosophy	**I**ndicate general objectives	**G**enerate plans	**N**ail down evaluation plan
Step 1	Step 2	Step 3	Step 4	Step 5	Step 6

What knowledge and skills will enable your audience to change their behavior? Again, being mindful of what you learned about your audience, find out about your audience's knowledge and skills related to the goal behavior. This includes skills needed to choose and prepare foods, as well as goal setting and self-monitoring. If possible, use information from your audience; however, the research literature may be equally helpful in identifying facilitators. After you've listed the facilitators in the left column of the table, identify the facilitating determinants from psychosocial theories to which they correspond in the right column.

Audience-Identified Facilitators	Psychosocial Determinant(s)
Teenage girls say they would eat fruits and vegetables if they knew how to prepare tasty snacks with them.	Food preparation skills
Teenage girls say they would eat fruits and vegetables at school if they received a daily reminder message on their phones.	Self-monitoring

Which motivators and facilitators will be useful for your session(s)? Keep your behavior change goal(s) in mind and go back through the two tables to identify which determinants you will use in your session(s). Indicate them with a highlight or a star.

Nutrition Education DESIGN Procedure

Decide behavior(s) — Step 1

Explore determinants of change — Step 2

Select theory & clarify philosophy — Step 3

Indicate general objectives — Step 4

Generate plans — Step 5

Nail down evaluation plan — Step 6

Step 3: Select theory and clarify philosophy.

Now that you have identified the psychosocial determinants that will motivate and facilitate your audience's achieving the behavioral goal, it is time to put them together in a theoretical framework that will guide your planning and evaluation. It is also important to reflect on your personal philosophy of nutrition education and see how it meshes with any other nutrition educators you may be collaborating with during your session(s).

Use the Select Theory and Clarify Philosophy Worksheet to help you select a theory model for your session(s) or intervention and describe your personal philosophies related to nutrition education in general as well as the goals of your session(s) or intervention.

What theory (or combination of theories) will guide your educational session(s)? Compare the determinants you identified from your audience in Step 2 to the theories in Chapters 4 and 5 and choose the one(s) most representative of the determinants you highlighted in Step 2.

How can your theoretical framework be visually represented? Modify the theory or theories you chose to be suitable for your audience based on your determinants from Step 2 in order to create a theory model. Below draw a visual of the theory model to show the flow of how your determinants relate to each other to help your audience achieve your behavior change goal(s).

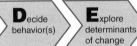

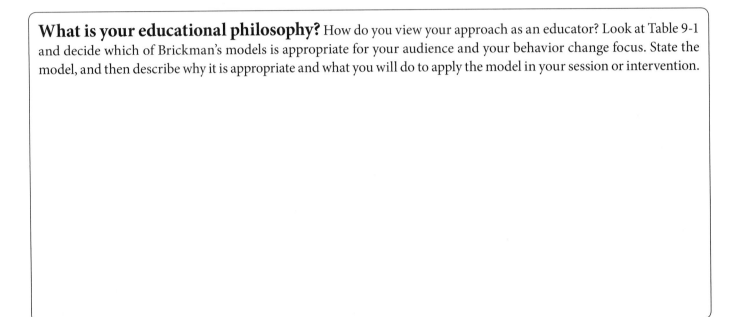

What is your educational philosophy? How do you view your approach as an educator? Look at Table 9-1 and decide which of Brickman's models is appropriate for your audience and your behavior change focus. State the model, and then describe why it is appropriate and what you will do to apply the model in your session or intervention.

What is your perspective about food and nutrition? Look at the section in Chapter 9 titled "Articulating the Intervention's Perspectives on How Nutrition content Will Be Addressed," and in this section write about your perspectives on the food and nutrition content issues you will need to consider in your session(s) or intervention.

Nutrition Education DESIGN Procedure

Decide behavior(s)	**E**xplore determinants of change	**S**elect theory & clarify philosophy	**I**ndicate general objectives	**G**enerate plans	**N**ail down evaluation plan
Step 1	Step 2	Step 3	Step 4	Step 5	Step 6

Step 4: Indicate general objectives.

Translating your behavioral theory into educational objectives to guide your session planning is essential. Remind yourself of your behavior change goal(s) and use your theoretical framework as a guide to work through this step and develop general objectives for your session(s). These objectives will also guide your evaluation plan.

Note that you need one set of general objectives for each behavior change goal. If you are planning only one behavior change goal (e.g., to increase fruit and vegetable consumption) you will have only one set of general motivating and facilitating objectives, whether you devote one or several sessions to the same goal.

Use the Step 4 Indicate General Objectives worksheet to help you develop the overarching educational objectives for your one session or several sessions devoted to the same behavior as well as the practical considerations necessary for it to be a success.

> **Which of the behavior change goals from Step 1 do these general educational objectives address?**

> **What general motivational objectives will guide your session(s) or intervention?** First, list the motivational theoretical determinants you identified in Step 3 in the left column of the table, below. Then, in the right column, use the stem provided to write a general objective for each of the motivational determinants. Carefully consider which verb appropriately expresses your objective. Use the word banks provided on the following page to help you write your objectives.

Motivational Psychosocial Determinant	General Educational Objective Participants will be able to [verb]...
Perceived social norms	Participants will be able to persuasively argue to their peer group why they should eat more fruits and vegetables.

Nutrition Education DESIGN Procedure

Decide behavior(s)	**E**xplore determinants of change	**S**elect theory & clarify philosophy	**I**ndicate general objectives	**G**enerate plans	**N**ail down evaluation plan
Step 1	Step 2	Step 3	Step 4	Step 5	Step 6

What general facilitating objectives will guide your session(s) or intervention?

Now list the facilitating theoretical determinants and write a general objective for each. Continue to use the word banks to help you consider which verb appropriately expresses your objective.

Facilitating Psychosocial Determinant	General Educational Objective Participants will be able to [verb]…
Food and nutrition skills	Students will be able to prepare appealing fruit and vegetable snacks.

Cognitive Verbs	
Remember	List, record, state, define, name, describe, tell, recall
Understand	Explain, describe, summarize, classify, discuss, compare, illustrate
Apply	Sketch, perform, use, solve, construct, role-play, demonstrate, conduct
Analyze	Test, distinguish, critique, appraise, calculate, measure, debate
Evaluate	Review, appraise, justify, argue, conclude, assess, rate, defend
Create	Develop, plan, collect, build, construct, create, design, integrate

Affective Verbs
Express, value, feel, appreciate, care, defend, challenge, judge, question, adopt, advocate, justify, cooperate, persuade, approve, choose, endorse, dispute

Psychomotor Verbs
Cut, prepare, cook, choose, measure, demonstrate, assemble, produce, adjust, locate, arrange, conduct, manipulate, perform, sort, draw, construct

Nutrition Education DESIGN Procedure

Decide behavior(s) — Step 1
Explore determinants of change — Step 2
Select theory & clarify philosophy — Step 3
Indicate general objectives — Step 4
Generate plans — Step 5
Nail down evaluation plan — Step 6

Step 5: Generate educational plans.

In this step, you use everything you have learned about your audience to generate educational plans for sessions that will help your audience attain your behavior change goal(s). Generate one educational plan for each of your sessions. You use your theory model and general educational objectives to create activities that are engaging, interesting, and meaningful for your audience. This is also the time to take stock of the practical aspects of working with your specific audience.

Use the Step 5 Generate Educational Plans worksheet as an organizational guide to help you design each of your educational sessions and translate theory into practice. You first use the planning matrix tool to outline your session. Then you convert the matrix outline into a narrative teaching format to use with your audience.

What are the practical considerations? Think about the practical considerations that will play a role in how you operationalize your objectives when you begin planning your session(s). When possible, use information from the audience itself; however, the research literature may also be helpful in completing this step.

Audience Trait	Description
Educational level or schooling	
Physical/cognitive level	
Literacy and numeracy skills	
Preferred learning style	
Special needs	
Emotional needs	
Social needs	

Resources Needed	Resources Available
Time	
Space	
Equipment	
Administrative support	
Other	

Nutrition Education DESIGN Procedure

Decide behavior(s)	**E**xplore determinants of change	**S**elect theory & clarify philosophy	**I**ndicate general objectives	**G**enerate plans	**N**ail down evaluation plan
Step 1	Step 2	Step 3	Step 4	Step 5	Step 6

What is the behavior change goal from Step 1 for this session?

What general educational objectives will you address in this session? Which motivational and/ or facilitating objectives from Step 4 will guide your session?

Planning matrix to outline your session: What activities will you do to guide your audience to your educational objectives? Use the determinants and general objectives you have selected to achieve the behavior change goal of this particular session to think about the specific objectives you will need to guide the creation of activities. As you think about your specific objectives and start planning activities, sequence the activities according to the four Es: Excite, Explain, Expand, and Exit. Place the determinants where you think they would best fit into the sequence. Enter this information into columns 1 and 2. Next, refer to Tables 11-1 and 12-1 in the text and choose the behavior change strategy that is best suited to leveraging the motivating and facilitating determinants for your audience and the flow of your lesson. Enter the strategy into the third column. Then, write the specific educational objective for this chosen strategy in column 4. Finally, in column 5, briefly describe the activities you will use with your audience to achieve the specific objective.

Sequencing: 4Es	Determinant(s)	Strategy*	Specific Objective	Activity/Activities

*Strategies are similar to behavior change techniques used in health psychology (e.g., Michie et al., 2013), and procedures described by Baranowski (2009).

Nutrition Education DESIGN
Procedure

| **D**ecide behavior(s) | **E**xplore determinants of change | **S**elect theory & clarify philosophy | **I**ndicate general objectives | **G**enerate plans | **N**ail down evaluation plan |
| Step 1 | Step 2 | Step 3 | Step 4 | Step 5 | Step 6 |

Planning matrix to outline your session (Continued)

Sequencing: 4Es	Determinant(s)	Strategy	Specific Objective	Activity/Activities

Educational plan in narrative teaching format for delivery to your audience. What is your detailed procedure for delivering the session?

Use the planning matrix outline to design the session in detail. Describe the procedure for each activity in the order in which it will occur during the session. Often motivational determinants correspond with the Excite and Exit part of the session, while facilitating determinants correspond to the Explain and Expand parts of the session. However, each audience and session is different; it is often important to include motivational determinants within the Explain and Expand parts of the session. Don't forget to include how long you expect each activity to take! You should provide a brief overview of the entire session and the necessary materials at the beginning of the session plan. Use the case study as an example.

Write out your narrative teaching plan for your educational session on the following page.

Nutrition Education DESIGN
Procedure

Decide behavior(s)   **E**xplore determinants of change   **S**elect theory & clarify philosophy   **I**ndicate general objectives   **G**enerate plans   **N**ail down evaluation plan

Step 1   Step 2   Step 3   Step 4   Step 5   Step 6

Catchy title:

Behavioral goal:

Overview (teaching point):

General educational objectives:

Materials:

Procedure:

Excite

Explain

Expand

Exit

Nutrition Education DESIGN Procedure

Decide behavior(s)	**E**xplore determinants of change	**S**elect theory & clarify philosophy	**I**ndicate general objectives	**G**enerate plans	**N**ail down evaluation plan
Step 1	Step 2	Step 3	Step 4	Step 5	Step 6

Educational plan for an additional session.

What is the behavior change goal from Step 1 for this session?

What general educational objectives will you address in this session? Which motivational and/or facilitating objectives from Step 4 will guide your session?

Planning matrix to outline your session: What activities will you do to guide your audience to your educational objectives? Use the determinants and general objectives you have selected to achieve the behavior change goal of this particular session to think about the specific objectives you will need to guide the creation of activities. As you think about your specific objectives and start planning activities, sequence the activities according to the four Es: Excite, Explain, Expand, and Exit. Place the determinants where you think they would best fit into the sequence. Enter this information into columns 1 and 2. Next, refer to Tables 11-1 and 12-1 in the text and choose the behavior change strategy that is best suited to leveraging the motivating and facilitating determinants for your audience and the flow of your lesson. Enter the strategy into the third column. Then, write the specific educational objective for this chosen strategy in column 4. Finally, in column 5, briefly describe the activities you will use with your audience to achieve the specific objective.

Sequencing: 4Es	Determinant(s)	Strategy	Specific Objective	Activity/Activities

* Strategies are similar to behavior change techniques used in health psychology (e.g. Michie et al., 2013), and procedures described by Baranowski (2009).

Nutrition Education DESIGN
Procedure

| **D**ecide behavior(s) | **E**xplore determinants of change | **S**elect theory & clarify philosophy | **I**ndicate general objectives | **G**enerate plans | **N**ail down evaluation plan |
| Step 1 | Step 2 | Step 3 | Step 4 | Step 5 | Step 6 |

Planning matrix to outline your session (Continued)

Sequencing: 4Es	Determinant(s)	Strategy	Specific Objective	Activity/Activities

Educational plan in narrative teaching format for delivery to your audience. What is your detailed procedure for delivering the session?

Use the planning matrix outline to design the session in detail. Describe the procedure for each activity in the order in which it will occur during the session. Often motivational determinants correspond with the Excite and Exit part of the session, while facilitating determinants correspond to the Explain and Expand parts of the session. However, each audience and session is different; it is often important to include motivational determinants within the Explain and Expand parts of the session. Don't forget to include how long you expect each activity to take! You should provide a brief overview of the entire session and the necessary materials at the beginning of the session plan. Use the case study as an example.

Write out your narrative teaching plan for your educational session on the following page.

Nutrition Education DESIGN Procedure

Decide behavior(s) — Step 1
Explore determinants of change — Step 2
Select theory & clarify philosophy — Step 3
Indicate general objectives — Step 4
Generate plans — Step 5
Nail down evaluation plan — Step 6

Catchy title:

Behavioral goal:

Overview (teaching point):

General educational objectives:

Materials:

Procedure:

Excite

Explain

Expand

Exit

Nutrition Education DESIGN Procedure

Decide behavior(s)	**E**xplore determinants of change	**S**elect theory & clarify philosophy	**I**ndicate general objectives	**G**enerate plans	**N**ail down evaluation plan
Step 1	Step 2	Step 3	Step 4	Step 5	Step 6

Step 6: Nail down evaluation plan.

Of course, you will want (and possibly be required) to show how effective your educational sessions were in achieving your objectives. By planning an evaluation before you begin your sessions, you will ensure success. Don't be afraid to go back and tweak your session plans after you nail down your evaluation plan in order to make sure they are perfectly aligned.

As you work through your evaluation plan, first determine what the outcomes would be if you are successful in achieving your general educational objectives and behavioral goal(s). Then decide how to measure those outcomes.

Use the Nail Down Evaluation Plan worksheet to help you design your evaluation plan.

How will you know if your audience achieved your objectives? Copy your general educational objectives and paste them into column 1. Then complete column 2 with the appropriate methods to help you determine if your objectives have been met. Finally, complete column 3 with questions you might ask your audience as part of your evaluation.

General Educational Objective (Theoretical Determinant)	Method	Sample Question(s) to Evaluate Outcome
Participants will have increased confidence in cooking vegetables at home. (Self-efficacy)	Survey	How confident are you that you can cook a healthy vegetable recipe at home? (not at all confident, somewhat confident, confident, very confident)

Nutrition Education DESIGN
Procedure

Decide behavior(s)	**E**xplore determinants of change	**S**elect theory & clarify philosophy	**I**ndicate general objectives	**G**enerate plans	**N**ail down evaluation plan
Step 1	Step 2	Step 3	Step 4	Step 5	Step 6

How will you know if your audience achieved your behavior change goal(s)?

Copy your behavior change goal(s) and paste them into column 1. Then complete column 2 with the appropriate methods to help you determine if your goal(s) have been met. Finally, complete column 3 with questions you might ask your audience as part of your evaluation.

Behavior Change Goal	Methods	Sample Question(s) to Evaluate Outcome
Participants will drink fewer sweetened beverages.	Food frequency questionnaire	How many sugary drinks, such as soda, sweetened iced tea, and fruit drinks, did you drink yesterday? (fill in number _____)

How will you know if the issue of concern has been improved?

This is only applicable for multi-session interventions. Record the issue(s) of concern you identified in step 1 in column 1. Then complete column 2 with the appropriate methods to help you determine if your issues of concern have been improved. Finally, complete column 3 with questions you might ask your audience as part of your evaluation.

Issue of Concern	Methods	Sample Measurement(s) to Evaluate Outcome
Childhood obesity	Anthropometric measurements	Height (pre-post); Weight (pre-post)

Possible Methods
Survey, Interview, Focus group, Dietary recall, Food frequency questionnaire, Food diary, Group discussion, Projects, Worksheets, Group show of hands in response to questions, Participant engagement, Participant responses, Anthropometric measurements, Physiological parameters, Observation

Nutrition Education DESIGN Procedure

Decide behavior(s)	**E**xplore determinants of change	**S**elect theory & clarify philosophy	**I**ndicate general objectives	**G**enerate plans	**N**ail down evaluation plan
Step 1	Step 2	Step 3	Step 4	Step 5	Step 6

How did your session go? Use the prompts in the table below to think about how you might gather information for the process evaluation of your educational session. Consider your audience and the amount of time you have to gather this information. This step is especially important if you plan to teach a similar lesson or present to a similar audience in the future.

Process Component	Methods	Sample Question(s)
Did you complete your session?		
Did you follow your plan?		
Was your audience satisfied with the session?		
What did the audience think could be improved?		
Other:		

What sources did you use to complete the Nutrition Education DESIGN Procedure?
Include your reference list or bibliography here.

Congratulations!
You've completed the Nutrition Education DESIGN Procedure.
Good luck teaching and evaluating your sessions!

Using the DESIGN Procedure to Promote Environmental Supports for Behavior Change and Taking Action

OVERVIEW

This chapter describes how to use the six-step DESIGN Procedure to create plans for increasing environmental support for participants to engage in the behavior change goals targeted by the intervention. The focus is on providing supportive activities at various levels of a social ecological model: the interpersonal level involving social support; the environmental settings level involving institutions, organizations, and community; and the policy, social structures, and system level. The information in Chapter 6 will be especially helpful to you with this process.

CHAPTER OUTLINE

LEARNING OBJECTIVES

At the end of the chapter, you should be able to:

- Describe general types of activities that can be used to address potential environmental determinants of the behavior change goals targeted by the intervention

- Recognize the importance of collaboration with decision-makers and policymakers

- Select from the potential environmental influences on the behavior change goals identified in Step 1 those that are to be targeted

in the intervention to increase interpersonal and policy, system, and environmental support for taking action

- Design specific activities to address the relevant environmental support objectives based on current nutrition education research, theory, and existing evaluated programs

- Develop a plan for evaluating the interpersonal and policy, system, and environmental support activities

Introduction: Promoting Social, Policy, and Environmental Supports for Intervention Behavior Change Goals

A fifth grade student has participated in several nutrition education sessions in class about eating more fruits and vegetables. The sessions were exciting and he decides he will eat his vegetable in the school lunch. He also picks up an apple at lunch. The apple is loose on his tray and falls off as he walks to his table. There is no place to wash it so he puts it into his pocket to eat later. The vegetable is "mystery vegetable," olive green, mushy, and does not smell good, so he does not eat it. When he gets home, he realizes that he lost the apple. So there went his good intentions to eat his fruits and vegetables at lunch!

Clearly, in addition to motivation and skills, individuals need environments that support healthy behaviors. This represents the third component in our conceptual framework for theory-based nutrition education, consisting of: (1) enhancing motivation to act, (2) facilitating the ability to act, and (3) promoting environmental supports for action. The aim for the third component is for the healthful choice to be an easy choice, made so by identifying or creating opportunities for action and reducing barriers in the environment.

It is increasingly clear that many of the food-, nutrition-, and physical activity-related issues of key concern are not easily addressed by nutrition educators working alone. In order to address issues such as preventing overweight, decreasing chronic disease risk, decreasing food

insecurity and malnutrition, increasing breastfeeding, increasing intakes of fruits and vegetables, and increasing consumption of foods that are sustainably produced, we must work in collaboration with others because changes in behavior require environmental support as well as individual action.

Social ecological models suggest that these determinants, which are external to the individual, can be seen as consisting of several levels of influence on behaviors and range from the interpersonal to the institutional and community to the policy and systems levels. These expanded levels of influence provide potential leverage points and venues for nutrition education. These levels of influence are conceptualized in different ways (McLeroy et al. 1988; Gregson et al. 2001; Green and Kreuter 2005; Story et al. 2008; U.S. Department of Health and Human Services [DHHS] 2010). One conceptualization is provided by the U.S. Dietary Guidelines (DHHS 2010). (These are described in detail in Chapter 6.)

FIGURE 14-1 is a modification of the U.S. Dietary Guidelines' social ecological model to show the many levels and sectors of influence on people's food and activity choices and the different nutrition education-related strategies that are needed within each of these levels to support behavior change:

- *Intrapersonal- or individual-level factors*, where psychosocial strategies are used to address beliefs or outcome expectations, motivations, emotions, self-efficacy, perceived norms, and behavioral capability or knowledge and skills

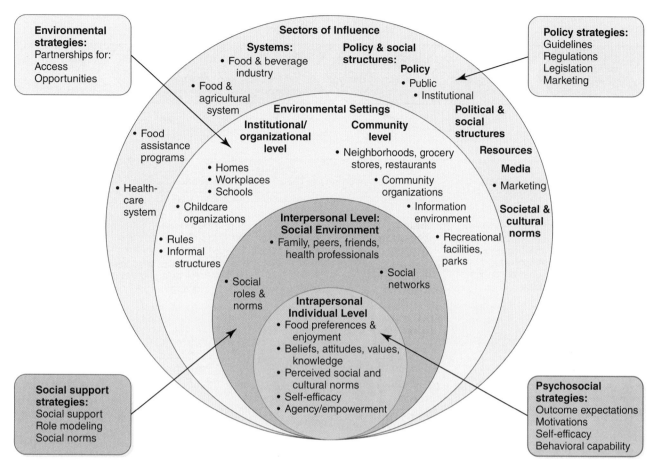

FIGURE 14-1 Social ecological model: nutrition education strategies at different levels of action.

Data from Dietary Guidelines for Americans, 2010. U.S. Department of Agriculture and U.S. Department of Health and Human Services. www.dietaryguidelines.gov.

- *Interpersonal-level factors*, where strategies are needed within individuals' social networks to provide role modeling, social support, and appropriate social norms

- *Environmental settings*, which involve institutional/ organizational-level and community-level factors, where partnerships and collaborations can help to increase access and opportunities for participants to implement the behavior change goals of the intervention

- *Sectors of influence*, which involve policy, social structures, and systems where guidelines, regulations, and marketing can help make the behavior change goals of the intervention an easy choice

In reviewing the mission of your program or intervention and resource considerations, you or your nutrition education team may decide that in collaboration or partnership with others, you will have the resources and skills to design activities or components that will provide social, environmental, and policy supports for the behavior change goals of the intervention in addition to designing individual-level direct and indirect nutrition education activities. For example, you may have the opportunity to increase social support for the intended audience by creating support groups for the intervention participants, working with peer educators, developing a family component to support school- or worksite-based programs, and creating informational environments that reinforce behavior and change social norms. Or you may be able to seek out and work with community groups or policymakers and decision-makers in institutions, agencies, and communities to improve the opportunities and access for your audience to engage in the behavior change goals of your intervention and to develop policies that encourage and reinforce the targeted healthful eating and physical activity practices.

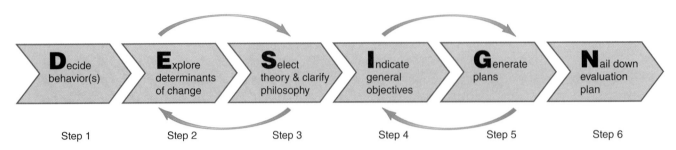

| | Step 1 | | Step 2 | | Step 3 | | Step 4 | | Step 5 | | Step 6 |

Inputs: Collecting the Assessment Data		Outputs: Designing the Theory-Based Intervention				Outcomes: Evaluation Plan
Tasks: • **Decide** behavior change goal(s) of the program, based on: • Analyzing issues and behaviors of concern for audience	*Tasks:* • **Explore** policy, system, and environmental supports for behavior change goals	*Tasks:* • **Select** components or channels • **Select** appropriate theories or models for levels of intervention • **Clarify** program philosophy	*Tasks:* • **Indicate** policy, system, and environmental support objectives	*Tasks:* • **Generate** policy, system, and environment plans: • Activities to address the determinants of change	*Tasks:* • **Nail down** outcome evaluation plan • Determine tools to measure outcome(s) • **Plan** process evaluation
Products: Statement of pogram behavior change goal(s)	*Products:* List of environmental/ policy supports for behavior change goals	*Products:* List of components or channels Theory model(s) for program components Statement of program philosophy	*Products:* A list of policy, system, and environmental objectives for your program	*Products:* Support plans that link determinants and objectives, and strategies	*Products:* Evaluation plan List of indicators and tools to measure outcome(s) Procedures and measures for process evaluation

FIGURE 14-2 Nutrition Education DESIGN Procedure for policy, system, and environment supports for behavior change.

The following collaborators or partners may prove helpful, and often crucial, for planning supportive environmental and policy strategies (wherever relevant to your program): principals and school superintendents; food service providers in schools and workplaces; community and government agencies, such as public health departments or departments of education; religious institutions; existing task forces or coalitions; community organizations related to food and nutrition, such as food recovery programs, food banks, soup kitchens, and food security and hunger organizations; after-school organizations; sustainable food systems organizations; gardening associations; or other nonprofit organizations interested in food, physical activity, and health. This chapter takes you through the six-step DESIGN Procedure, now adapted for planning activities related to environment and policy. The procedure is described in detail in Chapters 7–13.

These tasks and products for each of the six steps are summarized in **FIGURE 14-2**. A case study is presented at the end of this chapter to illustrate the steps. The case study is the same one presented in Chapter 7 and followed through Chapters 8–13.

Step 1: Deciding Program Behavior Change Goals for Audience by Assessing Issues and Behaviors of Concern

In Step 1 you identify the behavior change goals for your intervention based on an analysis of issues of concern that are considered serious and prevalent enough to justify the expenditure of time and resources. You also identify for whom these issues are of greatest concern. Once you have decided on the behavior change goals of your intervention, these goals remain the same whether your intervention is to be delivered in group settings or through various media, or whether you are planning social, environmental, and policy support activities for the participants in the intervention. Hence this step is exactly the same one you completed in Chapter 7. A brief summary of the procedure is provided here but read Chapter 7 for full details. Likewise, the case study illustrating how to conduct this step is shown in detail at the end of Chapter 7. The Step 1 Decide Behavior Change or Action Goal(s) Worksheet is in the Workbook at the end of Chapter 13. Step 1 consists of three sets of activities:

- Who is your audience?
- What can you learn about the issues and behaviors of your audience from general sources?
- What can you learn about the issues and behaviors of your specific audience?

WHO IS YOUR AUDIENCE?

It is important to be clear who your audience is and to conduct a careful assessment of this audience. Your audience can be teens, Head Start children, low-income families, employees at a worksite, those with diabetes in an outpatient clinic, athletes, members of a fitness club, or seniors at a congregate meal site—just about anyone. In many cases, the intended audience is already determined for you by others, such as by the mission of the agency or organization in which the nutrition education will be conducted or by some funding source. Otherwise, the choice of audience is usually based on greatest need or on degree of interest.

WHAT CAN YOU LEARN ABOUT THE ISSUES AND BEHAVIORS OF YOUR AUDIENCE FROM AVAILABLE GENERAL SOURCES?

- *In terms of issues of concern*: You can learn about the issues facing audiences similar to yours, such as health issues, issues related to the food system, social and societal issues related to food, or other issues, through sources such as research literature reviews, health surveys, community organizations, national mortality and morbidity data, and government and expert panel reports. This information provides the rationale for your sessions or program.

- *In terms of behaviors of concern*: You can learn about behaviors of similar audiences that contribute to these issues of concern though the research literature, consumer surveys by supermarket chains or restaurant associations, government food consumption surveys, government dietary recommendations, and so forth.

WHAT CAN YOU LEARN ABOUT THE ISSUES AND BEHAVIORS OF YOUR SPECIFIC AUDIENCE?

- *In terms of both issues of concern and behaviors that might contribute to them*: You can obtain information about your specific audience through focus group discussions, in-depth interviews of key individuals, observations, or surveys. You should also identify current behaviors that are already assets that can be encouraged to promote health and well-being, and ask about their interests and desires for the program.

DECIDE ON THE BEHAVIOR CHANGE GOALS OF THE PROGRAM FOR YOUR AUDIENCE

Based on your assessments, choose one or a few major behaviors, actions, or practices to target in your program. These become the *behavioral change goals of your program*. These behaviors or practices are stated in terms of *changes* or *actions* the program or session(s) seek to facilitate for your audience to achieve. **Note: Enter the information about your audience and your behavioral change goals in the Step 1 Decide Behavior Change or Action Goal(s) Worksheet at the end of this chapter.**

Step 2: Exploring Environmental Supports for Behavior Change

With the targeted and specific behavioral change goals of the program clearly set, your next step is to identify the interpersonal social environments, environmental settings, and policies and social systems that make it easier or more difficult for your audience to act on them. Understanding these environmental determinants will permit you to embark on collaborations with providers of food or services, institutions, government agencies, and community organizations in order to facilitate and enlarge the audience's opportunities for action.

How to assess *intra-personal individual-level influences* on behavior, such as motivations, attitudes, preferences, knowledge, and skills, is described in Chapter 8. In this chapter we focus on assessing the other levels and sectors of influence. Conducting such an environmental analysis will help you develop appropriate activities. The following provide examples of assessment activities; use those that are relevant to your program.

INTERPERSONAL SOCIAL ENVIRONMENT

- *Family environment.* If your primary audience is adults, find out who is responsible for buying food and for preparing it. Do they eat with others whose needs must be considered, such as children, spouses, partners, and/or other family members? What degree of family support is there for the targeted behaviors? How could support be increased? In what formats would they like this support? For example, through workshops, newsletters, email, text messaging, videos sent home, or websites? For youth, similar questions can be asked.

- *Social networks and social support.* Does your primary audience receive support from their peers (e.g., other parents, coworkers, others in the community) and from other social networks (e.g., religious groups, cultural associations) to maintain the desired behavior after it has been adopted? What kind of support do they receive and from whom: emotional, instrumental, informational, and feedback? Do they use social media? If so, how? Also inquire about *potential* social supports: How could you or the nutrition education intervention help them acquire better social supports for enacting the targeted healthful behaviors? Would they be interested in a self-help social support group, a buddy system, or support though social media?

ENVIRONMENTAL SETTINGS: INSTITUTIONAL- AND COMMUNITY-LEVEL SUPPORT

- *Access and opportunities for food needed to carry out the targeted behavior change goals.* Find out whether the foods the intended audience will need in order to make changes in the targeted behaviors or practices are available and accessible in their neighborhoods, workplaces, or school cafeteria. For example, are school meals attractive and supportive of your program behavioral goals? If you have targeted fruits and vegetables, are they easily accessible in workplaces and

the stores or shops in the community at an affordable price? If you are working on food sustainability issues: Is there a farm-to-school or farm-to-cafeteria program? You might also want to survey how many farmers' markets are available and accessible to your intended audience and whether these accept Supplemental Nutrition Assistance Program (SNAP) electronic benefit transfer cards.

- *Access and opportunities in the physical environment.* Is the built environment conducive to carrying out the behavioral goals of your program? You or your team can draw a map of the community showing the location and type of grocery stores (especially supermarkets), corner stores, fast food outlets, restaurants, farmers' markets, recreational facilities, and parks. If that is not possible, at least walk around the neighborhood and see what there is. Review this map: Is good-quality, fresh produce available at a reasonable price? Are there restaurants and food vendors that carry targeted foods at an affordable price? How walkable are the streets in the neighborhood? Are there safe and attractive parks or recreational facilities nearby, such as basketball courts or gyms? Are these affordable?

- *Community capacity and empowerment.* Is the group interested in advocacy to improve their food and activity environment? If so, what prior experiences have they had in working with groups to change their environment? What skills do they have in organizing groups, building coalitions, and planning and executing advocacy? What skills would they like to acquire?

SECTORS OF INFLUENCE: POLICY, SOCIAL STRUCTURES, AND SYSTEMS

Policy

Investigate institutional and public policies that may affect the behavioral goals of your program. These policies will depend on the setting of your program, such as schools, institutions, or communities.

- *Policies related to food and activity in workplaces that might facilitate or impede the healthful behaviors targeted by your program.* What policies does management have in relation to the health of its employees? For example, is there employer sponsorship of health initiatives or employer permission to use worksite communication networks to encourage healthy behaviors? Does the institution provide employees with flex time so that they can participate in health promotion activities? Are there policies about healthy food selections in the cafeteria, if they have one? Does the institution, as the default option, serve water from the tap (if safe) at official functions rather than bottled water? This would be supportive of your intervention if drinking tap water instead of bottled water is one of your behavioral goals for ecological reasons. What policies need to be modified or enacted that your program and partners can influence?

■ *Policies related to food and activity in schools that might facilitate or impede the healthful behaviors targeted by your program.* Does the school have policies related to food and physical activity? In the United States and in some other countries, schools are required to have such policies. The health promoting school is an example (WHO 1996, 2013). If so, how well are the school's wellness or health-promotion policies being implemented? Is the wellness committee or health promotion group meeting regularly? Are the appropriate and required stakeholders on the committee and taking action? Does the food offered in the school conform to policy? Consider: What kinds of food are served in the lunchroom and used in school fundraising, in the classroom as rewards, and in celebrations? Do beverages and snacks in vending machines or school stores conform to policy? What still needs to be done and how can your program assist?

■ *Public policies related to food and activity that might impede or facilitate the healthful behaviors targeted by your program.* What policies of local or state government relevant to your program goals need to be, or can be, modified or enacted? Examples might be required labeling of sweetened drinks or of calorie counts in fast food restaurants if consuming smaller portions of these was one of you behavioral goals. How can you and your collaborators assist in the process?

Social Structures: Communication and Marketing Environment

■ *Information environment of intervention setting.* What is the information environment of the setting in which the intervention itself will take place (such as the school or community center)? For example, what foods are displayed in posters in rooms, hallways, cafeterias, or grocery stores? Are there policies on advertisements about food and drinks in public spaces? How could

the information environment be changed to be more supportive of the targeted behaviors?

■ *Marketing.* What kinds of marketing about food are especially targeting your intended audience (e.g., sweetened beverage billboards in low-income neighborhoods or at local sporting events)? What actions can you and your partners take to encourage more healthful marketing practices?

Food- and Health-Related Systems

■ *Food programs.* What food assistance programs are available to the intended audience? What food system policies are in place that support your intervention goals? How can you and your collaborators work with the intended audience to influence the legislation or policies about these programs, such as through letters, calls, emails, or personal visits to legislators?

■ *Healthcare system.* Do the intended audience members have access to the healthcare services they need for their diet-related disease conditions, such as diabetes or hypertension? How might you and your collaborators work with the intended audience to influence policy related to access to these dietary services?

METHODS FOR CONDUCTING THE POLICY, SYSTEMS, AND ENVIRONMENT ANALYSES

Data concerning potential environmental and policy factors can be obtained from quantitative and qualitative methods such as the following: literature review of similar settings; review of policy documents, existing data, surveys, checklists, and environmental health index assessments; observation of availability of food and active living opportunities in settings that are relevant to the behavioral goals of your program (grocery stores, farmers' markets, workplace, school, and so forth); and focus group discussions and interviews of key informants. In the United States, assessment tools are available from the government for conducting self-assessments in schools (School Health Index, http://www.cdc.gov/healthyyouth/shi/), worksites (Worksite Health ScoreCard, http://www.cdc.gov/dhdsp/pubs/docs/HSC_Manual.pdf), and grocery stores (Nutrition Environment Measures Survey in Stores, NEMS–S, http://www.med.upenn.edu/nems/measures.shtml). Geographic information system data can also generate useful information for community mapping.

Step 3: Selecting Program Components and Appropriate Theory

You are now ready to select how many and which program components you will design. Your choice will depend heavily on the scope of the intervention possible given the resources available to you and your findings from Steps 1 and 2.

SELECT HOW MANY AND WHICH COMPONENTS

Answers to the following questions may be helpful as you are considering how many and which components to develop:

1. *What do the research literature and best practices say are effective types of components or channels to use in programs with this audience for the behavioral goal(s) of your program that you identified in Step 1?* Review the research evidence on evaluated programs to find out what components have been used and proven to work. Also look into evaluated programs produced by various government and other professional organizations. Programs with children and youth usually involve school curricula as the primary component with environmental and policy support activities directed at parents, the school food and activity environment, and the school food service. After-school programs are often accompanied by

work with family, peers, and relevant community institutions. With adult employees, environmental and policy activities are often directed at making the work environment more health promoting; there may also be a family component.

2. *What resources will you have for the program?* How many nutrition education personnel will be available for this program? How many personnel from your partner organizations will be available? What skills do you collectively possess? What is your time frame? You will need to allow time to develop the program, so the more components you have, the more time you will need.

3. *Do you have all the partners or collaborators you need to provide the desired environmental and policy support activities for your behavioral goals?* These may be from the institution, community, or government agencies.

4. *What products will you need to produce?* Each component will require that you develop products to carry out the needed activities, such as educational plans, materials, communication messages, training manuals, electronic media visuals, and websites.

Examples of potential program components and products are shown in **TABLE 14-1**. **BOX 14-1** describes the guidelines for promoting healthy eating and physical activity in schools published by the U.S. Centers for Disease Control and Prevention (CDC), and we can see that they suggest the use of multiple components.

Table14-1 Potential Program Components and Implementation Products: Examples

Program Components	Potential Program Products
School-Based Programs	
Classroom component	Classroom curriculum or manual with lesson plans/activities for all the sessions
	Student activity sheets and homework
	Audio and video resources
	Computer and website activities
	Incentives and rewards
	Snack preparation and taste-testing or cooking recipes
	Gardening materials
Teacher professional development sessions	Teacher professional development protocol or manual
Family involvement component: ■ Educational sessions ■ Other activities	Family education manual for all the sessions Family educational session materials Family activities done by family and youth at home Newsletters and other mailed information Recipes and tip sheets for family activities Family fun nights protocols

School environment (through collaborations)	
■ School food service changes	School food service/cafeteria professional development manuals
	Menu modification manual
	If there is to be a farm-to-school program then a procurement manual needs to be developed
■ School food policies	School food environment assessment tools
	School Wellness Policy Council's (or other committee) recruitment and activity protocols
	School Wellness Policy manuals
■ School informational environment	Classroom, hallway, and cafeteria posters
	Announcements over the school's public announcement system, where relevant
Family component	Family newsletters, activity sheets, recipes, and tip sheets
	Messages through social media and mobile devices
Workplace Programs	
Worksite educational component	
■ Kickoff event	Protocol for kickoff activities
	Materials for kickoff activities
■ Educational sessions	Manual of lessons/activities for the sessions
	Activity sheets, handouts
■ Activities	Health fair protocol
	Food demonstration protocol
	Height/weight measurement equipment and protocol, if relevant
	Nutrition quizzes
■ Information distribution	Brochures and self-assessment with feedback materials
	Tip sheets and recipes
Worksite environment component (through collaborations)	Worksite food environment assessment tools
	Employee councils' recruitment and activity protocols
■ Worksite food service offerings	Recommended menu offerings/modification manual
■ Catering policies	Catering policy document
■ Information environment	Nutrition information in cafeterias (signage) and on vending machines
Community Programs	
Community educational component (N *sessions*)	Manual with protocol or educational (lesson) plans for sessions/activities for the N sessions
	Activity sheets, handouts
	Snack preparation and taste-testing recipes
	Cooking classes: protocols for teaching skills, recipes
	Incentives and rewards
Social marketing component	Social marketing messages and materials
	Recruitment materials for venues to increase access and opportunities
Farmers' market component	Manual with protocol for conducting farmers' market tours and cooking demonstrations
	Recipes and handouts

BOX 14-1 School Health Guidelines to Promote Healthful Eating and Physical Activity

Based on the available scientific literature, national nutrition policy documents, and current practice, the CDC provides the following broad recommendations for ensuring a quality nutrition program within a comprehensive school health program:

- *Policy:* Use a coordinated approach to develop, implement, and evaluate healthy eating and physical activity policies and practices.

- *Environment:* Establish school environments that support healthy eating and physical activity.

- *School meals:* Provide a quality school meal program and ensure that students have only appealing, healthy food and beverage choices offered outside of the school meal program.

- *Physical activity:* Implement a comprehensive physical activity program with quality physical education as the cornerstone.

- *Health education:* Implement health education that provides students with the knowledge, attitudes, skills, and experiences needed for healthy eating and physical activity.

- *Comprehensive health services:* Provide students with health, mental health, and social services to address healthy eating, physical activity, and related chronic disease prevention.

- *Family and community involvement:* Partner with families and community members in the development and implementation of healthy eating and physical activity policies, practices, and programs.

- *Employee health:* Provide a school employee wellness program that includes healthy eating and physical activity services for all school staff members.

- *Professional development for staff:* Employ qualified persons, and provide professional development opportunities.

Source: Centers for Disease Control and Prevention. 2011. School health guidelines to promote healthy eating and physical activity. *Morbidity and Mortality Weekly Report* (Recommendations and Reports); 60(5):1–71.

SELECT APPROPRIATE THEORIES AND APPROACHES FOR PROMOTING SOCIAL, POLICY, SYSTEMS, AND ENVIRONMENTAL SUPPORTS FOR ACTION

The social ecological model provides a framework for organizing the many influences on people's eating practices in a way that is useful to provide us with an understanding of the points of leverage and *where* we might intervene. It is not a theory, however. It does not tell us what the determinants are at each level and sector of influence, how the determinants predict behavior change, and *how* to intervene. For that, we have to draw on a number of other theories that address how change might happen at each level and which are particularly suited to which level of intervention. Some of these are described in detail in Chapter 6. For example:

- *Intrapersonal level:* Psychosocial theories such as the health belief model, theory of planned behavior/reasoned action approach, social cognitive theory, self-determination theory, health action process approach, and other self-regulation theories and other appropriate theories

- *Interpersonal/social support level:* Social cognitive theory, and social support and social networks theories

- *Environmental settings for action involving institutions/organizations and communities:* Diffusion of innovation theory within organizations and communities, partnership and collaboration development, community capacity building, and community action approaches

- *Sectors of influence involving policy and systems:* Education and advocacy approaches with decision-makers and policymakers to modify or create policies and systems to be supportive of healthy eating and active living

Some interventions are primarily directed at making changes at a specific level, such as changing school meals to make them more healthful or adding fruit and vegetable carts on the streets in low-income neighborhoods where few stores carry produce. These activities are conducted at the environmental settings level. These will use theories of change that are appropriate for that level of intervention only. Other interventions work to change community level and public policy only. These strategies are described in more detail elsewhere (Green and Kreuter 2005; Glanz, Rimer, and Viswanath 2008).

The DESIGN Procedure focuses on interventions that target specific behavior changes that seem warranted because of a pressing health, food system, or social issue, and that aim to assist people to make these changes. Thus, you may want to make changes at several levels of influence but with the clear understanding that these changes are focused on the primary aim of assisting a given audience to make the behavior changes being targeted by your intervention. For example, the primary behavior change goal may be to assist children to eat more fruits and vegetables. To make this behavior easier, you may want to provide workshops to families on effective parenting practices, work with school food service staff to prepare fruits and vegetables in school meals so that they are attractive to eat, and work with corner stores next to the school to stock more healthful snacks for children to purchase on the way home from school.

Using Theories at Different Levels of Intervention Directed at Targeted Behavior Change

An example of this is the Collaboration for Health, Activity, and Nutrition in Children's Environments (CHANCE) program within the Expanded Food and Nutrition Education Program (EFNEP) in New York State aimed at reducing childhood obesity. The program is described in detail in Chapter 6. In summary, the behavior change goals of the program are for children to eat more fruits and vegetables, to consume fewer sweetened drinks and snacks, and to be less sedentary and more active. To accomplish these goals, the program developed a parent workshop series of eight sessions for parents of children aged 3–11 years, called Healthy Children, Healthy Families: Parents Making a Difference (Lent et al. 2012). It teaches parents and families the food and nutrition information and skills they need to provide healthy foods to their children (*Paths to Success*) and parenting skills that enable parents to help their children eat these foods (*Keys to Success*). The workshop series

uses psychosocial theories for facilitating behavior change and parenting styles theory to encourage appropriate parenting practices.

To make it easier for families to make the recommended food-related behavior changes and parenting practices, CHANCE also includes activities at different levels of influence. At the institutional level, activities include providing training for agency staff who serve children (including day care and Head Start staff) to encourage offering healthy snacks, reducing TV time, increasing active play, and modeling healthy behaviors. At the community level, activities include developing collaborations with other agencies and institutions that serve children to work together to help children adopt these behavioral goals. At the food environment level, activities include working with corner store owners to encourage and support them in stocking healthy choices and displaying them attractively. The parent workshop curriculum is available to other EFNEP programs around the country through a diffusion of innovations approach (https://fnec.cornell.edu/Our_Initiatives/CHANCE.cfm).

Using a Unifying Theory Model for Different Levels of Intervention Directed at Targeted Behavior Change

For the intervention you are designing, the theories to use to guide the development of activities may differ for each of the levels and sectors of influence that you choose to address in order to provide support for the behavior change goals of your intervention. However, there are also ways to provide a unifying theory model for the more focused purpose of intervention as proposed in the DESIGN Procedure. Social cognitive theory in particular can easily be used within a social ecological context to provide a more unified theory.

Social cognitive theory (SCT) states that behavior is the result of personal, behavioral, and environmental factors that influence each other in a dynamic and reciprocal fashion. This is called *reciprocal determinism*. SCT is described in more detail in Chapter 5. In particular, the environmental component can include many of the levels of influence of the social ecological model, such as institutional/organizational factors, community factors, and even policy factors. The theory includes a number of determinants of behavior, and these are described in Table 5-1.

Table 14-2 Use of Social Cognitive Theory as a Unifying Theory for Several Levels of Intervention

Activity	Social Cognitive Theory: Component (and Construct)	Social Ecological Model Level or Sector of Influence
School administrators decide to institute garden in school	Environment: reciprocal determinism	Policy and systems
School administrators decide that each class will experience the garden at least once a month	Environment: reciprocal determinism	Policy and systems
Local foods are provided in the cafeteria	Environment: reciprocal determinism	Environmental setting: institutional
School sponsors a community tasting	Personal: expectancies	Environmental setting: community
Teachers model by eating school lunch including fruit and vegetables	Personal: social modeling, positive reinforcement	Interpersonal level: social support
Farmers visit cafeteria or classroom on a regular basis	Personal: expectancies	Interpersonal level: social support
Taste tests are performed	Personal: expectancies, positive reinforcement	Intrapersonal level
Food is prepared and shared in class	Personal: expectancies, behavioral capability, self-efficacy	Intrapersonal level

Berlin and colleagues have shown that SCT can be used to develop farm-to-school (FTS) programs that involve several of the levels of the social ecological model (Berlin et al. 2013a, 2013b). The behavior change goal is for youth to incorporate more healthful local foods into their diets. The authors note that the SCT determinants can be applied to this behavior change goal with the following objectives:

- *Outcome expectations:* Youth will have beliefs about the positive outcomes or benefits of eating a diet that incorporates healthful, local foods.

- *Outcome expectancies:* Youth will value the outcomes of eating a diet of healthful, local foods.
- *Behavioral capability:* Youth will have the knowledge and skills needed to incorporate healthful, local foods into their diet.
- *Environment:* The environment will provide opportunities to eat healthful, local foods.
- *Self-efficacy:* Youth will have increased confidence in their ability to choose and eat healthful, local foods.
- *Reinforcement:* Responses (by youth or others) to youth's eating healthful, local foods will increase their likelihood of eating them again.
- *Self-regulation or self-direction skills:* Youth will be able to consciously decide to eat healthful, local foods and monitor and adjust how they are doing.

In terms of specific activities, the use of SCT can help to address several levels and sectors of influence. Some examples from Berlin and colleagues (2013b) are shown in **TABLE 14-2**.

Step 4: Indicating Environmental Support Objectives for the Behavior Change Goals of the Program

From the policy, systems, and environmental factors that you identified in Step 2, select those that you will realistically be able to target in the intervention to increase access and opportunities to your audience for the targeted behavior change goals of your program.

WRITING GENERAL ENVIRONMENTAL SUPPORT OBJECTIVES: THE CASE STUDY AS EXAMPLE

First, write *general* environmental support objectives for changes in the interpersonal/social environment and in policy, systems, or the larger environment to increase the opportunities of the intended audience to engage in the intervention's behavior change goal or goals.

The case study described at the end of the chapter involves three components to support the classroom intervention. The general objectives for these components include the following:

- *The school food service* will provide attractive and appealing fruits and vegetables in school meals and other food venues.

- *The school will implement policies* that ensure that the food and activity environment promote health (for example, vending machines and school stores, if present, will carry water and healthy items, rather than sweetened beverages or packaged, highly processed snacks).
- *Parents* will decrease the availability of sweetened drinks and packaged snacks for their children at home and increase the accessibility of fruits and vegetables.

WRITING OBJECTIVES SPECIFIC TO EACH LEVEL OR SECTOR

FIGURE 14-3 shows how nutrition education can be directed at various levels and sectors of influence on diet-related behavior change using the logic model: the individual level; the interpersonal level; the institutional, organizational, and community level; and the social structures, policies, and systems level (Chipman 2014). The objectives at both the individual and interpersonal levels are educational in nature and address personal determinants of behavior change or action, such as beliefs, attitudes, affect, and skills, with outcomes for individuals that can be achieved within a short-, medium-, and long-term time frame. The objectives at the other levels are directed at environmental determinants of behavior change but are also designed to influence your audience members, in this case by making the healthy action be the easier action through changes in policy, systems, and social structures.

For each of these levels of intervention, some objectives can be achieved in the short-term, while others in the medium-term and long-term. As shown in Figure 14-3, at the individual and interpersonal levels, the short-term objective is to enhance motivation and skills, the medium-term objective is to use the enhanced motivation and skills to change behaviors, and the long-term objective is to reduce disease risk, improve health, and improve other food-related outcomes.

For the institution, organization, and community level, the short-term objectives are to develop partners, and with them, identify challenges and opportunities for making environmental changes that will support the intervention's behavior change goals. The medium-term objectives are to write plans for making these changes, and the long-term objectives are for these plans to be implemented and have the intended positive effect.

For the policy, social structures, and systems level, the short-term objectives are to work with policymakers and decision-makers to identify and define issues that need policy actions to support the intervention's behavior change goals. The medium-term objectives are to work together in collaboration to initiate action, and the long-term objectives are to actually revise or adopt policies and social system changes to make the goal's behaviors easier to do.

Writing Objectives for Interpersonal-Level Social Environment Supports

Social support can be an important environmental determinant of individuals' eating patterns. If your program is to be in a worksite, community center, WIC clinic, or outpatient clinic, your objectives for interpersonal, social environment factors may be to create social support groups for those in the program or to create a buddy system to support daily walking for health (where participants select a friend to walk with).

If you are working with school-aged children, parents and family members can influence children's willingness and ability to take recommended action because they are providers of food and serve as role models, consciously or not, through their parenting practices. Hence, a parent/family component can be planned to assist parents to be more supportive of their children's attempts to eat healthfully. Parents or family members are external to the students and thus serve a supporting role. At the same time, they represent a new audience for nutrition education. If you plan on workshops with parents, you will need to design sessions for them, involving general and specific *educational* objectives. Use the process described in Chapters 7–13. Remember that designing newsletters to be sent home with students and other activities with parents will also involve a clear statement of objectives and a clear theoretical base.

As shown in the case study, a parent component has as its own *behavioral goals*: Parents will make a variety of fruits and vegetables available and accessible to their children, decrease their purchases of sweetened drinks and packaged high-calorie snacks, and engage in physical activity with their children. General *educational* objectives of the parent component are then written for each of the parental support behaviors based on selected determinants of the behaviors.

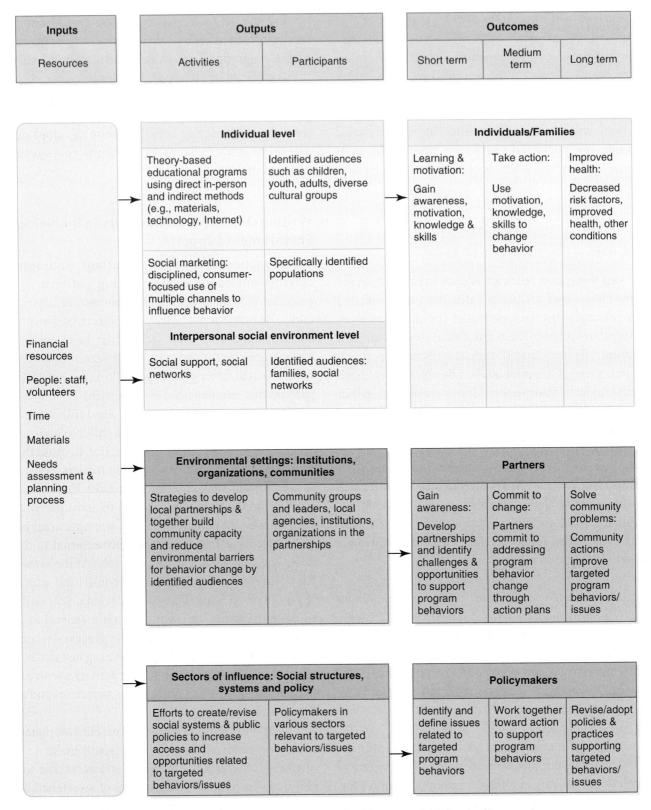

FIGURE 14-3 Community nutrition education logic model framework addressing multiple levels of intervention.

Modified from Community Nutrition Education (CNE) Logic Model Overview, Version 3: 2014. Helen Chipman, National Program Leader, Food and Nutrition Education, NIFA/USDA.

See the case study behavioral goals, general educational objectives, and lesson plan for the parent/family component for one session later in this chapter.

Writing Objectives for Organizational- or Community-Level Environmental and Policy Supports

School Example

To make the school environment more supportive of the behaviors targeted by the program, some long-term support objectives might be the following:

- *Social environment:* School will increase social modeling of healthful eating by valued celebrities.
- *Food environment:* School will provide many opportunities for students to taste fruits and vegetables in the cafeteria and other venues; school stores will replace high-calorie, highly processed packaged snacks with healthier options.
- *Policy:* School will implement policies for not using food for fundraisers or as rewards for student achievement or behavior.
- *Media/information environment:* School will develop and display posters of teens eating healthful foods.

To reach these long-term objectives, short-term objectives will be awareness of the importance of these school-wide actions, and medium-term objectives will be commitment to action. See the Step 4 Indicate Environmental Support Objectives Worksheet in the case study at the end of this chapter for examples of specific objectives for the school environment component.

Community Example

- *Social environment:* Peer educators will be trained to facilitate ongoing social support groups initiated by the program.
- *Food environment:* A farmers' market or mobile market will be initiated in the community neighborhood; the grocery store most frequented by the intended audience will stock more high-quality fresh fruits and vegetables at affordable prices.
- *Policy:* The street outside selected schools will be closed 1 day a week from 4:00 to 6:00 PM so that children and families can play there.
- *Media/information environment:* Program developers will work with collaborators to place posters advertising fruits and vegetables in grocery stores and on billboards.

Step 5: Generating Plans to Increase Interpersonal Social Support

Nutrition educators can promote supportive social environments using strategies suggested by social cognitive theory and social support and social network theories. Within families, social modeling, as delineated by social cognitive theory, can be used to provide support for the behavior change goals of your program. Nutrition educators can use social network theory to strengthen existing social networks to make them more supportive of the food- and nutrition-related behavior change goals of your program, such as involving the family in increasing breastfeeding rates and duration, developing new networks that are supportive of participants' desire to take action, and providing media or informational support as reinforcements and cues to action. These activities can be considered to be interpersonal-level support strategies. See Chapter 6 for more details.

MAKING EXISTING NETWORKS MORE SUPPORTIVE

You can design activities to encourage members of participants' current social networks to be more supportive of the behavioral goals of the programs. These networks might include parent associations in schools, employee associations at workplaces, or groups that meet regularly in communities and organizations. Social support can also involve members connecting with each other using social media. Work with participants to design these activities.

Parental Support and Role Modeling

For programs directed at preschool or school-aged children in school settings, parents are external to the students and are hence part of students' external environment. Work with parents to design these activities.

Educational Sessions

The most general approach is to design sessions with parents so that they can support their children's attempts to eat healthfully through their roles as providers of food and as role models, consciously or not, and through their parenting practices. See Chapter 2 for more details on the role of parenting. In this case, parents represent a new "audience" for whom general and specific educational objectives need to be written and educational activities designed in a process similar to that described earlier.

(See Chapters 7–13.) In our case study with middle school students, the intervention involved a parent component, and the same six steps were used to generate the educational session plans. One such educational plan and one newsletter are shown later in this chapter.

Alternative Channels of Communication

In most communities, parents are very busy, and getting parents to attend nutrition education sessions may not be feasible. You will need to use alternate channels and design alternate educational activities that will fit into their busy schedules, using newsletters and perhaps technologies such as text messaging, email, social media, or websites. Carefully determine the educational objectives of these communications. Are they designed to stimulate awareness and interest? Provide food- and nutrition-related knowledge and skills? Elicit parental support for your program? Or to increase the accessibility at home of the foods targeted by your program?

Home Activities

For programs in elementary schools, it is most effective to develop activities that children can do at home that require parental participation. Families can accumulate points for these activities, for which they can receive incentives and reinforcements. Newsletters with activities, recipes, discount coupons, and information on the benefits of the targeted behaviors can be sent, and calendars with monthly eating tips can be distributed. You can provide taste tests, media displays, and activities at parent–teacher organization meetings and hand out colorful brochures. Again, the educational objectives of these materials should be clear: Is their purpose to motivate, to provide knowledge and skills, or to do both? Which item or activity does which?

Family Support for Adults

In workplaces and outpatient clinics, it may be possible to provide educational activities for families to help them create a home environment that is supportive of participants' attempts to engage in needed or desired actions, such as a type 2 diabetes management diet or eating diets that are lower in saturated fat. Activities that have been found to be effective are written learn-at-home programs distributed to participants at the workplace, family newsletters, and family activities related to program goals that can be incorporated into workplace family holiday parties or picnics. Use of newer technologies, such as email, text

messaging, and social media may be useful in today's busy world. For each of these activities, goals and objectives need to be developed so that the purposes of the activity are clear.

Peer Educators as Social Support

Peer educators have been used in a variety of settings, such as in schools, with low-income families through EFNEP, with older adults, and for breastfeeding promotion. The role of peer educators is not only to teach sessions and serve as models, but also to provide social support. You will need to provide professional development wherein you help peer educators understand the purposes and content of the program. They are a new audience to educate, and hence you will need to determine a set of behavioral goals and educational objectives for their training and develop appropriate theory-based educational strategies.

DEVELOPING NEW SOCIAL NETWORKS THAT ARE SUPPORTIVE OF CHANGE

Social support is incorporated into many health interventions through the development of new social groups, such as weight control groups at work, HIV support groups at a health center, cooking classes, or behavioral

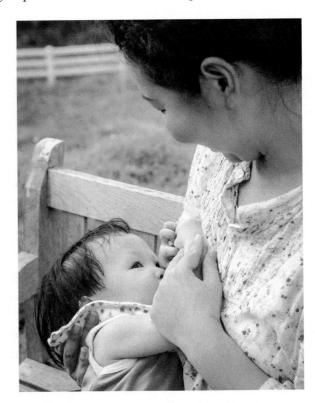

Breastfeeding mothers need peer and social support.
© parinyabinsuk/Shutterstock

change sessions with participants in a program. Programs can also initiate new social networks in which individuals participating in the intervention can help each other (such as forming walking groups, buddy systems, or social network groups).

Support Groups

Nutrition programs frequently create social support by providing regular structured occasions for participants to meet and support each other. Such structured social support was identified in a review of nutrition education as one of the key elements that contributed to effectiveness (Ammerman et al. 2002). Weight loss interventions, such as Weight Watchers, routinely incorporate social support groups. Interventions in schools, workplaces, and communities also have incorporated social support groups.

Social Support Group Sessions

Social support group sessions are not just a matter of getting a group together and talking. Write educational objectives for the sessions that are directed at psychosocial determinants of behavioral goals and design activities for each objective. In other words, develop an educational plan. However, you implement it through facilitated dialogue and mutual support. These are described in detail in Chapter 17. The structure or agenda usually involves the following: individuals share how they did since they last met in terms of successes and challenges (focus on successes); you introduce the focus of the session; group members assist each other from their own wealth of experience; you provide content where necessary and design learning tasks to promote active engagement and maintain support; you provide worksheets, handouts, food tasting, or cooking demonstrations when feasible and appropriate; and time is set aside for the development of action plans or goal setting for the next session. In essence, you follow the 4 E sequence described in chapter 11: excite, explain, expand, and exit. If you will not be the group leader, design a manual for the group leader that includes all of this information.

During the session, your role is to be a facilitator to guide the discussion. The participants are experts on their lives, even though you may be an expert on food and nutrition information. (Even here, participants can be very knowledgeable.) They come with prior experience and expertise. Invite them to share with each other and create dialogue. Build on the strengths of the group members, not their deficits.

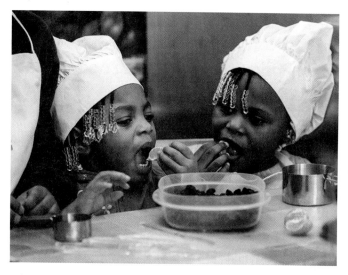

Schools can provide opportunities for children to try new foods.
Tim Reiter. Courtesy of Food Bank For New York City.

Mutual Support

You can also foster social support by encouraging program participants to help each other through such strategies as forming buddy systems or walking clubs; creating an email listserv or social media group to share ideas, experiences, and resources; and going out to eat together and practicing learned behavioral skills.

CREATING INFORMATIONAL SUPPORTS FOR PROGRAM BEHAVIORAL GOALS

Information in public forums can serve as an environmental support by providing cues to action. For example, you can work with collaborators and decision-makers to institute point-of-choice labeling of targeted foods such as fruits and vegetables or lower-fat foods in grocery stores or workplaces, distribute key chains that have program messages printed on them, hang posters on walls, and place flyers or brochures on tables in settings where program participants eat, such as cafeterias.

Information in public spaces can help establish social and community norms that are supportive of the behavioral goals of the program. For example, posters about breastfeeding in pediatricians' offices or posters on eating fruits and vegetables in restaurants, company cafeterias, health centers, and community centers can encourage people to see these behaviors as the social norm. Posters about taking the stairs can be placed in workplaces. Billboards in the community can also help to establish norms and serve as cues to action.

Step 5: Generating Plans for Institutional- and Community-Level Policy, Systems, and Food Environment Activities

The role of nutrition educators is to identify access and opportunities in various environmental settings of your intended audience and to develop partnerships and collaborations so that together you can make the healthy choice the easy choice in these settings. In the short run, you want to gain the awareness of decision-makers and policymakers about the importance of the behavioral goals of your program, and then get their commitment and ultimately, work together to achieve these behavioral goals.

FOOD POLICY, SYSTEMS, AND ENVIRONMENTAL ACTIVITIES IN SCHOOLS

Wellness Policy Council or Nutrition Committee

Legislation in the United States now requires every local school district that participates in the federal school meals program (most schools) to develop and implement a wellness policy. See Chapter 6 for details. It is likely that the school's wellness or nutrition policy is supportive of the behavioral goals of your program.

Although school districts have developed such policies, some plans may not be implemented fully in each school (Story et al. 2009). Policies also need to be evaluated and updated from time to time (Institute of Medicine [IOM] 2007). Nutrition educators can serve as a valuable resource.

If your school district does not have a similar policy, or it is not functioning, you may incorporate the following strategies in assisting schools in implementing, revising, or updating a wellness policy to support healthy eating goals including those of your program.

- *Assessing the school food environment.* An accurate description of current food-related practices and policies provides a framework for discussion and decision making, permits the school in which you are working to devise an appropriate action plan to implement its wellness policy, and provides a means by which to monitor progress. One useful assessment tool is the School Health Index (SHI) from the CDC (http://www.cdc.gov/healthyyouth/shi/). It seeks information on broad policies such as the degree of commitment to

nutrition and physical activity, quality meals, and a pleasant eating experience. It is considered best that the school wellness council or nutrition committee members conduct this assessment. You may help the group develop an assessment tool (or monitoring tool if a policy is already in place) and administer it.

- *Developing a policy implementation plan.* Whether implementing a policy or revising it, the group's task is now to analyze the school's food and nutrition assessment data that have been collected, come up with a shared vision, identify areas needing improvement, and develop action plans. The Institute of Medicine's nutrition standards are helpful here (IOM 2007). Your role as the nutrition educator is to provide technical assistance in the form of relevant research data and to help the group think through issues and make choices.

- *Putting the plan into action.* The team may come up with very creative, manageable, and meaningful activities that are supportive of your program's behavioral goals. For example, in one study, the nutrition advisory council set the policy that instead of using high-fat, high-sugar foods as rewards for students, teachers would use "healthy food" coupons that students could redeem in the school cafeteria for baked chips, fruit, or low-fat desserts. The council also would produce and display posters advertising healthy choices (Kubik, Lytle, and Story 2001). Your role is to provide technical assistance and advice.

Changes in School Meals

All schools are interested in children having access to quality meals that they will eat and a pleasant atmosphere in which to eat them (http://www.schoolnutrition.org). In the United States, strict standards have been set for the kinds of foods to serve in school meals. If you are planning a classroom program and would like the school meals to be more supportive of your program's behavioral goals, plan to meet with the school food service manager to discuss how you might collaborate. Perhaps the school food service staff is already providing the foods you are targeting but needs help with promotion. The Smarter Lunchroom approach (http://smarterlunchrooms.org) may be desirable because it does not change what is served but how it is served. It seeks to increase the convenience, attractiveness, and normative nature of healthy foods. For example, it suggests having menus with attractive color photos of the fruits and vegetables served or having fresh fruit displayed attractively in bowls or baskets. (See Chapter 6 for details.) View the process as a collaboration between persons who have different but complementary knowledge and skills that are needed to enhance healthful student eating.

If the schools in your country rely on outside vendors to provide meals at recess or lunch, the suggestions for worksites may work well. An effective program in Mexico City provides some helpful suggestions for strategies to use (Safdie et al. 2013). It is described in detail in Nutrition Education in Action 6-2 in Chapter 6.

Use of Local Foods in Schools: Farm-to-School Programs

Many schools are introducing salad bars using fresh produce from local farmers' markets or local farms in farm-to-school programs (http://www.farmtoschool.org). These programs are initiated locally. You may want to consider promoting these options if they are relevant to your program. Farm-to-school programs usually also provide experiential learning opportunities by having farmers visit classrooms, sponsoring educational events at farmers' markets, and making field visits to farms. Schools can fulfill their mission to provide wholesome, nutritious foods that children want to eat, and farmers have access to a new market. Information on the many activities in different states can be found at the National Farm to School Network website (http://www.farmtoschool.org) and in **NUTRITION EDUCATION IN ACTION 14-1**.

School Gardens

Schools are increasingly seeing the relevance and importance of having school gardens in which to grow vegetables. Children learn where food comes from and become more interested in nutrition. If gardening is an important supportive activity for your program, you may want to develop coalitions with knowledgeable individuals or groups to initiate and maintain such gardens if you do not have the expertise to do so within your own team. See http://www.edibleschoolyard.org for more information.

POLICY, SYSTEMS, AND FOOD ENVIRONMENT ACTIVITIES IN WORKPLACES

Many of the strategies described for schools also apply to environmental support activities in workplaces. However, changes in the foods served are usually more difficult to implement because food service operations are generally managed by external, for-profit companies, which do not necessarily share the interest of the employer in improved employee health. Changes in policy related to employee health may also require time.

If your program will be conducted in a workplace, you can include the following strategies in your plan for the foods sold:

- *Build collaboration and foster buy-in.* Make presentations, meet with, and educate key workplace managers and food service decision-makers about the importance of your program's goals.
- *Use a phased approach: start with simple changes first.* In terms of foods served, work with the manager to identify a short list of items currently served that meet your criteria for individual foods that support your program's behavioral goals (e.g., fruits and vegetables). Indicate these with signs and your logo. If these are well received and it is clear that these changes do not have a negative financial impact, the food service managers may be ready to make recipe modifications. Here, you can provide technical assistance for making changes.
- *Promote employee advisory committees.* Active participation of workplace employees is vital. Depending on the scope of your program, you may help to form a nutrition advisory committee made up of employees and management that will provide ongoing feedback and suggestions about the kinds of changes they would like in food service and in other areas related to health, such as creating health fairs featuring the behavioral goals of your program, group walks at lunch time, or incentives for active living that may include funds toward membership in a fitness center. Committee members can take over your functions for long-term institutionalization of these changes.

You can also work with collaborators to change workplace culture and policy for catered foods for committee meetings, lunches, and so forth:

- Workplace will provide only tap water (where it is safe) in pitchers flavored with slices of fruit such as oranges, strawberries, cucumbers, or other fruits or vegetables; no sweetened drinks.
- Throw-away utensils will be reduced to the extent possible.
- Baked sweet items will take health into consideration.
- Further changes can be added, as appropriate for the setting.

NUTRITION EDUCATION IN ACTION 14-1 Farm-to-School Programs Connect Schools with Local Farms

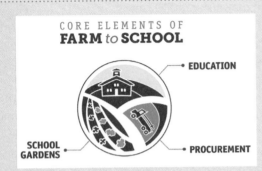

National Farm to School Network.

Farm-to-school programs are programs in which schools buy and feature farm-fresh foods, such as fruits and vegetables, eggs, honey, meat, and beans, in their menus; provide students experiential learning opportunities through class visits to farms, gardening, and recycling programs; and incorporate nutrition education into their activities. Farm-fresh salad bars are often offered as part of the National School Lunch Program, and local foods are often featured in the cafeteria or in fundraising events. Thus, farmers and schools develop partnerships so that local farmers have access to the school market and, at the same time, participate in programs designed to educate children about local farms and agriculture.

Legislation titled "Access to Local Food and School Gardens," which was part of the Child Nutrition and WIC Reauthorization Act of 2004, permits schools to compete for grant funds to help school food service personnel develop procurement relationships with local farmers and equip their kitchen facilities to handle local foods. The program also supports agriculture-based nutrition education, such as school gardens, to teach students where their food comes from. There are farm-to-cafeteria programs in about 39,000 schools in 50 states involving about 21 million students that not only feed children fresh, local food, but get them excited about it.

Results of an evaluation showed positive impacts on many aspects of the school, among them:

- *Student impacts.* Improvements in student knowledge, attitudes, and behavior, such as choosing healthier options in the cafeteria, eating more fruits and vegetables at school and home, modifying daily exercise routines, and increasing social skills and self-esteem
- *Teacher impacts.* Positive changes in their diets and lifestyles
- *Food service operations.* Generally positive impacts on quality of foods offered, increased knowledge and interest of staff, increased participation rates, and higher labor costs, but no clear indication of whether overall costs increased
- *Farmer impacts.* Increased income from schools, diversification of market, and increased collaboratives or cooperatives to supply schools
- *Parent benefits.* Gains in interest and ability to improve family diets and help children make healthier choices as well as improved shopping for healthy and local foods
- *Community benefits.* Increased interest in purchasing local foods and awareness of foods served in school cafeterias

Sources: National Farm to School Network (http://www.farmtoschool.org); Joshi, A., and A. M. Azuma. 2008. *Bearing fruit: Farm to school program evaluation resources and recommendations.* Occidental College, CA: National Farm to School Network, Center for Food and Justice; and UNC Research Summaries. 2011. University of North Carolina and National Farm to School Network (http://www.farmtoschool.org/files/publications_376.pdf).

POLICY, SYSTEMS, AND FOOD ENVIRONMENT ACTIVITIES IN COMMUNITIES

Increasing policy, systems, and food environment supports at the community level for the behavioral targets of your intervention will most likely require collaboration with several to many other groups who have similar goals to those of your program. There are many possible theoretical frameworks for working with communities. Some of these are discussed in Chapter 6. An appropriate theoretical framework for our purposes here is fostering collective efficacy and empowerment.

Collective Efficacy and Community Action Plans

Collective efficacy is the belief of groups and community members that they have the capacity to take collective action to create change in their environment. Collaborations can lead to a sense of collective efficacy. Where you and your partners or collaborators have similar goals, the group can together make community action plans to address specific issues or to achieve specific objectives (somewhat like goal setting for individuals). When the group is successful at bringing about change on one issue, the members feel self-efficacious and become ready to take on other issues.

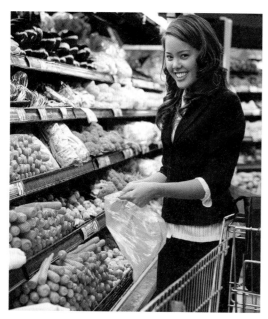

Visually appealing produce displays in grocery stores can sway shoppers.

© Stephen Coburn/Dreamstime.com

In the short run, you and your collaborators want to gain the awareness of decision-makers and policymakers about the importance of the behavioral goals of your programs, then gain their commitment, and ultimately, work together to achieve these goals.

DESIGNING COMMUNITY-LEVEL ACTIVITIES

Active participation of community members in all activities is crucial—from planning to implementing to evaluating. Consequently, as described for institutional activities in schools and workplaces, your first activity is to locate decision-makers in other organizations—whether these are grocery stores or community gardens—discuss your program with them and seek strong collaborations. This collaborative group can decide on strategies. The following strategies can be considered, to the degree they are relevant for your program.

- *Provide point-of-purchase information.* You can collaborate with grocery stores relevant to your program and provide posters, brochures, and shelf labels for foods targeted by your intervention (Story et al. 2008). Shelf labels can enhance awareness of the foods and increase use of the information. Point-of-purchase information can also be used in restaurants and other places where food is served.
- *Provide coupons at stores and farmers' markets.* Your program may issue coupons for program participants to use in selected stores that are redeemable for foods

relevant to your intervention, such as low-fat milk. Your program would need to pay for these. You may also be able to participate in government farmers' market coupon programs for various low-income populations. These have increased low-income shoppers' attendance at farmers' markets and can be used as an environmental support to your program.

- *Work with community food assistance organizations.* Many community organizations are involved in providing food assistance to communities, such as food recovery or food gleaning programs, food banks, and community kitchens or soup kitchens. You may be able to link activities within your educational program to such programs in your community. If your nutrition education sessions or program is being provided through these organizations, then make at least some of the foods available in these settings supportive of your program's behavioral goals. You may wish to develop policies regarding which kinds of foods the organization is willing to accept for redistribution to those in need to ensure that they are wholesome and nutritious. America's Second Harvest (http://www.secondharvest.org) is a national food bank network of more than 200 regional member food banks and food rescue organizations.
- *Link with community-supported agriculture (CSA).* You may be able to link individuals in your educational program to community-supported agriculture. CSA helps to support family farms while providing city dwellers, particularly those in low-income neighborhoods, with access to high-quality, locally grown, affordable produce. During the winter and spring, the CSA farmer sells shares in his or her farm's upcoming harvest to individuals, families, or institutions. The share price goes toward the cost of growing and distributing a season's worth of produce and paying the farmer a living wage. Generally, each week, from June through November, the CSA farmer delivers the week's share to a central neighborhood distribution site—usually a community center or house of worship. Members collect their food at their neighborhood sites. Organizations in your community may be able to link your program participants with local CSA farmers.

An example of the kinds of multilevel activities conducted within a community is provided in **NUTRITION EDUCATION IN ACTION 14-2**. Rock on Café was a grassroots effort community program to achieve sustainable systems changes in school lunch programs through partnerships.

NUTRITION EDUCATION IN ACTION 14-2 Rock on Café

Rock on Café was a grassroots community program to achieve sustainable systems changes in school lunch programs through partnerships. It was part of a larger program called Steps to a Healthier New York and involved four counties and 15 school districts, with the educational cooperative Board of Cooperative Educational Services (BOCES) as the lead organization.

Assessment Information

- The three leading *health issues of concern* for Steps to a Healthier New York were diabetes, obesity, and asthma.
- The *behaviors or practices* that contributed to these conditions were identified as poor nutrition, physical inactivity, and tobacco use.

The Intervention

- The *intervention theoretical model* was the social ecological model, along with social marketing principles.
- The *nutrition education program objectives* were based on theory:
  1. *Individual level:* Educating students, parents, and food service directors (FSDs).
  2. *School level:* Repackaging healthy options, including content, preparation and presentation, and restriction of foods low in nutrition value, occurred at the school level.
  3. *School and community social norms:* Involving school and community role models in the advertisements to be made in order to make healthy food choices the acceptable norm.
  4. *Regional policy to change food environment:* Food procurement, menu planning, and branding.

Evaluation Results

School-level impacts:

- Purchases of fresh fruit and vegetables increased by 14%.
- School meals consistently met the 30% fat guidelines and better.
- School lunch participation went up 3%.

Parent impact:

- Parents that thought the school lunch was a healthy option increased approximately 7% from 38% to 45%.

School food service impact:

- All FSDs rated the program as good to excellent.
- Use of a registered dietitian and consolidated food procurement were rated as most valuable.

Overall impact:

- Team building, organizational learning, community partnerships, and social marketing all contributed to the success and likelihood of long-term sustainability of the changes.
- *The intervention components and processes* were as follows:

Timeline and Major Activity	Intervention Components	Intervention Processes
Year 1: Program planning and team building	■ Regional planning team ■ Regional food procurement initiative ■ Dietitian services contracted	■ Secure support of FSDs, school superintendents ■ Conduct needs assessment ■ Establish short- and long-term goals
Year 2: Creating capacity with initial participation and training	■ Education for FSDs ■ Electronic analysis of school foods served ■ Standardize lunch menus	■ Student surveys and taste testing ■ Creating new recipes ■ Staff development and training
Year 3: Main intervention	■ Social marketing/branding ■ Key stakeholders' involvement ■ Education for children and parents	■ Acquire support of community partners ■ Launch public relations campaign to spread message ■ Social marketing (stickers, posters, aprons, menu boards) ■ Data monitoring

Source: Johnson Y., R. Denniston, M. Morgan, and M. Bordeau. 2009. Steps to a Healthier New York: Achieving sustainable systems changes in school lunch programs. *Health Promotion Practice* 10:100S–108S.

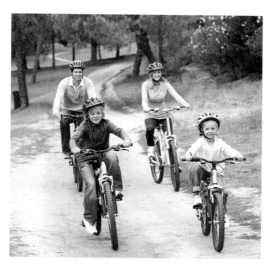

Making biking trails available and accessible increases opportunities for people to be active.

© iStockphoto/Thinkstock

Step 5: Generating a Sequenced Plan for Implementation

We have defined nutrition education as a combination of educational strategies, accompanied by environmental supports, designed to facilitate the voluntary adoption of food choices and other food- and nutrition-related behaviors conducive to health and well-being delivered through multiple venues, involving activities at the individual, institutional, community, and policy levels. The activities that we have described can now be organized and sequenced for implementation in a way that enhances behavior change and action and complements any educational activities that you have planned with the intended audience. Maybe your program has selected several goal behaviors that can be addressed more or less independently, or the behaviors may build on each other and hence need to be sequenced. Just as with individual sessions, it is most effective to start with motivational component activities and then move on to those that build on your initial activities.

CASE STUDY AS EXAMPLE OF SEQUENCED PLAN

Case Study Components

The case study about middle school youth provides an example of a sequenced plan. It is described in detail in Chapter 7 and again at the end of this chapter. *Four behaviors* were selected: increasing intake of fruits and vegetables, increasing physical activity, decreasing daily intake of sugar-sweetened beverages, and decreasing consumption of highly processed, packaged, energy-dense snacks.

The nutrition education team decided that the program would consist of *three components*: a classroom component, a parent component, and changes in the school environment. The intervention is summarized in the logic model diagram within the Step 3 Select Intervention Components and Appropriate Theory case study worksheet at the end of this chapter. The *classroom component* consists of 10 sessions: one introductory and one conclusion and two sessions for each of the four behaviors. The sessions are designed to be somewhat independent of each other, though it was felt that the activities for the session on sweetened beverages were more dramatic and should be taught first. The *parent component* consists of two in-person sessions for parents and two newsletters sent home with the students. The *school environment component* consists of activities directed at decision-makers, the school food environment, social modeling, organizational food policy, and the media or informational environment. See the case study at the end of this chapter for details.

For the *parent component*, the two workshop sessions are planned to focus on parenting practices to encourage increased consumption of fruit and vegetables and decreased consumption of sweetened beverages. The two newsletters focus on decreasing consumption of highly processed, packaged, high-calorie snacks and increasing physical activity.

The educational plan for one session—on fruits and vegetables—and one newsletter—on processed packaged snacks—are shown at the end of the chapter. These were both generated based on using the DESIGN Procedure, this time with the parents as the audience

For the *school environment* component, the team decided to focus on:

- *Interpersonal social support environment*: Increasing the decision-makers' awareness, motivation, and implementation of the intervention's behavior change goals (that are also recommended by the U.S. Dietary Guidelines); social modeling by teachers and celebrities
- *School setting*: Changes in school offerings in the lunchroom and taste testing opportunities
- *Organizational food policy*: Activation of school wellness policy council; guidelines for foods to be used in the classroom and for reward purposes in the classroom
- *Media or information environment*: Posters and signage in school cafeteria and hallways

Table 14-3 Implementation Schedule for the Intervention Components in the Case Study

Activities Before Intervention

- Meet with administrators/decision-makers to inform, motivate, and obtain buy-in and enthusiastic support
- Meet with parent association about parent workshops
- Attend wellness policy council meeting to discuss intervention and how it can help the council in its work
- Provide professional development for teachers teaching the curriculum sessions
- Train food service staff on foods targeted by the intervention

Intervention Component and Activities	Week 1	Week 2	Week 3	Week 4	Week 5
Classroom sessions (two times per week)	X	X	X	X	X
Parent/family workshops		X		X	
Parent/family newsletters			X		X
Celebrity assembly	X				
Wellness policy council meeting	X				X
Wellness activities (cafeteria taste tests, recess fun activity)		X			X
School garden visit by class		X		X	
Information environment: posters and signage	X	X	X	X	X
School meals (ongoing)	X	X	X	X	X
School garden maintenance (ongoing)	X	X	X	X	X

Case Study Sequencing of Components

The sequence of the program components was planned as follows and is also shown in **TABLE 14-3**:

- *School administrators and teachers*: Presentations and discussions to initiate awareness, motivation, and commitment to providing the program in the school, or to obtain "buy-in;" took place before the intervention itself
- *Classroom sessions:* To be two times a week for 5 weeks
- *Social support and modeling*: Celebrity visit: week 1
- *Parent sessions*: During weeks 2 and 4; *parent newsletters* in weeks 3 and 5
- *Media and information environment*: Posters and signage: all 5 weeks plus an additional 5 weeks afterward

You and your team will want to carefully think through and plan the implementation schedule for your program.

Step 6: Nailing Down the Evaluation Plan

The final step in the DESIGN Procedure is to nail down an evaluation plan. After putting so much time and effort into planning and implementing your program, you,

your collaborators, and other stakeholders will want to know how effective it is. The basic principles of evaluation described in Chapter 13 apply here as well.

Figure 14-3, described earlier, provides a framework for evaluating nutrition education that addresses multiple levels and sectors of influence that can be used to evaluate the policy, systems, and environmental support components of your program. Some of the outcomes can be achieved in the short-term, while others may take longer to achieve. These outcomes are based on the objectives you stated for your program in Step 4. Collecting the needed data will usually require the collaboration of various individuals and groups that have decision-making power in that environment, such as school administrators, workplace and institutional managers, community organizations, and food providers.

Tools to measure environmental and policy changes are emerging, such as tools to evaluate the quality of school wellness policies (Schwartz et al. 2009) or quality of foods in stores and restaurants such as the Nutrition Environment Measures Survey (Glanz et al. 2007, http://www.med.upenn.edu/nems/measures.shtml). However, indicators and measures of program effectiveness in terms of changes made in environment and policy are usually very specific to each program. Some examples are shown in the tables below but you will need to develop specific ones for your program.

EVALUATING INTERPERSONAL-LEVEL SOCIAL SUPPORT

TABLE 14-4 describes examples of the possible objectives and tools/instruments/measures that can be used to evaluate the impact of a program on interpersonal-level social support provided by parents to their children and by coworkers and administrators in workplaces. Some

of these measures or instruments are quantitative and others qualitative. The quantitative instruments can be administered before and after the program; changes in scores on these instruments are indicative of the impact of the program on these outcomes.

EVALUATING POLICY, SYSTEMS, AND ENVIRONMENTAL SUPPORTS AT MULTIPLE LEVELS

In schools, the food environment is more controlled than it is in workplaces. The intervention, and hence

Table 14-4 Evaluating Interpersonal-Level Support of Healthful Behaviors: Examples		
Support Strategy	**Objectives to Achieve Outcomes**	**Tools or Instruments for Evaluating Outcomes**
Parents/Households		
Behavior change	Parents/family members will increase availability and accessibility of targeted healthful foods for their children.	■ Parents indicate from a list whether healthful foods targeted by the program are present in the home and offered at meals (e.g., Marsh, Cullen, and Baranowski 2003).
	Parents will develop and implement policies and practices related to child eating behaviors.	■ Parents indicate from a list their policies with respect to children's tasting new foods and choosing how much to eat; questionnaire about parenting practices around feeding: encouragement to eat, setting boundaries, rewarding eating (e.g., Blisset 2011).
Outcome expectations (perceived benefits)	Parents will have increased understanding of the impact of fruits and vegetables on health.	■ Knowledge instrument (written or oral) on role of various nutrients in F&V in health and disease (multiple choice).
Role modeling	Parents/adults in household will serve as role models for their children by increasing consumption of healthy foods targeted by the intervention.	■ Parents report quantity and frequency of personally eating a list of fruits and vegetables (e.g., Reynolds et al. 2002).
Worksites		
Social support	Coworker and/or family will provide support for targeted healthful behavior changes.	■ Individuals complete surveys; for example, on whether coworkers, family, or social support group members never, seldom, sometimes, or often: ■ Compliment their attempt to eat healthfully ■ Bring in healthful foods or fruits or vegetables for them to try ■ Encourage them to eat more healthful foods (Sorensen, Stoddard, and Macario 1998)
Social networks	The number of social support groups and high degree of functioning within groups will increase.	■ Observations of support group functioning and checklists ■ Qualitative interviews of group participants and group facilitators

Table 14-5 Evaluating Institutional-Level Policy, System, and Food Environment Supports: Examples

Strategy	Objectives	Tools or Instruments for Outcomes
Food Environment		
Provision of healthful foods in food service	Food service personnel or food vendors will follow recommended purchasing and preparation methods to provide healthful food supportive of intervention behavior change goals.	■ Interviews and observations using checklists to identify how many, which, and how often recommended practices are carried out (e.g., salad bars) ■ Review of purchase records
	Food quality reflects changes recommended by intervention.	■ Analysis of planned and actual menus (computer nutrient/food composition programs) ■ Observation of food services on-site
Food-related activities in the cafeteria	Workplace food service personnel or vendors will conduct food-related activities in the cafeteria.	■ Checklist completed by staff on number of activities per month ■ Review of quality of foods promoted: checklist or observation
Provision of targeted healthful food items in school or organization stores	Guidelines for organization stores will be developed and implemented; there will be an increased number/proportion of targeted healthful foods in stores.	■ Review of guidelines (process) ■ Count of number and/or proportion of healthful items available in stores
Food from local farms or local processors	School, workplace, or healthcare setting catering will use foods from local sources	■ Count of number and/or proportion of foods from local sources being served in cafeteria meals during appropriate season
School gardens	School will initiate and/or maintain a school garden.	■ Observation or survey: Was a garden initiated? Who maintains it? How is it supported financially? How involved are teachers using the garden?
Information Environment		
Supportive information environment for intervention behavior change goals	Positive and consistent messages about eating targeted healthful foods will be provided throughout the school or organization through informational materials.	■ Number of posters designed and posted; content consistent with program behavior change goals ■ Number of brochures, newsletters distributed ■ Survey of students/employees: number who read materials, degree of satisfaction, what learned
	Posters will promote stair walking in organization.	■ Number of posters displayed through an observed count; impact on number taking the stairs through a systematic procedure of observation, or a survey
Policy Environment or Organizational Climate		
Supportive organizational food policies for intervention behavior change goals	*Schools:* School administrator will commit to activating wellness policy council, with participation of a variety of stakeholders; school food services will develop and implement policies to encourage targeted foods.	■ Review of documents; interviews ■ Review of minutes of meetings; lists of participants; agendas ■ Mission statements; annual reports with a description of policies (existing and newly adopted) that have been implemented (number and degree of implementation)
	Worksites: Worksite policymakers will commit to creating employee advisory board; provide work time for employees to participate.	
Supportive organizational climate	Organizational climate will be supportive of intervention behavior change goals.	■ Survey instrument of participatory strategies, such as how active is board and how many activities conducted are supportive of program behavior change goals (e.g., Linnan et al. 1999; Ribisl and Reischl 1993) ■ *Schools:* Changes in scores on a school health index or score card ■ *Worksites:* Changes in scores on checklist of workplace policies and environment (e.g., Heart Check: Fisher and Golaszewski 2008)

Table 14-6 Community-Level Policy, System, and Food Environment Supports: Examples

Strategy	Objectives	Tools or Instruments for Outcomes
Increase community capacity to support intervention behavior change goals	Develop collaborations or partnerships; enhance commitment to address targeted behavior changes and actions (short-term). Collaboratives or partnerships will work together to initiate and implement specific actions to support intervention behavior change goals.	■ Number of organizations in the coalition or partnership ■ Scales to describe the extent and depth of the partnerships; contributions of each partner, effective functioning (Gregson et al. 2001) ■ Number of meetings held on intervention-targeted behavior change goals and actions (minutes of meetings, documentation); evidence of concrete written plans (short-term impact), evidence of implementation of plans (medium-term impact), evidence of increased community access to targeted healthful foods by audience (long-term impact)
Supportive information environment	There will be increased frequency of media coverage and community events (to enhance social norms for action).	■ Print media: Number of news articles, inches of column space times circulation ■ Electronic media: Minutes/seconds of airtime and monetary value of that time ■ Public relations events: Amount of materials disseminated
Supportive community food environment for intervention's targeted behavior change goals	Local grocery stores will carry and/or highlight foods supportive of intervention's targeted behavior change goals; labels and signage will be in place.	■ Data from grocery store association or organization on how many grocery stores now carry targeted foods ■ Observations at the sites using checklists to evaluate how many targeted healthful foods are highlighted and/or have labels and signage.

the evaluation, can be more formal and systematic. In workplaces, the changes usually involve adding food options to existing menus and making some specific changes rather than implementing systemic changes. It is possible to change media or informational environments and hence social norms, for example, by placing walking prompts in stairwells. The number of people taking the stairs in a given time can provide an estimate of impact. **TABLE 14-5** describes possible objectives and instruments to measure change for institutional environmental supports. **TABLE 14-6** lists possible objectives and measures for community food environment and policy supports.

Criteria of Effectiveness

For each of the measures you choose to evaluate the program, you also need to decide the level of change that you consider necessary to judge effectiveness.

For example, is the criterion of success whether fresh fruits and vegetables are available every day or just some days? Should the criterion be the availability of low-fat options in all worksite cafeteria meals or some? What percentage of increase would be considered success for the use of SNAP electronic benefits transfer cards at community farmers' markets?

Summary

Nutrition education programs can increase social support for the audience and work with partners and collaborators to promote policy, food environment, and community activities that increase support for intervention participants to engage in the nutrition- and food-related behaviors targeted by the program. You can develop programs to encourage family support and the food environments of intervention sites such as schools, Head Start programs, workplaces, community centers, and congregate meal sites for older adults to make healthful foods available and accessible as well as encourage and reinforce the behavior change goals targeted by the intervention you are designing.

Use the DESIGN Procedure to design the social support, policy systems, and environmental components of your program.

In Step 1 you *decide* on the behavior change or action goals of the intervention. This step is common to the design of both the intervention's *individual-level* direct and indirect nutrition education activities and the intervention's *social, policy, systems, and environmental support* components.

In step 2 you *explore* the social support, and policy, systems, and environmental factors that may facilitate the intervention's behavior change goals.

In step 3, you *select* how many and which components you will design and the theory base for each. You also clarify your intervention philosophy and your perspectives on food and nutrition content.

In step 4, you *indicate* the overall general objectives for the program involving several components.

In step 5, you *generate* and sequence plans to address the interpersonal, organizational, and community factors influencing the behavior change goals of your intervention to make them more supportive.

In step 6, you *nail down* an evaluation plan.

With families and others related by social networks, you can use indirect venues such as newsletters with activities, recipes, and information on the benefits of the targeted behaviors or social media, or direct venues such as workshops, facilitated group discussions and social support groups.

In schools, school-wide food-related policies can be developed to address food and beverage availability, vending machine contents, and school store inventory as well as school cafeteria offerings to provide students the opportunity to have easy access to the healthful food choices being promoted by your intervention and to see healthful food practices modeled.

In workplaces, healthful alternatives can be made available in the cafeteria and in vending machines and can be promoted. In communities, access and opportunities to enact the healthful behavior change goals of you intervention can be increased with policy and system change activities.

In all settings, you will work in collaboration or partnership with others and with decision-makers to make healthful choices the easy and normative choices. The active participation through community building of school and neighborhood community members, worksite employees, and leaders must be incorporated into any intervention. Indeed, community empowerment and collective efficacy are high priorities. Adopting these comprehensive approaches enhances the likelihood of improving the effectiveness of your nutrition education intervention.

Case Study: The DESIGN Procedure in Practice

The ongoing case study group is middle school youth. As you recall, for space reasons we address only one of the intervention's behavior change goals: increasing the intake of fruits and vegetables. The case study worksheets at the end of this chapter show how the six-step DESIGN Procedure was used to generate the environmental support plans for the intervention. The support plans encompass several aspects of the environment of the middle school students who are receiving the 10-session curriculum: interpersonal support by parents, teachers, and other school staff; the school food and information environment and food-related policies; and activities in the immediate neighborhood of the school. The intervention is also providing support to the students in the form of a parent/family component that is educational in nature: two workshops and two newsletters. A sample program of activities to address the school environment is shown in the case study at the end of this chapter, and the family component is described on the next page.

Changing the school food environment means working with decision-makers in the school setting to create a healthy food environment for the middle school youth. The case study at the end of the chapter states some potential general environmental and policy support objectives and then describes activities that can be conducted to achieve these objectives, involving social support, changes in school meals, school-wide food policy, and school information environment.

The family component is a special case. It focuses on helping family members learn about the behavioral changes being targeted in the curriculum for their children and building their parenting skills to be more supportive

CASE STUDY　Parent/Family Component: Educational Session Plan on Fruits and Vegetables

Helping your child to love fruits and vegetables

Behavioral goal: Parents/family members will use appropriate parenting practices to support their children eating fruits and vegetables.

General educational objectives:

- Parents will understand and value the importance of eating a variety of fruits and vegetables for their children (perceived benefits).
- Parents will demonstrate skills in making fruits and vegetables easily accessible to their children (behavioral capability).
- Parents will develop appropriate parenting skills that will facilitate their children eating fruits and vegetables (skills).
- Parents will demonstrate commitment to using appropriate parenting skills to facilitate their children eating fruits and vegetables (behavioral intention).

Overview (teaching point): Appropriate parenting practices can help encourage children to eat a variety of fruits and vegetables.

Materials

A variety of fresh whole fruits and vegetables of different colors and attractively displayed (or colorful photos if fresh not available); tip sheets and simple recipes for vegetable dishes; tip sheet for how to use appropriate authoritative parenting practices; action plan sheets

Procedure

Excite

Personalized self-assessment*: List fruits and vegetables eaten (perceived risk**).

Show the array of fruits and vegetables of different colors and ask them how many they have tried, which ones they like, and which ones their children like or do not like. Give them a worksheet with these words on it: breakfast, after school, dinner, and snack. Ask them to indicate in one column how much their child ate of fruits and vegetables on these occasions. Ask them in the next column to guess how much their children should be eating each day. Ask them to compare their child's intake to recommendations for that age (4 cups). Discuss any surprises.

Explain

Information on positive outcomes*: Brainstorm benefits of fruits and vegetables for their children (outcome expectations**).

Brainstorm and list benefits on chart paper. With enthusiasm, explain why they are good for their children (and for them). Or use exciting photos or online video if Internet is available.

Expand

Self-efficacy through facilitated dialogue*: Parents share success stories in getting their children to eat fruits and vegetables (self-efficacy**).

Using a solutions approach, have parents share their success stories in getting their children to eat fruits and vegetables, particularly vegetables. Share feelings. What seems to be common? What principles or tips come from them?

Behavioral capability: Stimulating thinking about appropriate parenting practices.

Discuss what are some appropriate parenting practices for encouraging children to eat fruits and vegetables, such as:

- Show by example—let them see you enjoying eating fruits and vegetables.
- Get creative in the kitchen to make fruits and vegetables that are healthy and appealing.
- Place washed fruit on counter or table ready to eat.
- Cut up vegetables and store in an easily accessible place in the refrigerator so youth can easily see and pick up and eat.
- Offer the same foods for everyone; stop being a short order cook. Set boundaries but offer options within the boundaries and ask child to help with planning meals.
- Reward with attention, not food.
- Eat meals together, and focus on each other at the table. Turn off the television and hold the phone calls. Enjoy conversation and food.
- Offer choices between healthy options such as "Which would you like for dinner, broccoli or cauliflower?" instead of "Would you like broccoli for dinner?"

Facilitated group discussion*: Challenges and ways to overcome them (self-efficacy**).

Have the group discuss challenges they expect when they try these parenting practices and how they would overcome these challenges.

(Continues)

CASE STUDY **Parent/Family Component: Educational Session Plan on Fruits and Vegetables (Continued)**

Exit

Action goal setting*: Planning for specific actions (goal setting**).

Have parents go back to the worksheet they completed at the beginning and review where they could add or encourage their child to eat fruits and vegetables. Parents then select two to three very specific actions they will take and complete an action plan for exactly when, where, and how they will make fruits and vegetables easily available, and what parenting practices they will use to encourage their child to eat them.

* = The behavior change strategy used

** = The determinant addressed by the activity

(See Tables 11-1 and 12-1.)

CASE STUDY **Parent Component: Newsletter on Processed Packaged Snacks**

Taking Control: Eating Well and Being Fit

Family Newsletter | Small-sizing processed, packaged snacks makes a big difference.

Why Care About Your Child's Snack Choices

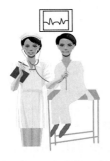

Snacks typically play a big role in the life of middle school students. They have active, busy lives and are often on the run from morning until night. Additionally, if they are growing they may be hungry much of the time. However, the snacks that are typically easily available in our food environment can be putting adolescents' health at risk. More and more adolescents are being diagnosed with conditions such as high levels of bood fat, high levels of blood sugar, and high blood pressure. *(Outcome expectations: Perceived risk)*

Did you know...

- A snack of three chocolate peanut butter cups has over 4 teaspoons of fat. The recommendation is to not exceed 13 teaspoons a day. They also have 8 teaspoons of sugar, and the recommendation is to not exceed 12½ teaspoons a day.

You can see how snacks can easily add on extra fat and sugar in the diet. Having smaller portions of processed packaged snacks can help adolescents do what they want to be able to do today, and keep them healthy into the future. *(Perceived benefits)*

Great Ways to Small-Size Processed, Packaged Snacks and Add Snacks that Pack in the Nutrition Adolescents Need

Look over the tips below and model these practices with your child so that she or he will take on the same behaviors when making snacks choices. *(Social modeling)*

- When given the choice between several sizes of a snack, such as chips or cookies, your child can choose the small size or split with a friend. (We suggest no more than one small snack each day.)

- When buying snacks at a convenience store, your child can try snacks such as granola bars that usually have less sugar and fat than other snacks.

- Help your child to cut up fruit or vegetables in the morning and place in a sealed container. Also have fruits and vegetables easily available at home. This way your child will have snacks with lots of good nutrients that are naturally low in fat and sugar.

- Have your child eat balanced meals so that he or she gets filled up with healthful foods at mealtime and thus will be less likely to be grabbing for snacks.

(Knowledge and skills)

For more information about Taking Control. Eating Well, and Being Fit, stop by the parent room any time!

of these behavior changes. Thus, the family component involves an educational intervention, this time with parents as the audience, with the behavioral change goal for parents being to enhance their parenting behaviors in order to be supportive of their child. The same six-step DESIGN Procedure used to generate the youth educational plans for group sessions was used to generate the parent/family educational plans for group sessions. Because family members are busy, the family component consists of only two group educational sessions—one directed at supporting youth's fruit and vegetable consumption and another at supporting them in reducing intakes of sweetened beverages—and two newsletters—one on packaged, processed, high-calorie snacks and one on physical activity. These can be delivered in person through their child or via email or snail mail, depending on their choice.

For illustrative purposes, the case studies present the educational plan for one group workshop session for family members on how to encourage fruit and vegetable intakes by their child and an example of a newsletter for family members on processed, packaged snacks.

Your Turn: Completing the Six-Step DESIGN Worksheets—A Focus on Social, Policy, Systems, and Environmental Supports

Intervention activities directed at increasing the access and opportunities for taking healthful action through policy, systems, and environmental change can take many different forms. The DESIGN Procedure Workbook provided at the end of this chapter takes you through the six-step process for designing intervention activities that provide interpersonal as well as environmental and policy support to your audience for your intervention behavior change goals. These activities can complement your educational activities with your audience to enhance overall effectiveness.

Questions and Activities

1. The social ecological model describes various levels of influence on dietary behaviors that need to be addressed for behavior change to be effective. Distinguish between the kinds of strategies used at each of these levels. What is the role of nutrition educators at each of these levels? Where and how do you see yourself in these roles?

2. Describe how you might make existing social networks more supportive for (a) children and (b) adults.

3. Describe several key features for designing a social support group for your intended audience so that it will likely be effective.

4. How would you select the appropriate theory to use for an intervention if it has several components at several levels of influence?

5. How might collaborating with other organizations be useful in your work as a nutrition educator? What are some challenges you may experience? How might you overcome these challenges?

6. For an intervention that you plan to conduct that consists of several components, what are some challenges you might face in evaluating impact? How might you overcome these challenges?

7. Discuss some challenges to evaluating an intervention that consists of several components. How might you address these challenges?

References

Ammerman, A. S., C. H. Lindquist, K. N. Lohr, and J. Hersey. 2002. The efficacy of behavioral interventions to modify dietary fat and fruit and vegetable intake: a review of the evidence. *Preventive Medicine* 35(1):25–41.

Berlin L., K. Norris, J. Kolodinsky, and A. Nelson. 2013a. Farm-to-school: Implications for child nutrition. Food System Research Collaborative, Center for Rural Studies, University of Vermont. *Opportunities for Agriculture Working Paper Series* 1:1.

———. 2013b. The role of social cognitive theory in farm-to-school-related activities: implications for child nutrition. *Journal of School Health* 83:589–595.

Blissett, J. 2011. Relationships between parenting style, feeding style and feeding practices and fruit and vegetable consumption in early childhood. *Appetite* 57(3):826–831.

Centers for Disease Control and Prevention (CDC). 2011. School health guidelines to promote healthy eating and physical activity. *Morbidity and Mortality Weekly Report* 60(RR-5):1–71. http://www.cdc.gov/mmwr/pdf/rr/rr6005.pdf Accessed 5/30/15.

Chipman, H. 2014, February. Revision 3 of the CNE Logic Model. Food and Nutrition Education, NIFA/USDA.

Fisher, B. D., and T. Golaszewski. 2008. Heart Check lite: modifications to an established worksite heart health assessment. *American Journal of Health Promotion* 22(3):208–212.

Glanz, K., B. K. Rimer, and K. Viswanath 2008. *Health behavior and health education: Theory, research, and practice.* San Francisco: Jossey-Bass.

Glanz, K., J. F. Sallis, B. F. Saelens, and L. D. Frank. 2007. Nutrition Environment Measures Survey in stores (NEMS-S): Development and evaluation. *American Journal of Preventive Medicine* 32(4):282–289.

Glanz, K., and A. L. Yaroch. 2004. Strategies for increasing fruit and vegetable intake in grocery stores and communities: Policy, pricing, and environmental change. *Preventive Medicine* 39(Suppl. 2):S75–S80.

Green, L. W., and M. M. Kreuter. 2005. *Health promotion planning: An educational and ecological approach.* Fourth ed. Mountain View, CA: Mayfield Publishing.

Gregson, J., S. B. Foerster, R. Orr, et al. 2001. System, environmental, and policy changes: Using the social-ecological model as a framework for evaluating nutrition education and social marketing programs with low-income audiences. *Journal of Nutrition Education* 33:S4–S15.

Institute of Medicine (IOM). 2007. *Nutrition standards for foods in schools: Leading the way towards healthier youth.* Washington, DC: National Academies Press.

Kubik, M. Y., L. A. Lytle, and M. Story. 2001. A practical, theory-based approach to establishing school nutrition advisory councils. *Journal of the American Dietetic Association* 101:223–228.

Lent, M., R. F. Hill, J. S. Dollahite, W. S. Wolfe, and K. L. Dickin. 2012. Healthy Children, Healthy Families: Parents Making a Difference: A curriculum integrating key nutrition, physical activity, and parenting practices to help prevent childhood obesity. *Journal of Nutrition Education and Behavior* 44:90–92.

Linnan, L. A., J. Fava, B. Thompson, K. Emmons, K. Basen-Engquist, C. Probart, et al. 1999. Measuring participatory strategies: instrument development for worksite populations. *Health Education Research* 14(3):371–386.

Marsh, T., K. W. Cullen, and T. Baranowski. 2003. Validation of a fruit, juice, vegetable availability questionnaire. *Journal of the American Dietetic Association* 35:93–97.

McLeroy, K. R., D. Bibeau, A. Steckler, and K. Glanz. 1988. An ecological perspective on health promotion programs. *Health Education Quarterly* 15:351–377.

Reynolds, K. D., A. L. Yaroch, F. A. Franklin, and J. Maloy. 2002. Testing mediating variables in a school-based nutrition intervention program. *Health Psychology* 21:51–60.

Ribisi, K. M., and T. M. Reischl. 1993. Measuring the climate for health at organizations. Development of the worksite health climate scales. *Journal of Occupational Medicine* 35(8):812–824.

Safdie, M., L. Levesque, I. Gonzalez-Casanova, D. Salvo, A. Islas, S. Hernandez-Cordero, A Bonvecchio, J. A. Privera. 2013. Promoting healthful diet and physical activity in the Mexican school system for the prevention of obesity in children. *Salud Publica Mexico* 55(suppl 3):S357–S373.

Schwartz M., A. Lund, H. Grow, E. McDonnell, C. Probart, A. Samuelson, and L. Lytle. 2009. A comprehensive coding system to measure the quality of school wellness policies. *Journal of the American Dietetic Association* 109(7):1256–1262.

Sorensen, G., A. Stoddard, and E. Macario. 1998. Social support and readiness to make dietary changes. *Health Education Behavior* 25:586–598.

Story, M., K. M. Kaphingst, R. Robinson-O'Brien, and K. Glanz. 2008. Creating healthy food and eating environments: Policy and environmental approaches. *Annual Review of Public Health* 29:253–272.

Story, M., M. S. Nanney, and M. B. Schwartz. 2009. Schools and obesity prevention: Creating school environments and policies to promote healthy eating and physical activity. *Milbank Quarterly* 87(1):71–100.

United States Department of Health and Human Services. 2010. *Dietary Guidelines for Americans.* www.health.gov/dietaryguidelines/ Accessed 8/14/14.

World Health Organization (WHO). 1996. *Local Action: Creating Health Promoting Schools* (WHO/NMH/HPS/00.3). Geneva, Switzerland: Author.

World Health Organization (WHO). 2013. What is a health promoting school? http://www.who.int/school_youth_health/gshi/hps/en/ Accessed 6/4/15.

The Nutrition Education DESIGN Procedure
for Environmental Support Activities

Nutrition Education:

Linking Research, Theory, and Practice

Isobel R. Contento

with contributions from
Pamela Koch and Marissa Burgermaster
Teachers College Columbia University

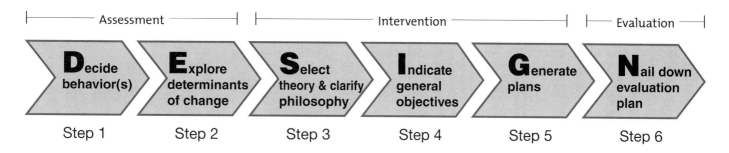

Assessment		Intervention			Evaluation
Decide behavior(s)	**E**xplore determinants of change	**S**elect theory & clarify philosophy	**I**ndicate general objectives	**G**enerate plans	**N**ail down evaluation plan
Step 1	Step 2	Step 3	Step 4	Step 5	Step 6

Nutrition education is a valuable part of improving the health and well-being of people everywhere. The Nutrition Education DESIGN Procedure provides a simple and systematic way to link behavioral theory with your creativity as a nutrition educator to generate educational plans that are engaging, evidence-based, and meaningful in promoting healthful eating.

During the course of six easy steps, you will learn a good deal about your audience and use that information to design group sessions, anywhere from one session to a multi-session intervention. First, you will examine your audience's issues and behaviors of concern and their assets and decide on the behavior change focus of your session(s) or intervention. Next, you will seek out information about how the audience might effectively be motivated to change their behavior as well as what information and skills they need to learn in order to be empowered to do so. Then, you will use the information you have gathered to choose an appropriate behavior change theory to guide your session or intervention design. At this point you will also reflect on your personal perspectives on nutrition education. Next you will indicate the objectives for your session(s) or intervention and generate the educational plans you will use to teach your session(s) or intervention. Finally, you will conclude the procedure by developing a plan for evaluating your session(s) or intervention.

Throughout the procedure you should refer to corresponding chapters in *Nutrition Education: Linking Research, Theory, and Practice*. As you learn about your audience through research literature, websites, and the stakeholders themselves, be sure to cite these information sources as appropriate in the bibliography at the end of the workbook.

Nutrition Education DESIGN Procedure

Decide behavior(s)	**E**xplore determinants of change	**S**elect theory & clarify philosophy	**I**ndicate general objectives	**G**enerate plans	**N**ail down evaluation plan
Step 1	Step 2	Step 3	Step 4	Step 5	Step 6

Step 1: Decide behavior change or action goal(s).

Before you design any nutrition education intervention, whether it is a few sessions or a larger intervention with several components, it is important to learn about your primary audience. From this you will be able to determine the behaviors and issues upon which to focus your intervention. This assessment is conducted in Step 1, and the process is described in detail in Chapter 7.

Use the Decide Behavior Change or Action Goal(s) Worksheet to restate some of the key information from your Step 1 worksheet in Chapter 7.

Who is your audience? E.g., moms, teens, older adults, diabetics, Head Start teachers

7th and 8th graders in a public, urban middle school

What is your behavior change goal?

*Students will increase fruit and vegetable consumption.

Students will decrease sugar sweetened beverage consumption.

Students will decrease fast food consumption.

Students will increase physical activity.

*For the purposes of this workbook case study, only this behavior will be addressed. The entire case study intervention involves all four of these behaviors. An intervention with multiple sessions and/or components may address one or more of the potential behavior changes, depending on the audience and the length of the intervention.

How would adopting this behavior benefit your audience? What issues of concern will be made better if your audience reaches your behavior change goal(s)?

Increasing fruit and vegetable consumption will address childhood obesity, which has implications for chronic disease reduction, including cancers and heart disease. It will also make them healthier in the present by providing the vitamins and minerals they need. Furthermore, if students are taught to purchase local, seasonal produce whenever possible, it will support the sustainability of the food system as well as fair wages for food workers.

Nutrition Education DESIGN Procedure

Decide behavior(s) / **E**xplore determinants of change / **S**elect theory & clarify philosophy / **I**ndicate general objectives / **G**enerate plans / **N**ail down evaluation plan

Step 1   Step 2   Step 3   Step 4   Step 5   Step 6

Step 2: Explore environmental determinants of change.

After you decide the behavior change goal(s) of your intervention, in Step 2 you will find out as much as possible about policy, systems and environmental factors that may support participants to take on the behavior change goals. The social ecological model provides you with the framework to ask the questions and organize the answers.

Use the Explore Environmental Determinants of Change Worksheet as a guide to help you identify and select the support factors that relate to your intervention behavior change or action goal(s).

What can you learn about your audience's sociocultural environment? What can you learn about your audience's social and cultural context by talking with them and visiting the neighborhood?

There are approximately 1,750 students in the school. Based on the last census, the community in which the intervention will be taking place is ethnically diverse. The median household income is $32,000 and the median family income is approximately $40,000. Roughly 20% of the population is below the poverty level. All of the students live with a parent or other adult caregiver. Sixty percent report having input on household groceries. Sixty percent have regular responsibilities at home ranging from chores to taking care of younger siblings. Generally both parents work. The school is well-kept and has good physical education resources. Outside of school, 40% are involved with organized sports, and 50% take part in after school activities associated with the school (e.g., baseball, art club, yearbook). They are not too enthusiastic about the school's food service and in particular they do not like how vegetables are cooked. The school's wellness policy council does not meet regularly and the food store carries many highly processed and packaged high-sugar, high-fat snacks.

What can you learn about the policy, systems and environmental (PSE) assets of your audience? What existing policies, systems and environmental factors support the behavior change goal(s) of your intervention?

The school does have a school garden, and there are some enthusiastic, health-conscious teachers. The administrators are interested in the health of the children but do not have much time to initiate or follow up on health promotion efforts. There is a strong parent–teacher association, and parents have expressed interest in being able to keep their children healthy.

Nutrition Education DESIGN Procedure

Decide behavior(s)	**E**xplore determinants of change	**S**elect theory & clarify philosophy	**I**ndicate general objectives	**G**enerate plans	**N**ail down evaluation plan
Step 1	Step 2	Step 3	Step 4	Step 5	Step 6

What changes need to be made in the audience's environment to support the intervention's behavior change goals?

Find out how your intervention, in collaboration with others, could change the policy, systems, and environmental supporting factors listed below to facilitate your intended audience in performing your behavior change goals. You may use information from the audience itself as well as the research literature and other sources to complete this step.

Interpersonal/Social Support	Type of Support
Parents will be better able to help their children eat better if they can share their experiences with each other.	Social support
Parents are interested in the health of their children and like workshops where they can share information with each other.	Social support
They are very busy but would be willing to attend group meetings if it is not just a lecture and is facilitated by someone who is culturally similar.	Social support, social modeling
Teachers often drink sweetened drinks in the classroom.	Social support, social modeling (negative)

Environmental Setting Support	Type of Support
Fruit is made less expensive than overly processed packaged snacks in worksite cafeteria.	Provision of healthful food service
Fruits and vegetables offered in the school lunch need to be much more appealing for students to eat them.	Provision of healthful food service
Conducting food tastings multiple times in the cafeteria would motivate children to eat better.	Food-related activity in the cafeteria
It would be helpful to have colorful, attractive motivating posters on cafeteria walls and school corridors to encourage eating fruits and vegetables.	Information environment

Policy/System Support	Type of Support
School wellness council needs to be activated to develop healthful food policy.	Organizational food policy
The school's wellness policy council needs to become more active and come up with policy for the kinds of foods that can be sold and used in the classroom.	Organizational food policy
One specific person or committee needs to be in charge of the school garden so it is well kept.	Organizational food policy
Classes are not required to visit the garden, so it is not well integrated with the school curriculum. It is important to link the garden to learning to promote healthful eating.	Organizational food policy

Nutrition Education DESIGN Procedure

Decide behavior(s) — Step 1
Explore determinants of change — Step 2
Select theory & clarify philosophy — Step 3
Indicate general objectives — Step 4
Generate plans — Step 5
Nail down evaluation plan — Step 6

Step 3: Select intervention components and appropriate theory.

In Step 3, you identify the components that will make up your nutrition education intervention. Additionally, you lay out the theoretical and philosophical bases for your intervention.

Use the Select Intervention Components and Appropriate Theory Worksheet to help you select appropriate policy, systems, and environmental components that will support your audience in taking on the behavior change goals and actions of your intervention.

What program components will you include in your program? List and/or diagram the components of your program. For example, in addition to group sessions you might have newsletters and point of purchase information. You may also have activities to change policy, systems, and/or the food and activity environment; these are additional components.

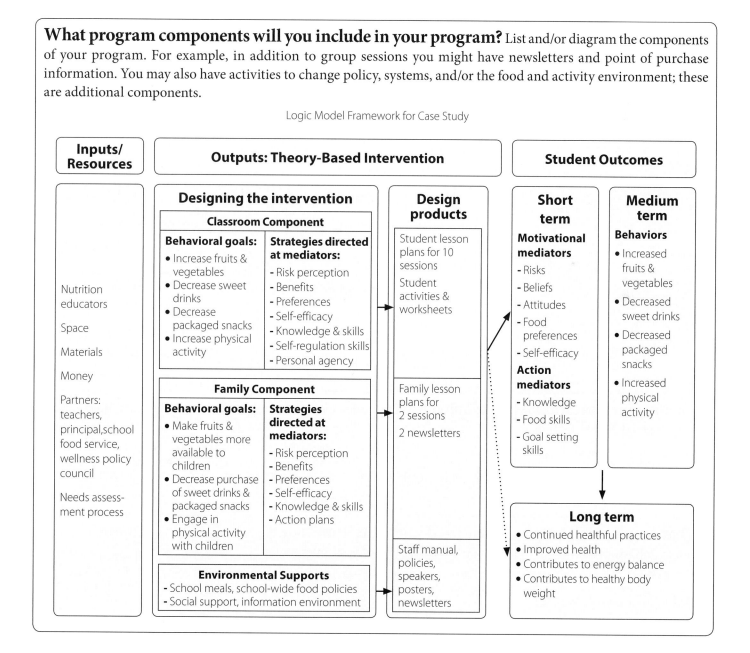

Logic Model Framework for Case Study

Nutrition Education DESIGN Procedure

Decide behavior(s) — Step 1
Explore determinants of change — Step 2
Select theory & clarify philosophy — Step 3
Indicate general objectives — Step 4
Generate plans — Step 5
Nail down evaluation plan — Step 6

What is the conceptual framework for your program? That is, what theory or theories will guide your program? Look back at policy, systems, and environmental supports you identified in Step 2 and indicate whether you will use different theories for each level of the intervention or combine elements from different theories to form an integrated theory-based framework or model.

Social cognitive theory, with policy system and environmental change at several levels of intervention incorporated into the environment component of the theory

How can your framework be represented? Draw a diagram of your model or conceptual framework, if possible, showing the determinants of behavior change you will address and how they relate to one another and your behavior change.

Theoretical Framework for Case Study Environmental Supports

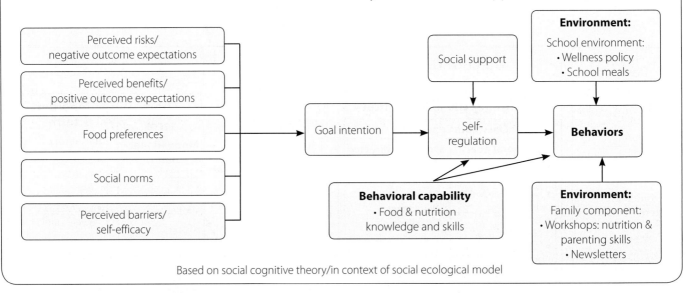

Based on social cognitive theory/in context of social ecological model

What is your educational philosophy? Briefly describe your philosophy of nutrition education interventions as applied to this intervention.

We, as nutrition educators, believe that youth are responsible for their health and have the power to make healthful food and activity choices, but that they need the necessary understanding, motivation, and tools to take charge in today's difficult environment. We also believe that it is the responsibility of the school and home to provide an environment that is supportive and makes healthful options available.

What is your philosophy about food and nutrition? Briefly provide your perspective on nutrition content and issues relevant to the behavior change goal(s) of your intervention.

We believe children should be taught to eat foods that are minimally processed, naturally nutrient dense, and fresh and local to the extent feasible given resource and availability constraints. Also, the issue of weight will not be addressed directly; instead, healthful eating and activity patterns will be emphasized.

Nutrition Education DESIGN
Procedure

| **D**ecide behavior(s) | **E**xplore determinants of change | **S**elect theory & clarify philosophy | **I**ndicate general objectives | **G**enerate plans | **N**ail down evaluation plan |
| Step 1 | Step 2 | Step 3 | Step 4 | Step 5 | Step 6 |

Step 4: Indicate environmental support objectives.

In Step 4, you will write objectives that you need to guide the design of environmental support activities.

Use the Indicate Environmental Support Objectives worksheet to help you develop the overarching objectives for all your environmental support components.

> ## Which of the behavior change goals do these environmental support objectives address?
> Restate your intervention's behavior change goal(s) here.
>
> Students will increase fruit and vegetable consumption.

What general environmental support objectives will guide your support activities? Using the key determinants or strategies from your theory model or conceptual framework, write general objectives for your overarching policy, systems, and environmental support activities for all components directed at your behavior change goal.

Environmental Support Strategy	General Support Objective
Food environment	The school will promote healthy foods throughout the school.
Social support	The school will support the parents in learning about nutrition and parenting styles.
Social support	The school will promote positive role models for eating a healthy diet.
Food environment	The intervention will work with school food service to provide many opportunities for youth to taste fruits and vegetables.
Food environment	School food service will provide more fruits and vegetables in meals, attractively prepared and tasty.
Information environment	The school's postings, newsletters, and other communications will be supportive of eating fruits and vegetables.
Organizational food policy	School administrators will promote and support maintenance of the school wellness council.
Organizational food policy	School administrators will promote and support maintenance of the school garden.
Community food environment	The neighborhood around the school will provide healthier food options for children and families.

Nutrition Education DESIGN Procedure

Decide behavior(s)	Explore determinants of change	Select theory & clarify philosophy	Indicate general objectives	Generate plans	Nail down evaluation plan
Step 1	Step 2	Step 3	Step 4	Step 5	Step 6

Step 5: Generate plan for environmental supports.

These pages of the Step 5 worksheet are devoted to designing the interpersonal as well as policy, systems, and environmental (PSE) support plans for the various environmental/policy components included in your logic model. Generally, these components consist of activities directed at changes in one or more facets of the environment or policy to make them more supportive of your program's behavior change goals.

Use the Step 5 Generate Plan for Environmental Supports Worksheet as a planning tool to outline your support activities. You should have one support plan for each intervention component you stated in Step 3. For example, one for the "school environment" and one for "collaboration with other agencies/organizations" if you plan on these components to be supportive of nutrition education sessions or indirect education activities.

Look over your general support objectives in Step 4. Pick those that apply to a given component and use them as a starting point for more specific objectives and activities for that component. You may not address all the levels indicated for each component. Use only those tables below that are relevant to your intervention.

Which of the behavior change goals do these support educational objectives address? Restate your intervention's behavior change goal(s) here.

Students will increase fruit and vegetable consumption.

What activities will you do to achieve your interpersonal support objectives?

Interpersonal-Level Support Strategy	Specific Support Objective	Activity/Activities
Social support	Teachers will be supportive of children's drinking fewer sweetened beverages.	Teachers will be encouraged to drink water instead of sweetened beverages in class and provide positive reinforcement to children drinking water instead of sweetened beverages.
Social support	Staff will encourage children to eat the fruits and vegetables at lunch.	When food is served, school food service staff will smile and make encouraging remarks to students.
Social support	Parents will offer fruits and vegetables and engage in appropriate parenting practices.	Parent association will negotiate with local EFNEP office to offer hands-on and participatory parent workshops in school.
Social support	Students will have relatable health role models.	Bring in local celebrities for school assembly to talk about why they choose healthy eating patterns.

Nutrition Education DESIGN
Procedure

Decide behavior(s)	Explore determinants of change	Select theory & clarify philosophy	Indicate general objectives	Generate plans	Nail down evaluation plan
Step 1	Step 2	Step 3	Step 4	Step 5	Step 6

What activities will you do to achieve your PSE support objectives? Think about how you might address PSE supports at an institutional and a community level.

Institutional-Level PSE Support Strategy	Specific Support Objective	Activity/Activities
Food environment	Vegetables will be prepared in appealing ways.	Training workshops and handouts with tips for school food service personnel.
Food environment	Youth will taste appropriately prepared vegetables.	Surveys to find out how youth like vegetables to be prepared; work with school food service to conduct taste testings in the cafeteria.
Information environment	Eating fruits and vegetables will become a more normative behavior.	Food service staff, administrators, and teachers install colorful, attractive, motivating posters on cafeteria walls and school corridors.
Organizational food policy	The school wellness council will develop guidelines for in-school foods supportive of increased fruit and vegetable consumption.	Decision-makers will be educated about the importance of healthful eating for learning; technical assistance for developing guidelines.
Organizational food policy	School administrators will promote and support maintenance of the school garden.	Staff appointed and provided time to maintain garden; teacher professional development on integrating garden activities into curriculum.

Community-Level PSE Support Strategy	Specific Support Objective	Activity/Activities
Supportive community food environment	Corner stores near school will offer healthful snacks.	Intervention will work with corner stores to identify healthful alternative snacks for youth before and after school that are feasible and profitable.
Supportive community food environment	Community will eat from the school garden.	Parent association will organize and promote a weekend taste testing of items from the school garden.

Nutrition Education DESIGN Procedure

Decide behavior(s) — Step 1
Explore determinants of change — Step 2
Select theory & clarify philosophy — Step 3
Indicate general objectives — Step 4
Generate plans — Step 5
Nail down evaluation plan — Step 6

Step 6: Nail down evaluation plan.

In Step 6, you use the Nail Down Evaluation Worksheet to plan the evaluation of the environmental support activities for your intervention.

How will you know if you achieved your support objectives? Copy your general support objectives and support strategies and paste them into column 1. Then complete column 2 with the appropriate methods to help you determine if your objectives have been met. Finally, complete column 3 with questions you might ask your audience as part of your evaluation. You may use the research literature to find a validated tool or instrument or you may create your own.

Interpersonal Support Objective (Strategy)	Method	Sample Question(s) to Evaluate Outcome
Intervention will create social network groups for participants. (Social networks)	Interview	How does volunteering together with other parents in the garden influence how you talk with your children about food?
Staff will encourage children to eat the fruits and vegetables at lunch. (Social support)	Cafeteria observation	Did food service workers verbally encourage students to take fruits and vegetables?
Parents will offer fruits and vegetables and engage in appropriate parenting practices. (Social support)	Survey	Yesterday, did you offer your child a vegetable at breakfast? at lunch? at dinner?

Institutional PSE Support Objective (Strategy)	Method	Sample Question(s) to Evaluate Outcome
Food service managers will follow recommended purchasing and preparation methods to provide healthful foods. (Food environment)	Content analysis	What proportion of ingredients purchased this month were fruits and vegetables?
Vegetables will be prepared in appealing ways. (School food environment)	Cafeteria observation	Was vegetable dish visually appealing? Was vegetable dish palatable?
The school wellness council will develop guidelines for in-school foods supportive of increased fruit and vegetable consumption. (School food policy)	Content analysis	Review in-school food guidelines.

Nutrition Education DESIGN
Procedure

Decide behavior(s)	**E**xplore determinants of change	**S**elect theory & clarify philosophy	**I**ndicate general objectives	**G**enerate plans	**N**ail down evaluation plan
Step 1	Step 2	Step 3	Step 4	Step 5	Step 6

How will you know if you achieved your support objectives? (continued)

Community PSE Support Objective (Strategy)	Method	Sample Question(s) to Evaluate Outcome
Establish partnerships with stakeholders in the neighborhood.	Interview with Principal	What neighborhood groups does your school partner with?
Corner stores near school will offer healthful snacks. (Community food environment)	Observational checklist	How many fruit or vegetable offerings are available?
Commuity will eat from the school garden. (Community food environment)	Photographs	Photographs from community events at school garden.

Possible Methods
Survey, Interview, Focus group, Participation/attendance records, Observations, Content analysis of relevant documents

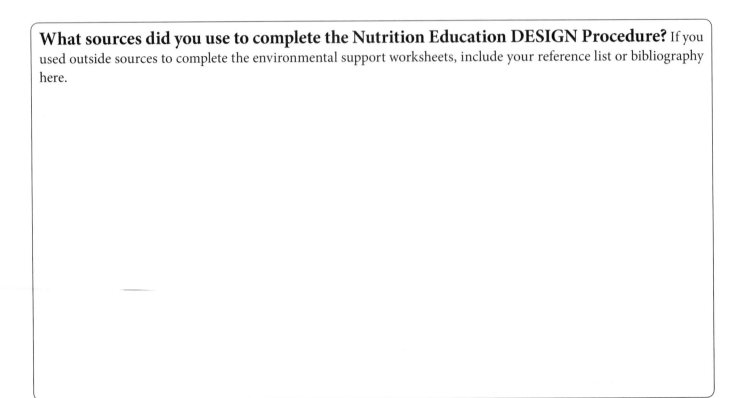

What sources did you use to complete the Nutrition Education DESIGN Procedure? If you used outside sources to complete the environmental support worksheets, include your reference list or bibliography here.

Congratulations!

You've completed the Nutrition Education DESIGN Procedure for Environmental Support Activities.

Good luck teaching and evaluating your sessions!

The Nutrition Education DESIGN Procedure
for Environmental Support Activities

Nutrition Education:

Linking Research, Theory, and Practice

Isobel R. Contento

with contributions from
Pamela Koch and Marissa Burgermaster
Teachers College Columbia University

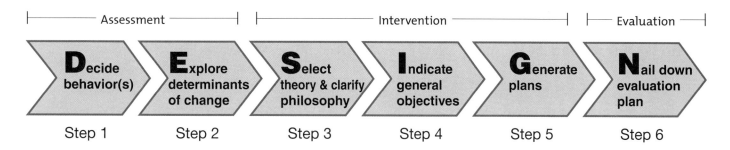

Nutrition education is a valuable part of improving the health and well-being of people everywhere. The Nutrition Education DESIGN Procedure provides a simple and systematic way to link theory and evidence with your creativity as a nutrition educator to generate effective plans for conducting your intervention or program. These plans can be for educational sessions to achieve the behavioral goals of your program or for environmental activities that are supportive of these behavioral goals. In this workbook you will generate plans for providing environmental support activities for the behavioral goals of your intervention or program. In general you will work with collaborators to conduct these activities.

During the course of six easy steps, you will learn a good deal about your audience and use that information to generate your plans. First, you will examine your audience's issues and behaviors of concern and their assets and decide on the behavior change focus of your intervention. Next, you will seek out information about the changes that need to be made in the audience's environment to support these behavior change goals. Then, you will select how many and which components you will use and the appropriate theory or framework to guide your intervention. At this point you will also reflect on your personal perspectives related to education and nutrition content. Next you will indicate the general support objectives for your intervention, and then generate the environmental support plans directed at interpersonal, institutional and community levels of support. Finally, you will conclude the procedure by developing a plan for evaluating your intervention.

Throughout the procedure you should refer to Chapter 14 in *Nutrition Education: Linking Research, Theory, and Practice*. As you learn about the environmental factors influencing your audience through research literature, websites, and stakeholders themselves, be sure to cite these information sources as appropriate in the bibliography at the end of this the workbook.

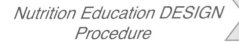 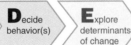
Step 1: Decide behavior change or action goal(s).

Before you design any nutrition education intervention, whether it is a few sessions or a larger intervention with several components, it is important to learn about your primary audience. From this you will be able to determine the behaviors and issues upon which to focus your intervention. This assessment is conducted in Step 1, and the process is described in detail in Chapter 7.

Use the Decide Behavior Change or Action Goal(s) Worksheet to restate some of the key information from your Step 1 worksheet in Chapter 7.

Who is your audience? E.g., moms, teens, older adults, diabetics, Head Start teachers

What is your behavior change goal?

How would adopting this behavior benefit your audience? What issues of concern will be made better if your audience reaches your behavior change goal(s)?

Nutrition Education DESIGN Procedure

Decide behavior(s)	**E**xplore determinants of change	**S**elect theory & clarify philosophy	**I**ndicate general objectives	**G**enerate plans	**N**ail down evaluation plan
Step 1	Step 2	Step 3	Step 4	Step 5	Step 6

Step 2: Explore environmental determinants of change.

After you decide the behavior change goal(s) of your intervention, in Step 2 you will find out as much as possible about policy, systems and environmental factors that may support participants to take on the behavior change goals. The social ecological model provides you with the framework to ask the questions and organize the answers.

Use the Explore Environmental Determinants of Change Worksheet as a guide to help you identify and select the support factors that relate to your intervention behavior change or action goal(s).

What can you learn about your audience's sociocultural environment? What can you learn about your audience's social and cultural context by talking with them and visiting the neighborhood?

What can you learn about the policy, systems and environmental (PSE) assets of your audience? What existing policies, systems and environmental factors support the behavior change goal(s) of your intervention?

Nutrition Education DESIGN Procedure

Decide behavior(s)	**E**xplore determinants of change	**S**elect theory & clarify philosophy	**I**ndicate general objectives	**G**enerate plans	**N**ail down evaluation plan
Step 1	Step 2	Step 3	Step 4	Step 5	Step 6

What changes need to be made in the audience's environment to support the intervention's behavior change goals? Find out how your intervention, in collaboration with others, could change the policy, systems, and environmental supporting factors listed below to facilitate your intended audience in performing your behavior change goals. You may use information from the audience itself as well as the research literature and other sources to complete this step.

Interpersonal/Social Support	Type of Support
Parents will be better able to help their children eat better if they can share their experiences with each other.	Social support

Environmental Setting Support	Type of Support
Fruit is made less expensive than overly processed packaged snacks in worksite cafeteria.	Provision of healthful food service

Policy/System Support	Type of Support
School wellness council needs to be activated to develop healthful food policy.	Organizational food policy

Nutrition Education DESIGN Procedure

Decide behavior(s) — Step 1

Explore determinants of change — Step 2

Select theory & clarify philosophy — Step 3

Indicate general objectives — Step 4

Generate plans — Step 5

Nail down evaluation plan — Step 6

Step 3: Select intervention components and appropriate theory.

In Step 3, you identify the components that will make up your nutrition education intervention. Additionally, you lay out the theoretical and philosophical bases for your intervention.

Use the Select Intervention Components and Appropriate Theory Worksheet to help you select appropriate policy, systems, and environmental components that will support your audience in taking on the behavior change goals and actions of your intervention.

What program components will you include in your program? List and/or diagram the components of your program. For example, in addition to group sessions you might have newsletters and point of purchase information. You may also have activities to change policy, systems, and/or the food and activity environment; these are additional components.

Nutrition Education DESIGN
Procedure

Decide behavior(s) | **E**xplore determinants of change | **S**elect theory & clarify philosophy | **I**ndicate general objectives | **G**enerate plans | **N**ail down evaluation plan

Step 1 | Step 2 | Step 3 | Step 4 | Step 5 | Step 6

What is the conceptual framework for your program? That is, what theory or theories will guide your program? Look back at policy, systems, and environmental supports you identified in Step 2 and indicate whether you will use different theories for each level of the intervention or combine elements from different theories to form an integrated theory-based framework or model.

How can your framework be represented? Draw a diagram of your model or conceptual framework, if possible, showing the determinants of behavior change you will address and how they relate to one another and your behavior change.

What is your educational philosophy? Briefly describe your philosophy of nutrition education interventions as applied to this intervention.

What is your philosophy about food and nutrition? Briefly provide your perspective on nutrition content and issues relevant to the behavior change goal(s) of your intervention.

Nutrition Education DESIGN Procedure

Decide behavior(s)	**E**xplore determinants of change	**S**elect theory & clarify philosophy	**I**ndicate general objectives	**G**enerate plans	**N**ail down evaluation plan
Step 1	Step 2	Step 3	Step 4	Step 5	Step 6

Step 4: Indicate environmental support objectives.

In Step 4, you will write objectives that you need to guide the design of environmental support activities.

Use the Indicate Environmental Support Objectives worksheet to help you develop the overarching objectives for all your environmental support components.

Which of the behavior change goals do these environmental support objectives address?
Restate your intervention's behavior change goal(s) here.

What general environmental support objectives will guide your support activities? Using the key determinants or strategies from your theory model or conceptual framework, write general objectives for your overarching policy, systems, and environmental support activities for all components directed at your behavior change goal.

Environmental Support Strategy	General Support Objective
Food environment	The school will promote healthy foods throughout the school.

Nutrition Education DESIGN Procedure

Decide behavior(s) — Step 1
Explore determinants of change — Step 2
Select theory & clarify philosophy — Step 3
Indicate general objectives — Step 4
Generate plans — Step 5
Nail down evaluation plan — Step 6

Step 5: Generate plan for environmental supports.

These pages of the Step 5 worksheet are devoted to designing the interpersonal as well as policy, systems, and environmental (PSE) support plans for the various environmental/policy components included in your logic model. Generally, these components consist of activities directed at changes in one or more facets of the environment or policy to make them more supportive of your program's behavior change goals.

Use the Step 5 Generate Plan for Environmental Supports Worksheet as a planning tool to outline your support activities. You should have one support plan for each intervention component you stated in Step 3. For example, one for the "school environment" and one for "collaboration with other agencies/organizations" if you plan on these components to be supportive of nutrition education sessions or indirect education activities.

Look over your general support objectives in Step 4. Pick those that apply to a given component and use them as a starting point for more specific objectives and activities for that component. You may not address all the levels indicated for each component. Use only those tables below that are relevant to your intervention.

> **Which of the behavior change goals do these support educational objectives address?** Restate your intervention's behavior change goal(s) here.

> **What activities will you do to achieve your interpersonal support objectives?**

Interpersonal-Level Support Strategy	Specific Support Objective	Activity/Activities

Nutrition Education DESIGN Procedure

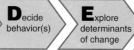

D ecide behavior(s)	E xplore determinants of change	S elect theory & clarify philosophy	I ndicate general objectives	G enerate plans	N ail down evaluation plan
Step 1	Step 2	Step 3	Step 4	Step 5	Step 6

What activities will you do to achieve your PSE support objectives? Think about how you might address PSE supports at an institutional and a community level.

Institutional-Level PSE Support Strategy	Specific Support Objective	Activity/Activities

Community-Level PSE Support Strategy	Specific Support Objective	Activity/Activities

Nutrition Education DESIGN Procedure

Step 1	Step 2	Step 3	Step 4	Step 5	Step 6
Decide behavior(s)	**E**xplore determinants of change	**S**elect theory & clarify philosophy	**I**ndicate general objectives	**G**enerate plans	**N**ail down evaluation plan

Step 6: Nail down evaluation plan.

In Step 6, you use the Nail Down Evaluation Worksheet to plan the evaluation of the environmental support activities for your intervention.

How will you know if you achieved your support objectives? Copy your general support objectives and support strategies and paste them into column 1. Then complete column 2 with the appropriate methods to help you determine if your objectives have been met. Finally, complete column 3 with questions you might ask your audience as part of your evaluation. You may use the research literature to find a validated tool or instrument or you may create your own.

Interpersonal Support Objective (Strategy)	Method	Sample Question(s) to Evaluate Outcome
Intervention will create social network groups for participants. (Social networks)	Interview	How does volunteering together with other parents in the garden influence how you talk with your children about food?

Institutional PSE Support Objective (Strategy)	Method	Sample Question(s) to Evaluate Outcome
Food service managers will follow recommended purchasing and preparation methods to provide healthful foods. (Food environment)	Content analysis	What proportion of ingredients purchased this month were fruits and vegetables?

Nutrition Education DESIGN Procedure

Decide behavior(s)	Explore determinants of change	Select theory & clarify philosophy	Indicate general objectives	Generate plans	Nail down evaluation plan
Step 1	Step 2	Step 3	Step 4	Step 5	Step 6

How will you know if you achieved your support objectives? (continued)

Community PSE Support Objective (Strategy)	Method	Sample Question(s) to Evaluate Outcome
Establish partnerships with stakeholders in the neighborhood.	Interview with Principal	What neighborhood groups does your school partner with?

Possible Methods
Survey, Interview, Focus group, Participation/attendance records, Observations, Content analysis of relevant documents

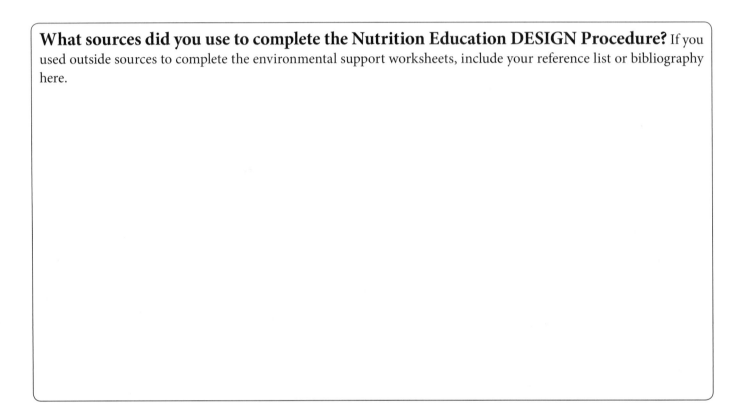

Nutrition Education DESIGN Procedure

Decide behavior(s) — Step 1
Explore determinants of change — Step 2
Select theory & clarify philosophy — Step 3
Indicate general objectives — Step 4
Generate plans — Step 5
Nail down evaluation plan — Step 6

What sources did you use to complete the Nutrition Education DESIGN Procedure? If you used outside sources to complete the environmental support worksheets, include your reference list or bibliography here.

Congratulations!

You've completed the Nutrition Education DESIGN Procedure for Environmental Supports.

Good luck presenting and evaluating your support activites!

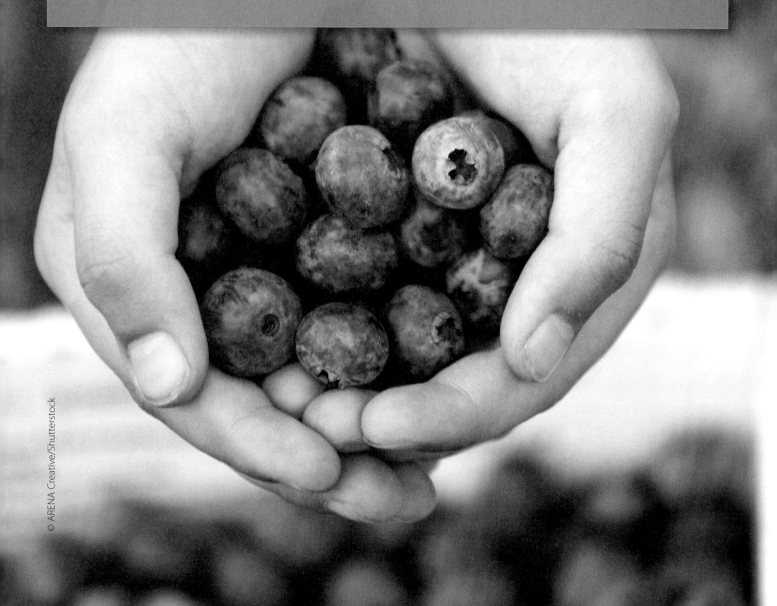

PART III

Research and Theory in Action: Delivering Nutrition Education in Practice

CHAPTER 15

Delivering Nutrition Education Effectively in Group Settings

OVERVIEW

This chapter begins a new section of the book on the nuts and bolts of how to deliver nutrition education effectively for a variety of audiences through direct education in group settings and indirect education using a variety of other channels such as social marketing, visual or written materials, or Internet activities. This chapter provides an overview of communication principles that are important for delivering nutrition education effectively and then focuses on practical methods for working successfully with groups based on understanding audience learning styles and appropriate instructional methods. Chapter 16 focuses on implementing nutrition education through a variety of other channels that might accompany group sessions as well as social marketing and Chapter 17 focuses on working with diverse age, cultural, and literacy population groups.

CHAPTER OUTLINE

- Delivering nutrition education effectively: the nuts and bolts
- Communicating with your audience: basic principles
- Understanding and applying learning theory: learning approaches and learning styles
- Understanding and applying instructional design theory
- Creating environments for learning
- Methods of instruction/teaching: practical ways to activate learning and enhance behavior change
- Conducting the group sessions: from sequencing instruction to nuts and bolts of delivery
- Summary

LEARNING OBJECTIVES

At the end of the chapter, you should be able to:

- Describe basic principles of communication for nutrition education
- Apply learning theory and learning style research in delivering nutrition education
- Use information on group dynamics to more effectively deliver nutrition education
- Describe key features in conducting facilitated group discussions and dialogues
- Link educational plans to effective delivery in group sessions.

Delivering Nutrition Education Effectively: The Nuts and Bolts

This section of the book builds on the information in previous chapters. Part I of the book examines the evidence base for effective nutrition education, concluding that it is most likely to be successful when it focuses on behavior change within the context of cultural eating patterns, family practices, and social networks, uses theory as a tool to enhance motivation and facilitate the ability to change behavior or to take action, and increases opportunities for action. Part II of the book takes you through a step-by-step DESIGN Procedure to plan your nutrition education sessions and to increase policy, system, and environmental support for the behavioral goals of your intervention.

Now that you have designed the nutrition education intervention, including its behavioral goals, educational objectives, theory-based education strategies and activities; have laid out your evaluation plan; and are ready to conduct the nutrition education, how exactly do you proceed when you meet with your group or when you lay out your educational materials? Part III is designed to answer that question. It describes exactly how to deliver the intervention in practice through a variety of channels such as group sessions, printed materials, and other media in a way that is motivating and useful. Conducting group activities and developing other supportive activities require numerous skills—even after the intervention content and activities have been carefully planned. Wonderfully designed nutrition education sessions can be ruined by poor delivery. This does not mean that wonderful delivery will turn a poorly designed session into an effective one, but it does mean that *how* you actually deliver the sessions is extremely important.

This chapter focuses on working with groups. The next chapter focuses on implementing nutrition education through a variety of other channels that might accompany group sessions, such as supporting visual media, written materials, grocery tours, health fairs, Internet activities, social marketing, and other venues.

Although the design and delivery of nutrition education are described in different sections of the book, you will want to go back and forth between sections. For example, as you think about how exactly you will conduct the sessions or deliver what you have designed, you may find that you need to go back to Step 5 of the DESIGN Procedure to make changes in your educational plans to make them more in line with your delivery methods. Because all interactions among people involve communication, communication is at the heart of nutrition education. This chapter thus begins with a brief description of communication and its importance.

Communicating with Your Audience: Basic Principles

How much time do you spend each day talking or communicating with other people? If you are like other adults, you spend about 70% of your waking hours talking with or communicating with others. With the rapid rise in popularity of email and social media, such communication is often mediated as opposed to face-to-face. It is estimated that, on average, teens spend 3–7 hours per day communicating through social media such as texting, tweeting, Facebook, and so forth. These are all forms of communicating. Communication consists of very complicated processes; this chapter has space to describe only briefly its chief features.

As nutrition educators, we are constantly communicating, verbally or nonverbally, whether we are aware of it or not. The moment we meet with our audience, we have started to communicate. These communications greatly influence whether our delivery of nutrition education is successful or not.

Communication is one of those terms we use frequently and yet might have a hard time defining. The word comes from the Latin *communis*, meaning "common." In general it refers to all methods of conveying thought and feeling between individuals. Most definitions have in common the notions that communication is the process of sending and receiving messages and that for a transmission of messages to be successful, a mutual understanding between the communicator and the recipient must occur. Communication refers to what is expressed verbally or nonverbally; it applies to articulated words and to unvocalized feelings. In a broad sense, then, communication includes all methods that can convey thought or feelings and describes interactions between individuals and groups as well as between various media and people.

The term *interpersonal communication* is often used to describe the communication context that involves direct, face-to-face interaction among people, whether one-on-one or in small groups. The term *mediated communication* is often used to describe the communication that occurs

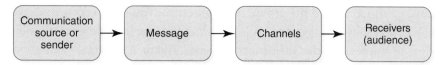

FIGURE 15-1 Basic communication model.

through some nonpersonal channel such as television or radio, printed materials, telephone, advertising, emails, internet, or social media.

We begin with a model that captures the basic elements of communication, and then expand on this model for the nutrition education context. This model states that communication involves the following components arranged in the following sequence, as shown in **FIGURE 15-1**:

- Communication source, or sender
- Message (sent through one or more channels)
- Channels
- Receivers (audience)

In the case of nutrition education, the *communication source* or *sender* is the nutrition educator, who sends a message (which can be as simple as "Eat more fruits and vegetables" or much more complex, such as how to help parents get their children to eat healthfully) through *channels* such as lecturing, making a presentation, leading a group discussion, newsletters, interactive media, email, internet, or mass media campaigns to *receivers*, who are the audience for whom you are planning your educational sessions: groups of low-income mothers of young children, seniors in a government-sponsored congregate meal program, outpatients at a diabetes clinic, college athletes, those living with HIV/AIDS at a community center, or teens in an after-school program. These individuals attend to the message in your session, comprehend it, process it cognitively and affectively, and act on it by either accepting it or rejecting it. "Message" in this context refers to food or nutrition content, which can consist of simple messages about the behavioral change goals of your intervention (Eat Your Colors) or more complex messages about a food or nutrition issue, stated in a specific and simple way in order to be understandable by your audience.

This basic model is clearly unidirectional, with a message being sent by a source to receivers, who receive the message somewhat passively. This model applies well to presentations and lectures, where there is very little interaction among group members. However, it does not

capture the richness and complexities of interactions among individuals in groups that influence message processing. In group discussion, all individuals take turns being the sender and the receiver through the channel of speaking. After exploring the basic components of this model, the chapter then describes how the communication process is modified by complex interactions in social settings, where much of deliberate nutrition education occurs.

COMMUNICATION SOURCE CHARACTERISTICS

In nutrition education, you are the sender or source of the communication, as we have noted. From the outset, recognize that just as individuals cannot not behave, so, too, in any situation involving social interaction, individuals cannot not communicate. This means that you, as the nutrition educator, are communicating at all times, regardless of whether you are conscious of it or whether the communication is intentional or successful, from the moment the group sets eyes on you until the time you leave. Communication of the message is more likely to be effective if nutrition educators have the following characteristics.

High Credibility

Nutrition educators are more likely to have high credibility if the audience perceives them as being competent and trustworthy. *Competence* refers to having the skill, knowledge, and judgment relevant to the issue. *Credibility* can be extrinsic, which refers to the audience's perception of the source before the message is delivered (e.g., by virtue of the nutrition educator's position or reputation), or intrinsic, which refers to the image of authoritativeness that you create as a direct result of how you deliver your session.

To increase credibility, then, when you introduce yourself or are introduced you need to let the audience know your professional qualifications and experience so that they recognize your *competence*. This needs to be done with sensitivity: you should not be boastful or self-serving, but you should not be overly modest either. The audience needs to know that you are qualified to lead the group. It will help them relax and feel that they are in good hands. How you come across during the session also influences your credibility and trustworthiness. For instance, if your tone is authoritative and you are organized, the audience will be much more convinced than if you sound tentative and are disorganized.

Trustworthiness refers to nutrition educators coming across as having no ulterior motives for the opinions they offer or the actions they advocate. That is, they have "good motives." To ensure an audience's trust, you need to make clear to audience members that you are not using the occasion to sell something to them. If you do represent your own business or practice or a given group, corporation, or industry, you need to indicate this clearly to the audience up front.

Dynamism and Passion

One of the keys to success in delivering nutrition education is to be passionate and enthusiastic. Communication sources or senders of messages are more effective when they are likable or attractive in the sense of having an attractive and dynamic personality and being seen as healthy. This is especially true when the audience is not initially motivated. Show your passion for the issue you are talking about! Express friendliness and warmth. Make your enthusiasm contagious.

Common Ground and Understanding of the Audience

Effectiveness is enhanced if the audience perceives that the nutrition educator has some common ground with the audience or at least a sense of affinity with them. Communication specialists point out that because emotion always influences decisions, the audience must sense that the communicator understands their problems and cares. Empathy, or affinity with the audience, is called for, not sympathy, which can be patronizing. Audiences need to feel that they are respected.

Thus, you are more effective if you establish some common ground by initially expressing some views that are also held by the audience and by demonstrating understanding of the opinions and lives of group members. For example, while teaching the skill of reading food labels, you may want to acknowledge how confusing and time-consuming reading food labels can be (a personal story can be very powerful here). Then, go on to provide the necessary label-reading skills. In discussing parenting

practices, you can express understanding and respect for what the (parent) audience members face on a day-to-day basis. Again, a personal story about your own children or children you have worked with can be very helpful. It is important to be authentic, however. Using the latest hip language with a group of teenagers, for example, when it is obvious that this is not congruous with who you are and how you would normally speak, will only make the teenagers think you are phony.

Cultural Competence

When you work with diverse cultural groups, you are more effective when you are knowledgeable about their culture; demonstrate awareness, respect, and acceptance of the group's cultural beliefs and practices; and are comfortable with and able to work within the values, traditions, eating patterns, and customs of the participants' community.

> Your passion for the issues and behavior change goals of the intervention, your dynamism as you deliver the message, genuine positive regard and respect for your audience, and cultural sensitivity are all crucial ingredients for the success of nutrition education.

MESSAGE CHARACTERISTICS

Every communication has a *content aspect*, which is the manifest or overt information being conveyed, in our case, consisting of food- and nutrition-related motivational information (perceived barriers, self-efficacy, and so forth) or information to facilitate behavior change. These messages are the words you speak, the message you are trying to convey, or the illustrations and pictures you present. Every communication also has an implied or *metacommunication aspect*, which is information about the information, whether this is conveyed consciously or not. In verbal communications it could be your tone of voice or facial expressions. In the case of printed messages, metacommunication could be conveyed through the pictures you use, the layout, and the ordering of content. This meta-level information helps the audience interpret whether the nutrition educator thinks the information is really important, engaging, or burdensome, or whether the nutrition educator is being humorous or serious.

Making the Message Motivating and Easy to Understand: Elaboration Likelihood Model

The content of our messages or educational plans can be easy or difficult to process and inviting or off-putting based on how we deliver the content. The elaboration likelihood model of communication (ELM) proposes that individuals differ in their motivation and ability to thoughtfully process educational messages or reasons for change, and yet thoughtful processing of such messages is more likely to lead to behavior change and action (Petty and Cacioppo 1986; Petty, Barden, and Wheeler 2009). (See Chapters 4 and 11 for more details.)

To increase the *motivation* of the audience to process the messages in your educational plan, make the messages:

- Unexpected or novel
- Memorable
- Meaningful
- Culturally appropriate
- Stated in terms of what participants will gain from taking action, as well as what they will lose by not taking action
- Involve humor, warmth, or other attributes as appropriate for a given audience

To increase the *ability* of the audience to process the messages in your educational plan, here are some tips:

- Make your messages straightforward and clear.
- Repeat or reinforce them.
- Present the messages with a minimum of distractions.

The use of emotion-based messages through materials and activities has been shown to be especially effective (McCarthy 2005). These tips apply whether you deliver the messages through mass media, brochures, newsletters, or in a group setting.

FIGURE 15-2 shows a couple of the Pick a Better Snack and Play Your Way messages for children from the Iowa Nutrition Education Network campaign. Note that the messages are behavior-focused, specific, easy to understand, and expressed in very few words. The graphics are bold and attractive. They convey the idea of exuberance and enjoyment and that the actions are easy and fun to perform. These represent the metacommunication aspect of the messages.

Nonverbal Communication Accompanying the Message

When you deliver nutrition education in person, nonverbal communication always accompanies the verbal message and is often more influential than the verbal communication. Receivers (your audience) learn to trust their interpretations of the nonverbal messages because they know that these cannot be consciously selected or controlled by the sender. Indeed, communication experts believe that the image the nutrition educator projects may account for more than half of the total message conveyed to a group at first meeting. Nonverbal communication includes facial expressions, tone of voice, eye contact, gestures, and touch. Nonverbal cues, particularly facial expressions and tone

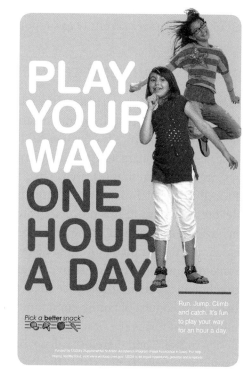

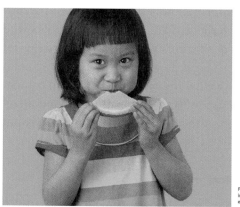

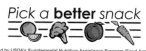

FIGURE 15-2 Campaigns to promote healthy lifestyles: Pick a Better Snack: How Easy is That? and Play Your Way: One Hour a Day campaigns.

Courtesy of Iowa Department of Public Health.

of voice, can express acceptance and support for group members or convey judgment and disapproval.

Nonverbal cues can indicate whether you are working *with* the group to state barriers and identify ways to overcome them or simply manipulating them to come up with the solutions. Educators are often judgmental and do not know it; however, the audience is very quick to pick up on it. For example, a nonjudgmental tone is straightforward and sounds provisional instead of dogmatic or defensive. Tone of voice and mannerisms can also express whether you respect the group and consider yourself a member or whether you feel superior. Compare expressions such as "You may not be able to grasp this, but believe me, I have been doing this for 10 years and it works," with "That sounds like a good idea. I have worked with others who found it did not work for them, but you are the one who must be satisfied with the eating pattern. So, you can experiment and find whether it works for you. Let us know how it goes." As you work with groups when you deliver your educational plans, be very aware of the nonverbal messages that you are transmitting.

Nonverbal communication also accompanies verbal communication through nonpersonal channels, such as videos, media campaigns, websites, posters, and newsletters. The graphics, colors, visual images, and music or sounds all convey information. Therefore you must select all of these features carefully to support the message.

RECEIVER OR AUDIENCE CHARACTERISTICS

Identifying the characteristics of the audience is extremely important in any health communication model. This is done through a process of assessment of audience interests, needs, and characteristics, sometimes called formative research or marketing research. This is why the DESIGN Procedure for planning theory-based nutrition education devotes two steps to this process. In Step 1, you assess the behaviors and practices of the audience, and in Step 2, you assess the determinants of these behaviors, such as their stage of emotional readiness to change and which social psychological factors influence their food-related practices in the context of family, community, and culture. This information forms the basis of the educational plans you design in Step 5 and therefore will not be repeated. The following are a few characteristics that are likely to affect how audience members may attend to, comprehend, and react to the message of the educational plans that you designed.

Personal Motivation to Attend to the Message

Audience members are predisposed to react to messages in a particular way based on their own experiences, beliefs, attitudes, and habits. Successful communication takes into account these predispositions and the reasons behind them. That is, communication is more effective if the message is personalized or tailored to the predispositions, outcome expectations, attitudes, needs, and assets of the audience, as has been emphasized previously, to increase motivation to process your message. In addition, the messages need to be tailored to, or based on, the cultural backgrounds of your audience. (See Chapter 17 for details.) As noted earlier, these personalized messages should be meaningful and memorable.

Educational Skills

Audience members' skills in processing the message also influence the effectiveness of the communication. Receivers must understand and process a message before it can have an effect on their attitudes or behaviors. Thus, receivers' abilities to listen, read, think about, or understand the nutrition concepts you wish to communicate are important considerations when designing and delivering the message of your educational plan. Make the message clear and straightforward for the given audience, but never condescending. This is especially important for low-literacy audiences.

Life Situation

Sometimes other urgent or important matters are going on in the lives of receivers that may interfere with their willingness and ability to process messages. This interference is often referred to as noise. As researchers have noted, cognitive information is filtered through psychological states (Achterberg 1988). Audience members who are sick or in pain or who are anxious and worried cannot pay attention to messages as well as those who are calm and well. This means that the messages or session content and methods you use must gain the attention and affect the comprehension of the audience, taking into account such interference.

Learning Style Preferences

Participants' preferred learning styles influence how much attention they pay to a message. For example, in the context of group sessions, listening to you lecture may be the

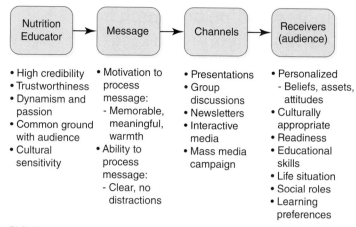

FIGURE 15-3 Summary of key features of each of the communication process components.

last thing a group of adolescents will want to do, whereas a cadre of executives may be perfectly comfortable listening to your message and may indeed prefer this mode of communication. These learning styles are explored in greater detail later in this chapter.

Social Roles and Life Course

The social status roles of the audience also influence response to the message. These roles are behaviors expected of people because of their position in society—for example, the role of "mother," "busy executive," and so forth. Audience members must feel that the message is appropriate for their role in society. The messages must also seem relevant to people at different stages of their life course, such as student, young working adult, parent of young children, parent of grown children, or older adult.

Summary

A summary of the basic features of the communication process is shown in **FIGURE 15-3**.

COMMUNICATIONS IN SOCIAL CONTEXT

The complexity of food- and nutrition-related behaviors and the social nature of communication has led to a more complex understanding of nutrition communications (Gillespie and Yarbrough 1984). The social context of communications also affects their reception in various ways.

The receivers' reference groups may influence response to the message. People are socially organized, with formal

or informal group memberships or reference groups. These can be peers, family, and others whose opinions are valued by audience members. Research indicates that the response to messages is a social phenomenon that involves not only what the audience members think of the messages, but also what trusted others, such as family members, close friends, or coworkers, think of the message. That is, individuals' responses are influenced by what they think others will think of their new opinions or actions. For example, teenagers will be more likely to change beverage choices if they think the change would be acceptable to their peers.

Communication Is a Two-Way Street

The nutrition educator and the receivers both provide inputs into the communication process. Communication is a two-way, not a one-way, street. The nutrition educator designs the sessions, but the audience provides inputs—more formally through the needs assessment process (as in Steps 1 and 2 of the DESIGN Procedure), and always during the sessions themselves. This is often called feedback. As you saw earlier, people cannot not communicate. This means the audience in a group setting cannot not communicate to the nutrition educator as well. Even in a very structured situation such as a lecture class, it has been found that when students in one half of the class look bored, pass notes, and start having side conversations and those in the other half are fully alert and interested and asking questions, the instructor will soon direct all of his or her attention to the latter half of the class. The audience has thus shaped the behavior of the communicator. See **FIGURE 15-4**.

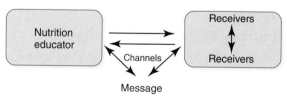

Communication in Social Context

- Communication in action is dynamic!

- The sender and receiver are always influencing each other and this influences the message.

- Receivers are constantly being influenced by what *others* say and by what *they think others will think* of the message.

FIGURE 15-4 Communication is interactive.

Communication Is Interactive

Complex interactions among individuals influence outcome. These interactions may be of two types: between the audience and the communicator and between audience members and their reference groups or peers. These complex interactions influence acceptance or rejection of the communication. The nutrition educator and the audience communicate with each other verbally or nonverbally, consciously or unconsciously, and these interactions influence outcome, as noted earlier. Others also influence audience members in the group. For example, if the reference group norm for teens is that answering the nutrition educator's questions during question-and-answer periods is not cool, then you will need to find other ways to engage students, such as small group discussions or projects.

Consequently, messages and group sessions are more likely to be effective if interactions between the communicator and the audience and between the audience members and their peers are built into the communication process. For example, women are more likely to adopt breastfeeding if they think this practice will be acceptable in the eyes of their peers. Here, a group process whereby women can share their perceptions and feelings with others would enhance breastfeeding adoption and maintenance. Successes and challenges can be shared, and mutual learning can take place. Indeed, Freire's dialogical method of critical consciousness-raising (Freire and Shor 1987) or Vella's method of facilitated dialogue (Vella 2002) may be very suitable in certain circumstances. In this process, educators or communicators pose questions and engage in dialogue with the group to facilitate understanding of the causes, consequences, and possible solutions of problems identified by the group. These issues are discussed in greater detail later in this chapter.

Implications for Nutrition Education

One clear implication of understanding the communication process is that it is extremely important for nutrition educators to become good communicators. For this to occur, it is helpful to understand exactly how receivers (the audience) process your message and how best to communicate with them. This means understanding how people learn, knowing the learning styles of your audience and selecting educational or instructional methods for communicating effectively with your audience. These are the issues we will explore next.

Understanding and Applying Learning Theory: Learning Approaches and Learning Styles

UNDERSTANDING LEARNING THEORY

How people come to know things has been the subject of intense interest and discussion ever since the time of Plato, who thought that knowledge arises from the *workings of the mind*, though we do acquire sensory information from the world, and Aristotle, his student and successor, who thought that the *external world* is the basis of people's impressions and knowledge. These two approaches still echo in today's theories of learning. Psychology, as a field of study, came into being when it was concluded that the study of human consciousness was a legitimate area of scientific investigation, and how people learn has certainly been part of that. Numerous studies and theories have been developed since these early beginnings, and the neurophysiological bases of our mental processing systems have also been investigated.

Learning theories are conceptual frameworks that range from those that are primarily *behaviorist*, positing that learning comes from stimuli and reinforcements from the outside world and focuses on observable aspects of learning; to *cognitive*, positing people are rational information processors focusing on brain-based learning such as thinking, memory, knowing, and problem-solving; to *social cognitive*, which says that learning is a cognitive process that takes place in a social context, which supplies both modeling of the behavior by others and reinforcements, and thus involves the interaction of personal, behavioral and environmental factors; to *cognitive and social constructivist*, where learning is seen as an active, constructive process in which the learner actively constructs or builds new ideas or concepts; to theories that attend to *motivation and emotions* and those that focus on *self-regulation* or self-directed learning and behavior in a supportive environment.

We can see that there is no one definition of learning. The one that most closely aligns with the focus on behavior change and the social psychological and social ecological approach used in health education and promotion and in nutrition education is an *integrated approach*, in which learning is seen as the process that brings together cognitive, affective or emotional, and environmental influences for acquiring, enhancing, or making changes in one's knowledge, skills, values, and world views (Illeris 2003, 2009). Some would add that this process involves practice and experience and results in an "an enduring change in behavior, or in the capacity to behave in a given fashion" (Schunk 2011). Illeris proposes a model of learning that integrates the *cognitive processes of learning*, with its focus on content—knowledge, understanding, and skills through acquisition and elaboration of information through various brain mechanisms; the *incentive dimension* with its focus on motivation, emotion and volition; and the *social dimension or the situational aspect* with its focus on action, communication, and cooperation, in which the environment influences the learner but the learner also influences the environment. Nutrition education can use this *integrated approach* to learning theory, and it can also bring in other theories related to the learning process as appropriate for the population with which we are working, such as developmental theory when working with children or adult learning theory when we design educational activities for adult groups.

IMPLICATIONS FOR LEARNING APPROACHES: ACTIVE AND COOPERATIVE LEARNING

Clearly, in an integrated approach to learning, mere presentation of information such as getting up in front of an audience to tell what we know will not result in learning. The dynamic engagement of the participants with the content, derived from motivation and volition (or active choice), is essential—whether mental, emotional, or physical engagement. Learning thus involves an interaction between learners (communication receivers/intervention participants) and the activities that educators have designed. Consequently, nutrition education must involve *active learning* (described in detail later in this chapter).

In addition, because learning also involves interaction with the social world, cooperative learning is more likely to be effective in most settings. Here, as nutrition educators, we develop activities that provide opportunities for small groups to engage in learning activities together. This maps onto the social cognitive theory approach that is widely used in nutrition and health education. This theory is described in detail in Chapter 5. Here, behavior is seen as the result of the interaction among motivation, knowledge, skills, and the environment (Bandura 1986, 2004). It also maps onto self-determination theory, which states that key factors, such as a sense of autonomy, competence, and relatedness to others, are essential to growth and learning (Deci and Ryan 2008).

Research provides evidence that there are advantages to using an active, cooperative approach. Neuroimaging and neurochemical investigations show that under normal conditions, information in the form of auditory or visual information flows into the brain, where it is received by a structure called the amygdala. Here, the information is imbued with emotional meaning and linked to previously stored knowledge (Salamone and Correa 2002). This information, now enhanced with emotional and relational data, is then processed and stored for later use and executive function. When people engage in well designed, emotionally meaningful, and authentic cooperative learning activities in which they feel that their individual learning styles, skills, and talents are valued, this flow of information into storage and use is facilitated (Hermans et al. 2014). In contrast, when individuals are repeatedly placed in learning situations perceived to be stressful (speaking up in a group, making presentations), memory processing, consolidation, or retrieval are impaired (Juster, McEwen, and Lupien 2010).

In addition to enhancing emotional meaningfulness and storage of information, positive learning experiences stimulate greater release of dopamine, a neurotransmitter (brain chemical) associated with increased memory storage, comprehension, and executive function (Waeiti, Dickinson, and Schultz 2001; Puig et al. 2014). Successful cooperative group activities, involving social collaboration, motivation, expectation of success, and authentic praise from peers, engages the brain's reward system and creates conditions that enhance dopamine release (Kohls et al. 2013). Furthermore, active constructive thinking stimulated by analyzing issues, discussion, drawing group charts and diagrams, and so forth encourages the integration of information in multiple brain sites, which, in turn, enhances comprehension.

For all these reasons, we are more likely to be effective in bringing about learning and behavior change as nutrition educators if we use hands-on *and* minds-on activities, particularly those that incorporate well-designed positive and collaborative group experiences.

Because learning is seen as the interaction among dozens of different functional areas in the brain, it may be that each area has a relatively different importance for any particular person. Thus people may differ in how they learn, resulting in possible multiple intelligences (Sternberg 1985;

Gardner 2001). That means we will need to vary how we provide nutrition education to our audiences.

UNDERSTANDING LEARNING STYLES: KOLB'S MODEL

One of the receiver/program participant characteristics to keep in mind, therefore, is that individuals may have different learning styles. A given audience may have one predominant learning style, but more likely, the group will include people with different learning styles. This means that different types of learning activities are needed within each session to accommodate these differences. The various DESIGN Procedure features emphasized in Step 5 took learning style into consideration, although it was not stated. (See Chapters 11 and 12 for details.)

There are several ways to organize learning styles (Waring and Evans 2014). One way was proposed by Kolb, based on his research of the experience of learning (Kolb 1984). Kolb proposes that individuals differ in the way they understand their experience of, and adapt to, the world, and that these variances can be placed on a continuum of *perception*. At one end of the continuum are the sensing/feeling individuals who project themselves onto the current reality of each experience by sensing and feeling their way around. Conversely, people on the thinking end of the continuum tend to analyze experiences logically through their intellect. People do move back and forth on the continuum, but most have a comfortable "hovering place." Each of these two kinds of perception has strengths and weaknesses. Both are valuable. Learners need both perspectives. See **FIGURE 15-5**.

The second way in which people learn differently is in how they *process* experiences and information. When confronted with learning new things, some people watch and reflect first to filter the experience through their own value system. Other people jump in and act immediately, saving the reflection for later, if at all. Watchers need to internalize; doers need to act. Neither way is better, but rich learning involves both.

When these two kinds of *perceiving* and *processing* are looked at together, a four-quadrant learning style model is formed (Figure 15-5).

- *Imaginative learners* process information reflectively and process it by intuiting and feeling. They want the world to be a meaningful place for them and therefore strive to connect personally to the content they are learning. They believe in their own experience and are interested in people and culture.
- *Analytic learners* perceive information abstractly and process it reflectively. They learn by thinking through concepts and pay attention to expert opinions. They are industrious and thrive in traditional classrooms and nutrition education lecture settings. Verbally skilled and avid readers, analytic learners sometimes see ideas as being more fascinating than people.
- *Commonsense learners* perceive information abstractly and process it actively. They learn by applying theories to practice and are avid problem solvers. They need to know how things work and wonder how (and if) what they learn in a nutrition education session can be of immediate use to them.
- *Dynamic learners* perceive information concretely and process it actively. They learn by trial and error and are enthusiastic about new things. They are at ease with people and enjoy taking risks and wrangling with change. Dynamic learners pursue interests through a variety of avenues, and therefore the structure of formal nutrition education sessions seems limiting to them.

Kolb (1984) suggests that each session or series of sessions include learning activities that address each of these learning styles in the following sequence: concrete

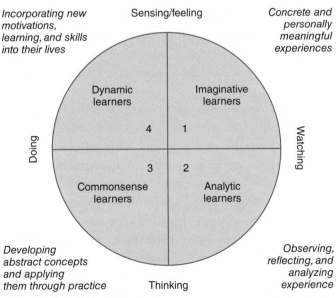

FIGURE 15-5 The four major learning styles and educational activities appropriate to each.

Modified from Kolb, D. A. 1984. *Experiential Learning*. Englewood Cliffs, NJ: Prentice Hall.

experiences, observations and reflections, formation of abstract concepts and generalizations, and testing the implications of concepts in new situations (Table 15-1).

Note that as nutrition educators, we tend to teach according to our own learning style preferences, so we should be aware of our preferences and ensure that we deliver nutrition education in ways that will reach individuals with different learning styles and enrich their repertoire of ways of learning (and perhaps our own at the same time!).

Understanding and Applying Instructional Design Theory

UNDERSTANDING INSTRUCTIONAL DESIGN THEORY

As we have noted, learning is about an interaction between learners and the activities educators design. So *learning* is what intervention participants do, while *education* is what the nutrition educator does. Such education is often referred to as *instruction*, although many use the term *teaching* as synonymous with instruction. Sometimes the term *pedagogy* is also used, described as the science and art of teaching. Instruction has been defined as "anything that is done purposely to facilitate learning" (Reigeluth and Carr-Chellman 2009). Whereas sometimes there is a distinction between *instruction* as something done to learners (i.e., learners are passive) and *construction* as something done *by* learners (i.e., learners are active), more recent views are that instruction includes constructivist methods and self-directed learning as well as more traditional views of instruction such as lecture or direct instruction. Thus the term *instruction* represents a larger enterprise than teaching in the traditional sense. We will use the term *instruction* as what nutrition educators do, recognizing it is *not* simply getting up in front of a group and lecturing. It includes the numerous activities that were described in great detail in Chapters 11 and 12. Consequently, we will use the term *educator* rather than teacher.

Designing our instruction or educational sessions requires us to consider many factors:

- Using principles of good instruction or teaching
- Sequencing instruction or educational activities
- Addressing the three domains of learning
- Considering the learning styles of the participants in our sessions or intervention

Using Principles of Good Instruction or Teaching

Considerable research and debate have been devoted to what is considered to be good instruction (Gagne 1985; Reigeluth and Carr-Chellman 2009). One summary (Merrill 2009) proposes that good instruction consists of the following principles: *activation*, where the instruction activates what learners already know and provides opportunity for them to share previous experiences; *demonstration*, where instruction provides demonstration of skills through media appropriate to the content and engages learners in peer discussion; *task-centered*, where instruction should involve a progression of increasingly difficult tasks; *application*, where learners have the opportunity to apply what they have learned through coaching, corrective feedback, and peer collaboration; and *integration*, where instruction should integrate new learning into previous knowledge, skills, and behavioral repertoire and create, invent, or explore personal ways to use their new learning.

Good instruction also involves *meaningful learning*. Ausubel (2000) focuses on how to meaningfully anchor learning so that it is internalized and retained in people's cognitive structures for use. The cognitive and motivational-affective factors influencing this process are important, among them the use of *advance organizers* where the material to be covered is described so that new information can be scaffolded onto prior learning.

Sequencing the Instruction/Educational Activities

Instructional design theory is consequently concerned with not only the components of instruction but also how instruction is sequenced during the learning experience. The specific educational activities conducted with a group are often called *events of instruction* (Gagne 1995; Merrill 2009). The sequence of events proposed by Merrill consists of a four-phase cycle, based on the principles described above: activation, demonstration, application, and integration. This instructional sequence of events is similar to one advocated by Gagne (1985) that was modified by Kinzie (2005) for use with health promotion programs, which is used as the basis of how to design an educational plan described in Step 5 of the DESIGN Procedure. (See Chapter 11.) We can see that there is considerable agreement on how to sequence learning.

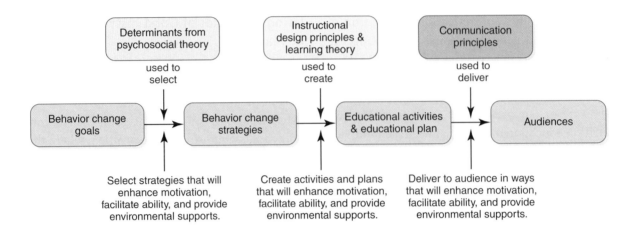

Addressing the Three Domains of Learning and Instruction

Effective instruction addresses the three major domains in which learning occurs—the *cognitive, affective,* and *psychomotor* (Beatty 2009). These are described in detail in Chapter 10. Recall that in designing our nutrition education sessions, we need to ensure that our educational activities not only address each of these domains, but that we also consider the level of complexity within each of these domains. For example, *levels of thinking* can range from simple knowledge to the more complex tasks of analysis, evaluation, and synthesis (Bloom et al. 1956); *levels of affective or emotional engagement* can range from only receiving the instruction to valuing and internalizing values (Anderson and Krathwohl 2000); and *levels of psychomotor skills* can range from observing to imitating to being able to modify the action to improve the outcome. Designing educational activities that address a range of these learning tasks makes for more effective and lively nutrition education.

Considering Learning Styles

To design effective nutrition education, we also need to take into account the learning styles of our participants, described earlier in this chapter.

APPLYING INSTRUCTIONAL DESIGN THEORY: TEACHING AROUND THE CYCLE

We can use these principles from learning theory and instructional design theory in the field of education to deliver nutrition education that is based on social psychological approaches to motivating and facilitating dietary change. Stated another way, we can make our social psychological theory–based nutrition education more effective if we design our sessions or intervention *activities* to operationalize our theory-based motivators and facilitators using the principles of good instruction and applying them to all three domains of human learning, sequence the events of instruction (or educational activities) appropriately, and take into account the different learning styles of our participants. The sequence of developing and delivering nutrition education sessions can be summarized as follows (see also the above diagram):

> **Choose behavioral change goal → identify psychosocial theory–based determinants of behavior change → select determinant-based strategies → create educational objectives and activities based on learning theory and instructional theory from education → sequence into an educational plan and deliver using good communication principles,** as shown schematically in the diagram above.

Here, we describe how to use the model of Kolb (1984) to build our sessions around instructional/educational activities that address the cognitive and affective domains and different learning styles. These activities are described in more detail in **TABLE 15-1**. Note that here we are suggesting instructing (teaching) around the cycle.

1. The sessions can begin with *concrete experiences* to activate learning by focusing on sensing and feeling, making the session personal and relevant to the participants. This can be through use of trigger films, observations, demonstrations, and explorations of their own prior knowledge, attitudes, or behaviors through an activity. This is called self-assessment in earlier chapters. (*Sensing/feeling*)

TABLE 15-1 Learning Activities to Address Each Learning Style

What does using the learning style approach look like in terms of instructional activities? Use activities to address all the learning styles by "teaching around the cycle."

Quadrant and Learner Type	Focus	Educational Activities
Quadrant 1: Imaginative learners		
Creating a concrete experience	*Focus on sensing and feeling.* Activate knowledge by making learning meaningful. The focus is on the learners and how they can connect to themselves what is being learned. The aim is motivation of learners.	Relevant trigger films, demonstrations, hook questions, brainstorming, observations, games, self-assessments
Quadrant 2: Analytic learners		
Observing, reflecting, and analyzing experience; integrating reflective analysis into concepts	*Focus on watching/reflecting.* Assist learners to gain knowledge by introducing needed content. Learners reflect on prior experience from quadrant 1 and develop concepts and skills. The aim is to facilitate ability to take action.	Discussions, mini-debates, journals or logs, thinking questions, analyses of pros and cons, mini lectures (graphs and charts, pictures, summaries), readings
Quadrant 3: Commonsense learners		
Developing abstract concepts and/or skills; practicing skills	*Focus on thinking.* Assist learners to examine how they can apply what they have learned. The aim is to provide opportunities for practice.	Making or completing graphs/charts, drawings, conclusions; case studies; writing activities; "minds-on" worksheets
Quadrant 4: Dynamic learners		
Practicing and adding something of oneself; analyzing application for relevance or usefulness	*Focus on doing.* Encourage creativity and self-expression by asking group members to take what they have learned and practiced and expand on it in their own way. The aim is to challenge the group to incorporate new motivations, learning, and skills in an ongoing way into their lives.	"Hands-on" activities; contracts, commitments, or action plans; developing products or videos, puzzles and/or skits, and simulations; field study; field visits

2. The second part of the session or program can involve addressing *motivational (why-to) knowledge* for the audience to observe and reflect on, such as the latest scientific information about the benefits of taking action. This could be a mini-lecture, incorporating graphs and visuals where appropriate. Together, these two sections of the sessions will increase interest and motivation. (*Watching*)

3. The next part can focus on developing *abstract concepts and skills* through activities in which the individuals begin to form their own understandings of the issues related to taking action, such as through needed how-to knowledge and skills. Opportunities to practice need to be applied. (*Thinking*)

4. Finally, the group can take steps to *apply* the new motivations, learning, and skills gained in an ongoing way into their lives, such as by setting goals for specific actions they will take. (*Doing*)

As you can see, Kolb's instructional sequence is very similar to the sequence of Gagne (1985; Gagne et al. 2004),

as modified by Kinzie (2005) for health promotion activities and used as the basis of Step 5 of the DESIGN Procedure. (See Chapter 11 for details.) It is also similar to other contemporary models for sequencing instruction (Merrill 2009). We designate this sequence for use in nutrition education as follows:

- **Excite:** Gain attention. *Use an attention-getter that is personally relevant for your audience about the behavior change goal(s) of your session. Can involve risk assessment.*

- **Explain:** Present stimulus or new material that is motivational and tailored to the prior knowledge and experience of the audience. *The focus is on perceived benefits for why-to take action, affective attitudes and feelings, and barriers.*

- **Expand:** Provide guidance and practice to engage in actions, with a *focus on functional knowledge and skills, that is, how-to take action. Use credible social models.*

- **Exit:** Apply and close. *Enhance application, goal setting skills, and action planning, and provide supports.*

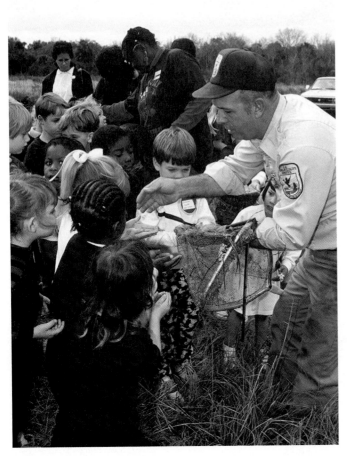

For younger children, a trip to a farm to see how vegetables and fruits are produced may be a great way to create a more hands-on learning experience.

Courtesy of John and Karen Hollingsworth/U.S. Fish & Wildlife Service.

At this point you may wish to review the educational plan(s) you developed in Step 5 of the DESIGN Procedure. (Refer to Chapters 11 and 12.) Ensure that you incorporated activities directed at all three domains of learning and at different learning styles and that you sequenced your educational activities appropriately.

Creating Environments for Learning

As nutrition educators who seek to motivate and facilitate behavior changes, we need to include additional considerations for learning and behavior change. Most of nutrition education occurs in group settings and often with adults. Hence we also want to understand the dynamics of how groups function and also how to create safe learning environments.

Kurt Lewin, who is considered a leading developer of the field of social psychology and who made profound contributions to the understanding of motivation of behavior, as noted earlier in the book, is also generally considered to be the founder of modern group dynamics. His work on field dynamics or field theory has had enormous influence on the understanding of human behavior in the context of others.

LEWIN ON GROUP DYNAMICS

Lewin emphasizes that individuals' beliefs, attitudes, and habits are intimately related to those of the groups to which they belong. Humans, who always live in groups, are constantly involved in dynamic interactions with others. These interactions can be symbolic or can be affective and emotional in nature. In his view, the group is not the sum of its members. It is a structure that emerges from the interaction of behaving individuals who constantly and dynamically adjust to each other to form a "field" (Lewin 1951). The result of this mutual adaptation is a set of ever more complex patterns of behavior within the group. Neither the individual nor the group structure has an independent existence—they are mutually and dynamically dependent on each other, resulting in a set of group dynamics (Lewin 1935, 1947). These principles apply to those living in families as well.

Group Decision Method for Changing Food Habits

Lewin conducted a series of experiments on changing people's food beliefs and attitudes (or values, as he called

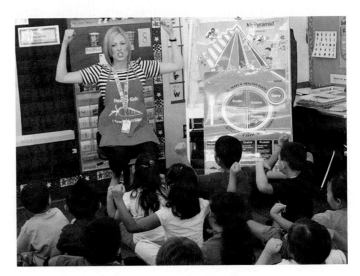

A key feature of effective communication is enthusiasm and dynamism.

Courtesy of UC CalFresh.

them) and food habits. During World War II when meat was scarce, he and his collaborators conducted several studies to compare "the relative effectiveness of a lecture method and a method of group decision for changing food habits" (Lewin 1943). These studies were experimental in nature and carefully controlled for leader effect and socio-economic and ethnic differences.

Increasing Organ Meat Consumption

In one study with housewives, Lewin compared these two ways of encouraging people to eat organ meats (kidneys, sweetbreads/brains, and beef hearts), purposely chosen because they are normally rejected. The lecture used health, status, and patriotic appeals, followed by handouts with recipes. The second method involved a short presentation by the leader, which also linked the problem of nutrition to health, status, and the war effort. There was ample opportunity for the women to discuss why they rejected these meats and to share experiences with each other. They then identified ways to overcome barriers (with ideas from the leader if needed). Next, the group members were ready to make a decision about whether to try one of these meats the following week using the recipes provided. They verbalized their decision to the others. Of the women in the lecture-only setting, only 10% served one of the recommended foods, whereas of those who had an opportunity to discuss and make a group decision, 52% served the recommended foods.

Whole Wheat Bread Consumption

Lewin conducted a similar study with a different audience—college students—emphasizing whole grain bread. In this case, he compared a "request" to the students to eat more whole grain bread instead of white bread with group decision and obtained similar results (Lewin 1943). His work suggests, therefore, that group dynamics are important and that a democratic social climate, in which group members have the opportunity to be involved in making decisions for themselves, is more conducive to social change than other social climates. He emphasized that the method was one of *group decision* rather than just *group discussion* because closure in terms of decision making was considered important to the approach, along with public commitment. Such commitment made in the context of supportive peers was a motivating factor to make good on one's commitment to oneself. As Lewin noted, no pressure tactics were used; instead, "the group

setting gives the incentive for the decision and facilitates and reinforces it" (Lewin 1943).

Since then, there has been considerable research on group structure and development, group behavior, leadership issues, group learning, and group development in a variety of settings, such as education, worksites, and communities. There have also been numerous professional conversations about the appropriate roles of educators and group members, particularly in work with adults (Rogers 1969; Brookfield 1986, 2013; Vella 2002). All, however, agree that creating an emotionally safe learning environment is crucial.

CREATING SAFE LEARNING ENVIRONMENTS CONDUCIVE TO CHANGE

Many of the individuals nutrition educators work with want to make changes in their lives but are also afraid to do so. Food- and nutrition-related behaviors are embedded in so many other aspects of their lives that making a change in this one aspect may involve drastic changes in other aspects. Educators and psychologists (Rogers 1969; Freire and Shor 1987; Knowles, Holton, and Swanson 2011; Vella 2002) note that learning environments must be challenging enough to stimulate growth but also safe enough to allow people to grow and change in perspectives, knowledge, attitudes, motivation, and action. Cooperative learning is more effective than competitive learning in this context (Johnson and Johnson 1998). This means respecting that individuals come with a set of fears and defenses. It also means that the design of the sessions, the atmosphere in the room, and your approach to the situation should all signal that this is a safe space and time to learn and change. This feeling is especially important for adult learners in non-formal settings. Group leaders, such as nutrition educators, are often referred to as facilitators of such learning groups, rather than teachers or instructors.

Participants in any group bring with them a set of fears. The following list describes a few of them. **BOX 15-1**, based on work by Sappington (1984), discusses how you can address these fears to make the learning environment safe for participants.

- *Outcome fears.* These include participants' fear that they will not get what they want, that the information and activities may not be relevant to their personal needs, that there will not be enough time, and that the session will go over time.

BOX 15-1 Creating a Safe Learning Environment

The following lists present ways to reduce audience fears and create a safe learning environment.

Outcome Fears

- *Provide a welcoming start.* Make sure the room is comfortable in terms of light, heating, and ventilation. Arrange the setting or seating to be appropriate to the learning situation. Conscious decisions need to be made about whether to arrange seating in a circle or half circle (more intimate than rows), around tables, and so forth. Have coffee or tea out if appropriate, and nametags.

- *Greet the group and introduce yourself.* If appropriate to the setting and size of the group, have the group members introduce themselves as well.

- *Set the time frame.* Let the audience know approximately how long the session will last.

- *Make your competence and experience clear, either through prior material you hand out or through your introduction.* This will make the group feel confident in your being able to provide a valuable experience for them.

- *State the objectives of the session clearly and provide a brief overview of the agenda or activities.* This will make the participants feel assured that the material will be relevant to their needs and that the activities are well organized.

Interpersonal Fears

- *State ground rules about how individuals will relate to each other.* Ask the group to contribute so that all are comfortable with the rules. Key ground rules are to respect each other and the facilitator and to listen to each other.

- *Design activities to be done first in pairs and then in small groups.* Do this before having a large group discussion.

- *As the facilitator of the group, provide nonjudgmental responses to individual contributions.* By listening carefully to the feelings behind the questions and comments, you can gauge the fear or safety level in the individual and the group. Model the desired behavior and use warm, accepting humor where appropriate.

Evaluation Fears

- *Validate each response either verbally or by writing responses on newsprint.*

- *Provide nonjudgmental responses.* For example, rather than saying that what a group member said was "not quite accurate," thank the person for bringing up that point because it is something that many others might also be thinking, and then say, "The latest information on that point is . . .".

- *Provide constructive feedback.*

Internal Fears

- *Be respectful of each individual.*

- *Validate individuals' past experiences.*

- *Use genuine dialogue as the approach.* Ask open-ended questions and listen to responses in order to allow for a free-flowing exchange of ideas so that all group members can learn from each other.

- *Interpersonal fears or social concerns.* These are often the greatest barrier in group settings to significant learning and change. They include fear of embarrassment, looking stupid or incompetent to peers or to the nutrition educator, criticism by others in the group, being called on when one is not ready, judgment of one's beliefs or positions, feeling vulnerable, unfamiliarity with others in a new group, or competition with others.

- *Evaluation fears.* These include fear of failure at the tasks that have been chosen and fear that one's verbal responses are not correct.

- *Internal fears.* The deepest fears that group participants often bring are those that challenge their self-concept. Fear of incompetence or inadequacy arises from a genuine fear of not being able to do what is suggested. Changing would suggest that previous beliefs, attitudes, or actions were inferior or bad.

In general, safe environments are created when people feel respected; when their feelings are honored, their self-worth is assured, and their fears are overcome; and when the "delights of growth outweigh the anxieties of growth." Building safe learning environments is a crucial part of facilitated group discussion and dialogue, which is described later.

UNDERSTANDING GROUP DYNAMICS IN NUTRITION EDUCATION SESSIONS

Even if you have designed engaging activities and wish to incorporate group discussion, you can confront situations that consistently plague instructors and group discussion leaders. If you are not ready to face spontaneous aspects of group dynamics, you may find yourself distracted, frustrated, or even becoming hostile. Defuse the anxiety by considering ahead of time how you will respond in some situations you might face, such as those shown in **BOX 15-2**. These situations can be issues of authority (yours) and power (the audience's). The following list presents some ways you might handle these situations. In facilitated discussions or dialogues of groups that have met for some time, members of the group may take on many of the following roles.

- *Quiet members.* It is important to respect all individuals in the group in terms of whether they wish to participate in discussions or not. They may be shy, or their quietness may be cultural. However, silence may also be a reflection of boredom, indifference, or a person's sense of superiority, timidity, or insecurity. Thus, it is important for you to figure out why group members are silent. If they are shy or insecure, it is helpful to provide activities such as icebreakers, brainstorming, or working in pairs or small groups. You can also reinforce and praise each attempt they make to speak up in the group. Sometimes quiet members really wish to speak up and will do so if you give them some encouragement, using smiles, nods, and perhaps asking them to respond. If they have blank expressions, it would be unwise to invite them to participate.

- *Dominant or talkative members.* The most common problem facilitators have is what to say to those who are overly dominant and talkative. It is important to handle the situation carefully because what you do will have an impact on all the others in the group. It is crucial to treat individuals with respect and not to humiliate or embarrass them. Being disrespectful is not only hurtful for the individual, but also makes others in the group feel unsafe and uncomfortable.

BOX 15-2 Give Your Session a Fair Trial: Be Aware of the Effects of Group Dynamics

You know your content. You have designed activities that are based on theory and research and are engaging, interactive, and fun. But you may still confront situations that have plagued instructors and discussion leaders forever. If you are not ready to face spontaneous aspects of group dynamics, you may find yourself distracted and frustrated. Defuse the anxiety ahead of time by considering how you would handle each of these chronic instructional problems if they come up:

1. Only a few people are on time. When should you begin?
2. People arrive late (missing critical content or instructions).
3. One person dominates the session.
4. People do other work while you are presenting.
5. Some refuse to join the activity.
6. Many tangents are raised.
7. Someone wants to link every issue to a long personal story.
8. A heated argument erupts over a content issue.
9. People leave early or exit the room frequently.
10. Someone thinks he or she should be teaching the session rather than you.
11. Someone nods off.
12. Two people chat continuously at the back of the room or within the circle.
13. Some people are much more informed on the topic than you.
14. You are asked a string of questions you cannot answer.
15. Some people let it be known that the only reason they are there is because they are required to be.

Source: Morin, K. 2008. Presentation at Teachers College, Columbia University, New York.

Several techniques may be effective in dealing with dominant or overly talkative participants. Some people are overly talkative because they are insecure and repeat themselves because they are not sure that the points they are making have been understood. If this is the case, you might interrupt them gently but firmly by thanking them for their response, paraphrase concisely what they have said or reflect their feelings so that they feel they have been understood, and then turn to others for responses. Usually these participants will stop talking because they feel they have been understood.

Others are talkative because they enjoy talking or they believe that they can raise their status within the group by sharing information. They will not stop talking even when you or others in the group have paraphrased what they said or reflected their feelings. In this case, you might want to acknowledge their contributions and then say that short comments are easier for others to follow and that lengthy comments tend to lose people. If the pattern persists, you may need to talk with the participant privately. Talkative group members are often unaware of the fact that others may not appreciate their lengthy comments.

- *Distractors or disrupters.* These individuals may carry out side conversations or make side comments to the group or frequently get up and leave the room, disrupting the group, whether the nutrition educator is presenting or leading the discussion or others are talking. Generally, you should not embarrass members who are engaged in side conversations if these are brief and intermittent. If the conversations are disrupting, you might stop talking and ask the individuals involved an easy question or ask them to share their thoughts with the group. If the disruptions persist, you should speak with them in private and point out that their behavior distracts and disrupts learning and is disrespectful of others.
- *Complainers.* Some participants are always complaining about some aspect of the group or about the physical surroundings. Acknowledge them and thank them for their concern. Ask them for suggestions for alternate approaches. Indicate that you will explore their suggestions and then be firm about staying on track. If the complaining persists, take the individuals aside and talk with them privately.
- *Digressers.* These group members constantly digress from the main issues of the discussion or activities

by talking about matters unrelated to the issues. You can respond by saying, "What you say is interesting, but let's get back to . . .". Or you can very neutrally ask, "How does this relate to what we are talking about?" Or again, "This is interesting, but given our time constraints, we can discuss these issues later if we have time."

- *Resistors.* These individuals say that whatever is being proposed by you or the others can't be done, or they just can't do it. This response may stem from fear or insecurity. Acknowledge their feelings and indicate that all change is difficult and that they can take one step at a time. If possible, partner them with someone else in the group who can provide support.
- *Know-it-alls.* Some group members may indicate that they know more than you and keep correcting you. Acknowledge that they seem to know a lot. You might ask them about their sources of information. Even if you believe the source is very questionable, ask them what makes them believe the source. Remain questioning and probing. You might also ask the others in the group to respond. It may be effective for you to place such persons in some leadership role.
- *Wisecrackers.* Some degree of humor may be helpful in the group. However, you will need to determine when the humor stops being helpful in relieving tension and starts interfering with group learning. This usually occurs when more attention is focused on the person who is making the wisecracks than on what is being said. You can say to the person, with a smile and in a tone that suggests that you appreciate what he or she has said, that it is time to get back to the issues. If the wisecracks continue, you may have to say it again, but with a firm tone.
- *Latecomers.* If one or two individuals are late for an ongoing group or learning situation, you may ignore it. However, if they are consistently late, you may need to say something such as, "I know it is not always easy to get here on time, given the traffic and your situation, but I do want to remind us all that learning works best when we are all here from the beginning of the group session. It is also respectful of the others who may have made considerable effort to be here on time." If lateness persists for some individuals, you may want to talk with them privately to find out what the issues are for them. If the entire group consistently arrives late, you will need to carefully examine your own hidden

messages to the group. Perhaps you do not start or end on time. This may convey the message that the group is not that important and thus not worth being on time for. This will arouse considerable resentment, particularly from those who make an effort to be on time. It may be interpreted as disrespect for group members' time.

Methods of Instruction/Teaching: Practical Ways to Activate Learning and Enhance Behavior Change

You have already designed learning experiences for nutrition education group sessions in Step 5. The following discussion concerns how to deliver the educational experiences that you have planned. These are sometimes called *methods of instruction*.

INSTRUCTIONAL METHODS FOR IMPLEMENTING LEARNING EXPERIENCES

With a thorough understanding of communication principles and learning styles and also how to handle group dynamics, you are ready to explore in greater depth the many different instructional formats that you can use to deliver the nutrition education plans you have designed, such as lectures, demonstrations, hands-on learning tasks, or group discussions. Each has advantages and disadvantages. These various formats are described in the following subsections.

Lecture: Sage on the Stage

Lecture is still the predominant educational delivery method used today. It is how most people were taught, and many educators tend to teach as they were taught. During lecturing, group participants play a passive role as learners while the leader assumes the role of expert. As noted earlier, people remember only 10% of what they hear, so lecturing is not considered the most desirable method for reaching the public. A survey found that a group of mothers in the Women, Infants and Children (WIC) program, struggling with complex issues regarding getting their children to develop healthful eating patterns, gave lectures a very low rating.

The lecture method should not be ruled out entirely, however. It can be useful in classroom settings when presenting new information that students will be required to master later on or at professional meetings when new information is presented to participants. In addition, lecture may be the preferred style for some types of learners. For example, one study examined the usefulness of social cognitive theory–based strategies such as taste testing, role playing, brainstorming, and goal setting to improve business executives' away-from-home eating behaviors (Olson and Kelly 1989). The study found that these busy business executives hated the use of hands-on behaviorally based activities. They were already interested in making changes in their eating practices and wanted the necessary how-to information delivered quickly and compactly. Activities just took too long. This affirms the importance of finding out audience learning style preferences in the needs analysis in Step 2.

Mini-lectures. Generally, lecture works best when it is delivered in short, palatable bites. The average person can listen for no longer than 10 minutes before needing to stop to process the information being taken in. Visuals such as charts, graphs, and pictures enhance the presentation of vital information while helping to accommodate learners who are not keen on the lecture as a viable mode of delivery. Analytic learners may be amenable to a longer lecture, whereas dynamic learners will begin to squirm after the first 5 minutes. Of course, listening to an engaging nutrition educator on an issue of interest will make any lecture seem shorter.

Mini-lectures can be embedded in an otherwise activity-based session. For example, a mini-lecture is very useful during the part of the session in which scientific evidence of perceived outcomes of behavior, both positive and negative, is presented. Likewise, a mini-lecture may be useful for providing evidence-based information about effective actions for reducing risk or improving health, whether personal, community, or environmental.

Active Learning Through Activities and Learning Tasks

Activities and experiences can heighten learning in a way that no passive learning can. Indeed, as noted before: "I hear—and forget; I see—and remember; I do—and understand." In addition, you know from earlier in this chapter that active learning not only increases awareness, but also enhances motivation. The doers—dynamic and commonsense learners—prefer hands-on learning.

This includes the many activities and learning tasks that you might design for your participants, such as calculating fat or sugar content in foods, completing checklists, sorting items into categories, completing worksheets comparing foods in terms of cost and nutritional content, or analyzing local restaurant menus for the most healthful meals. If it is feasible, other learning experiences might be food taste testing, cooking or simple food preparation, grocery store tours, and visits to farms or farmers' markets. Refer to Table 15-1 for active methods that can be used with groups.

Providing worksheets for the activities, handouts, tip sheets, and follow-up materials is very helpful to participants, because they can read the reinforcing materials at their own pace and use them to put the messages of your sessions into action. How to make these engaging and effective is described in Chapter 16.

Discussions

Discussions are one of the most constructive strategies for learning. In traditional schooling, a quiet classroom was considered a productive one. However, higher-order thinking skills require complex cognition, which is facilitated by individuals verbalizing what they know, do not know, or want to know (Johnson and Johnson 1998).

As a nutrition educator, you can encourage group participants to talk to each other. For example, use the enthusiasm that participants have for each other to promote learning. Passive learning, such as listening to the nutrition educator talk, does not employ the richer cognitive processes that promote memory, elaboration, or attitudinal changes. Imaginative learners in particular enjoy discussions regarding "what if" questions, analytic learners prefer "why" questions, and commonsense learners prefer "how" questions; dynamic learners appreciate all three perspectives.

Brainstorming

Brainstorming is an effective method for getting groups of participants to generate lists in a creative way. Everyone has a creative streak in them, and educators need to get rid of the blocks that keep good ideas pent up. Establishing rules for brainstorming helps participants keep on track and feel safe enough to contribute. Dynamic and imaginative learners prefer brainstorming over passive learning

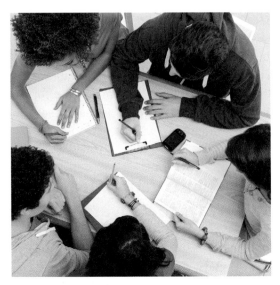

Brainstorming provides an effective, interactive way to involve everyone in a nutrition education lesson.

strategies. Brainstorming can be divided into two phases, for which the rules are as follows:

Phase One

- All critical judgment is ruled out; all ideas count.
- Wild ideas are expected; spontaneity, which comes when judgment is suspended, will flourish. Practical consideration is not important in this phase.
- Quantity, not quality, counts.
- Pool ideas and build on the ideas of others.

Phase Two

- Apply critical judgment—evaluate proposed ideas for feasibility.
- As a group, decide on the one or two best options if the group is interested in taking action.

Brainstorming can be useful in nutrition education for such purposes as generating a list of barriers to eating healthfully among teenagers, ways to get children to eat more healthfully, or easy meals for working mothers to prepare.

Demonstrations, Including Cooking Demonstrations

Demonstrations can serve many functions. They can be used to show how something is done. They can also serve a motivational role and help the group explore ideas and attitudes. Often they serve both functions. For example, cooking demonstrations can teach skills. At the same time, they reduce the barriers to action for the participants and thus enhance their motivation and likelihood to take action. Other demonstrations do not specifically teach skills but are designed to enhance motivation. For example, you can spoon out the amount of fat or sugar in some popular fast foods and sweetened beverages. This will mean bringing the target foods to the sessions. Consider bringing empty wrappers of the demonstration foods because the audience may want to know what you plan to do with the food after you are done. Saying you will throw it away gives the message that you are comfortable with wasting food (not an appropriate message for any audience and especially inappropriate for a low-income audience). Or they may ask if they can take it home, which of course undermines your latent message.

Conducting demonstrations means that you must have all the materials you need at the site or must bring them with you. It has often been said that a major qualification for a nutrition educator is the willingness to take materials (sometimes bulky and awkward) with you to sites, including food or food ingredients. Those with cars often find that their trunks are full. Those in inner cities using public transportation find other means. For example, one nutrition educator uses a suitcase on wheels to bring needed materials to sites: one that is large enough to include a portable butane stove plus a few needed pots and pans, utensils, paper towels, and so forth. She takes it in taxicabs and buses. A second major qualification of a nutrition educator is the willingness to be flexible, that is, to use whatever is available to make the demonstration work. For example, if you want to show how blood vessels can get clogged during a lifetime of eating high-saturated-fat foods, you may not

be able to purchase the demonstration materials. But you can buy some clear tubing in a hardware store (to serve as the blood vessel), solid cooking fat, some food coloring, a funnel, and a large bowl. You can place some of the fat in the tubing to block it partially (you do not want to block all of it), dissolve red food dye in water, and pour it through the funnel into the tube, with the large bowl ready to catch the colored water.

It is important to practice demonstrations ahead of time to know that they will work under the circumstances of your session. This is especially important for demonstrating food preparation skills.

Debates

Debates offer a lively vehicle for highlighting the two sides of an issue. There is much controversy in the area of food and nutrition, as you are aware. Instead of lecturing about the pros and cons of a given matter, have participants research each side and then go at it in the session. All learners will enjoy a good debate, but the doers—dynamic and commonsense learners—will probably prefer to do the debating, whereas the watchers will be content to sit and absorb the show. Good issues for debate might include whether to take dietary supplements, whether children should drink low-fat milk, and how to introduce healthy foods into the home.

Facilitated Group Discussion: From Sage on the Stage to Guide on the Side

Guided discussions can range considerably in the degree to which the nutrition educator exerts leadership. You may

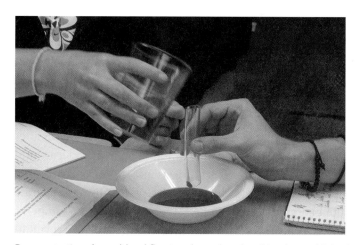
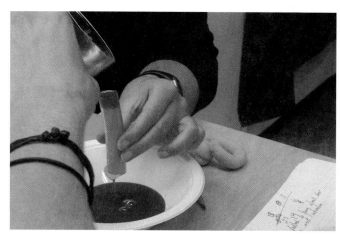

Demonstration shows blood flowing through a clear blood vessel (plastic tubing) and one clogged from unhealthy eating patterns.

Courtesy of Pamela Koch, EdD, RD.

make presentations with added activities; these would not be considered facilitated discussions. Or you may design sessions with open-ended questions and discussion but following a specific lesson plan. Or you may provide mini-lectures interspersed with guided discussion. These approaches are the most widely used and are appropriate for many group settings. There are group learning situations in which the entire session is devoted to a facilitated discussion. These adult group learning settings are described variously as *facilitated group discussions, facilitated dialogue,* or *learner-based education* (Abusabha, Peacock, and Achterberg 1999; Sigman-Grant 2004; Husing and Elfant 2005), which vary somewhat in the degree of leadership provided by the nutrition educator. This approach is described in greater detail in Chapter 17.

No matter whether the entire session is a facilitated group discussion or consists of mini-lectures interspersed with guided discussion, the role of the facilitator is to guide the group unobtrusively and to encourage interaction among members. You can do this by addressing questions posed to you by one of the group members, by saying things such as, "Do you have any reactions to that or suggestions, Maria?" You can also look away from the speaker in the group as he or she attempts to make eye contact with you. The speaker will soon get the idea that he or she should look to others for responses. A good way to increase group interaction, especially at first, is to use the following technique: tell the group that after a given person speaks, he or she will pick the next person who wishes to speak, who will then pick the next person, and so forth.

The facilitator also needs to know when and how to take control. This depends on the degree of leadership you have decided is appropriate for the given group. Although an authoritarian approach can stifle group discussion, being too uncertain, timid, or laissez-faire can make the group feel unsure of itself and undermine your authority in the group. You can retain your authority while setting up an open, safe, and democratic social climate. When the group goes off track, you can gently bring it back by saying something such as, "Those are important issues, but the issue we are addressing today is *x*."

Summary

The instructional strategies described here are effective, diverse methods that promote learning across the learning styles spectrum and address the three domains of learning. Most of them involve active participation in which group participants step beyond the role of passive sponges. Important in each of these approaches is for the nutrition educator to evaluate whether the task involves purely hands-on work or whether there is indeed a thinking, minds-on dimension serving the learning objectives that you have stated in your educational plans.

Conducting the Group Sessions: From Sequencing Instruction to Nuts and Bolts of Delivery

THE OPENER

As the group leader or facilitator, you will be sized up by the audience from the moment you enter the room. It is important that their first impressions of you are positive. You should arrive early; meet the audience as they come in; and smile, chat, and look confident whether you feel that way or not. This relaxes the audience or group and makes them want to listen to what you have to say. It also helps establish that you have an attractive, dynamic personality. When the session begins, take a moment to look at the audience, smile, and make eye contact here and there with audience members. This establishes that you are interested in the audience, not just in what you want to say.

It is important to create a safe learning environment by continuing to develop rapport with the audience through looking at them and being comfortable with them. This gives permission for the audience to ask questions and make comments, or participate in group discussion.

THE SESSION

Room Arrangements

Another reason to arrive early is to check out the physical arrangement and technology in the room. Depending on the size of the group and the physical setup of the room, you may have the opportunity to arrange the seating to encourage effective learning in that setting. Decide whether you want to rearrange the seating to be in a circle, around tables, or some other arrangement. If you will be using audiovisual materials, be sure you know how to operate the equipment you will be using. Check out the temperature settings. If you will be using flip charts or newsprint to record group responses, make sure you have the markers you need. Make sure your handouts are ready to distribute.

Your Educational Plan in Hand

It is important to create an arrangement that allows you to connect with the audience, so check out where to put your materials and educational plan notes. You could use a table on which to place your materials. What, then, to do with your educational plan with the needed notes to lead the group? You may be able to see your notes from the table, or keep them in your hand. You may find it useful to place your lesson plan sections on cards that you can hold in your hand. For a facilitated group discussion it is still important to have your educational plan visible to you.

Nervousness and Anxiety

You should never share your internal feelings of nervousness or anxiety. Others cannot see or feel your anxiety unless you bring it to their attention by saying such things as how nervous you are, how intimidating the audience seems, or that you did not have a chance to prepare. Even if asked, do not acknowledge your fright. The group wants to learn and enjoy, and a safe learning environment is established when you seem relaxed and comfortable. When audience members are aware of the leader's fragility or stage fright, they become nervous in sympathy and start worrying for you instead of focusing on your message or the activities you have planned. The best way to reduce nervousness and anxiety is to be well prepared and to rehearse your presentation ahead of time.

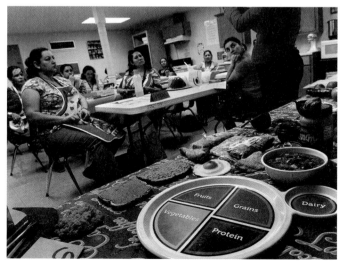

Group nutrition education using appropriate visuals can be helpful for facilitating behavior change.

© Michael S. Williamson/The Washington Post via Getty Images.

Time Management

Paying attention to how you are doing in terms of your educational plan and the time available for your presentation is crucial. However, you should find a way to monitor the time without your audience being aware of it. Looking constantly at your watch can give many unintended messages, such as that you can't wait for the session to be over or that you are afraid you are going to go over time. Place a timepiece where you can see it unobtrusively.

Language and Diction

The language you use needs to be clear, vivid, and appropriate. The audience members cannot go back to figure out something you said, as they could if they were reading a book or piece of printed material. Therefore, what you say has to be clear and understandable the first time around. Use familiar words and the active voice instead of passive voice to the extent possible. The language you use should also be appropriate to the occasion (formal or informal) and to the audience. To be effective, the words, idioms, and style of your mini-lectures or presentation must be suitable to the group, culturally appropriate, and nonsexist. The language you use should also be appropriate for you. As noted earlier, you have to be authentic to who you are; you can't be someone else—telling jokes or using hip language when these can be seen as forced and inconsistent with your personality and background. You can work out a style that is effective for you.

Your diction is also important. Your credibility with the audience is influenced by your diction. When you misarticulate words, such as saying "wanna" for "want to" or "wilya" for "will you," and mispronounce words, such as "revelant" for "relevant" or "nucular" for "nuclear," the audience may develop negative impressions of you. Likewise, the use of ums, ahs, "likes," and "you knows" between words can grate on the audience. Listen to yourself speak when you rehearse, and train yourself to speak with clear diction in settings such as these.

Voice, Volume, Pitch, and Rate of Speaking

No matter what kind of voice you were born with, you can learn to make good use of what you have to make effective group presentations or lead group sessions. Adjust your volume to the acoustics of the room. You want the individuals at the back of the room to hear you, but you do not want to shout. Your natural pitch could be high or low, but your speaking will be livelier when you vary your pitch by going up and down as you emphasize a point or ask a question. By varying your pitch (these variations are called inflections), you convey a variety of emotions and come across as dynamic, as opposed to when you speak in a monotone. Your inflections reveal whether you are being sincere or sarcastic, angry or anxious, and interested or bored. Enthusiasm about what you are saying goes a long way.

Pacing the rate (or speed) at which you speak is also important. If you speak too slowly, you may bore your audience. But if you speak too fast, the audience may not be able to keep up with your ideas. They may also get anxious because they suspect you are anxious. Indeed, people do tend to speed up when they are nervous. Pay attention to your pacing and practice a speed that seems appropriate for the audience. Pause from time to time at the end of a section for a point to sink in or for the audience to catch up with you. People need time to process information. Because your mind can go much faster than your speaking, scan the group for "feedback" as you speak. Do they appear bored or puzzled? You might adjust what you are saying to fit your feedback.

Provide Signposts and Summarize Periodically

Provide signposts as to where you are in the speech, saying, for example, "first . . . ," "second . . . ," and so on. Use signposts to emphasize important points you want to make as well. You can say things such as, "The most important thing to remember about *x* is . . ." or "Above all, you need to know . . .". Summarizing periodically is also very helpful, both in your own presentation and the group discussion. As you begin the second main point, you could summarize in one sentence the key idea of the first point before proceeding.

Nonverbal Communication

As noted previously, nonverbal communication can be as powerful as the verbal communication it accompanies. Your personal appearance, facial expressions, gestures, bodily movement, and eye contact all convey information to the audience, and you want this information to be favorable so that the audience will focus on your message and not on you.

Listeners always see speakers before they hear them. There is evidence that how a speaker dresses and is groomed affects a speaker's credibility and reception

considerably. The Madonnas and Einsteins of the world can get away with looking or wearing whatever they wish; the rest of us cannot. The main point is that you want the audience to focus on the message and activities you have designed, not on your personal appearance and grooming. So, check out the setting before you go to judge what will be appropriate to the audience and setting and to who you are. Professional but not too formal works in many settings. Remember that you will also be seen as a representative of the nutrition education profession.

When and how much to move can present a challenge. You can look for opportunities to break the invisible barrier between presenter and audience, so moving toward the audience or moving around a little can be helpful. However, pacing back and forth, fidgeting with your notes or with coins in your pocket, or playing with your hair are signs of nervousness and can be distracting. At the other end of the spectrum, standing rigidly in the same place can also signal nervousness. Pay attention to what you do, and practice coming across as confident. Saying to yourself, "I like the audience and the audience likes me" can be helpful.

What to do with your hands can be problematic. Clasp them behind your back? Put them in your pockets? Let them hang at your side? How much should you gesture? There are no rules about this, and people are all comfortable with different ways of holding their bodies and with when and how to gesture. The best way to think about this issue is that whatever you choose to do should appear natural and should not distract from your message.

Eye contact with the group helps you to establish a bond with the group. Look at individuals, not at some space between people, and move your eye contact from person to person around the entire room. Don't focus only on one side of the room or only on those who look most interested. How you look at the audience is also important—pleasantly, personally, and with sincerity. You want to convey that you are pleased to be there, that you have something important to say, and that you want them to believe that the message is important.

THE CONCLUSION: CLOSURE AND ACTION PLANNING

The conclusion of the session is extremely important. The audience needs to have a sense of closure. Its main purpose is to reinforce group participants' commitment to the main behavioral goal(s) of the session. This usually means some kind of action goal setting activity or action plan. This is probably already in the educational plan you developed in Step 5 of the DESIGN Procedure. Always allow enough time for this. Otherwise, the audience is left feeling a lack of closure and will be uncertain of what they should be doing. A strong closure contributes greatly to effectiveness of the session.

CO-LEADING GROUP SESSIONS

Often two people will be involved in leading the group session. This has many advantages: you can prepare together, and each brings special strengths. This is likely to increase the quality of the group experience. When you are co-leading, you can draw energy from each other. By interacting with each other, you are likely to be more lively and enthusiastic. In addition, many of the tasks described earlier can be shared. Thus, while one person is speaking, the other can be monitoring the audience and keeping track of time and how the content is being covered. Co-presenters can also help each other out if necessary. If one gets off track or goes blank, the other can jump in. Experienced co-leading educators have suggested the following formats for how two educators can work together (Garmston and Bailey 1988):

- *Tag team.* In the tag-team format, one person speaks and then the other does. This method is especially useful for those who do not regularly co-lead together or when there is considerable material to cover and it is easier for each person to become an expert for each segment.
- *Speak and add.* In the speak-and-add format, one person is the main educator or group facilitator and the other is the support person. The main educator is in charge of the content and decides when and how to proceed. The support person adds information when it seems useful or appropriate.
- *Speak and chart.* In the speak-and-chart format, the lead person presents content and elicits responses from the audience, and the support person records the information on newsprint or some other format. Both educators must be clear about their roles, and the support person must be able to record the ideas of the lead or the audience quickly and without comment.
- *Duet.* In the duet format, both educators are up front together and each presents content or leads discussion in small chunks of about 2 minutes each. The

presentation thus goes back and forth. The presenters stand 5–7 feet apart, but look at the audience and each other to cue each other in. They may move toward each other when they speak and move back when they are not speaking. This works best when the two people are experienced educators or have rehearsed carefully.

CASE EXAMPLE ILLUSTRATING INTEGRATION OF PSYCHOSOCIAL BEHAVIOR CHANGE THEORY AND EDUCATIONAL LEARNING AND INSTRUCTIONAL DESIGN/TEACHING THEORIES

A case example of the integration of psychosocial behavior change theory, and educational learning and instructional design theories in delivering a nutrition education session is shown in **NUTRITION EDUCATION IN ACTION 15-1**. The determinants of behavior change being addressed by each activity are shown in bold italics.

DELIVERING NUTRITION EDUCATION WORKSHOPS

The term *workshop* is used to describe many different kinds of group sessions. Usually, the term refers to some kind of professional development activity, but this is not always the case. Generally, workshops run longer than presentations or group discussions do, but not always. They also usually involve more than one leader—but again, not always. What they do have in common is that they involve active participation of the group members. Workshops usually consist of a number of the activities described earlier in this chapter: presentations, group discussions, and group activities, which will not be repeated here.

The workshop can be structured somewhat like a presentation or group discussion in the sense of having an introduction, a body, and a conclusion. The workshop usually begins with a group introductory activity or icebreaker to establish a safe environment and sense of cohesiveness. If the group is small enough, you can ask participants to state what they most want from the experience. This is then followed by an overview of the objectives of the workshop, the main issues to be covered, and expectations.

You can deliver the main body of the workshop using a variety of formats to address all of the learning styles discussed earlier. This involves a sequence proposed

NUTRITION EDUCATION IN ACTION 15-1 Case Example: Linking Educational Plan to Effective Delivery in a Nutrition Education Session

You are What You Drink: Educational Plan for After School Session with Adolescents
(based on theory of planned behavior)

Behavioral goal: Adolescent girls will replace consumption of soda and other highly sweetened beverages with increased water consumption.

General educational objectives: Adolescent girls will be able to:

- Describe the risks and costs of sweetened beverage consumption and the benefits of drinking water. (*Outcome expectations*)
- Evaluate current consumption of sweet drinks. (*Outcome expectations/self-assessment*)
- Identify barriers to decreasing consumption of sweetened drinks. (*Outcome expectations/perceived barriers*)
- Express positive attitudes toward increased water consumption. (*Attitudes*)
- State intention to reduce consumption of sweetened beverages and increase consumption of water. (*Behavioral intention*)

* Determinants from the theory of planned behavior addressed by activities are in **bold italics** below.

Educational plan for one group session derived from the behavior-focused and psychosocial theory-based DESIGN Procedure	Learning theory and instructional design theory principles from education for delivering session
1. Introduction, overview, ground rules (5 mins).	Nutrition educators look at the group with warm smiles; are dressed casually but neatly. Seating arranged around tables, name tags (safe learning environment); introduction to foster credibility and common ground; tone of voice enthusiastic, manner dynamic; title of session and what will be addressed = advance organizer (Ausubel); presentation style: duet.
Hi, I am Sarah and I am Judith. We are nutrition educators from the Health Center at NoName University and we are here today to discuss nutrition topics that are important to you based on the information you gave us when we visited you before. We are going to look at one way we can improve our health – reducing our intake of sugary drinks and increasing water consumption. We will look at why this is important and the ways to do that. We recognize how difficult it is to eat healthy, including us too, so we are really excited to be here to share what we know. We want this to be a fun and informative afternoon. Some ground rules: respect comments and opinions of others and listen, you will not be tested on the material. Session will be 90 minutes.	
	Most activities address both affective and cognitive domain learning; and target higher levels of thinking (Anderson & Krathwohl) and higher degrees of affective engagement (Krathwohl).
Excite: Gain attention	
2. Fill out worksheets: *Self-assessment* Log of beverage consumption yesterday (5 mins).	Self-assessment is motivating; activate learning principle (Merrill), concrete experience especially for imaginative learners (Kolb); active learning.
3. Demonstration of amount of sugar in drinks: *Outcome expectations/ perceived risk* (10 mins).	Perceived risk = motivational why-to information; visual and memorable; watching and reflecting especially for analytic learners. Addresses affective as well as cognitive domains.
- We brought in six different drinks that are commonly found in corner stores and that you might often choose to drink (sodas, sports drinks etc). Raise your hands if you wrote that you drank one of these drinks yesterday.	
- Ask volunteer to come up to measure amounts of sugar in each of the drinks: Then let them know the actual amount.	
Explain: Present new material	
4. Use worksheets to assess personal sugar consumption in drinks (5 mins) *Outcome expectations/ personalizing risk.*	Self-assessment compared to recommendations is motivating; personally meaningful learning (Ausubel) concrete experience; (Kolb) active learning.

5a. Brainstorm and record on newsprint health risks of high sugar beverage consumption (6 mins): Outcome expectations/ negative.	Motivational why-to information; active learning; leaders validate each comment and give on-judgmental responses and call on people by name (safe learning environment); presentation style: speak and chart.
■ Calories, dental caries, lack of nutrients such as calcium; one bottle per day = 72 pounds of extra sugar a year.	
5b. Brainstorm and record on newsprint benefits of drinking water (6 mins): *Outcome expectations/ positive.*	Motivational why-to information; active; safe learning environment (Sappington), presentation style: speak and chart.
■ Vital nutrient, hydration, no calories, good for performance during exercise, no cost, no additives.	
6. Use worksheets to assess cost of drink consumption (10 mins): *Personal norms.*	Meaningful, active learning; especially for analytic and commonsense learners.
Students use the drink log to calculate how many bottles they throw away per week, per year (300 bottles); dollar costs per week and per year Report to group.	
■ Personal norms: value cost in terms of money, chemical fallout from factories making the bottles, landfill.	
Expand: Provide guidance and practice	
7. Discuss barriers to change (10 mins): *Perceived behavioral control).*	Application (Merrill), active meaningful learning (Ausubel), good for commonsense learners (Kolb); small sub-groups for safe learning environment (Sappington); presentation style: duet.
■ Divide group into two sub-groups: those who are high-level sugar beverage consumers discuss barriers to reducing consumption and record on newsprint. Low-level consumers describe their helpful strategies. Sub-groups share with total group.	
■ Barriers to reduce sweet drinks may include: taste, caffeine addiction, habit, popular, only drink in house, normal drink.	
Exit: Apply and close	
8. Action goal-setting process (10 mins): *Behavioral intention/ implementation intentions.*	Integration principle, peer engagement (Merrill); public commitment (Lewin); safe learning environment (Sappington); presentation style: duet.
Hand-out "My Commitment" sheet, with some drink choices. Ask them to mark each goal they want to work on (commit to) in the coming week. Also, flip over the sheet to see the calendar on the back of the commitment. Use this calendar to keep track of their progress. Once the goals are chosen, sign the form showing their commitment. Have one of the others sign as a witness. Ask for people to share their action goal if they feel comfortable doing so.	
9. Distribute water bottles and instructor wrap up (5 minutes).	Nutrition educators' positive regard and respect for audience may help implementation of action goals.
Thank everyone for participating, hand out water bottles, and point out the water fountain nearby.	

in the instructional procedure—teaching around the learning cycle—described earlier in this chapter. This is the same as the 4 Es sequence of instruction. (See description in Chapter 11.) Thus, there should be exciting, concrete, hands-on experiences to open the session or self-assessments to investigate the audience's own prior knowledge, attitudes, or behaviors (Excite); mini-presentations of needed information (Explain); time for work in groups to develop skills (Expand); and opportunity to apply the skills in their professional or personal lives (Exit).

The conclusion should be carefully planned to bring a sense of closure to the workshop, to summarize what has been accomplished, and to provide an opportunity for the group members to state how they plan to use the information and skills in the future.

Summary

Working with groups is at the heart of nutrition education. This chapter describes many ways for nutrition educators to work with groups. Different methods work for different audiences, different situations, and different purposes. The aim in all cases, however, is for the method used to be effective in communicating the behavior change messages you designed in such a way that the group becomes motivated to actively contemplate your message and to take action when appropriate. Effective communication involves understanding the communication process and the factors that influence it. Working with groups requires understanding different learning styles and how best to create a safe and challenging learning environment for all. It also requires understanding group dynamics and being able to manage difficult situations. Organizing your session to reflect effective instructional design principles will help to make your session more effective. Your passion for the issues and behavior goals of your intervention, and your enthusiasm in delivering your message, will be absolutely crucial for success.

At this time, you may wish to review the educational plan(s) you designed in Step 5 of the DESIGN Procedure to see if you incorporated the principles and understandings described in this chapter on learning theory, learning styles, instructional theory, and creating environments for learning. (Step 5 is covered in Chapters 11 and 12.) Combining these approaches integrates behavioral nutrition theory, learning theory and learning styles research, group dynamics and creating safe and effective learning environments, and instructional design principles. Such an integration is likely to increase the effectiveness of your nutrition education.

Working with groups is challenging and hard work, both in planning and delivery. However, working with groups can also be very rewarding for you, the nutrition educator, and a great experience for participants and is likely to enhance their motivation and facilitate their ability to take action when the environment is safe and the learning experience is carefully planned and effectively and enthusiastically delivered.

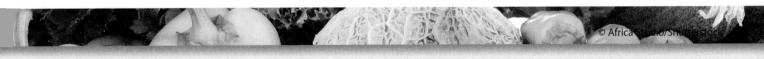

© Africa Studio/Shutterstock.

Questions and Activities

1. Think back to an occasion in a professional setting when you presented an idea for a group to consider and act on. Analyze your interaction in terms of the purpose of your communication and the effect on your listeners. Were you successful in your communication? Why or why not?

2. On a sheet of paper, create a table with two columns. Label one "Characteristics that make nutrition educators effective communicators in a group setting." Label the other one "Characteristics that make nutrition educators ineffective communicators in a group setting." In each column, list and briefly describe what you think are the five most important characteristics for that category. Candidly review your current strengths and weaknesses in terms of these characteristics. Pick three you would most like to improve.

3. Describe four learning styles that have been identified by some educators. Which kind of learning style best describes you? What can you do to make a group learning experience effective for different kinds of learners?

4. Compare and contrast the following methods for delivering nutrition education to groups: lectures, demonstrations, debates, and facilitated group discussions.

5. Review your current skills related to the methods described in the previous question: Which ones are you most comfortable using? Which would you like to become better at? How would you proceed to hone your skills in these methods?

6. List four things you could do to create a safe learning environment for a group of adults. Would you plan the

same way if the group was an after-school program made up of upper elementary school children? Explain.

7. If you were the leader of a group, how would you handle the following kinds of group members? Quiet members, complainers, those who dominate the conversation, digressers, those engaged in side conversations, and those who are consistently late.

8. What are some key features for holding the attention of a group?

9. Why is the introduction to a presentation or group session so important? What are its key components?

10. Rehearse in front of the mirror the group session you are planning to lead. What do you think you are conveying nonverbally?

11. List all the ways you can enhance your credibility as a nutrition educator when you lead a group or make a presentation.

References

Abusabha, R., J. Peacock, and C. Achterberg. 1999. How to make nutrition education more meaningful through facilitated group discussions. *Journal of the American Dietetic Association* 99:72–76.

Achterberg, C. 1988. Factors that influence learner readiness. *Journal of the American Dietetic Association* 88:1426–1428.

Anderson, L. W., and D. R. Krathwohl, editors. 2000. *A taxonomy for learning, teaching, and assessing: A revision of Bloom's taxonomy of educational objectives.* Boston: Pearson.

Ausubel, D. P. 2000. *The acquisition and retention of knowledge: a cognitive view.* New York: Springer Science+Business.

Bandura, A. 1986. *Foundations of thought and action: A social cognitive theory.* Englewood Cliffs, NJ: Prentice Hall.

———. 2004. Health promotion by social cognitive means. *Health Education and Behavior* 31(2):143–164.

Beatty, B. J. 2009. Fostering integrated learning outcomes across the domains. In *Instructional-design theories and models. Volume III. Building a common knowledge base*, edited by C. M. Reigeluth and A. A. Carr-Chellman. New York: Routledge.

Bloom, B. S., M. D. Engelhart, E. J. Furst, W. H. Hill, and D. R. Krathwohl. 1956. *Taxonomy of educational objectives. Handbook I: The cognitive domain.* New York: David McKay.

Brookfield, S. 1986. *Understanding and facilitating adult learning: A comprehensive analysis of principles and effective practices.* San Francisco: Jossey-Bass.

———. 2013. *Powerful techniques for working with adults.* San Francisco: Jossey-Bass.

Deci, E. L., and R. M. Ryan. 2008. Facilitating optimal motivation and psychological well-being across life's domains. *Canadian Psychology* 49:14–23.

Freire, P., and I. Shor. 1987. *A pedagogy for liberation: Dialogues on transforming education.* New York: Bergin and Garvey.

Gagne, R. W. 1985. *The conditions of learning and theory of instruction.* Fourth ed. New York: Holt, Rinehart, & Winston.

Gagne, R., W. W. Wager, J. M. Keller, and K. Golas. 2004. *Principles of instructional design.* Boston: Cengage.

Gardner, H. E. 2011. *Frames of mind: The theory of multiple intelligences.* New York: Basic Books.

Garmston, R., and S. Bailey. 1988. Paddling together: A co-presenting primer. *Training and Development Journal* 1:52–56.

Gillespie, A. H., and P. Yarbrough. 1984. A conceptual model for communicating nutrition. *Journal of Nutrition Education* 17:168–172.

Hermans, E. J., F. P. Battaglia, P. Atsak, L. D. de Voogd, G. Fernández, and B. Roozendaal. 2014. How the amygdala affects emotional memory by altering brain network properties. *Neurobiology of Learning and Memory* 112:2–16.

Husing, C., and M. Elfant. 2005. Finding the teacher within: A story of learner-centered education in California WIC. *Journal of Nutrition Education and Behavior* 37(Suppl. 1):S22.

Illeris, K. 2003. *Three dimensions of learning: Contemporary learning theory in the tension field between the cognitive, the emotional and the social.* Malabar, FL: Krieger.

———. 2009. The three dimensions of learning and competence development. In *Contemporary learning theories*, edited by K. Illeris. London: Routledge.

Johnson, D. W., and R. T. Johnson. 1998. *Learning together and alone: Cooperative, competitive, and individualistic learning.* Fifth ed. Englewood Cliffs, NJ: Prentice Hall.

Juster, R. P., B. S. McEwen, and S. J. Lupien. 2010. Allostatic load biomarkers of chronic stress and impact on health and cognition. *Neuroscience and Biobehavioral Reviews* 35(1):2–16.

Kinzie, M. B. 2005. Instructional design strategies for health behavior change. *Patient Education and Counseling* 56:3–15.

Knowles, M. S., E. F. Holton, and R. A. Swanson. 2011. *The adult learner: The definitive classis in adult education and human resource management development.* Seventh ed. Burlington, MA: Butterworth-Heinnemann/Elsevier.

Kohls, G., M. T Perino, J. M Taylor, E. N. Madva, S. J. Cayless, V. Troiani, et al. 2013. The nucleus accumbens is involved in both the pursuit of social reward and the avoidance of social punishment. *Neuropsychologia* 51(11):2062–2069.

Kolb, D. A. 1984. *Experiential learning.* Englewood Cliffs, NJ: Prentice Hall.

Krathwohl, D. R., B. S. Bloom, and B. B. Masia. 1964. *Taxonomy of educational objectives: The classification of educational goals. Handbook II: Affective domain*. New York: David McKay.

Lewin, K. 1935. *A dynamic theory of personality*. New York: McGraw-Hill.

———. 1943. Forces behind food habits and methods of change. In *The problem of changing food habits* (National Research Council Bulletin 108). Washington, DC: National Academy of Sciences.

———. 1947. Frontiers in group dynamics. I. Concept, method, reality in social science: Social equilibria and social change. *Human Relations* 1:5–41.

———. 1951. *Field theory in social science: Selected theoretical papers*. New York: Harper.

McCarthy, P. 2005. Touching hearts to impact lives: Harnessing the power of emotion to change behaviors. *Journal of Nutrition Education and Behavior* 37(Suppl. 1):S19.

Merrill, M. D. 2009. First principles of instruction. In *Instructional-design theories and models. Volume III. Building a common knowledge base*, edited by C. M. Reigeluth and A. A. Carr-Chellman. New York: Routledge.

Olson, C. M., and G. L. Kelly. 1989. The challenge of implementing theory-based intervention research in nutrition education. *Journal of Nutrition Education* 22:280–284.

Petty, R. E., J. Barden, and S. C. Wheeler, 2009. The elaboration likelihood model of persuasion: Developing health promotions for sustained behavioral change. In *Emerging theories in health promotion practice and research*, edited by R. J. DiClemente, R. A. Crosby, and M. C. Kegler. San Francisco: Jossey-Bass.

Petty, R. E., and J. T. Cacioppo. 1986. *Communication and persuasion: Central and peripheral routes to attitude change*. New York: Springer-Verlag.

Puig, M. V., J. Rose, R. Schmidt, and N. Freund. 2014. Dopamine modulation of learning and memory in the prefrontal cortex: Insights from studies in primates, rodents, and birds. *Frontiers in Neural Circuits* 8.

Reigeluth, C. M., and A. A. Carr-Chellman. 2009. Understanding instructional-design theory. In *Instructional-design theories and models. Volume III. Building a common knowledge base*, edited by C. M. Reigeluth and A. A. Carr-Chellman. New York: Routledge.

Rogers, C. 1969. *Freedom to learn*. Columbus, OH: Merrill.

Salamone, J. D., and M. Correa. 2002. Motivational views of reinforcement: Implications for understanding the behavioral functions of nucleus accumbens dopamine. *Behavioral Brain Research* 137:3–15.

Sappington, T. E. 1984. Creating learning environments conducive to change: The role of fear/safety in the adult learning process. In *Innovative higher education*. New York: Human Services Press.

Schunk, D. H. 2011. *Learning theories: An educational perspective*. Sixth ed. Boston, MA: Allyn and Bacon/Pearson Education.

Sigman-Grant, M. 2004. *Facilitated dialogue basics: A self-study guide for nutrition educators—Let's dance*. University of Nevada, Cooperative Extension, NV.

Sternberg, R. J. 1985. *Beyond I.Q.: A triarchic theory of human intelligence*. Cambridge, UK: Cambridge University Press.

Vella, J. 2002. *Learning to listen, learning to teach: The power of dialogue in educating adults*. Hoboken, NJ: Jossey-Bass.

Waeiti, O., A. Dickinson, and W. Schultz. 2001. Dopamine responses comply with basics assumptions of formal learning theory. *Nature* 412:43–48.

Waring, M., and C. Evans. 2014. *Understanding pedagogy: Developing a critical approach to teaching and learning*. London: Routledge.

CHAPTER 16

Media Supports and Other Channels for Nutrition Education

OVERVIEW

This chapter provides an overview of the various kinds of media that can be used to support group education, such as visuals, written materials, videos, and Web-based online images. This chapter also describes how indirect nutrition education can be delivered through various channels such as printed materials, telephone, email, digital devices and social media, mass media strategies, and social marketing activities.

CHAPTER OUTLINE

- Introduction
- Using supporting visuals in group sessions and oral presentations
- Developing and using written materials
- Educational activities using a variety of channels
- Mass media and social marketing activities
- Using new technologies
- Summary

LEARNING OBJECTIVES

At the end of the chapter, you should be able to:

- Apply design principles for developing supporting visuals for group sessions and oral presentations, and state guidelines for their use
- Develop appropriately written materials for use in nutrition education
- Describe how to deliver nutrition education through activities such as cooking, supermarket tours, and health fairs
- Understand key principles of health communications and social marketing
- Implement nutrition education social marketing activities as a member of a team
- Describe the use of newer technologies for nutrition education using the Internet and digital and social media venues

Introduction

A nutrition educator has been asked to speak to a class of teenagers about healthy eating. Based on her assessments, she decides that sugar intake will be the behavioral focus. She begins the session by showing the group a number of sweetened drinks familiar to this audience of varying sizes: regular soda, energy drinks, sports drinks, sweetened teas, and fruit drinks. She asks them to estimate how many teaspoons of sugar are present in each drink. She does this as follows. Using a teaspoon, she asks a volunteer to begin to spoon out sugar from a container she brought into a clear plastic cup until the audience tells the volunteer to stop. There are gasps in the group when they see how much sugar is present in their favorite drinks.

An old saying tells that one picture is worth a thousand words. People understand what speakers say, find it more interesting, and remember more when visual and other media are used in addition to the verbal message. However, as noted earlier, people remember only about 20% of what they hear and about 50% of what they see and hear, while they remember as much as about 90% when they are actively involved in talking about it as they do something. Today's audiences have grown up in the television and computer ages and are used to obtaining information visually as well as orally or in text form. About 99% of households have a television, and adults spend an average of 20 hours per week watching. Some four out of five households have computers and spend several hours each day using them, particularly young people. People browse the Internet, watch videos, and see advertising when online or on billboards. They are used to being bombarded with information and persuasion from a variety of high-quality media sources. These media affect all age groups.

Using visual aids and written supporting materials with presentations or group discussions is thus important for nutrition education. These supporting media might include slides, real objects such as food packages, handouts, online videos or images, or other materials. When the supporting materials are of high quality, they will enhance your credibility, make you seem more prepared, and enhance the effectiveness of your message. Supporting visual media are especially important for low-income groups who may have limited reading ability and for those whose first language is not English. When real foods are used and tasted, the addition of other senses, such as sight and touch, as well as smell and taste, enhances the message.

Channels other than group sessions can also be important for delivering nutrition education messages, such as health fairs, newsletters through worksites or community organizations, billboards, **social marketing** media campaigns, social media, or Web-based interventions. These channels are becoming increasingly important as people have less and less time to attend group sessions.

This chapter describes the use of visual and written media as supporting aids for group sessions as well as the use of other channels to deliver supporting nutrition education for the group intervention. These can be used in conjunction with the group-based educational intervention that you developed through the DESIGN Procedure in Chapters 7–13 and as part of the environmental supports intervention you developed in the DESIGN Procedure in Chapter 14.

Using Supporting Visuals in Group Sessions and Oral Presentations

Humans are visual creatures. When news stories on television or smartphones about events such as tsunamis, hurricanes, or earthquakes are accompanied by visual images, particularly those showing the suffering of individuals, the impact is dramatic. Often before the news program is over, relief organizations are deluged by calls from viewers wanting to make a donation.

Using supporting visuals or visual aids in nutrition education has many advantages, chief among them being that they make your message clearer and more lively. You can outline the main points on your visual (e.g., slide, flip chart), and thus help the audience or group follow the key messages you wish to convey. Or you can show real objects or pictures, or present a graph of the statistics that you are quoting. These will make the message more vivid. Using supporting visuals also stimulates interest. And, of course, your audience will be more likely to remember your message. In the scenario at the beginning of the chapter, the teens will be more likely to remember how much sugar is in some common beverages because of the demonstration, and this may help them in their drink choices. The next subsection discusses various visual media that you can use. Consider the following questions as you choose which to use:

- Who is the audience? What kinds of visual media are most appropriate for this audience? For example, a low-literacy audience may need different kinds of visuals than a highly educated audience.

- What does the audience prefer?
- What is the setting? Will you be in the front of a long room in which people in the back will be able to see slides but not real objects such as foods?
- What is the size of the audience—10, 25, 50, or 100 or more? Some visuals, such as food models, work well only with a small audience, whereas others, such as slides, can work with larger audiences.
- What equipment is available in the room?
- What length of time do you have? What kinds of visuals will fit into that time frame? For example, a DVD may take too long, but you could use excerpts.
- How much time do you have to prepare the visuals?
- What skills do you have to develop the visuals that you need? Can someone else assist you? Or are the needed visuals already available?

TYPES OF SUPPORTING VISUALS

You can use a variety of visuals to support and reinforce your message, ranging from real foods to slides.

Real Objects: Foods and Packages

Showing real foods or packages can have a dramatic impact and make your behavioral goals clearer. For example, a session on the importance of eating a variety of fruits and vegetables can begin with bringing in an array of differently colored fruits and vegetables and asking the audience if they can identify them or have tasted them. You can also bring in a variety of packaged food products for a session on label reading or as examples of highly processed packaged snacks to eat less of. Or you can bring in a variety of foods from the farmers' market to show foods from local sources. Real objects are especially useful for showing portion sizes of different items, such as sodas or small, medium, and large sizes of movie-theater popcorn.

It is best to bring in empty packages and containers (such as empty soda cans and popcorn buckets), particularly for the less healthful items: they are easier to carry, you do not have to worry about the foods perishing, and you do not have to decide what to do when individuals want to take the items home! To avoid distraction for the audience, it is best to keep these kinds of visuals out of sight until you are ready to show them. It is also useful to bring in cups and measuring spoons if you want to show serving sizes of foods.

- *Advantages:* Realistic; dramatic; enhances motivation; improves understanding of the message and increases retention. Objects and packages are portable.
- *Disadvantages:* Some foods are perishable; not suitable for groups larger than 15–20 members.

Models of Foods and Other Nutrition-Related Objects

Models of foods are actual-sized, realistic, three-dimensional models made of plastic or rubber. They are especially useful for showing the sizes of servings of foods recommended by dietary guidelines and for foods that are perishable, such as meats (e.g., hamburger, chicken). Other kinds of models can also be used, such as models of the heart or of clogged arteries.

- *Advantages:* Food models are realistic, portable, and can show actual portion sizes of foods. Other models can be selected to illustrate complex organs or processes.
- *Disadvantages:* Cannot be seen in groups larger than 15–20 members.

Poster Boards

For many settings, there may be no facilities for hanging or projecting visuals, such as in a gym or lunchroom. Poster boards prepared ahead of time can be very effective. Pictures from magazines or empty packages of various kinds of food items can be mounted onto poster boards for display. You may also be able to glue on pockets, in which you can place various pictures or cards of items that you can pull out to show as you need. You can also display pie charts, bar graphs, and line graphs. You may develop a collection of these poster boards to use for sessions focusing on different behaviors.

How exactly to keep poster boards standing presents a challenge that must be resolved before the occasion. A sturdy grade of poster board or foamcore and a method to keep it standing can be devised, such as on tables, chairs, or propped up against the walls.

- *Advantages:* Inexpensive; portable; very helpful when there is not much equipment in the room.
- *Disadvantages:* Fragile when carried; limited amount of information; cannot be used with large groups; can get worn with repeated use.

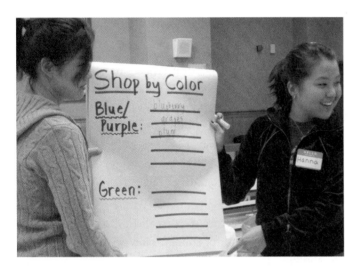

Flip charts are an inexpensive and easy way to engage your audience.

Courtesy of Program in Nutrition, Teachers College Columbia University.

Flip Charts

A flip chart with a display easel is very useful in a setting without much equipment. Flip charts consist of large pads of newsprint sheets that are fastened or glued together at the top. Write on the newsprint with crayon or felt-tip pens that do not bleed through the paper. Use a dark-colored pen, and write large enough for everyone in the group to read. You can prepare the sheets ahead of time to contain graphs, pie charts, written outlines, clip art, and so forth. Each sheet is flipped over at the top when you have finished showing the information. Flip charts are particularly useful for group brainstorming activities. The ideas can be recorded and then the sheets torn off and attached to a wall or blackboard for all to see. The sheets can also be taken away after the meeting. Use of different-colored pens can be very helpful.

- *Advantages:* Inexpensive; prepared flip charts can be reused from group to group; appropriate in informal settings such as senior centers or community programs where there is no equipment or suitable space for other visuals; audience friendly, particularly when information is being collected from the group; information collected during the session can be preserved.
- *Disadvantages:* Cannot be seen in groups larger than 20–25 members; inconvenient to carry; requires someone to write clearly and quickly if it is being used to capture ideas of a group; prepared flip charts can get worn with repeated use.

Chalkboard

The chalkboard, too, can serve as a visual aid. It can be very useful if you write legibly and large enough for all to see and can spell well. However, it is important not to turn your back to the audience and talk to the board. It also takes time to write on the board, so you need to practice talking and writing at the same time, while facing the audience as much as possible during the process.

- *Advantages:* Inexpensive; easy to use; may be all that is available in certain settings.
- *Disadvantages:* Presenter often talks to the board; takes time to write material; poor handwriting reduces effectiveness.

Slides (PowerPoint, Freelance, Persuasion, Presentation)

Increasingly, those making presentations or working with groups use computer software programs to create images involving just about everything from text to graphs, charts, and tables (**FIGURE 16-1**). Photographs can also be scanned in with high fidelity. There are ways to include animation, sound, and video clips, allowing for multimedia presentations. The images are sharp and multicolored and can be made any size you need. The presentation can be printed out on paper and used as a handout at the beginning of the session for the audience to follow along or distributed at the end as reinforcement.

It is best to use colors and graphics on the slides that can be seen without turning off the lights. This usually means dark letters on a light background, not the white letters on blue background often used in nutrition or medical professional updates. This helps you maintain contact with the audience. Make the slides visually compelling (**FIGURE 16-2**)—use of high technology does not automatically make a presentation interesting. Most programs now offer many design templates to choose from, and you should exploit these options.

It takes considerable time to learn how to use the software; design the text, graphs, and charts; import images from other sources; and organize all these in a way that is appropriate. Give yourself plenty of time to create the visuals. Arrive early and run through your presentation before the audience or group arrives. In addition, always carry a backup mini-drive. If you have printed out your slides as handouts, you can use the handouts as the basis of your talk if the equipment fails. Finally, be prepared to give your presentation or conduct the group session without the slides if you have to.

- *Advantages:* PowerPoint-type slides provide high-quality lettering, charts, and graphics. Careful use of

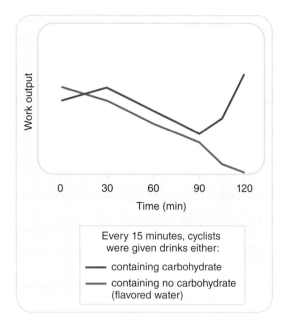

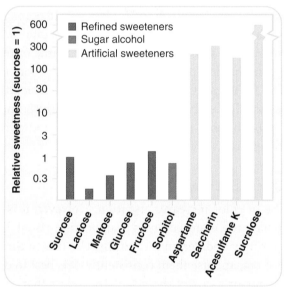

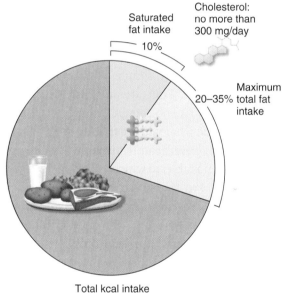

FIGURE 16-1 Example of effective line chart, bar graph, and pie chart presentations.

color and animation can enhance motivation. Your presentation can be saved to a mini-drive and easily transported from your home or office to the place of the group session. Slides are relatively easy to create once you have learned the program.

■ *Disadvantages:* The necessary equipment is expensive and not always available in field settings for nutrition education such as senior centers, after-school settings, or community group education, whether in high-income or low-income countries. Use of slides can distance you from the audience, especially when the room is dark and you cannot see the audience. It is easy to put too much information on a slide.

DESIGN PRINCIPLES FOR PREPARING SUPPORTING VISUALS

You have probably experienced the presenter who begins a presentation by saying, "I know that you can't read this, but . . .". You wonder why the presenter even bothered with the supporting visual! Whatever the form of the supporting visuals you are preparing, following certain guidelines will help you make them effective (Smith and Alford 1989; Knight and Probart 1992; Raines and Williamson 1995). Public speaking expert Lucas (2011) provides useful guidelines that have been adapted here for use in nutrition education.

Two Great Ways to Get More Healthy!

Make half your plate fruits and vegetables

To help manage your weight and prevent diseases such as cancer, heart disease and type 2 diabetes.

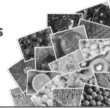

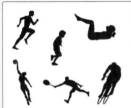

Do physical activity everyday

To help your body stay toned, increase energy level, improve concentraion, and prevent chronic diseases.

FIGURE 16-2 Example of effective slide presentation.

Courtesy of Pamela Koch, EdD, RD.

Clear and Simple Supporting Visuals

Supporting visuals should be simple, clear, and directly relevant to your message. They are aids, not the centerpiece. Use only as many real objects and models as are necessary to help visualize what you are talking about. Make slides, flip charts, and overhead transparencies concise; use the fewest words possible, to which you will add as you speak. Thus, the visual will contain much less information than you will actually present: it should not be something that you will read word for word and say nothing else. Each slide or overhead should present only one idea or one set of ideas. It is suggested that the number of words be limited to between 20 and 36. Some have recommended "the rule of six," which is to use no more than six lines of text and no more than six words per line (Raines and Williamson 1995). This may be overly restrictive, but the principle is not to load the slide with information from margin to margin.

Reproductions of tables and graphs from journal articles or books are rarely effective. Such tables are meant to be studied at the reader's leisure while being held about a foot or so away. They cannot be processed and understood in the few seconds available during a presentation or group session, particularly for low-literacy audiences. Unless you are presenting to a professional audience, simplify the tables and graphs and render them boldly so that they can be understood quickly, as shown here for the line and bar graphs and pie charts.

Computer software programs provide numerous different background formats from which to select. However, use simple designs only. When you make supporting visuals too busy or complicated or you put too much information on them, you are more likely to confuse your group than enlighten them.

Supporting Visuals Large Enough for the Audience to See

Presenters often have the urge to put a lot of information on the supporting visuals and hence to make the information too small. Remember, though, that if no one can see it, it is not only useless, but also may provoke annoyance from the audience.

For computer-generated slides, use font sizes that can be read from the back of the room when projected. It is recommended that for titles you use font sizes of 36 points; for subtitles, 24 points; and for the text, 18 points. Making fonts bold may increase readability. Capital letters are suitable for short titles of five to six words or fewer, but a combination of capital and lowercase letters is preferable for longer titles. All caps are more difficult to read, especially for those of lower literacy (Smith and Alford 1989). Number lists or use bullets, and underline words for emphasis. Keep paragraphs short.

Choice of Colors

Use of color increases attention. However, it is possible to have too many colors in a supporting visual. Use color sparingly and design it carefully. Use one to three colors at most, and use them consistently. It is best to decide on the major focus of the visual and select that color first. An effective practice is to select dark lettering or print on a light background. Some argue for using a dark background, particularly dark blue. In this case the graphics and lettering should be larger and white, or some strongly contrasting, bright color such as yellow. Do not use black on blue. The biggest danger in using a dark background is that the lettering and graphics may not be bright enough to see. In addition, a dark background usually requires that the room lights be dimmed, which means you lose touch with your audience.

Appropriate Fonts

Most computers come with dozens, if not hundreds, of different fonts or typefaces that you can use. It is best to choose those that are simple and easy to read. Also, limit the number of different fonts you use in any given presentation. For example, use a squarer font in capitals for the title and a rounder font for the text. The rounder fonts are usually called serif because they have little feet. The squarer typefaces are called sans (from the French meaning "without") serif, or without feet. A third style is called decorative and includes all those that do not belong in the other two categories.

The following list presents some common fonts and their appropriateness.

More Effective	Less Effective
Times or Times New Roman (serif)	*Lucinda Handwriting*
Arial (sans serif)	Harrington
Helvetica (sans serif)	Chalkboard

GUIDELINES FOR USING SUPPORTING VISUALS WITH AN AUDIENCE

Having selected or designed your supporting visuals with care, you need to give careful consideration to how you will use them when you are with your group. You want to ensure that you use them effectively to get your message across.

Ensure That Your Audience Will Be Able to See Your Visuals

When you plan on using visuals such as poster boards, be sure to arrive early so that you can identify where to place them so that everyone can see. Will you have access to easels? If not, where can you place your visuals so that they will not fall over? If you are using objects, where can you place them so that everyone in the audience can see? If you are using slides or overheads, do not stand in front of them and block the vision of the audience.

Show Your Supporting Visuals at the Appropriate Time

If you are using real objects such as food, food models, or food packages, do not show them to the audience until you are talking about them with the group. Leave them in cardboard boxes or bags until you are ready, or cover them up if you need to place them on a table in front of the audience. The same is true of poster boards or flip charts.

Ensure that a blank sheet or a sheet with the title of the session is facing the audience as they come in. Likewise, for slides and transparencies, use a title slide as the audience or group enters, and introduce a blank (for slides) or cover up a transparency when you are not using the visuals. When you are finished, cover them up or put them away in order not to distract the audience.

Maintain Contact with Your Audience at All Times

When you use overhead transparencies, slides, or poster boards, you might often find yourself facing the visuals and not your audience. Be sure you only glance at the visuals and continue talking to your audience so that you maintain eye contact with them.

Use Handouts and Materials Appropriately

You may have only one visual, such as a photo or object that you want to pass around while you speak. However, doing so will cause you to lose the attention of those who currently have the object in their hand and are looking at it, and distract all the others who are wondering about it. In most settings, it is best to pass out materials such as handouts at the end. If you make handouts for everyone and wish to hand them out at various times, do so at strategic points and allow time for all individuals to receive them before proceeding. Recognize, however, that these actions may be distracting.

Developing and Using Written Materials

Written materials in this context refers to short printed pieces such as handouts, flyers, brochures, tip sheets, booklets, and recipes that will be used with your intended nutrition education audience. Printed materials have many advantages compared with the other media described so far. Printed materials can be kept. Whereas messages in the visual media fly by, people can read and digest printed information at their own pace and refer back to it over time. Printed media can provide information that can be read in private. Many individuals may be reluctant to ask questions in a group setting or to discuss issues they have. However, they may be eager to receive information provided in handouts or brochures that they can take home. And, of course, printed materials can reinforce information discussed in a group setting or provided in a presentation.

The design of written materials should involve similar considerations to those of the six-step DESIGN Procedure used to design the group intervention itself. Many of the guidelines described earlier for designing supporting visuals apply to supporting printed pieces as well. This section highlights guidelines that may be useful for nutrition educators who are developing simple supportive materials. The advent of desktop publishing makes it possible for most people to develop and design a variety of materials that are pleasing to the eye and of good quality. However, the services of a graphic designer, professional writer, or editor may be necessary to ensure high quality in the design and readability of written materials.

PLANNING THE PRINTED PIECE

The effectiveness of printed materials is improved if you have clear answers for the following questions for each printed piece:

- *What is the primary purpose for each printed piece?* If you could accomplish just one goal, what would it be? Is this a promotional piece designed to generate interest in the group program, or is it an information piece that will be used in conjunction with the program? You should be able to say, "The primary purpose of this flyer is to get people to come to the group nutrition education session" or "The purpose of this poster is to make eating a variety of colors of fruits and vegetables seem cool to teens." In other words, is the purpose to enhance motivation to take action and activate decision making (why-to information), or is the material to be used to reinforce the session by providing food and nutrition information that facilitates skills acquisition (how-to information), or is it some combination of both? Which personal determinants of behavior change are addressed? In the example just given with teens, the purpose is to enhance motivation by addressing social norms, a primary theory construct in both social cognitive theory and theory of planned behavior.
- *What are the secondary purposes?* A printed piece usually has more than one goal. However, when you try to accomplish several goals, you risk not accomplishing any of them very well. So, think carefully

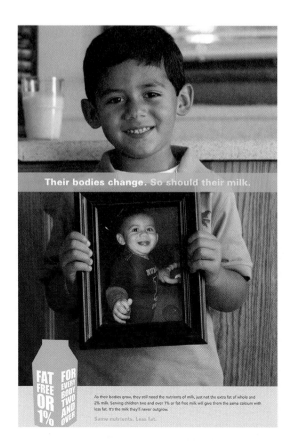

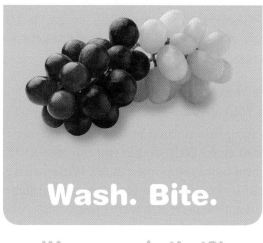

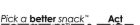

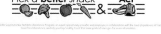

FIGURE 16-3 Two posters with highly visual, clear messages directed at parents (top, to serve low-fat and non-fat milk to children over the age of 2; bottom, to encourage children to eat fruits and vegetables by example).

Courtesy of Iowa Department of Public Health.

about which goal is your primary purpose and which purposes are secondary. If you have a secondary purpose, you may want to consider a format that makes this clear—perhaps by using smaller lettering or positioning it lower on the page. Remember that there are also unstated purposes, which are the impressions you want people to get from reading your printed piece. Posters for teens hung up or placed in the cafeteria, for example, may indicate that the school is concerned about teens' health and welfare. A common unstated purpose is for a printed piece to help the reader see you as professional and credible or to see your organization or agency as a leader in the field.

■ *What actions or behaviors do you want the audience to take?* What do you want individuals to do as a result of reading your piece? Individuals are more likely to take action if you lay out specific suggestions for what actions they can take. For example, in a brochure on cancer risk prevention, do you want the individuals to go to a medical facility to get screened? Then spell out how to do so. Do you want them to eat more fruits and vegetables? Then say so and tell them how to do so. Is your piece a policy document about actions a school can take to ensure a healthy school food environment? Then spell out what a school can do. What would you like the audience to do with the printed piece itself? Pass it on? Then say so. Put it on the refrigerator door or on a bulletin board? Say so.

■ *How will the printed piece be used?* Will the piece be used only in conjunction with the group intervention? Will it be used during the session and/or taken home? Or should it be able to stand alone?

■ *Who is the intended audience?* What is their background in terms of cultural or religious traditions? What is their age, sex, or educational level that might influence the nature and design of the piece? For example, individuals with low literacy skills will require different approaches than those with high levels of education. What does the intended audience prefer in terms of types of content and layout? A good needs analysis is extremely important here.

■ *What length do you need?* A common urge is to want to tell the audience everything in one printed piece. However it is important to be selective. Do you have enough to say to require a booklet, or will a brochure do? Will a flyer do instead of a poster? If you have too much information for one printed piece, consider breaking up the information into several different handouts, flyers, or brochures. Realize that with the advent of the Internet, attention spans for reading are getting shorter and shorter.

■ *What resources are available for this project?* The most frequently required resources are time, energy, and money. Needing a piece of printed material by a certain date will influence the nature of what you will be able to generate and produce. So, think through carefully what you are able to do given your time. Perhaps someone else can work on it or at least help you with it. Finally, most nutrition educators work with limited budgets. This calls for creativity and careful thinking. Perhaps instead of a poster, you could use a flyer, or perhaps a lighter weight paper will do.

■ *How will you evaluate the effectiveness of these materials?* It is important to obtain feedback on the materials, if not from written evaluation forms, then from asking the recipients of the materials. You may also discuss with other members of your team such questions as the following: Did the printed pieces fulfill their purpose? What did the readers learn from them? How much time, effort, and money did it take to produce them? Was it worth it? How can they be improved?

MAKING YOUR PRINTED MATERIALS MOTIVATING AND EFFECTIVE

You want your printed pieces to be effective with your audience. Some suggestions follow.

Tailor the Piece to Your Audience

Your audience will be more interested in your printed materials if they can immediately see that the information is relevant to them. This means that you need to know your audience well. A careful assessment, as outlined in Steps 1 and 2 of the Stepwise Procedure model for designing nutrition education, can provide you the information you need. This procedure is described in Chapters 7 and 8. In particular, you need to know the audience's food- and nutrition-related knowledge, their attitudes and values in relation to the issue in your printed material, their living situation, their cultural traditions and expectations, what magazines they read and what visual media they watch, and what their tastes are in terms of written materials.

Make the Writing Motivational and Reader-Friendly

Start with an Attention Grabber

It is important to gain and hold the attention of your readers just as you plan to do when designing educational plans or presentations for a live audience. Several ways to do this are by beginning your printed piece with one of the following:

- *An interesting anecdote or personal story.* Preferably, you should choose a story about someone similar to the audience and involving a situation familiar to them. "As a group of teens entered the school cafeteria last week, they were surprised to discover it had had a complete makeover and looked very cool."
- *A surprising fact or startling statistic.* "The rate of obesity is increasing. At current rates, all individuals in the United States will be overweight by the year *x*."
- *An intriguing question.* "Did you know that it has been estimated that one in three children today will develop diabetes during their lifetime?"
- *A checklist.* Create a checklist of foods or food-related behaviors addressed by the printed piece, such as a list of high-fat foods and fruits and vegetables. Ask readers to check off whether they eat them on most days. Come up with a score and tell them to read the rest of the printed material to learn how to eat a healthier diet.
- *A quiz.* Beginning with "Can you name five vegetables that are red or purple in color?" is likely to engage your readers.

Motivate the Reader

You are very interested in food, nutrition, and health, but you can't assume that the reader shares your enthusiasm! Describe the importance of the issue you are addressing, such as eating school meals. List the benefits of the actions you are writing about, such as eating breakfast or calcium-rich foods. Make clear to readers what is in this for them. Again, your needs assessment information from Step 2 is important here.

Put Important Information First

Assume that the reader will read just the first sentence, the first paragraph, or the first page. So place the most important information first rather than burying it in the middle of the document. Avoid lengthy introductions and long explanations at the beginning.

Be Simple and Direct

You are not writing a novel or poem. You are trying to communicate with the reader about important food- and nutrition-related information. So write simply and directly. To do this, consider the following tips:

- *Keep the words simple.* The field of nutrition is full of technical terms, and nutrition educators often use them when simple ones will do. Often the simplest words have the fewest syllables. For example, use *better* instead of *more advantageous,* and *use* instead of *utilize.*
- *Use the active voice rather than passive voice.* Active voice makes the writing more personal and lively. For example, instead of "The participants in our program will be provided with handouts," say "We will provide you with handouts."
- *Write strong sentences.* Vary the length of sentences, but generally keep them short. Varying the length of sentences changes the pace for readers and makes the writing more interesting. However, you should express only one idea per sentence. Long and complex sentences are difficult to understand and may discourage people, particularly those with low literacy, from reading. Aim for about 9 to 10 sentences per 100 words.
- *Keep paragraphs focused.* Begin sentences with the main topic. For example, say, "Watching your weight is very important when you have diabetes," rather than "When you learn that you have diabetes, it is important for you to watch your weight." Begin each paragraph with the topic sentence and keep the paragraph to one key idea or theme.
- *Aim for the right reading level.* Determine the appropriate reading level for your audience. In the United States, it may be best to aim for the fifth-grade reading level for most general printed pieces, and the third-grade level for low-literacy audiences. Computer programs will now provide information on the reading level, or readability scores, for the document you are writing. You can also calculate the **SMOG (Simple Measure of Gobbledygook)** score as follows: Take 10 sentences each from the beginning, middle, and last paragraphs of the document, then count how many words in these 30 sentences have three or more syllables (polysyllabic words). Look up the approximate grade level in **TABLE 16-1**. Readability is also influenced by concept density, so keep each paragraph to only one concept or message.

Table 16-1 Calculating Reading Levels: SMOG Conversion Table

Total Number of Words with Three or More Syllables	Approximate Grade Level (± 1.5 grades)
0–2	4
3–6	5
7–12	6
13–20	7
21–30	8
31–42	9
43–56	10
57–72	11
73–90	12
91–110	13
111–132	14
133–156	15
157–182	16
183–210	17
211–240	18

Data from McLaughlin, G. H. 1969. SMOG grading: A new readability formula. *Journal of Reading* 12:639–646.

- *Be professional and accurate.* Writing can take on many different styles, from humorous to chatty to serious. Regardless of style, use a professional tone in your writing. Being concise, clear, and readable will increase your credibility. Make sure your information is accurate.
- *Use a positive tone.* This does not mean you should be a Pollyanna. You know only too well that the news in the area of foods and nutrition is often dire. It means speaking to your readers in a respectful and positive manner. Being negative or condescending does not help you communicate your message.
- *Be consistent in your vocabulary, particularly for technical information.* For example, use hypertension or high blood pressure, but not both interchangeably.

Design Considerations

Make the written material look easy to read. The following tips can help:

- *Keep the document as short as you can.* If you say too much, the piece ends up looking crowded and difficult to read—and so it is not read.

- *Use more headings and keep them simple.* Break up the piece with more headlines and make them vivid and informative. This way, the reader who only skims the piece will get something out of it. Rather than "Introduction," use "An Overview of the Senior Program." Instead of "Picky Eaters," use "Ways to Handle Picky Eaters."
- *Use more paragraphs and make them shorter.* Short paragraphs make for easier reading, especially in brochures and flyers. Long paragraphs make the page look dense and may discourage readers.
- *Include adequate white (empty) space.* Many educators think of white space between paragraphs or in large margins as wasted space, waiting to be filled. However, it has been found that having adequate white space makes a piece easier to read. It is better to sacrifice some text than to have no white space.
- *Divide wide columns of text into two narrower columns for easier reading.* Lines that are too long strain the eye and make readers lose track of the content, whereas lines that are too short cause the eye to jump back and forth. A line length of 50 to 70 characters, as used in this text, is best because it is less tiring to the eye.
- *Make text left justified with a ragged right margin.* Left-justified text with a ragged right margin is easier to read because the ragged right profile helps the eye distinguish one line from the next. Full justification (lines that go to the same left and right margins) is difficult to read because it is hard to distinguish the lines and the eye has to adjust to different spacing between letters. Indenting the paragraphs is also important.
- *Use a simple font, especially with low-literacy audiences.* As emphasized earlier for designing visuals, using simple fonts and adequate font sizes can help the reader, particularly low-literacy audiences. Remember also that all capital letters are more difficult to read.
- *Use bullets where appropriate.* Bullets are useful when the information lends itself to a list. Tips, procedures, and things to do can all be listed with bullets. Bulleted lists break up the text and make brochures, handouts, and tip sheets easier to read.

FIGURE 16-4 shows a newsletter from the Iowa Fresh Conversations program of the Iowa Nutrition Network implemented with seniors. You can see that it exemplifies many of the tips described here: the objective is clear—a motivational piece about the benefits of snacking,

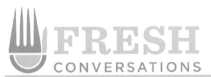

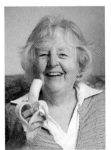

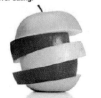

The Unexpected Benefits of
SNACKING!

Daily snacking is so common that we are just about eating one continuous meal a day! In fact only about four percent of Americans do not eat snacks. Smart snacking can be a great addition to our meal plans.

Healthy Snacks Rule

If you are likely to choose fruit for a snack you are part of a health trend to 'pick a better snack'. Fresh fruit is not only the most frequently consumed snack in the country (this a welcome surprise), it's also one of the fastest-growing snacks in popularity. Let's give that a big cheer! Americans on average ate fresh fruit as a snack more often than chocolate or potato chips. When you choose to eat healthy snacks you are taking control of your health.[1]

Snacking may provide as much as 25% of the calories you eat daily, making snacks as important as any meal you eat Just like the foods you choose for a meal, snacks help you reach the recommended servings of fruits, vegetables, whole grains, dairy and lean protein. Healthy snacking may keep you from being too hungry and over eating.

The BEST SNACKS come from whole foods like fresh, canned or dried fruits and vegetables, low-fat yogurt, low-fat cheese sticks, whole grain crackers, or nuts.

[1] Source: http://nm.com/ehall0386-hotstudy-fruit-america-c-favorite-snack

Snacking—A Balancing Act

Ideally, snacks are a nutritious bridge to the next meal. The key is to make sure that our bodies are not getting more calorie than needed. A way to do this is to aim for eating a 100 to 150 calories snack two to three hours after a meal.

FIGURE 16-4 Example of good printed material: Newsletter for older adults.

Courtesy of Iowa Department of Public Health.

accompanied by tips (i.e., involving both why-to and how-to information); it is very visually appealing, using a realistic photo of someone similar to the target audience expressing enjoyment; the text is written in several columns; it uses short paragraphs; headings and text fonts differ in size and color; and literacy level is appropriate, with few words over three syllables.

A Caution

Those working in programs for low-income families such as Head Start and Expanded Food and Nutrition Education Program (EFNEP) in the United States have found that participants do not judge all program activities to be equally enjoyable or effective. Tips can be found in **BOX 16-1**.

Educational Activities Using a Variety of Channels

Nutrition educators engage in many activities in addition to conducting discussion groups, making presentations, and developing supporting written and visual materials. These include such activities as organizing health fairs and grocery store tours and conducting cooking classes. For all of these activities, plan ahead using the principles and procedures outlined in the DESIGN Procedure described for group sessions. These principles and procedures are described in Part II of this book.

PLANNING THE ACTIVITY

The effectiveness of these activities is improved if you are clear about the following:

- *What is the specific purpose of the activity?* The educational objectives of the activity should be clear. You should be able to say: "The purpose of this activity is to teach skills in food selection (or in cooking) so that the audience is able to follow the behavioral change goals of the intervention." In other words, is the purpose to enhance motivation to take action and activate decision making (emphasizing why-to take action) or is it to provide food and nutrition information and facilitate skills acquisition for those already motivated (emphasizing how-to take action), or is it some combination of both? What theoretical framework is being used? Which personal determinants of behavior change will you address?

- *What actions or behaviors do you want the audience to take?* Is the behavioral outcome of the activity, such as a health fair, for the audience to become aware of and attend the full program you are offering? Is it a freestanding educational activity with specific behavioral goals? An example may be that you organize a health fair at which participants can be screened physiologically for a condition, such as blood pressure or percent body fat, or screened using a behavioral checklist, such as for their intake of fruits and vegetables. This screening may be followed by handouts about what to do. Thus, spell out clearly what you wish the action outcomes to be for the activity.

BOX 16-1 **Helping Low-Income Consumers Achieve the Goal to Eat More Fruits and Vegetables: Tips for Nutrition Educators**

More Effective and Enjoyable Ways to Promote Fruit and Vegetable Consumption

Taste Testing and Cooking

- Provide tasters with the recipe and demonstrate the preparation steps.
- Offer ways to prepare culturally appropriate "old favorites" in healthy ways.
- Offer the opportunity to taste new and unusual fruits and vegetables.
- Provide hands-on educational activities to help incorporate fruits and vegetables into meals and snacks.

Recipe Flyers or Booklets

- Limit the number of ingredients (preferably no more than five).
- Ingredients should be low-cost and usually on hand.
- Limit the number of steps; they should be quick and easy to do.
- Do not include steps that use lots of pots and pans.
- Do not use terms that people might not understand.
- Include a picture of how it should turn out.
- Include tips for how to get the best buys when shopping for fruits and vegetables.
- Include tips related to meal planning.

Take-Home Items (Freebies) with Useful Information or Reminders

- Calendars (with reminders to eat fruits and vegetables, recipes, health information)
- Refrigerator magnets
- Magnetized shopping lists
- Tote bags

- Coffee mugs, or juice cups for kids
- Coloring books with recipes for kids
- Fruits and veggies (to make at home the recipes they tasted)

Less Effective Ways to Promote Fruits and Vegetable Consumption

Participants have made the following suggestions for incorporating these elements if you decide to use them.

Videos

- Show videos for no more than 5 to 10 minutes at a time.
- Select only videos that have "good actors" and "good music." People are very sophisticated consumers of visual media, so the quality of any visuals must be high.
- Use food demonstrations and taste testing or other hands-on activities in conjunction with the video.

Handouts or Brochures

- Discuss them with the group (don't just give to clients to take home).
- Make them colorful and appealing.
- Keep them simple, to the point, and useful to the clients.

Lecture-Style Presentations

- Use short mini-lectures only.
- Be an enthusiastic speaker with a positive attitude.
- Have personal experience with the topic.
- Avoid use of technical terms (but also do not talk down to the group).

GUIDELINES FOR NUTRITION EDUCATION THROUGH VARIOUS CHANNELS

Channels such as cooking experiences, health fairs, or grocery store tours are increasingly recognized as valuable channels for nutrition education to both motivate and facilitate dietary change. The following guidelines can help.

Cooking or Food Preparation as Nutrition Education

Just about everyone is interested in food, and participating in preparing food can be motivating. There is increasing evidence that cooking can be effective as a means of nutrition education beyond other hands-on, activity-based nutrition education activities (Liquori et al. 1998; Brown and Hermann 2005; Reicks et al. 2014). Consequently, nutrition education programs often include a session or part of a session, in which the participants cook or prepare some items that they then eat together. The following are some tips for conducting such activities.

Getting Started

Consider the following:

- *What are your educational objectives?* Be clear about the purpose or objectives of the food preparation activities. Hands-on without minds-on activity is not by itself educational. Do you wish to enhance motivation through the activity? For example, do you want to encourage children to try new foods? Or is it primarily a skills-building activity for people who are already motivated? Do you want to assist participants to learn new ways of making familiar recipes more healthful—for example, people who have been diagnosed with diabetes who want to know how to change what and how they cook?

- *What is the time frame?* What is the time frame that you have available for this activity? Is this a one-time session? How long is the session? Or will this be a series of cooking sessions with a consistent group? These differences will influence your selection of objectives, recipes, and activities.

- *Who is your audience?* Do they come from a variety of ethnic groups with different cultural backgrounds, or are they somewhat homogeneous? Are they low income? These considerations will influence your recipe development.

- *What is the group's cooking skills level?* For example, are you working with teens with few skills or experienced older women with many skills? In all cases, make clear to the group the relationship of this activity to the rest of the nutrition education session or set of sessions.

- *What are the facilities?* Is there a stove in the setting or will you have to bring a butane stove or hot plate? Are there any utensils? Check out the facilities ahead of time. If there are no cooking facilities and it is not possible for you to bring a heat source, you can still develop recipes that involve active food preparation, such as making a salad.

- *How large will the group be?* Will all of the group members participate in preparing the same recipe or will you have several cooking stations preparing different recipes?

- *What ingredients and materials will you need?* Materials include all the utensils you will need as well as all the food items you will need. When bringing perishable foods, you need to consider issues of food safety, such as travel time in terms of keeping items cold and leaving food out at room temperature for any length of time. You may need to consider a cooler or ice packs. If you have several stations, you may need several sets of utensils. If you have a lot of food materials, you will need sturdy boxes or suitcases on wheels.

Making the Cooking Experience Motivating and Effective

The following guidelines can help:

- *Tailor the experience to your audience.* Your audience will be more interested in food preparation if they can immediately see that the items being prepared are relevant to them, such as healthy and convenient snacks for teens or modifications of recipes for older adults. This means you need to know your audience well.

- *Make the cooking experience culturally appropriate.* One of the most visible and interesting ways in which people express their cultural and ethnic identity is through the foods they eat and the methods of preparing them. Hence, it is very important that the recipes you choose and the practices you recommend and teach take into consideration cultural differences between groups.

- *Test the recipes carefully ahead of time.* This will ensure that they will work—no matter how simple they seem to be. Test that they can be prepared in the setting in which the group will prepare them.

- *Always show respect for all participants.* Some may not like the recipes or have different levels of cooking skills, willingness to engage, and adventuresomeness in trying new foods. After all, preferences regarding food and eating are very personal. All participants bring valuable insights and past experiences to the table, and these should be honored.

- *Divide tasks into small group "assignments."* Each group may make a separate recipe or components of the same recipe.

- *Assemble all ingredients, materials, and utensils needed for each group ahead of time.* Place the ingredients for each group at a designated station or in a bag or box until you are ready to use them.
- *Review the recipes with the entire group.* Write the recipes on flip charts. If the group speaks English as a second language, record the recipe in their language of origin as well as in English. You may need to read the recipe, depending on the literacy level of the group.
- *Select the appropriate time within the session to do the food preparation activity.* You may lead a group discussion plus mini-lecture session first and conclude with the food activity as a skills development activity. Or you may have planned a series of cooking sessions for a group using food preparation as a primary form of nutrition education. In this case, interweave discussion of food and nutrition content with cooking, and provide motivational, why-to information as well as how-to food- and nutrition-related information. It is best not to talk too long before getting the group members started on the food preparation; provide information as you go along.
- Review responsible cooking practices with the group. These practices include the following:

  - Wash your hands before you begin, and wash them again if you cough, sneeze, or touch your hair or face.
  - Be careful with knives—even plastic knives.
  - Treat everyone with respect.
  - Cooking is most fun when everyone cooperates.
  - Listen carefully to the instructions and ask questions if you don't understand.
  - If you don't want to eat something, politely say, "No, thank you." Do not say it is gross or nasty—someone else may love the taste. With children, a common phrase is "Don't yuck my yum."

Conclude with eating together if that is possible or appropriate. Make the ambience pleasant. Some nutrition educators bring paper tablecloths, and even vases of flowers, so that the eating experience is enjoyable.

NUTRITION EDUCATION IN ACTION 16-1 provides information on CookShop as an example of a program that uses cooking in the classroom as a means of nutrition education (Liquori et al. 1998; Wadsworth 2005).

Conducting Grocery Store and Farmers' Market Tours

Tours of grocery stores or farmers' markets can be a wonderful experience for all ages. Such tours can be conducted in a variety of markets, ranging from small to large, and can serve many purposes.

Getting Started

Consider the following:

- *What are your educational objectives?* Be clear about the purpose or objectives of the supermarket or farmers' market tour. Do you wish to enhance motivation through this activity? Is it an application of other material learned? Or is it primarily a skills-building activity for people who are already motivated? You should have determined these objectives in Step 4 of the DESIGN Procedure. (See Chapter 10.) It is very important to be focused
- *Who is your audience?* Are they children or adults? This will make a difference in how the experience is structured. Are they of a particular ethnic or cultural group? Are they low in resources? Your audience assessment in Step 2 of the DESIGN Procedure can provide you with this information. (See Chapter 8.)

Planning the Tour

Get approval if the tour is to take place in a grocery store, especially if you are bringing a group of children. This usually involves asking the manager. The U.S. fruit and vegetable Eat More campaign encourages grocery stores to provide tours to children, and grocery stores are often happy to conduct them, seeing it as a good opportunity to encourage families to eat more fruits and vegetables and to generate positive community relations and media publicity. You will need to schedule a time that is convenient for the store as well as for your group. Approvals are not usually needed at most farmers' markets, although it is often helpful to inform the market manager ahead of time.

Develop an educational plan for the tour. This should be created as part of Step 4 of the DESIGN Procedure. Determine the specific educational objectives of the tour and design several activities to achieve them. For children and adults, develop activity sheets that they can complete while at the store or market. These may

NUTRITION EDUCATION IN ACTION 16-1 CookShop

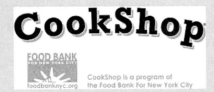

Courtesy of Food Bank for New York City.

CookShop, Food Bank for New York City's centerpiece nutrition education program, provides low-income New Yorkers of all ages with the knowledge and tools to adopt and enjoy a healthy diet and active lifestyle on a limited budget. Through hands-on workshops implemented in public schools and after-school programs and a citywide social marketing campaign, CookShop imparts nutrition and physical activity information, teaches cooking skills, and fosters enthusiasm for fresh and affordable fruit, vegetables, and other whole foods. It also provides an understanding of where food comes from, what goes into a nutritious diet and active lifestyle, how food and activity choices impact our bodies, and how to access healthy, affordable foods. Sites must apply to Food Bank to participate in the program, and once accepted, are provided with hands-on training, curriculum materials, and technical support to ensure consistent and successful implementation of the lessons. CookShop began in two New York City public elementary schools in 1995. Today the program includes several components reaching more than 40,000 participants with hands-on lessons and over 230,000 participants with social marketing messaging.

CookShop Classroom offers distinct curricula designed for elementary school children in kindergarten through fifth grade and after-school children aged 6–12 years. Lessons capitalize on students' natural curiosity and excitement by using sensory food exploration, cooking activities, and shared eating and physical activity experiences in the classroom. Materials feature colorful illustrations of key concepts, including pictures of farmers, plant parts, and food groups. The curricula are easily incorporated into lessons in math, literacy, science, and social studies, which creates stronger academic and behavioral change opportunities.

CookShop for Teens, also known as EATWISE (Educated and Aware Teens Who Inspire Smart Eating),

gives young people the knowledge and skills to make informed decisions about what they eat and drink, and how to live an active lifestyle. Designed as a peer education program, Food Bank provides high school students with training in nutrition and food issues, physical activity, media awareness, public speaking, and leadership skills, preparing them to become peer nutrition educators. Using this training, EATWISE peer educators then facilitate workshops in their high schools and community-based programs, connecting and engaging their schoolmates and communities with messages about healthy eating, enabling their peers—and themselves—to improve their own eating and physical activity habits. All EATWISE messages are promoted and reinforced through CookShop's social marketing campaign.

CookShop for Families is a complementary program offering workshops to the parents/guardians of children in public schools that participate in CookShop Classroom. The goal of this program is to engage entire families in making healthy choices together. Workshops complement the CookShop Classroom curricula, with an increased focus on skills such as reading food labels, meal planning, and understanding portion sizes, and feature simple, healthy recipes that use fresh, affordable ingredients. Adult participants receive take-home materials to promote whole family engagement in cooking and physical activities, providing practical skills and knowledge to make CookShop part of their families' daily lives.

Change One Thing is CookShop's social marketing campaign. It communicates nutrition education with succinct nutrition messages delivered through various methods, including advertising on radio, transit ads, in-school outreach, social media, and a new twist on the traditional ice cream truck that visits locations throughout the city bringing healthy recipes, snacks, drinks, and prizes. The campaign promotes the concept that eating healthy doesn't have to mean overhauling your diet or buying expensive "health food"; rather, change can start with just one healthy choice per day—*change one thing*.

Evaluation

Observation and research demonstrate that the greatest impact on student dietary change comes from classroom lessons that provide cooking and eating experiences and that are complemented by related experiences outside the classroom. CookShop focuses on common, inexpensive foods that are readily available in most neighborhoods and as part of Federal School Lunch Program menus.

More specifically, early evaluations of CookShop in the elementary school setting found cooking to be effective in improving intake of the targeted whole grains and vegetables, and a recent evaluation found that students, parents, and teachers all felt positively about the program. Students enjoyed the opportunity to try new foods; parents appreciated the fact that the program expanded their children's knowledge and awareness of healthy food options; and teachers valued CookShop's hands-on approach, its applicability to other school subjects, and its ability to engage students.

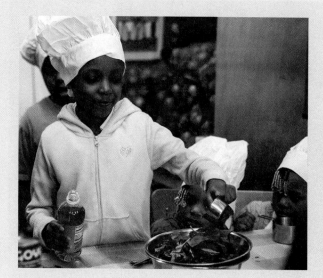

CookShop classroom.

Tim Reiter. Courtesy of Food Bank For New York City.

The CookShop program and its curriculum materials are developed and implemented by Food Bank for New York City, a nonprofit organization. Food Bank For New York City has been the city's major hunger-relief organization working to end hunger throughout the five boroughs for more than 30 years. Nearly one in five New Yorkers relies on Food Bank for food and other resources. Food Bank takes a strategic, multifaceted approach that provides meals and builds capacity in the neediest communities, while raising awareness and engagement among all New Yorkers. In addition, Food Bank's nutrition education programs and services empower more than 275,000 children, teens and adults to sustain a healthy diet on a low budget. More information about the program can be found on their website, http://www.foodbanknyc.org/cookshop.

include a scavenger hunt to find specific foods, such as low-fat items or specific fruits and vegetables. Or make the participants food detectives. Make the activities humorous or brain-twisters in order to provide interest and challenge.

Map out how you will proceed inside the store or market. Make arrangements for where your group can congregate while you give them information, and determine to what extent grocery store personnel will be involved.

Making the Experience Motivating and Effective

Make the tour a physically and mentally active experience. Do not just go from aisle to aisle talking about foods! In the store, carry out some verbal activities first. For example, a tour on fruits and vegetables can begin with questions such as "What colors do you see when you look at all these fruits and vegetables?" "Can you name a red fruit that you see? A green one?" and so forth.

Provide clipboards, or the equivalent, so that participants can complete written activities. Perhaps you could have them complete some kind of self-assessment relevant to the foods of focus. Then send them on a food investigation tour with a series of questions in their activity sheets. Assign points for completing various activities. The store may be willing to provide taste testing of some fruits and vegetables or of recipes made from them. This would result in a tour that challenges all the senses.

Make the tour informative and relevant to your audience. With adults in particular, the tour should teach skills as well as enhance motivation. Perhaps you can teach preparation methods for various vegetables and supply recipes, point out lower-fat versions of food products, introduce them to whole grains of various kinds, and so forth.

Clearly, there are many options for what you can do, limited only by what your group is interested in and your creativity.

Health Fairs

Many nutrition education programs find that holding a health fair is a useful activity, particularly in worksites, colleges, and community centers. As is the case for the activities described earlier, you need to start with a clear understanding of the specific purpose of the activity and of the actions or behaviors you want the participants to

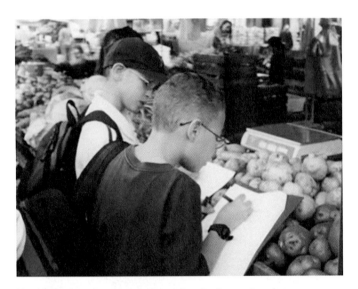

Nutrition education can be explored at the farmers' market.

Courtesy of Linking Food and the Environment, Teachers College Columbia University.

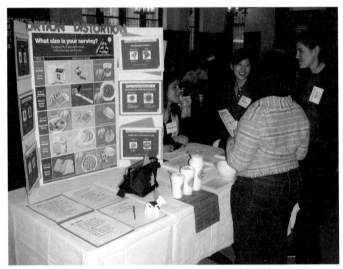

Nutrition education can be delivered through worksite health fairs.

Courtesy of Program in Nutrition, Teachers College Columbia University.

take as a result of participating in the health fair. Health fairs take some effort and planning, so you will have to start early. Develop a timeline based on the following considerations.

Getting Started

Be clear about the purpose or educational objectives of the health fair. Do you want the fair to attract attention as a kickoff event to motivate people to attend other activities of the program, such as group education or physical activity sessions? Or is it a standalone event where you want to motivate individuals to take a certain action and provide some skills on how to do it?

Planning the Health Fair

Consider the following:

- *Site.* Select or find a location. This may depend on how many people you think will attend and hence the space you will need. Will you have break-out activities? Can all of these be done in the same space, or will you need additional rooms?
- *Other potential participants.* Will program staff conduct all the activities or will you invite other similar agencies or groups to participate? For example, if the focus of the health fair is to increase fruit and vegetable consumption, you may want to ask personnel from a nearby hospital to conduct blood pressure screenings

as motivation. Or you may want someone from a local gym to demonstrate activities people can do in the home. This will help you decide how many tables you will need.

- *Raffles.* If you use raffles as a motivator to attend the health fair, you will need to seek out local vendors who can provide items for the raffle, such as membership to a gym. This will require letters and/or phone calls.
- *Activities.* Brainstorm the behaviors or issues you will focus on. Limit them depending on the scope of your fair. For each, decide on the central message. Each message or topic should have a table or booth on which you will display posters using a foamcore stand or something similar. You will need to develop quizzes, activities, and handouts. These need to be motivating and informative, using theory-based strategies as appropriate. They also need to be very short and doable at your table or booth.
- *Promotion and advertising.* You can promote the fair using a variety of approaches, such as posters displayed around the institution, postcards sent to various departments or to community groups, email messages sent to selected audiences, or a story in the institution's newsletter or local newspaper.

Making the Experience Motivating and Effective

Nutrition education staff or volunteers should have on nametags and be ready to greet attendees. Staff should be assigned to meet other vendors or participants and help them set up. The displays should look professional, attractive, and welcoming. The raffle products should be displayed all on one table so that attendees can see what they might get if they complete quizzes or other activities. Have someone take pictures so that they can be used as follow-up motivators if posted, for write-ups about the event, and for evaluation or documentation purposes.

Mass Media and Social Marketing Activities

A brief discussion of social marketing and mass media activities is included here because a mass media campaign or social marketing component often accompanies in-person, in-institution activities as part of a larger program. Activities often described as social marketing are really mass media nutrition communication campaigns. Nutrition mass media campaigns involve communication strategies to disseminate messages to targeted audiences through a variety of mass media channels such as newspaper articles, radio public service announcements (PSAs), or the Internet. Social marketing, on the other hand, is a complex enterprise that may or may not include mass media campaigns and involves the larger enterprise of marketing. It is described briefly here in terms of its use in nutrition education. Whether designing mass media campaigns or developing social marketing activities, nutrition educators usually work in collaboration with mass media or social marketing experts.

NUTRITION MASS MEDIA COMMUNICATION CAMPAIGNS

A mass media communication campaign is usually described as an intervention that intends to generate specific outcomes or effects, in a relatively large number of individuals, usually within a specified period of time, and through an organized set of communication activities (Rogers and Storey 1988; Institute of Medicine [IOM] 2002). Such campaigns are designed to reach large audiences using multiple channels. They usually require substantial resources in terms of money and effort. Campaigns seek to "influence the adoption of recommended health behaviors by influencing what the public knows about the behavior and/or by influencing actual and/or perceived social norms, and/or by changing actual skills and confidence in skills (self-efficacy), all of which are assumed to influence behavior" (IOM 2002). They are often part of social marketing programs. Such campaigns are sometimes conducted along with efforts to change the environment using a multiple-level, ecological model of health promotion.

The process of developing such campaigns involves consideration of the communication principles described in Chapter 15 and engagement in a systematic process somewhat similar to that described in the six-step nutrition education DESIGN Procedure used in this book. The process is as follows: (1) selecting the intended audience and specific behavioral outcomes, (2) conducting extensive formative research (needs assessment) with the audience, (3) choosing the message strategy and how the messages will be worded and executed, (4) selecting the channels and settings for dissemination, and (5) conducting ongoing monitoring and evaluation. Detailed instructions on how exactly to design and implement health communications can be found in documents such as *Making Health Communication Programs Work*, published by the National Cancer Institute (2004), and *Speaking of Health*, from the Institute of Medicine (2002). A review of studies found that health communication campaigns, generally aiming to increase awareness and enhance attitudes and motivation to act, can be effective in changing behavior if they are carefully and appropriately designed (Snyder 2007).

SOCIAL MARKETING

The term *social marketing* is defined in many different ways. Kotler and Zaltman (1971) first proposed that marketing principles could be applied to socially relevant programs, ideas, or behaviors. They saw social marketing as the design, implementation, and control of programs seeking to increase the acceptability of a social idea or practice of a target group. The term often refers to *a systematic planning process* that focuses on (1) consumer behavior (understanding the target group's values, attitudes, barriers, and incentives to change), (2) developing clear messages, (3) designing interventions, (4) implementing them, and (5) evaluating results on a continual basis. It also refers to *a particular conceptual framework* about how to bring about behavior change. The definitions have in common the notion that social marketing is a set of systematic procedures to promote personal and societal welfare.

The following subsections first describe the conceptual framework and then the social marketing process.

Conceptual Framework

Social marketing is based on the following set of considerations (Kotler and Zaltman 1971; Lefebvre and Flora 1988; Andreasen 1995; Rothschild 1999; Lee and Kotler 2011; Lefebvre 2011, 2013):

- Social marketing is applied to causes that are considered to be beneficial to both individuals and society.
- It seeks to promote the voluntary behavior of intended audiences in order to reduce risk or enhance health, not simply to increase awareness or alter attitudes.
- It does so by offering intended audience members reinforcing incentives and/or tangible consequences in an environment that invites voluntary change or exchange (more on this later).
- Social marketing is tailored to the unique perspectives, needs, and experiences of the intended audience with input from representatives of that audience.
- Social marketing strives to create conditions in the social structure that facilitate the behavioral changes promoted.
- Social marketing uses the processes and concepts of marketing.
- Social marketing is usually directed at individual behavior change but can also be directed at institutions and policies.

This section focuses on some central ideas and practices that are useful for nutrition education.

Self-Interest

Individuals are assumed to act in their own self-interest. Although there are many determinants of behavior beyond self-interest (Mansbridge 1990), it has been proposed that self-interest plays some role in most contexts of human interaction. Self-interest can be seen as similar to the concept of outcome expectations (or anticipated outcomes), a determinant in social psychological theory—people expect certain outcomes that are important to them from engaging in healthy behaviors, such as health or decreased risk of disease. Social marketers point out that nutrition education often emphasizes long-term rather than immediate outcomes, as in the example of urging people to increase their intake of calcium-rich foods to reduce the risk of

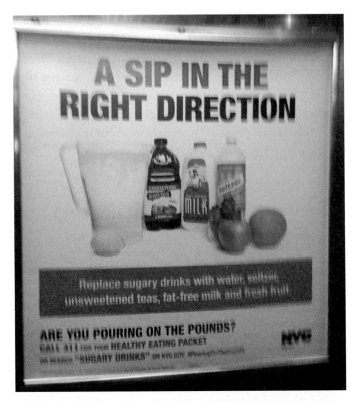

This sign in public transportation suggests that replacing sugary drinks with water is in their self-interest for preventing "pouring on the pounds."

Courtesy of New York City Department of Health and Mental Hygiene.

osteoporosis. Indeed, these long-term outcomes may be in conflict with more immediate outcomes based on self-interest. For example, people choose to eat unhealthy foods or not to be physically active because they have evaluated their life situations and have made their decisions based on their current judgment of their self-interest. Social marketing seeks to promote change by offering benefits that the intended audience perceives to be in their self-interest, as identified through thorough **market research** or needs analyses. That is, it offers "the benefits they (intended audience members) want, reducing the barriers they are concerned about, and using persuasion to participate in program activity" (Kotler and Roberto 1989, p. 24).

Exchange Theory

Central to social marketing is the notion of voluntary exchange of resources: one party gives up something in exchange for getting something from another party. In the case of nutrition education, this means that participants give up time, effort, convenience, or money in exchange for the benefits of enhanced physical health, improved psychological well-being, or a healthful, wholesome food system (Kotler and Zaltman 1971; Rothschild

1999). Social marketing seeks to make the exchange favorable for taking the targeted action by demonstrating that the benefits outweigh the costs of taking action, as does nutrition education. It should be noted that in the design of strategies for enhancing benefits and encouraging action, social marketing actually uses psychosocial theories as necessary tools, such as the health belief model, the theory of planned behavior, social cognitive theory, self-determination theory, or the transtheoretical model.

Focus on Intended Audience Members' Wants and Needs: Audience Benefit

The design of social marketing activities is based on what individuals or consumers want or need. Although evidence from research studies is important and best practices can be very useful, social marketing adds a strong focus on what specific audience members in a given community want and need. Hence it invests heavily in market research to find out about the specific perspectives, values, attitudes, interests, and needs of a given audience. This is similar to the needs analysis process described in Chapter 8. Social marketing also emphasizes pretesting potential materials, messages, and themes with the intended audience in order to refine the message based on their suggestions. If audience members influence the development of the program, it is more likely the intervention will be effective.

Segmentation of the Audience

To design messages and activities that are highly specific, social marketers try to segment, or subdivide, any broad category of individuals into more homogeneous subgroups using demographic criteria such as age, sex, income, and ethnicity; geographic criteria such as urban, suburban, and rural settings; psychological criteria such as motivations, readiness to change, or skill levels; and behavioral criteria such as the degree to which the group already practices the behavior of concern. Selection of which segment or subgroup to focus on can be based on various criteria, such as which group has the greatest need based on the size of the group and the incidence and severity of food- or nutrition-related conditions, which group is most ready to change, or which group has the most influence on others.

Tipping the Scales

Whereas education can increase awareness, promote active contemplation, enhance motivation, and teach food- and nutrition-related behavioral skills and self-regulation skills, social marketing goes beyond education by attempting to modify the relative attractiveness of the specific behavior as well. This is accomplished through the use of incentives and other benefits that positively reinforce the behavior and through the reduction of barriers or costs associated with the behavior, thereby tipping the scales in favor of the behavior, according to Rothschild (1999). Social marketing focuses on providing direct, immediate, and tangible benefits that are reinforcing. It also attempts to reduce both personal barriers, such as beliefs and expectations, and external barriers by making the environment favorable for the appropriate behavior. In the case of an intervention to increase the consumption of fruits and vegetables, social marketers not only provide educational messages through a variety of media, but also reduce barriers by such activities as increasing the availability of fruits and vegetables in schools, working with grocery stores to lower prices, or providing coupons that participants can redeem at stores.

Key Elements in Planning Social Marketing

The social marketing planning process systematically addresses the 4 Ps of the "marketing mix" considered by commercial marketers (Kotler and Zaltman 1971; Maibech, Rothschild, and Novelli 2002; Lee and Kotler 2011).

Product

Product refers to what is exchanged with the intended audience for a price. The product may not be a tangible item but a service, practice, or intangible idea such as health. For the product to be "buyable," people must first perceive that they have a problem and that the product being offered is a good solution. Here, formative research is important to unveil consumers' perceptions about the problem and how strongly they feel that they can do something to solve the problem. Thus, products are desired behaviors, benefits of these behaviors, and any tangible objects and services offered to support the behaviors.

The core product can be a *health idea or behavior* that is of benefit to individuals. For example, the idea can be improved health, or the behavior can be eating five to nine servings of fruits and vegetables daily. *Supporting products can be material items*, such as coupons for fruits and vegetables at farmers' markets, or a service such as a Women, Infants and Children (WIC) clinic or nutrition education classes (but not the materials used in the classes—these are described later in this chapter and fall in a different category). In designing a program, you have to be very clear about what exactly your product is. If it is a behavior, you need to find out from the intended audience what behaviors they see as realistic, effective, practical, or easy to do. You should also be specific: Is the product the behavior of eating *more* fruits and vegetables or eating a specific amount such as 4.5 cups a day or more?

Price

Price refers to the barriers or costs to the consumer associated with obtaining the product, such as adopting the desired behavior, and any monetary and nonmonetary incentives, recognition, and rewards used to reduce the costs. Costs can include the economic costs of eating more fruits and vegetables as well as the inconvenience and increased time involved in the preparation of healthful foods, or perhaps the psychological costs of learning new ways of eating. Social marketing recognizes that decisions to act are based on considerations of both benefits and costs. Individuals ask themselves, "What will I gain if I engage in this behavior, and what will it cost me?" Often individuals fail to take action not because they do not recognize the benefits, but because the costs are too high.

Social marketing thus seeks to increase the benefits and decrease the price or barriers of engaging in the behavior of concern (Andreasen 1995; Rothschild 1999; Lee and Kotler 2016). It does this by addressing the internal determinants of behavior discussed earlier in the book, such as perceived risk, beliefs about outcomes of taking action, knowledge, social norms, and self-confidence or self-efficacy. Social marketing also addresses external barriers such as policy, access, skills, and cultural trends by attempting to create conditions in the social structure and environment to facilitate the actions being promoted. More simply said, it attempts to make the more healthful behavior the easy behavior.

In the case of promoting fruits and vegetables to low-income mothers of young children, the benefits might be the good health of their children or wanting to enhance their children's educational opportunities and performance. Internal barriers might be lack of time and cooking skills or confusion about portion sizes for their children. External barriers might include the high cost of healthful foods such as fruits and vegetables. The

Supplemental Nutrition Assistance Program (SNAP) and coupons for farmers' markets would be ways to reduce external barriers.

Place

Place refers to where and when the product will reach the consumer. In the case of intangible products, it is the place where the audience will receive the information. This may mean researching which media channels are most effective for reaching the intended audience. It may mean grocery stores, doctors' offices, schools, community centers, WIC clinics, or SNAP offices. Place can also refer to where you might offer program activities (such as classes) so that they are convenient to the intended audience. Social marketing seeks to increase the number of places where the product may be found, at the right times, and at the points at which audience members make their decisions. Behaviors must be easy to carry out; hence, placement must encourage the behavior. If increasing consumption of fruits and vegetables is the behavior, then the placement strategy might be to have information and messages conveniently located in the grocery store, workplace, or school lunchroom.

Promotion

The targeted audience members can be expected to voluntarily exchange their time, effort, and other resources if they are aware that the product, such as eating fruits and vegetables, offers them attractive benefits at a reasonable cost and can be practiced at convenient locations. The role of promotion is to create this awareness. For example, the More Matters campaign complements its efforts by placing the product (messages about fruits and vegetables) in the right places via a promotional campaign in the news media and point-of-purchase materials such as messages on grocery store bags. Promotion requires considerations such as the following:

- *What channels to use to reach the intended audience.* For fruit and vegetable consumption among low-income mothers of young children, the channels might be grocery stores, day-care centers, WIC clinics, Supplemental Nutrition Assistance Program offices, community centers, newspapers, and TV.
- *What types of messages might be effective.* The content of the messages will be based on your audience analysis or needs assessment. This is described in detail in Chapter 8. The nature of the message, such as whether

to use humor, emotion, or logical reasoning, should be based on your audience analysis. The tone of the messages should be positive, such as "We know it is hard, but we know that you want to make a change." It should also be respectful, fun, and personal. See Chapter 15 for more details.

Positioning and Branding

In addition to the standard 4 Ps, the *positioning* and *branding* of your product are also important to consider. Positioning is a psychological construct that involves the location of the product relative to products with which it competes. The product can be positioned in such a way to maximize benefits and minimize costs. Branding helps make people aware of the special features of the product. Positioning is difficult in nutrition education because it means having your product (message) outweigh that of the competitors. For example, it is very challenging to get teenagers to eat more fresh fruits and vegetables when they feel that the alternative products, such as high-fat, high-sugar snacks, taste much better. However, serving fruits and vegetables can be positioned as taking care of yourself, serving healthful meals to your family can be positioned as an act of love, and physical activity can be repositioned as a form of relaxation rather than as exercise (which some may view negatively).

The Best Bones Forever Campaign is an example of a social marketing campaign that uses primarily media and educational activities by many collaborating partners in communities. It is described in **NUTRITION EDUCATION IN ACTION 16-2**.

DESIGNING SOCIAL MARKETING ACTIVITIES

As you have seen, social marketing programs are tailored to the unique perspectives, needs, and experiences of the target audience and also seek to create conditions in the social structure and environment that facilitate the actions being promoted (Andreasen 1995; Lefebvre 2013; Lee and Kotler 2011). The set of procedures for designing social marketing is somewhat similar to that described in models of health communication and the six-step nutrition education DESIGN Procedure used in this book. In social marketing, these steps are usually referred to as formative research and planning, strategy design, implementation, and evaluation. The Centers for Disease Control and Prevention (CDC) provides resources on social marketing,

including a Web-based course and several case studies (CDC 2014a, 2014b).

To develop the social marketing campaign or activities, nutrition educators usually work in collaboration with health communication and social marketing experts by providing the food and nutrition content expertise. These experts are especially important in the formative research, message development, and planning stages. The process is fairly similar to the DESIGN Procedure and is summarized briefly here.

Formative research and planning involve setting goals, selecting the audience segment or subgroup to work with, and identifying the focus of the intervention (similar to DESIGN Procedure steps 1–3). The focus may be change in individual attitudes or behaviors, community norms, policies, or all three. The various channels are selected at this time, such as posters, classes, community events, changes in availability of the foods in stores, or policies in schools and workplaces. An environmental analysis is conducted and community participation is sought. Formative research seeks to understand the motivations, attitudes, and behaviors of the intended audience, as well as the audience's perceptions of the benefits and costs of taking the recommended action.

Strategy design includes designing the campaign message based on the formative research and pretesting the message using focus groups and surveys. The marketing mix, or 4 Ps, is selected at this time.

Implementation usually involves considerable collaboration with individuals and organizations in the community. This is described in greater detail in the next subsection. Funding and changes in social structures are sought so that the programs can be maintained over the long term.

Evaluation is important. There are many approaches, the simplest of which is to see whether the audience can recall campaign messages. Another measure is extent of exposure—the number of activities that audience members have attended, such as classes or workshops, live food demonstrations, or health fairs, or the number of materials they have taken home. These are what are called *process evaluation* measures, described in detail in Chapter 13. Measures of actual *outcomes* are also important; these include surveys of determinants of behavior change such as knowledge, beliefs, attitudes, behavioral intent, or stage of change and behavior change itself. Behaviors can be self-reported through a survey or by using monitoring data such as the

NUTRITION EDUCATION IN ACTION 16-2 **Best Bones Forever! Campaign**

Courtesy of Office on Women's Health, U.S. Department of Health and Human Services. Best Bones Forever! http://www.bestbonesforever.org

Best Bones Forever! is a U.S. national campaign directed at girls aged 9–14 years and their parents with the goal to increase calcium and vitamin D consumption and physical activity—habits that are important in the bone-building years of youth, particularly for girls. The campaign is a social marketing campaign that also takes a social ecological approach involving numerous community partners who implement the Best Bones Forever! messages into their existing health education activities.

Qualitative and quantitative formative research was conducted to understand the target audience's needs and wants, explore creative concepts and messaging, and guide creation of a brand that promises friendship and fun in exchange for bone-strengthening behaviors. Campaign creators then used social marketing principles, including the 4 Ps, to address the audience's opportunities, motivation, and ability to engage in target behaviors:

- *Opportunity and access* are provided by an ever-growing number of partners—this helps reduce barriers.

- Motivation is delivered through the *brand and campaign activities* that deliver fun.

- Ability is provided through *specific campaign components* by giving girls and their parents knowledge, skills, and self-efficacy to perform the behaviors.

The tag line to girls is: A bone health campaign for girls and their BFFs (best friends forever) to "grow strong together and stay strong forever!" The message to their parents is: Act now to help your daughter build her best bones forever!

The campaign includes:

- A website for girls about best for bones foods, recipes, physical activities, quizzes, and games with a focus on doing these with your BFFs
- Engaging materials for girls, such as a food and fitness diary
- Tools and resources for educators, community leaders, and healthcare professionals
- Activities for families
- Suggestions for parties and dance contests
- Activities for communities and partners

Evaluation

Building partnerships. The campaign used social marketing principles, including the 4 Ps, to build partnerships for the campaign. The campaign was successful in engaging partners in providing input into creating products and managing price and place as well as promotion.

Outreach. Numerous partners at the national and community level incorporated Best Bones Forever! messages into their health education efforts. A study of three communities found that they held community events and health fairs, made presentations to community and professional organizations, and promoted the message through local media coverage, performances, and school-based activities.

Impact on girls. A sub-study with girls and their families found that both girls and their parents significantly increased their knowledge of bone health, the importance they attached to consuming calcium and vitamin D–rich foods and preventing disease like osteoporosis, as well as their self-efficacy to engage in bone health–related behaviors.

Best Bones Forever! was developed and managed for 5 years by the Office on Women's Health in the U.S. Department of Health and Human Services. In November 2014, leadership of the campaign was transferred to American Bone Health (http://www.americanbonehealth .org), which had been a longtime partner of the campaign.

Source: Abercrombie, Sawatzki, and Doner Lotenberg 2012; Osborn et al. 2012; Sadler et al. 2013; and http://www.bestbonesforever.org; logo used with permission.

increase in sales of fruits and vegetables in grocery stores in the area or increased attendance at fitness classes and gyms.

An example of a statewide nutrition education and social marketing effort is Iowa Nutrition Network's Building and Strengthening Iowa Community Support for Nutrition and Physical Activity (BASICS) program described in **NUTRITION EDUCATION IN ACTION 16-3.**

IMPLEMENTING SOCIAL MARKETING ACTIVITIES

Social marketing often involves the mass media, but not always. Social marketing that uses mass media as the primary channel usually requires the collaboration of many individuals and organizations. Such campaigns can be local, community-wide, statewide, or national. After systematic planning has occurred, implementation still requires a considerable set of activities. Some potential practical methods for implementing social marketing are summarized here based on the literature and best practices of those who have been involved. These methods are useful to nutrition educators who are interested in incorporating mass media and community support components into their programs. The following suggestions are based on the experience of the Pick a Better Snack campaign in Iowa (Iowa Department of Public Health n.d.).

Media Activities

1. *Develop media partnerships.* Prior to the initiation of the campaign, actively solicit print, outdoor, and broadcast media partnerships to extend the reach of the campaign to audiences that would otherwise be out of the program's reach for financial reasons.

   - Meet with local television and radio station public service directors, station promotional managers, and print advertising managers to identify opportunities for partnerships.
   - Draw up a simple joint agreement that outlines how each partner will be identified in collaborative efforts, such as whose logos will be on media events. Such agreements avoid misunderstandings later on and engender trust.

2. *Introduce the campaign to the community.* You have only one shot to introduce your campaign. The challenge here is to make as big a splash as you can with a few simple messages and to get media coverage.

   - Plan a kickoff event such as a press conference. Select a site with a compelling visual element for broadcast media where a story can be told, such as at a farmers' market, grocery store, or after-school program.
   - Carefully develop two to four key messages to serve as the focus of the news conference or event.

3. *Sustain ongoing media relationships.* Work with local media to develop periodic articles or special features on the importance of your message, as did the Pick a Better Snack campaign.

   - Identify a few key reporters and news editors who are responsible for covering food or health issues and work on building a good working relationship with them. Contact them from time to time by phone or email with news about campaign events or article ideas. Follow up with information to support your story ideas. Or send them a draft of a potential article for them to modify.
   - Offer to serve as a resource for them on other food and nutrition issues.

4. *Plan an outdoor or public transportation campaign, if feasible.* Place your messages on billboards, bus benches, buses, subways, or bus shelters. These can be paid for or placed as public service announcements.

   - Work with outdoor media companies to identify the best locations for your intended audience and obtain cost estimates.
   - Outdoor media companies will frequently run billboards with public service announcements at no charge for the space. These may not be placed in prime locations, so negotiate with them about placement and duration.
   - Work with public transportation authorities to purchase or obtain free space for messages.

Community Outreach

1. *Develop a newsletter.* Develop a simple, inexpensive newsletter to keep key partners and targeted segments of the campaign's audience informed about your activities and progress.

   - The frequency of the newsletter will depend on your ability to develop a simple system for its regular development and distribution, but it should be at least quarterly.

NUTRITION EDUCATION IN ACTION 16-3 Building and Strengthening Iowa Community Support for Nutrition and Physical Activity (BASICS)

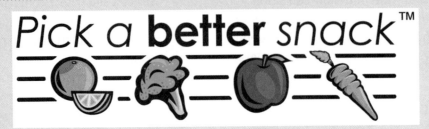

Courtesy of Iowa Department of Public Health.

The Building and Strengthening Iowa Community Support for Nutrition and Physical Activity (BASICS) program is a program of the Iowa Nutrition Network (INN). It is designed to improve fruit and vegetable and low-fat dairy consumption among elementary school children in schools with at least 50 percent participation in the free and reduced-price school lunch program. The intervention is designed to help nutrition educators working with the U.S. Department of Agriculture's (USDA's) Supplemental Nutrition Assistance Program (SNAP) and other programs to deliver science-based nutrition education to low-income children and their parents. The intervention focuses on key messages based on the Dietary Guidelines for Americans and uses a variety of behavior-focused strategies to promote these behaviors:

Youth-Specific Behavioral Goals

1. Children will choose to eat fruits and vegetables for snacks.
2. Children will choose to consume milk and milk products at meals and snacks, choosing low-fat or fat-free most often.

Parent-Specific Behavioral Goals

1. Model positive fruit and vegetable behaviors.
2. Offer fruits and vegetables to their child at meals and snacks.
3. Model positive milk behaviors.
4. Purchase and offer fat-free or low-fat milk and milk products for their family.

Developing the Messages

Extensive formative research and message testing was conducted leading to two campaigns:

Pick a Better Snack: Fruits and vegetables and physical activity campaign

- The goal is to decrease the barriers for eating fruits and vegetables as snacks, making the action easy to do with graphics (updated from previous campaign) showing photos of children enjoying eating fruit and vegetable snacks.

- All messages have the tag line: *How easy is that?* Examples are: Wash, Bite: *How easy is that?* for an apple or carrot; Slice. Eat. *How easy is that?* for an orange or other fruit; and so forth.

Their Bodies Change. So Should Their Milk. Low-fat milk campaign

- The goal is to motivate mothers of children 2 years and up to serve 1% or fat-free milk.

- The campaign message is easily comprehended and the emotional appeal is reflective, nostalgic, balanced with facts, and relatable to maternal emotion without any judgment. The campaign visual is of children holding photos of themselves as infants and toddlers.

The BASICS Program

The BASICS program delivers nutrition and physical activity education through a school-based program, consisting of monthly 30-minute lessons that are specifically designed for kindergarten through third-grade students. The lessons include activities such as food tastings, "I tried it!" stickers, and physical activity demonstrations. Family newsletters and fruit and vegetable/physical activity bingo cards reinforce the lessons with parents and caregivers.

Social Marketing Model

The Iowa Nutrition Network uses social marketing strategies to reinforce the classroom-based education using additional channels of communication:

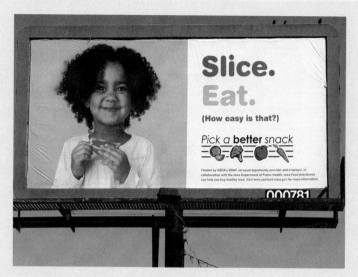 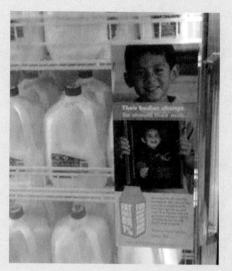

Billboard for Pick a Better Snack and point-of-purchase signage in a grocery store for Their Bodies Change. So Should Their Milk.

Courtesy of Iowa Department of Public Health.

Schools:

- Pick a Better Snack and Act posters and materials in the cafeteria

WIC centers for low-income preschoolers:

- Their Bodies Change. So Should Their Milk.

Communities:

- *Point-of-purchase signage and demonstrations* at supermarkets
- *Billboards* in SNAP-qualified low-income census tracts
- *Bus shelter signage*
- *Television and radio ads*
- *Family Nights Out*, a family event held at the participating child's school
- *Materials in schools* such as posters and banners
- *Materials at community organizations* such as WIC offices and YMCAs, including posters and window clings.

Evaluation

A thorough evaluation comparing those who received the intervention with those who did not found the following:

- *The BASICS program had significant impacts on fruit and vegetable consumption.* Compared to the comparison group, both BASICS and BASICS with community-based social marketing significantly increased children's average daily intakes of fruits and vegetables at home by 0.24 cups and 0.31 cups, respectively.
- *Children's at-home use of 1% and fat-free milk increased with BASICS Plus.* Children in families exposed to the BASICS Plus intervention, which included the social marketing campaign—"Their bodies change. So should their milk."—were 32 to 34 percent more likely to use low-fat (1%) or fat-free milk than whole or reduced-fat milk than children in the other two groups.

Source: Supplemental Nutrition Assistance Program Education and Evaluation Study (Wave II). Iowa Nutrition Network's Building and Strengthening Iowa Community Support (BASICS) for Nutrition and Physical Activity Program. Summary, Volume I Report, and Volume II Appendices. USDA, Food and Nutrition Service, Office of Policy Support. Nutrition Assistance Program Report. December 2013. http://www.fns.usda.gov/research-and-analysis.

- Because it will go to a variety of stakeholders, the newsletter should also include information relevant to the campaign, such as recipes and actionable ideas for taking the action promoted by the campaign.

2. *Collaborate with community organizations.* Collaborate with community organizations regarding events that would bring benefit to your program and the organization, such as farmers' markets, local food drives, broadcast media, and health fairs.

   - Work with a local farmers' market to organize an event that would both bring people to the farmers' market and bring awareness to the campaign messages. Demonstrate simple recipes reflecting the campaign action (such as eating more fruits and vegetables), decorate with campaign posters, and wear campaign-related t-shirts.
   - Work with other organizations at special events they may sponsor, such as community health fairs sponsored by local radio or TV stations.

3. *Place campaign literature in strategic locations.* Distribute program literature to the public in several health and medical services–related settings throughout the community.

   - Work with your local medical society leadership to encourage them to recommend to their members

that they participate by being willing to serve as distribution points for your campaign literature (such as posters, recipes, or bookmarks) to their clients.

- Distribute your written public service announcements to county medical groups for inclusion in their regular member newsletters.

Working with Schools

1. *Work with school food service staff.* Provide a campaign promotional package to food service directors for use in school cafeterias.

   - In this package include several posters and selected samples of point-of-sale materials to allow them to dress up the lunch line.
   - Encourage food service directors to periodically focus on the campaign for a week, such as to promote fruits and vegetables or low-fat milk that week.

2. *Coordinate with parent associations (PAs).* Solicit local schools' PAs to promote your goal behavior at their open houses, social events, and fundraising sales.

   - Have a booth at the parent association/school open house to raise awareness that the school is focusing on the campaign goal through its curriculum. Outline what parents can do at home to support the campaign's target goal.
   - Hand out samples of foods promoted by your campaign, as well as recipes, postcards, bookmarks, and so forth.
   - Seek parent association volunteers to promote imaginative after-school snacks, foods for sporting events, and school fundraisers (in place of bake sales) that support the campaign goals.

Grocery Store Activities

1. *Conduct in-store or farmers' market demonstrations.* Volunteer to conduct in-store food demonstrations in a local grocery store.

   - Work with the store manager to get approval to do a demonstration.
   - Demonstrate only one or two very simple ideas for the promoted foods; hand out recipes and other campaign material.

2. *Use incentive cards to encourage individuals to try promoted foods.* The campaign may develop incentives for children to eat certain foods, such as fruits

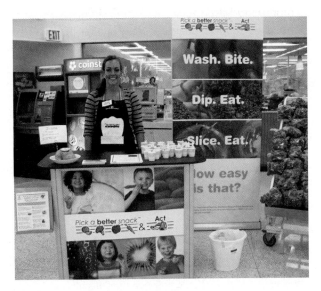

FIGURE 16-5 Iowa Pick a Better Snack campaign: Grocery store demonstration.

Building and Strengthening Iowa Community Support (BASICS) for Nutrition and Physical Activity, Iowa Nutrition Network. Supplemental Nutrition Assistance Program Education and Evaluation Study Wave II. 2013.

and vegetables, by handing out cards (through schools, WIC clinics, or other food-related settings) with activities printed on them for the whole family to do. When a family verifies that the activity has been completed, they can take the card to a participating grocery store or return it to the school to redeem it for an incentive. Focus group research has shown that "unfamiliarity" and fear of wasting food are frequently barriers to trying new foods. These cards can help families overcome their reluctance to try new foods. Incentives can also be free samples of campaign-related food items to help families overcome the barrier of fearing to purchase foods that their children will not eat.

- Develop a system for distribution of the educational incentive items.
- Work with store managers to develop a redemption procedure.

3. *Provide in-store signage.* Develop signs to identify the foods promoted by the campaign.
   - Set up criteria for classifying food items as qualifying as target foods. For example, if low-fat foods are a focus, define what you mean by low-fat. Come with a list of foods that qualify. Define what will qualify as a vegetable—canned, frozen, or fresh? What if it is in a prepared frozen meal? etc.

4. Work out with the store manager who will place the signs, who will monitor them, and who will change them as needed.

COMPARING SOCIAL MARKETING AND NUTRITION EDUCATION

Many years ago, an early social marketer, Richard Manoff (1985), who had achieved considerable success in improving nutrition in several developing countries, quipped at a Society for Nutrition Education meeting that "anything that works is social marketing; anything that does not is nutrition education." Others, on the other hand, criticize social marketing as too simplistic, and not promoting the critical thinking and reflection that are needed in making informed choices in a complex food system (Van Den Heede and Pelican 1995). The debate continues even as many nutrition education programs use social marketing activities as a component. On the other hand, there are many large-scale social marketing campaigns that believe that nutrition education is a component of social marketing.

This section compares the two endeavors on four features considered to be central to social marketing: it has a unique conceptual framework; it tailors messages and strategies to the unique perspectives, needs, and experiences of the target audience; it is a systematic audience-based planning process; and it goes beyond nutrition education by aiming to create conditions in the social structure and environment that reduce barriers and facilitate the actions being promoted.

Conceptual Framework

Two key concepts of social marketing are *self-interest* and *the exchange. Self-interest* can be seen as similar to the concept of outcome expectations (or anticipated outcomes), a determinant of behavior change common to many social psychological theories that we discuss at length in Chapters 4 and 5. That is, people will engage in a behavior if they believe that doing so will lead to outcomes they desire such as improved health, a sustainable and just food system, family cohesion, and so forth. This concept is widely used in nutrition education to enhance motivation. The concept of *exchange* is similar to consideration of benefits versus barriers of behavior change in many of the psychosocial theories described in Chapters 4 and 5 and operationalized in Chapters 11 and 12. Nutrition education, like social marketing, seeks to demonstrate that the benefits outweigh the costs of taking action (or the pros outweigh the cons). Indeed, social marketing often uses the psychosocial determinants of behavior change from theories familiar to nutrition educators to design its messages to enhance the exchange, such as the health belief model, the theory of planned behavior, social cognitive theory, and others.

Audience Focus

Social marketing's consumer or audience focus and emphasis on thorough formative research or audience analysis as a first step is similar to the needs assessment or audience analysis process that constitutes the first step in designing theory-based nutrition education. The contrast is in the level of importance given to this step. Social marketing spends considerable time and effort on this step in order to understand its audience and tailor its messages, whereas nutrition education programs often spend little time on this step. However, theory-based nutrition education also requires that a thorough needs analysis be conducted to identify the many mediators of behavior change, including motivators and reinforcers of action and barriers to change. Two chapters in this book are devoted to such assessments. In addition, social marketers also spend considerable resources on pretesting messages with potential audience members. Pilot testing is also always considered an important part of nutrition education. Still, social marketing does provide a good reminder about the importance of understanding the intended audiences.

Systematic Planning Process

As you examine the process of audience-based social marketing, you can see that it is not very different from the systematic process used in designing good health education or nutrition education. The steps in social marketing of formative research and planning, including a clear statement of objectives; strategy design, including strategy formation, and message and material development; pretesting; implementation; and evaluation and feedback are very similar to the steps of any systematic educational planning process, including the DESIGN Procedure for developing theory-based nutrition education used in this book. The use of the 4 Ps provides an interesting way to think of the strategy design process. Social marketers believe that nutrition education focuses only on "promotion" among the 4 Ps. This is often true. But our contemporary definition of nutrition education as being behavior-focused and theory-based is much more broad and a careful examination shows that these 4 Ps overlap many psychosocial theory variables. Social marketers do remind nutrition educators, however, to be more systematic in their planning process and to go beyond promotion in their strategies.

Reducing Tangible Barriers

Finally, social marketing is described as going beyond education by specifically modifying the relative attractiveness of the specific behavior. It does so by providing *tangible and immediate benefits* that are reinforcing and through reducing both *personal barriers*, such as beliefs and expectations, and external barriers by making the environment favorable for the appropriate behavior. For example, government social marketing programs can provide low-income consumers with coupons so that for every $5, let's say, they spend on fruits and vegetables at a farmers' market or grocery store they get an additional $2

to spend on fruits and vegetables. Theory-based nutrition education also seeks to increase the perception of benefits and decrease internal barriers, as has been described in great detail in this book.

Social Marketing, Nutrition Education, and the Social Ecological Model

Social marketing contributes a reminder to nutrition education to involve consumers or the public intensely in developing the program, to value their input, and to offer a sense of participant empowerment. Its set of planning ideas or tools, such as the 4 Ps, can also be very useful to nutrition education. The channels favored by social marketing, such as the mass media, offer the potential to reach a large portion of the population and to change the informational and normative environment. (Remember, though, that social marketing is not the same as a mass media campaign.)

On the other hand, nutrition education, when conducted with groups, goes beyond social marketing by providing a set of learning opportunities for the intended audience to develop and practice food- and nutrition-related cognitive skills, including critical thinking skills, as well as affective and behavior-specific skills that can assist individuals to make choices and take action on complex behaviors and issues. Venues such as facilitated group discussion also provide for social support and reinforcement of learning.

Finally, both nutrition education and social marketing are evolving. Lefebvre (2011) points out that in many settings, particularly in developing countries, social marketing tends to be synonymous with the offer of products and services, such as free testing and condoms for HIV prevention or free family planning clinics for birth control campaigns. In the United States, on the other hand, social marketing is synonymous with behavior change. Yet both are necessary—people must become motivated to use these products and services. Lefebvre (2011, 2013) argues that social marketing also can, and should, be directed at policymakers, opinion leaders, and the media, using communication principles to change markets and policies.

Nutrition education also increasingly incorporates environmental supports for action—including policy and system modification—as part of its programming, and thus decreases external barriers to action. The use of the social ecological approach is an example of this trend. This approach is described in Chapter 6. The two enterprises of social marketing and nutrition education thus share many characteristics, with both increasingly directed at individual behavior and at the environment. Indeed, social marketing can be used as one component of a multicomponent program that also includes nutrition education.

This integrated approach is sounding like the contemporary definition of nutrition education used in this book, which is that nutrition education uses behavior change theory and educational strategies, *accompanied by environmental supports*, to facilitate the voluntary adoption of behaviors conducive to health and well-being of self, community, and the planet.

Using New Technologies

Many technologically advanced communication channels show promise in nutrition education. *Nutrition informatics*, the intersection of information, nutrition, and technology, may be able to impact large audiences due to economic and dissemination benefits.

These technological advancements can be categorized in a variety of ways. For instance, types of electronic media for child health promotion have been classified into five categories: (1) *Web-based educational/therapeutic programs*, i.e., program content that is converted to Web format; (2) *tailored message systems,* i.e., programs that provide targeted information based on an individual's responses to questions; (3) *data monitoring and feedback,* i.e., programs in which an individual enters personal information over a period of time with feedback on improving behavior; (4) *active video games,* i.e., exercise games that require participants to be physical active; and (5) *interactive multimedia involving games,* i.e., videogames that promote behavior change (Baranowski and Frankel 2012). Among adults, digital and social media are popular.

For the purposes of this book, technology for nutrition education will be categorized by devices and then by tools and software programs available on these devices, since many instruments (e.g., computers and smartphones) can support the same or similar programs (e.g., social media platforms and tele- or Web-conferences).

It should be noted that development of nutrition education for all electronic media requires a systematic design process such as the DESIGN Procedure used in this book, involving selection of a clear behavior change goal; assessment of the key determinants that are motivators and facilitators of change; a statement of the objectives for the game, Web-based intervention, app, or social media intervention; and an appropriate match between the activity and the objectives and determinants of behavior change. One review of smartphone applications (apps) for diet and physical activity, for example, found that there was great variability in the degree to which the apps used theory-based behavior change *strategies* or *techniques* to accomplish their behavioral goals (Direito et al. 2014).

DEVICES

Many devices currently exist, but more are continually being developed. It is important for nutrition educators to stay up to date with popular technology in order to engage people where they are already spending much of their time.

Computers and Tablets

Computer use has skyrocketed over the past few decades. In 1983, only 10% of Americans had a home computer. However, 81% of Americans surveyed in 2014 reported using a laptop or desktop computer at home, work, school, or elsewhere. Interestingly, while desktop and laptop ownership is about equal (55–57%), desktop ownership is falling, while laptop use is rising (Pew Internet 2014a). Tablet usage is also becoming more popular among multiple generations for reading magazines and books, emailing,

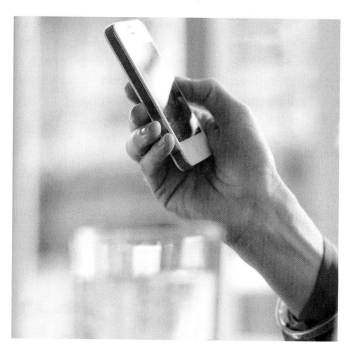

Apps for smartphones are being widely used for nutrition education.
© Bloom Productions/Getty Images.

playing online games, etc. Similar to computers, tablets are computer screens that accept input directly without using a keyboard. Currently, one in five American adults owns a tablet. By race, 34% of white adults and 29% of black adults owned a tablet computer in 2013 (Pew Internet 2014a).

Nutrition educators have much to gain from working with computers and tablets. For instance, education programs provided through a website on a computer or tablet, or social support from a social networking site have potential to change behavior.

Phones

Both landline and cell or mobile phones are included in this category. However, cell phones are increasingly becoming the primary and/or sole mode of phone communication. As of January 2014, 90% of Americans owned a cell phone and 58% of American adults owned a *smartphone,* i.e., a phone that offers advanced technological capabilities and Internet connectivity. With respect to demographics, 90% of white adults and 92% of black adults owned a cell phone in 2014, and 53% and 56% of white and black adults, respectively, owned a smartphone (Pew Internet 2014a). Due to their unique abilities and omnipresence, phones may provide novel health promotion strategies by being able to communicate directly with people (Bort-Roig et al. 2014).

Video Gaming Systems

About 2 in 5 American adults own a video gaming system, a device that is used for playing video games on a television. Some video games require a certain behavior, such as being physically active. These systems may be a new outlet for nutrition education, combining fun and active games with healthful behavior changes.

Personal Digital Assistants

Personal digital assistants (PDAs) are hand-held computers, usually used with a pen, that can be used in nutrition education, e.g., with data collection. One study found that a PDA program was effective in increasing vegetable and whole grain intake in mid-life and older adults (Atienza et al. 2008).

TOOLS FOR DEVICES

Websites

The World Wide Web offers many opportunities for nutrition education and indeed many programs provide

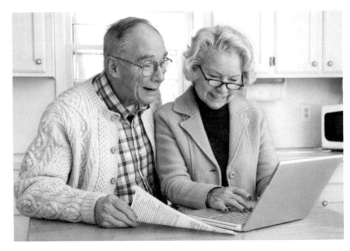

People of all ages use computers to find information and thus can be reached with online nutrition education programs.
© Creatas/Getty Images Plus/Thinkstock.

nutrition education directly to the public through this medium (Brug, Oenema, and Raat 2005; Kroeze, Werkman, and Brug 2006). The Web is indeed widespread; in January 2014, 87% of U.S. adults said they used the Internet. This has not always been the case, however. In 1983, 1.4% of American adults used the Internet, and by 1995, still only 3 out of 5 U.S. adults had even heard of the Internet (Pew Internet 2014a, 2014b).

Many people use the Web to find health information and look for websites with concise and accurate information (Hearn, Miller, and Fletcher 2013). A well-designed, attractive website that has accurate information from a credible source can be a very valuable method for getting nutrition messages out. Nutrition educators usually work with Web designers with specific skills to develop the programs, and thus this process may be expensive.

Websites can also be interactive with audiences of many generations. For instance, participants can log on to certain sections of a website to track their intake and activity. A 9-week, 5-a-Day Boy Scout achievement badge program—which involved troop activities and an Internet intervention—resulted in increased intakes of fruits and juice (Thompson et al. 2009). Also, a home-based, 8-week Internet intervention with girls improved fruit and vegetable intakes and physical activity (Thompson et al. 2008). In those over 40 years of age, short-term Internet-based programs have shown physical activity and nutrition benefits.

Further, websites can offer new means of nutrition assessment. For instance, a Web-based 24-hour recall measure, The Food Intake Recording Software System, displays 10,000+ food images, with additional images to assist in estimating portions, and can be used by children as young as third graders (Baranowski et al. 2014).

Webinars and Online Courses

Slightly different from websites are webinars and online courses. These modes of education provide seminars conducted over the Internet where many people can interact, ask questions, and share ideas. Webinars can be accessed through a website or by downloading certain software. One Web-based program was supplemented with webinar meetings where participants could engage in social support and social networking as well as be supported by a celebrity personal trainer. Participants lost more weight in the webinar group compared to those who did not have access to that feature (Hutchesson et al. 2013).

Social Media Platforms

Social media platforms, online applications that allow for the creation and exchange of user-generated content, include *collaborative projects* (e.g., Wikipedia), *blogs or microblogs* (e.g., Twitter), *content communities* (e.g., YouTube), *social networking sites* (SNSs) (e.g., Facebook), and *virtual gaming or social worlds* (e.g., Second Life) (Williams et al. 2014).

Americans of all generations are using social media platforms. Of those adults that are online, 71% and 18% have Facebook and Twitter accounts, respectively (Duggan and Smith 2013). About two-thirds of low-income, low-education, minority adults use social media (Lefebvre and Bornkessel 2013), suggesting this is a good way to reach them (Lohse 2013; Tobey and Manore 2014). Low-income parents describe their ideal social media site as trustworthy, safe, and relevant with colorful and concise content (Leak et al. 2014). Many children and adolescents are also using social media platforms, with 59% of children using them before the age of 10 (Lange 2014). Because of its widespread use, social media may be particularly useful in promoting nutrition-related behavior change. Social media can also provide a cost-effective way to increase user interaction, provide peer-to-peer support, and widen access to health interventions (Williams et al. 2014).

Facebook has been the most common social media platform used in nutrition education. Young adults who have been given access to secret Facebook groups used additional social support from each other and nutrition education personnel to increase physical activity and weight loss (Napolitano et al. 2013; Valle et al. 2013).

However, it is likely that social media components should be used as additional aspects of nutrition education interventions instead of solely relying on a platform to change behavior.

Email

Emails can be sent individually, to groups, or to large numbers via listservs for different purposes, such as reminding individuals of their nutrition and physical activity goals, or inviting them to participate in interventions. One study used email in a worksite. Batch emails were sent out inviting people to participate. Individuals completed a health assessment instrument on diet and physical activity and received immediate feedback. If they decided to continue, they were asked to choose to increase physical activity, increase fruits and vegetables, or decrease saturated fat, trans fat, and added sugar. They then received personalized small-step goals to choose to work on each week for 3 months. It resulted in significant improvements in diet and physical activity (Sternfeld et al. 2009). An advantage of email in a worksite setting is that the intervention comes to participants with little effort on the part of the participants once they sign up—the participant does not have to actively seek out the program.

Electronic and Digital Games

Electronic and digital games can be played on computers, tablets, phones, and video gaming systems. Video games provide extensive player involvement and are being explored for delivering health behavior change interventions in an engaging way (Baranowski et al. 2008, 2013; DeSmet et al. 2014). A theory-based psychoeducational game for fourth graders was highly effective in increasing fruit and vegetable intakes (Baranowski et al. 2003). Two serious video games for middle school youths, Escape from Diab and Nanoswarm, were able to teach goal setting skills (Thompson et al. 2007) and increase fruit and vegetable consumption (though not water consumption or physical activity) (Baranowski et al. 2011). In another serious game, Creature 101, middle school youth build avatars that live on another planet and are asked to care for creatures on that planet and assist them to eat more healthfully (Majumdar et al. 2013, 2015). It was effective at reducing consumption of sweetened drinks and processed snacks (see **FIGURE 16-6**). A randomized controlled study of a computer game with young adults found positive results on mediators and intentions to eat a healthy diet (Peng 2009).

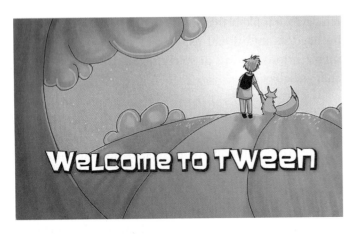

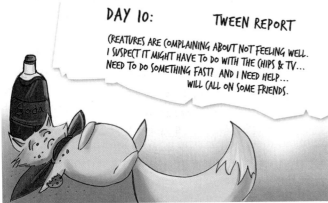

FIGURE 16-6 Creature 101 is a serious game for improving energy-balance–related behaviors in middle school children.

Majumdar, D., P. A. Koch, H. Lee, I. R. Contento, A. D. Islas-Ramos, and D. Fu. 2013. "Creature-101": A serious game to promote energy balance-related behaviors among middle school adolescents. Games for Health Journal 2(5):280–290.

Phone Calls and Teleconferences

While telephones themselves are not particularly advanced, they can still offer new nutrition education methods. For example, motivational interviewing over the telephone has shown some effectiveness. U.S. veterans increased their fruit and vegetable intake when motivational interview phone calls were used in nutrition education, compared to controls (Allicock et al. 2010). Members of black churches were also reached with telephone motivational interviewing with some success (Resnicow et al. 2001).

In addition to motivational interviewing, phones can be used for teleconferences. One study asked low-income overweight and obese mothers to join peer support group teleconferences as part of their intervention to prevent weight gain (Chang et al. 2014).

Apps

Smartphones and computers can download software called applications or apps that take many forms, such as podcasts (digital audio recordings) or tracking systems for food intake and physical activity expenditure. In one study, participants were instructed to use an intake and activity monitoring mobile app and listen to two nutrition education–related podcasts per week for 6 months. Participants successfully lost weight during this study (Turner-McGrievy and Tate 2011). Mobile apps are also being employed in school settings, such as in the 8-month multicomponent intervention with teenagers (Smith et al. 2014).

Text Messaging

Text messages through phones or hand-held computers have been found to be very useful in helping individuals self-monitor their diet and activity-related behaviors (Fjeldsoe, Marshall, and Miller 2009). Of those who currently own a cell phone, an estimated 81% have text-messaging capabilities. Some 70–92% of low-income individuals have *text-messaging* apps and Internet capabilities (Ahlers-Schmidt et al. 2011). After counseling or group sessions where individuals receive nutrition education, they can then receive messages, reminders, and tips daily, or even several times a day, depending on their choice. Messages through this channel have been useful for helping people lose weight or regulate their blood glucose level (Patrick et al. 2009; Newton, Wiltshire, and Elley 2009). Other studies have found text messaging useful for self-monitoring of sweetened beverage intake, physical activity, and screen time in children (Shapiro et al. 2008); for adherence to dietary recommendations in women (Glanz et al. 2006); and for support for youth with diabetes (Franklin et al. 2006).

Multimedia Soap Opera

A multimedia approach using a tailored soap opera and interactive infomercials that provided individualized feedback, knowledge, and strategies for lowering fat, based on stage of change, was effective (Campbell et al. 1999). Another multimedia soap opera approach was used to promote fruit and vegetable consumption, as well as promote English as a second language (ESL) to American immigrants (Martinez et al. 2013).

INDIVIDUALIZED MESSAGES

Individually tailored messages can enhance the effectiveness of communications through non-personal media such as letters, newsletters, and computers. In this approach, a targeted group—such as employees at a worksite or clients of a physician—is sent a questionnaire that asks them about their current practices with respect to the target behavior, as well as their beliefs, attitudes, social norms, perceived barriers, or state of change. They are then sent computer-generated letters that specifically address their own particular set of beliefs and practices. Thus, this approach addresses issues that are personally relevant to the target audience and the choices they have to make. Evidence suggests that such an approach may enhance effectiveness compared with general communications (Brug, Oenema, and Campbell 2003). Tailoring can also be based on the core values of a given cultural group, in addition to behavioral theory constructs, and has been found to enhance effectiveness (Kreuter et al. 2003, 2005).

Computer-tailored personal letters, newsletters, and magazines have been used with a variety of audiences: general practitioners' clients, healthy employees, healthy volunteers, retirees, members of health maintenance organizations, and church members.

Another channel that can be used is an interactive computer approach: one study used computers in the classroom for overweight prevention (Ezendam et al. 2007); another used touch-screen computers accompanied by in-person counseling and follow-up telephone counseling (Stevens et al. 2002). In addition, Web-based tailored messages and interactive approaches, such as nutrition assessment, goal setting, and monitoring, are becoming more popular among multiple age groups in nutrition education (Oenema, Brug, and Lechner 2001; De Bourdeaudhuij et al. 2007; Atkinson et al. 2009; Werkman et al. 2010; Mouttapa et al. 2011).

ADVANCED TECHNOLOGY WITH YOUTH

Because the current youth generation has grown up with advanced technology, using these methods can be engaging and has potential. As of 2013, 78% of teens aged 12–17 years had a cell phone and almost half (47%) of those were smartphones; one in four teens (23%) had a tablet computer, and nine in ten (93%) had a computer or had access to one at home (Pew Internet 2013). These numbers will no doubt grow even further. A systematic review and a meta-analysis of studies have concluded that computer-tailored personalized education improved desired energy-balance–related behaviors more than a generic classroom curriculum in schools (De Bourdeaudhuij et al. 2011; Delgado-Noguera et al. 2011).

Summary

Nutrition education for the public can be delivered through a variety of venues. This chapter describes some of the main channels and media you can use. It is important that you carefully determine your objectives when you use each of the channels and supporting materials. Sessions with groups are enhanced with the use of visuals, which can range from real foods and food packages to flip charts and slide presentations. Visuals should be interesting but simple. They should be clearly visible and appropriate in size so that you never have to say, "I know you can't read this, but . . .". Written materials such as brochures, flyers, and handouts are also widely used. If they are to be effective, however, you should carefully tailor each piece to your intended audience and make the writing motivational and reader-friendly. Written materials should be designed to look interesting and be easy to read. Other supporting channels include cooking or food preparation activities, conducting grocery tours, and planning health fairs.

This chapter also describes how nutrition educators can be involved in mass media communication campaigns as well as social marketing activities. Delivering nutrition education through these channels usually involves working with experts in these fields and within coalitions and collaborations. The principles of social marketing are described as well as many of the kinds of activities in which nutrition educators can participate as part of social marketing campaigns. It should be clear that there are numerous channels that you can use with any audience. This chapter had the space to describe only some of them. There are many more venues through which nutrition education can be delivered, and these are evolving very rapidly. It is important for nutrition educators to stay attuned to these developments.

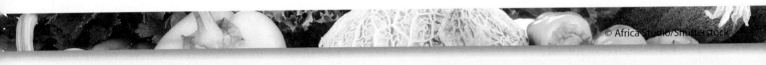

© Africa Studio/Shutterstock

Questions and Activities

1. What are the major advantages of using supporting visuals when working with groups?

2. What kinds of visuals might you use when working with groups? Describe how your choice might differ depending on your audience, such as teens in an after-school program or older adults at a senior citizen center.

3. List the design principles you would use to avoid having to say to a group, "I know that you cannot read this, but . . .".

4. Prepare a poster for use with a group that depicts one idea or theme. Write a description of your objectives for the visual and your intended audience. Write an analysis of your visual explaining how you used art and design principles to enhance quality.

5. You have prepared well for your session, your visuals are in place, and you are now in front of the group. Describe five guidelines for using the visuals in an effective manner.

6. Think of the last time you developed a printed piece. What objectives did you expect it to serve? Do you think it achieved your objectives? Why or why not?

7. How would you ensure that your printed materials are motivating and effective? Describe several specific ways of doing so.

8. You have decided that you will use cooking or food preparation as part of your nutrition education intervention. Based on what you have read, describe three guidelines to ensure a successful learning experience for your participants.

9. What purposes might be served by organizing nutrition education events at health fairs? Describe three tips to ensure that your purposes are met.

10. A central concept in social marketing is the concept of the "exchange." Describe this concept carefully.

11. Compare and contrast nutrition education and social marketing. How do they relate to each other?

12. Design social marketing to accompany the group sessions that you planned during the DESIGN Procedure. Indicate what exactly is the exchange in this setting and how you use the 4 Ps in your design.

13. Design an intervention with a social media component (e.g., Facebook). Indicate your target audience and strategies to encourage audience participation.

14. Choose a food or nutrition app that you like and use. Assuming it is designed to help you or your clients achieve some behavioral goal, carefully examine whether and how it uses theory variables to achieve behavior change.

15. You are thinking of developing a smartphone app that would help your audience drink fewer sweetened beverages each day. How might you use the DESIGN process to develop this app?

References

Abercrombie, A., D. Sawatzki, and L. Doner Lotenberg. 2012. Building partnerships to build the Best Bones Forever!: Applying the 4Ps to partnership development. *Social Marketing Quarterly* 18:55–66.

Ahlers-Schmidt, C. R., T. Hart, A. Chesser, A. Paschal, T. Nguyen, and R. R. Wittler. 2011. Content of text messaging immunization reminders: What low-income parents want to know. *Patient Education and Counseling* 85(1):119–121.

Allicock, M., L. Ko, E. van der Sterren, C. G. Valle, M. K. Campbell, and C. Carr. 2010. Pilot weight control intervention among US veterans to promote diets high in fruits and vegetables. *Preventive Medicine* 51(3–4):279–281.

Andreasen, A. R. 1995. *Marketing social change: Changing behavior to promote health, social development, and the environment.* San Francisco: Jossey-Bass.

Atienza, A. A., A. C. King, B. M. Olveira, D. K. Ahn, and C. D. Gardener. 2008. Using hand-held computer technologies to improve dietary intake. *American Journal of Preventive Medicine* 34:514–518.

Atkinson, N. L., S. L. Saperstein, S. M. Desmond, R. S. Gold, A. S. Billing, and J. Tian, 2009. Rural eHealth nutrition education for limited-income families: An iterative and user-centered design approach. *Journal of Medical Internet Research* 11(2):e21.

Baranowski, T., J. Baranowski, K. W. Cullen, T. Marsh, N. Islam, I. Zakeri, et al. 2003. Squire's Quest: Dietary outcome evaluation of a multimedia game. *American Journal of Preventive Medicine* 24:52–61.

Baranowski, T., J. Baranowski, D. Thompson, R. Buday, R. Jago, M. Juliano Griffoth, et al. 2011. Video game play, child diet, and physical activity behavior change: A randomized clinical trial. *American Journal of Preventive Medicine* 40(1):33–38.

Baranowski, T., R. Buday, D. I. Thompson, and J. Baranowski. 2008. Playing for real: Video games and stories for health-related behavior change. *American Journal of Preventive Medicine* 34:74–82.

Baranowski, T., R. Buday, D. Thompson, E. J. Lyons, A. S. Lu, and J. Baranowski. 2013. Developing games for health behavior change: Getting started. *Games for Health Journal* 2(4):183–190.

Baranowski, T., and L. Frankel. 2012. Let's get technical! Gaming and technology for weight control and health promotion in children. *Childhood Obesity* 8(1):34–37.

Baranowski, T., N. Islam, D. Douglass, H. Dadabhoy, A. Beltran, J. Baranowski, et al. 2014. Food Intake Recording Software System, version 4 (FIRSSt4): A self-completed 24-h dietary recall for children. *Journal of Human Nutrition and Dietetics* 27(Suppl. 1):66–71.

Bort-Roig, J., N. D. Gilson, A. Puig-Ribera, R. S. Contreras, and S. G. Trost. 2014. Measuring and influencing physical activity with smartphone technology: A systematic review. *Sports Medicine* 44(5):671–686.

Brown, B. J., and B. J. Hermann. 2005. Cooking classes increase fruit and vegetables intake and food safety behaviors in youth and adults. *Journal of Nutrition Education and Behavior* 37:1004–1005.

Brug, J., A. Oenema, and M. Campbell. 2003. Past, present, and future of computer-tailored nutrition education. *American Journal of Clinical Nutrition* 77(4 Suppl):1028S–1034S.

Brug, J., A. Oenema, and H. Raat. 2005. The Internet and nutrition education: Challenges and opportunities. *European Journal of Clinical Nutrition* 59(Suppl.):S130–S139.

Campbell, M. K., L. Honess-Morreale, D. Farrell, E. Carbone, and M. Brasure. 1999. A tailored multimedia nutrition education pilot program for low-income women receiving food assistance. *Health Education Research* 14:257–267.

Centers for Disease Control and Prevention. 2014a. Social marketing for nutrition and physical activity web course. http://www.cdc.gov/nccdphp/dnpao/socialmarketing/index.html Accessed 12/3/14.

———. 2014b. Case studies. http://www.cdc.gov/nccdphp/dnpao/socialmarketing/casestudies.html. Accessed 12/3/14.

Chang, M. W., S. Nitzke, R. Brown, and K. Resnicow. 2014. A community based prevention of weight gain intervention (Mothers in Motion) among young low-income overweight and obese mothers: Design and rationale. *BMC Public Health* 14(1):280.

De Bourdeaudhuij, I., V. Stevens, C. Vandelanotte, and J. Brug. 2007. Evaluation of an interactive computer-tailored nutrition intervention in a real-life setting. *Annals of Behavorial Medicine* 33(1):39–48.

De Bourdeaudhuij, I., E. Van Cauwenberghe, H. Spittaels, J. M. Oppert, C. Rostami, J. Brug, et al. 2011. School based interventions promoting both physical activity and eating in Europe: A systematic review within the HOPE project. *Obesity Research* 12(3):205–216.

Delgado-Noguera, M., S. Tort, M. J. Martínez-Zapata, and X. Bonfill. 2011. Primary school interventions to promote fruit and vegetables consumption: a systematic review and meta-analysis. *Preventive Medicine* 53(1–2):3–9.

Direito, A., L P. Dale, E. Shields, R. Dobson, R. Whitaker, and R. Maddison. 2014. Do physical activity and dietary smart-phone applications incorporate evidence-based behavior change techniques? *BMC Public Health* 14:646.

DeSmet, A., D. Van Ryckeghem, S. Compernolle, T. Baranowski, D. Thompson, G. Crombez, et al. 2014. A meta-analysis of serious digital games for healthy lifestyle promotion. *Preventive Medicine* 69:95–107.

Duggan, M., and A. Smith. 2013. Social Media Update 2013. http://www.pewinternet.org/2013/12/30/social-media-update-2013/ Accessed 4/14/14.

Ezendam, N. P., A. Oenema, P. M. van de Looij-Jansen, and J. Brug. 2007. Design and evaluation protocol of "FATaintPhat," a computer-tailored intervention to prevent weight gain in adolescents. *BMC Public Health* 12(7):324.

Fjeldsoe B. S., A. L. Marshall, and Y. D. Miller. 2009. Behavior change interventions delivered by mobile telephone short-message service. *American Journal of Preventive Medicine* 36(2):165–173.

Franklin, V. L., A. Waller, C. Pagliari, and S. A. Green. 2006. A randomized control trial of Sweet Talk, a text-messaging system to support young people with diabetes. *Diabetic Medicine* 23:1332–1338.

Glanz, K., S. Murphy, J. Moylan, D. Evensen, and J. D. Curb. 2006. Improved self-monitoring and adherence with hand-held computers: A pilot study. *American Journal of Health Promotion* 20:165–170.

Hearn, L., M. Miller, and A. Fletcher. 2013. Online healthy lifestyle support in the prenatal period: What do woman want and do they use it? *Australian Journal of Primary Health* 18(4):313–316.

Hutchesson, M. J., C. E. Collins, P. J. Morgan, and R. Callister, 2013. An 8-week web-based weight loss challenge with celebrity endorsement and enhanced social support: Observational study. *Journal of Medical Internet Research* 15(7):e129. DOI:10.2196/jmir.2540.

Institute of Medicine. 2002. *Speaking of health: Assessing health communication strategies for diverse populations.* Washington, DC: National Academies Press.

Iowa Department of Public Health. n.d. Pick a better snack. www.idph.state.ia.us/inn/Pickabettersnack.aspx Accessed 11/1/14.

Knight, S., and C. Probart. 1992. How to avoid saying "I know you can't read this but . . .". *Journal of Nutrition Education* 24:94B.

Kotler, P., and E. L. Roberto. 1989. *Social marketing: Strategies for changing public behavior.* New York: The Free Press.

Kotler, P., and G. Zaltman. 1971. Social marketing: An approach to planned social change. *Journal of Marketing* 35:3–12.

Kreuter, M. W., S. N. Kukwago, D. C. Bucholtz, E. M. Clark, and V. Sanders-Thompson. 2003. Achieving cultural appropriateness in health promotion programs: Targeted and tailored approaches. *Health Education and Behavior* 30:133–146.

Kreuter, M. W., C. Sugg-Skinner, C. L. Holt, E. M. Clark, D. Haire-Joshu, Q. Fu, et al. 2005. Cultural tailoring for mammography and fruit and vegetables intake among low-income African-American women in urban public health centers. *Preventive Medicine* 41:53–62.

Kroeze, W., A. Werkman, and J. Brug. 2006. A systematic review of randomized trials on the effectiveness of computer-tailored education and physical activity and dietary behaviors. *Annals of Behavioral Medicine* 31(3):205–223.

Lange, M. 2014. 59 percent of tiny children use social media. *New York Magazine*/The Cut. http://nymag.com/thecut/2014/02/over-half-kids-social-media-before-age-ten.html. Accessed 4/30/14.

Leak, T. M., L. Benavente, L. S. Goodell, A. Lassiter, L. Jones, and S. Bowen. 2014. EFNEP graduates' perspectives on social media to supplement nutrition education: Focus group findings from active users. *Journal of Nutrition Education and Behavior* 46(3):203–208.

Lee, N. R., and P. Kotler. 2016. *Social marketing: Influencing behaviors for good.* Fifth ed. Thousand Oaks, CA: Sage.

Lefebvre, R. C. 2011. An integrative model for social marketing. *Journal of Social Marketing* 1(1):54–72.

Lefebvre, R. C. 2013. *Social marketing and social change: Strategies and tools for improving health, well-being, and the environment.* San Francisco, CA: Jossey-Bass.

Lefebvre, R. C., and A. S. Bornkessel. 2013. Digital social networks and health. *Circulation* 127(17):1829–1836.

Lefebvre, R. C., and J. Flora. 1988. Social marketing and public health. *Health Education Quarterly* 15:299–315.

Liquori, T., P. D. Koch, I. R. Contento, and J. Castle. 1998. The CookShop program: Outcome evaluation of a nutrition education program linking lunchroom food experiences with classroom cooking experiences. *Journal of Nutrition Education* 30:302–313.

Lohse, B. 2013. Facebook is an effective strategy to recruit low-income women to online nutrition education. *Journal of Nutrition Education and Behavior* 45(1):69–76.

Lucas, S. E. 2011. *The art of public speaking.* 11th ed. New York: McGraw-Hill.

Maibech, E. W., M. L. Rothschild, and W. D. Novelli. 2002. Social marketing. In *Health behavior and health education: Theory, research and practice*, edited by K. Glanz, B. K. Rimer, and F. M. Lewis. San Francisco: Jossey-Bass.

Majumdar, D., P. A. Koch, H. Lee, I. R. Contento, A. de Lourdes Islas-Ramos, and D. Fu. 2013. "Creature-101": a serious game to promote energy balance-related behaviors among middle school adolescents. *Games for Health Journal* 2(5): 280–290.

Majumdar, D., P. A. Koch, H. Lee Gray, I. R. Contento, A. de Lourdes Islas-Ramos, and D. Fu. 2015. Nutrition science and behavioral theories integrated in a serious game for adolescents. *Simulation & Gaming*: 1–30. DOI: 10.1177/1046878115577163.

Manoff, R. K. 1985. *Social marketing.* New York: Praeger.

Mansbridge, J. J. 1990. *Beyond self-interest.* Chicago: University of Chicago Press.

Marcus, A. C., J. Heimendinger, P. Wolfe, D. Fairclough, B. K. Rimer, M. Morra, et al. 2001. A randomized trial of a brief intervention to increase fruit and vegetable intake: A replication study among callers to the CIS. *Preventive Medicine* 33:204–216.

Martinez, J. L., S. E. Rivers, L. R. Duncan, M. Bertoli, S. Domingo, A. E. Latimer-Cheung, et al. 2013. Healthy eating for life: Rationale and development of an English as a second language (ESL) curriculum for promoting healthy nutrition. *Translational Behavioral Medicine* 3(4):426–433.

Mouttapa, M., T. P. Robertson, A. J. McEligot, J. W. Weiss, L. Hoolihan, A. Ora, et al. 2011. The Personal Nutrition Planner: A 5-week, computer-tailored intervention for women. *Journal of Nutrition Education Behavior* 43(3): 165–172.

Napolitano, M. A., S. Hayes, G. G. Bennett, A. K. Ives, and G. D. Foster. 2013. Using Facebook and text messaging to deliver a weight loss program to college students. *Obesity (Silver Spring)* 21(1):25–31.

National Cancer Institute. 2004. *Making health communication programs work* (NIH Publication No. 04-5145). Bethesda, MD: National Cancer Institute, U.S. Department of Health and Human Services.

Newton, K. H., E. J. Wiltshire, and C. R. Elley. 2009. Pedometers and text messaging to increase physical activity: Randomized controlled trial of adolescents with type 1 diabetes. *Diabetes Care* 32(5):813–815.

Oenema, A., J. Brug, and L. Lechner. 2001. Web-based tailored nutrition education: Results of a randomized controlled trial. *Health Education Research* 16:647–660.

Osborn, E., M. D. Sadler, S. L. Saperstein, and D. Sawatzki. 2012. Physical activity in action: The *Best Bones Forever!* Let's Dance contest featuring Savvy. *Cases in Public Health Communication and Marketing* 6:65–86.

Patrick, K., F. Raab, M. A. Adams, L. Dillon, M. Zabinski, C. L. Rock, et al. 2009. A text-message–based intervention for weight loss: Randomized controlled trial. *Journal of Medical Internet Research* 11(1):e1.

Peng, W. 2009. Design and evaluation of a computer game to promote a healthy diet for young adults. *Health Communication* 24:115–127.

Pew Internet. 2013. Teens and technology 2013. Pew Research Internet Project. http://www.pewinternet.org/2013/03/13/teens-and-technology-2013/ Accessed 11/30/14.

———. 2014a. African Americans and technology use: Detailed demographic tables. Pew Research Internet Project. http://www.pewinternet.org/2014/01/06/detailed-demographic-tables/ Accessed 11/30/14.

———. 2014b. How the internet has woven itself into American life. Pew Research Internet Project. http://www.pewinternet.org/2014/02/27/part-1-how-the-internet-has-woven-itself-into-american-life/ Accessed 11/30/14.

Raines, C., and L. Williamson. 1995. *Using visual aids: The effective use of type, color, and graphics.* Revised ed. Menlo Park, CA: Crisp Learning.

Reicks M., A. C. Trofhloz, J. S. Stang, and M. N. Laaska. 2014. Impact of cooking and home food preparation interventions among adults: Outcomes and implications for future programs. *Journal of Nutrition Education and Behavior* 46(4):259–276.

Resnicow, K., A. Jackson, T. Wang, et al. 2001. A motivational interviewing intervention to increase fruit and vegetable intake through black churches: Results of the Eat for Life trial. *American Journal of Public Health* 91: 1686–1693.

Rogers, E. M., and J. D. Storey. 1988. Communications campaigns. In *Handbook of communication science*, edited by C. R. Berger and S. H. Chaffee. Newbury Park, CA: Sage.

Rothschild, M. L. 1999. Carrots, sticks, and promises: A conceptual framework for the management of public health and social issue behaviors. *Journal of Marketing* 63:24–37.

Sadler, M. D., S. L. Saperstein, E. Golan, L. Doner Lotenberg, D. Sawatzki, A. Abercrombie, et al. 2013. Integrating bone health information into existing health education efforts. *ICAN: Infant, Child, and Adolescent Nutrition* 5(3): 177–183.

Shapiro, J. R., S. Bauer, R. M. Hamer, H. Kordy, D. Ward, and C. M. Bulik. 2008. Use of text-messaging for monitoring sugar-sweetened beverages, physical activity, and screen time in children: A pilot study. *Journal of Nutrition Education and Behavior* 40:385–391.

Smith, J. J., P. J. Morgan, R. C. Plotnikoff, K. A. Dally, J. Salmon, A. D. Okely, et al. 2014. Rationale and study protocol for the 'Active Teen Leaders Avoiding Screen-time' (ATLAS) group randomized controlled trial: An obesity prevention intervention for adolescent boys from schools in low-income communities. *Contemporary Clinical Trials* 37(1):106–119. DOI:10.1016/j.cct.2013.11.008.

Smith, S. B., and B. J. Alford. 1989. Literate and semi-literate audiences: Tips for effective teaching. *Journal of Nutrition Education* 20:238C–D.

Snyder, L. B. 2007. Health communications campaigns and their impact on behavior. *Journal of Nutrition Education and Behavior* 39:S32–S40.

Sternfeld, B., C. Block, C. P. Quesenberry Jr., T. J. Block, G. Hussan, J. C. Norris, et al. 2009. Improving diet and physical activity with ALIVE: A worksite randomized trial. *American Journal of Preventive Medicine* 36(6):475–483.

Stevens, V. J., R. E. Glasgow, D. J. Toobert, N. Karanja, and K. S. Smith. 2002. Randomized trial of a brief dietary intervention to decrease consumption of fat and increase consumption of fruits and vegetables. *American Journal of Health Promotion* 16:129–134.

Thompson, D., T. Baranowski, J. Baranowski, K. Cullen, R. Jago, K. Watson, et al. 2009. Boy Scouts 5-a-Day badge: Outcome results of a troop and internet intervention. *Preventive Medicine* 49:518–526.

Thompson, D., T. Baranowski, R. Buday, J. Baranowski, M. Juliano, M. Frazior, et al. 2007. In pursuit of change: Youth response to intensive goal setting embedded in a serious video game. *Journal of Diabetes Science and Technology* 1:907–917.

Thompson, D., T. Baranowski, K. Cullen, K. Watson, Y. Liu, A. Canada, et al. 2008. Food, Fun, and Fitness, internet program for girls: Pilot evaluation of an e-health youth obesity prevention program examining predictors of obesity. *Preventive Medicine* 47:494–497.

Tobey, L. N., and M. M. Manore. 2014. Social media and nutrition education: The food hero experience. *Journal of Nutrition Education and Behavior* 46(2):128–133.

Turner-McGrievy, G., and D. Tate. 2011. Tweets, apps, and pods: Results of the 6-month Mobile Pounds Off Digitally (Mobile POD) randomized weight-loss intervention among adults. *Journal of Medical Internet Research* 13(4):e120. DOI:10.2196/jmir.1841.

Valle, C. G., D. F. Tate, D. K. Mayer, M. Allicock, and J. Cai. 2013. A randomized trial of a Facebook-based physical activity intervention for young adult cancer survivors. *Journal of Cancer Survivors* 7(3):355–368.

Van Den Heede, F. A., and S. Pelican. 1995. Reflections on marketing as an inappropriate model for nutrition education. *Journal of Nutrition Education* 27:141–145.

Wadsworth, K. 2005. From farm to table: The making of a classroom chef. Presented at the Society for Nutrition Education Conference, Orlando, FL.

Werkman, A., P. J. Hulshof, A. Stafleu, S. P. Kremers, F. J. Kok, E. G. Schouten, et al. 2010. Effect of an individually tailored one-year energy balance programme on body weight, body composition and lifestyle in recent retirees: A cluster randomised controlled trial. *BMC Public Health* 10:110.

Williams, G., M. P. Hamm, J. Shulhan, B. Vandermeer, and L. Hartling. 2014. Social media interventions for diet and exercise behaviors: A systematic review and meta-analysis of randomized controlled trials. *BMJ Open* 4(2):e003926. DOI:10.1136/bmjopen-2013-003926.

CHAPTER 17

Working with Diverse Age, Cultural, and Literacy Population Groups

OVERVIEW

This chapter provides an overview of strategies and methods to deliver systematically designed, behaviorally focused, theory-based nutrition education to various age and population groups.

CHAPTER OUTLINE

- Introduction
- Working with children and youth
- The adult learner
- Working with diverse cultural groups
- Low-literacy audiences
- Groups that differ by food-related lifestyle factors
- Summary

LEARNING OBJECTIVES

At the end of the chapter, you should be able to:

- Describe key features of the cognitive and emotional development of children and adolescents
- Deliver nutrition education activities that are appropriate to the developmental level of youth
- Conduct nutrition education activities that are based on adult education principles
- Describe key features of cultural competence, cultural sensitivity, and cultural appropriateness in the nutrition education context
- Demonstrate understanding of ways to deliver nutrition education activities that are culturally sensitive and appropriate
- Deliver nutrition education activities that are appropriate for low-literacy audiences
- Apply design principles for written and visual materials for use in nutrition education for low-literacy audiences

Introduction

At a nutrition education session, a group of mothers of young children sit in a circle, sharing their experiences of trying to provide healthful meals for their young children. They are animated and fully engaged with each other for an hour as they share challenges and successes. The educator facilitates the discussion unobtrusively and helps the group to come to closure about what they will do about this issue during the coming week.

Now try to imagine a group of preschoolers sitting in a circle and having a similar discussion for an hour, with little guidance from a nutrition educator. Totally impossible, of course! Clearly, the way nutrition education is delivered must be tailored to the group with which you are working. It is thus important to understand the differing characteristics of different population groups. Nutrition educators work in numerous settings: communities, healthcare settings, schools, food- and food-system–related community and advocacy organizations, and workplaces, among others. (See Chapter 1 for more details.) In addition, nutrition educators work with many diverse audiences, differing by age, sex, ethnicity, cultural background, religious affiliation, developmental stage, literacy status, socioeconomic status, geographic location, and so forth. They also work with many groups that have specific food- or nutrition-related issues, such as people with diabetes, pregnant and lactating women, and those who are overweight, to name a few.

This chapter focuses on audiences at different ages and stages of life, from different cultural backgrounds, and with different literacy levels. It provides some background information on each audience and makes suggestions regarding nutrition education delivery methods that are appropriate for each (Contento et al. 1995). Your intervention or session is more likely to be effective when you consider some of these differences in appropriate delivery methods at the time you are designing your educational plan or lesson plan through a systematic process such as the DESIGN Procedure. (See Chapters 7–14.)

Working with Children and Youth

Children are not little adults. Children are undergoing rapid physical, cognitive, and socio-emotional development. Hence, they have their own particular set of concerns and ways of viewing the world, and these change from the preschool years through adolescence. They are in the process of developing various cognitive structures and abilities, understandings of the world, motor skills, social skills, and emotional coping strategies that most adults take for granted. They develop these through their explorations of the world (Piaget and Inhelder 1969) and through social interaction with skilled individuals embedded in a sociocultural backdrop (Vygotsky 1962; Bronfenbrenner 1979). Understanding how children develop and how they learn about food and eating is crucial as you develop your educational plans or intervention in Step 5 of the DESIGN Procedure.

THE PRESCHOOL CHILD

The way young children view and experience the world is qualitatively different from that of adults. Child development research provides evidence that the cognitive world of preschool children is creative, fanciful, and free. However, they are becoming less dependent on their direct sensorimotor actions for direction of behavior and are increasingly able to function in a symbolic-conceptual mode in their thinking, for example, using scribbled designs to represent people, cars, houses, and other objects. They have some causal reasoning ability, but it does not lead to abstract generalizations or formation of logical concepts, as in older children or adults. Their attention span is short and they cannot distinguish between their perspective and that of another person. It is not surprising, then, that children younger than 4 years of age cannot consistently discern between television advertising and the informational content of programs. Children between 4 and 8 years of age can distinguish between television advertising and program content but do not effectively understand that the intent of television advertising is to persuade them.

Preschool children learn by manipulating the environment rather than by passive listening—that is, they learn by exploring, questioning, comparing, and labeling. Physical manipulation skills are being developed when children touch, feel, look, mix up, turn over, and throw things. Emotionally, exploration and the need to test independence are important during this time. They take on more initiative and are more purposeful. They are eager to learn, usually from other people: they observe parents, teachers, and other

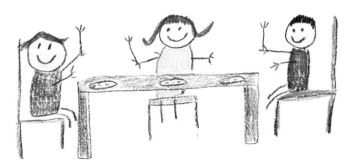

Family meals.
© Jon Schulte/Getty Images

children; they role play; and they start to accumulate and process information.

Young Children's Thinking About Food and Nutrition

Research on preschool children suggests that whereas 2-year-olds are only able to name or identify objects, 3- to 5-year-olds can begin to place them into categories such as size, color, and shape. In the food area, they can easily identify foods and are beginning to classify them. However, they classify foods based on observable qualities such as shape and color and easily identifiable features such as whether they are sweet or non-sweet foods, or whether they are meal items versus those that are more versatile including breakfast items and snacks (Michela and Contento 1984; Matheson, Spranger, and Saxe 2002). When asked in open-ended interviews, children know that food enters the body and leaves, but are not clear what happens there. They think that spinach, for example, goes unchanged into the muscles of Popeye (Contento 1981). However, they are curious about how things work and constantly ask the question "why," and start to develop some ideas about causal mechanisms. A study, described later, showed that when taught a conceptual framework to explain what happens to food, these young children can develop useful understandings (Gripshover and Markman 2013). They are also beginning to be able to relate foods to health: when asked what it means to be healthy, children mention "eating the right foods" as well as "big" and "strong." When asked what are the right kinds of foods, they name specific fruits and vegetables. Unhealthy foods named are high-fat, high-sugar snack foods (Singleton, Achterberg, and Shannon 1992).

When preschool children playing in toy kitchens were asked to make a meal for a research assistant, they demonstrated that they already had some knowledge of meal planning, food preparation, table preparation, food serving, eating, and cleaning up (Matheson et al. 2002). They also had notions about eating rules such as "You must eat a little bit of everything," "Eat it—it is good for you," and "This is mine and that's yours; you can eat whatever you want."

These observations suggest that nutrition education should not focus primarily on food group information but should instead emphasize conceptual frameworks, active methods, and play activities.

Young Children and Familiarity with Food

Children are not born with the natural ability to choose a nutritious diet; they have to learn to do so. The accumulating evidence from research suggests that early experience with food and eating has an impact on the development of food preferences and on the regulation of the amount of food eaten in several ways.

- *Familiarity with the food.* Very young children show a neophobic response, or reluctance to taste new or unfamiliar foods, a natural and protective mechanism that is one of the most common reasons for food rejection (Dovey et al. 2008). However, repeated exposures increase children's preference for a food or beverage (Birch 1999). A longitudinal study found that a large percentage of children's food preferences were formed as early as age 2 to 3 years and did not change over the 5-year period of the study, at which point the children were age 8 (Skinner et al. 2002). Other studies have shown that dislike of foods can be transformed into liking when children are repeatedly exposed to foods through tasting and eating (Wardle, Cooke, et al. 2003; Wardle, Herrara, et al. 2003; Savage, Fisher, and Birch 2007; Anzman-Frasca et al. 2012).

- *Association of foods with the physiological consequences of eating.* Very young children seem to be able to regulate the amount they eat based almost solely on their physiological reactions to foods (i.e., feeling full) (Birch 1987, 1999). As they get older, however, children eat substantially more when larger portions are offered, suggesting that the ability to respond solely to internal physiological cues decreases with age as external factors become more influential (Rolls, Engell, and Birch 2000; Fisher, Rolls, and Birch 2003). Indeed, they often learn to eat in the absence of hunger (Fisher and Birch 2002).

■ *Association of foods with the emotional tone of the social interactions that surround feeding.* Children come to prefer foods that are eaten in a positive emotional atmosphere (Birch 1987) as well as foods eaten by their peers. A survey of Head Start parents showed that their own positive nutrition-related attitudes were related to more pleasant family mealtimes, fewer negative mealtime practices, and less troublesome child eating behaviors (Gable and Lutz 2001). Head Start program mealtime environments and practices can thus contribute importantly to young children coming to like healthful foods.

■ *Learning and self-regulation.* As children develop the ability to identify which food cues are relevant in beginning, continuing, and ending eating, learning and self-regulation become extremely important. As noted previously, very young children seem to be able to regulate the amount they eat based primarily on their physiological reactions to food, but as they get older, external factors, including size of portions served, influence intake (DiSantis et al. 2013). The practices of parents and caregivers at home and preschool become influential as well: they are the providers of the food, they often influence the portion sizes offered, they serve as role models, they often prompt children to eat the healthy food and restrict the unhealthy food, and often provide rewards. The role of these parenting practices is complex, particularly in children of diverse ethnic and socioeconomic backgrounds (Contento, Zybert, and Williams 2005; Lin and Liang 2005; Hoerr et al. 2009; Rhee 2008; Blissett 2011; Pai and Contento 2014). However, the studies do support the recommended practice that it is the responsibility of the adults in families, day care centers, and schools to provide healthful foods, and it is the responsibility of the child to choose how much of these foods to eat, supported by non-controlling practices that encourage healthful eating but do not force consumption, accompanied by moderately restrictive practices about eating less healthful foods and snacks, all in a climate of emotional warmth and sensitivity to the child, is most likely to lead to healthy eating and a healthy weight (Satter 2008; O'Connor et al. 2009; Blisset 2011). From consistent practice in making choices from an array of healthful foods, children learn healthful eating patterns and develop the ability to regulate how much of these foods to eat.

Methods for Delivering Nutrition Education Appropriately to Preschool Children

What practical methods can you use, then, to increase the effectiveness of nutrition education for young children? Based on the information just discussed and on the research literature, the following methods of delivering nutrition education are likely to be useful.

Use Food-Based Activities

Food-based activities such as tasting parties, food preparation, and activities designed to engage the five senses with food are useful. Provide daily exposure to healthful meals and snacks to increase children's preferences for these foods. Nutrition educators note that meals and snacks provided at child care centers should be seen as the centerpiece of nutrition education and should be offered in a positive eating atmosphere.

Create Developmentally Appropriate Learning Experiences

Young children have certain cognitive skills that can be used in nutrition education. Programs also need to be tailored to children's emotional and motor developmental levels. Design activities that take into account the observations that 2- to 3-year-olds can name foods eaten at home or seen in the store and describe the tastes and textures of foods, whereas older preschoolers can classify foods by color and function, identify foods seen on TV, and learn reading skills along with food and nutrition by reading food-themed storybooks (Hertzler and DeBord 1994). In terms of the link between food and health, 2- to 3-year-olds can name body parts and tell the location of organs, such as eyes, and what they do. Older preschoolers can compare breathing and pulse rate when doing different activities and can state general connections between food and the body, for example, that carrots are good for your eyes.

Studies suggest that by age 5, young children have developed considerable knowledge about causal mechanisms based on intuitive theories they have developed from their own everyday observations (and their persistent question: "why?"), intuitive ideas, and cultural learning (Gropnik et al. 2001; Au et al. 2008; Gelman et al. 2009). An intervention that provided a conceptual explanatory framework to teach about the *mechanisms* for the functions of food in the body was effective in teaching important nutrition concepts and had some impact on behavior (Gripshover and Markman 2013). Here through storybooks read at snack time, children learned that variety is desirable (it is not healthy to eat just one kind of food) and that food contains tiny invisible nutrients that are extracted by the stomach and carried by blood to all parts of the body, where they are needed for all functions, both active (running) and inactive (thinking). The intervention did not provide specific instruction on healthy eating, but children did select more vegetables than the control group at snack time. This explanatory, mechanistic framework represents a "why-to" knowledge approach as opposed the often-used factual knowledge approach (which food goes into which food group) and appears to be motivational for behavior change in preschool children as for other age groups.

Apply Activity- and Play-Based Teaching Methods

Design activity-based teaching methods and play-based educational plans that build on children's naturalistic environments and interests. These activities should have clear messages so that they are "minds-on" as well as "hands-on." Studies show that where interventions had an impact on knowledge and eating practices, active participation by children in a nonthreatening environment was most conducive to success. Employ activities such as art projects, songs, jingles, role playing, stories, puppets, and puzzles. Curricula can focus on play. Toy kitchens or grocery stores provide opportunities for nutrition education. In addition, children can role play, trying new foods or practicing food safety behaviors in these contexts (Matheson et al. 2002). Children can work in school gardens or planter boxes in classrooms, learning about how food grows.

Focus on Behaviors

Identify specific children's behaviors to focus on, such as trying new foods, eating vegetables, or eating healthful snacks. Then work with parents and preschool staff to model eating healthful meals and snacks, offer foods to children in a positive social environment, and use rewards appropriately. For example, "trying new foods" was the behavior addressed in a social marketing campaign directed at preschoolers, called Food Friends. It used many of the kinds of activities described earlier: sensory activities that included "fruit and vegetable mystery bags,"

storybooks, opportunities to try new foods, and parental involvement (Young et al. 2004; Bellows and Anderson 2006; Bellows et al. 2006).

Encourage Self-Regulation

Parents and preschools can encourage the child's ability to self-regulate. It is the responsibility of families and preschools to provide children with healthful foods in appropriate settings and at appropriate times, but children should be able to choose how much to eat from among these foods. From this practice, children will learn to self-regulate the appropriate amounts of food to eat to satisfy hunger. These self-regulation skills will become increasingly cognitive, as well as biological in nature, as children develop cognitively and are exposed to, and have to make conscious choices from, an increasing array of foods, many of which are very attractive in a variety of nonhealthful ways. Children can be encouraged to pay attention to their hunger cues and to eat when they are hungry and to stop when they are full. These are cognitive activities, requiring conscious decisions.

Involve Parents and Families

Involving families either as major recipients of the program or in conjunction with the program offered to the preschool child is crucial for nutrition education of children this age (Ventura and Birch 2008). **BOX 17-1** lists the many core

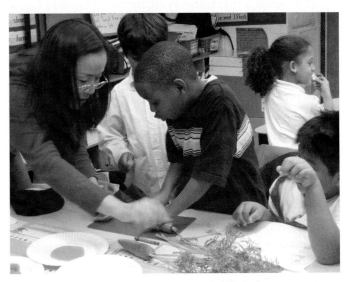

Food preparation helps young children develop motor skills and increases their liking for vegetables.

Courtesy of Program in Nutrition, Teachers College Columbia University.

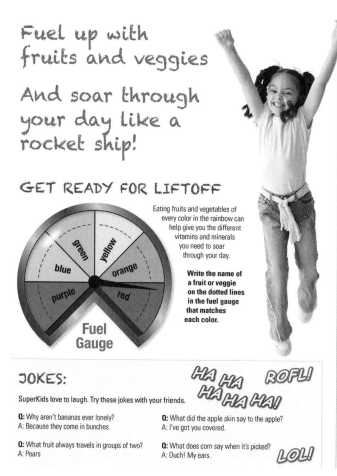

Fuel up with fruits and veggies

And soar through your day like a rocket ship!

GET READY FOR LIFTOFF

Eating fruits and vegetables of every color in the rainbow can help give you the different vitamins and minerals you need to soar through your day.

green yellow
blue   orange
purple red

Fuel Gauge

Write the name of a fruit or veggie on the dotted lines in the fuel gauge that matches each color.

JOKES:

SuperKids love to laugh. Try these jokes with your friends.

HA HA ROFL!
HA HA HA!

Q: Why aren't bananas ever lonely?
A: Because they come in bunches.

Q: What fruit always travels in groups of two?
A: Pears

Q: What did the apple skin say to the apple?
A: I've got you covered.

Q: What does corn say when it's picked?
A: Ouch! My ears.

LOL!

A core message for elementary school children is provided by the USDA.

U.S. Department of Agriculture, http://www.fns.usda.gov/core-nutrition/background.

healthy eating messages that the USDA suggests are appropriate for parents to use with their children. The USDA has also designed posters and other visual images to go with these messages. Some are for the children themselves and an example is shown here. Parents and teachers working together can make more of an impact through mutual reinforcement than either can alone. Studies with Head Start found that educating and encouraging parents was effective in increasing children's knowledge and reported consumption of more nutritious foods.

MIDDLE CHILDHOOD AND ADOLESCENCE

Children grow and change rapidly during the school years (Berk 2012). Middle childhood (ages 6–11) is a time of major cognitive development and mastery of cognitive, physical, and social skills. Children at this age are eager to understand people and the world around them. They like being physically active as their bodies grow steadily in muscle mass and strength and as they grow taller. They progress from dependence on their parents to increasing independence, with an increasing interest in developing friendships with others.

During adolescence (ages 12–19), growth accelerates, leading to dramatic physical, developmental, and social changes that can affect eating patterns. Diet quality declines as children move from childhood through adolescence. Their eating patterns put them at risk for current and future

---

BOX 17-1 Core Nutrition Messages for Children and Families (Selected)

For Mothers of Preschoolers

Role Modeling Messages

- They learn from watching you. Eat fruits and veggies, and your kids will, too.
- They take their lead from you. Eat fruits and veggies, and your kids will, too.
- Mom is a child's first teacher.
- Enjoy each other while enjoying family meals.
- Feed their independent spirit at meal times.

Cooking and Eating Together Messages

- Cook together. Eat together. Talk together. Make mealtime a family time.
- Make meals and memories together. It's a lesson they'll use for life.

- Let go a little to gain a lot.
- Help your child learn to love a variety of foods.

For Mothers of Elementary School–Age Children

Availability/Accessibility Messages

- Want your kids to reach for a healthy snack? Make sure fruits and veggies are in reach.
- When they come home hungry, have fruits and veggies ready to eat.
- Let your kids be "produce pickers." Help them pick fruits and veggies at the store.
- They're still growing. Help your kids grow strong. Serve fat-free or low-fat milk at meals.

(Continues)

BOX 17-1 **Core Nutrition Messages for Children and Families (Selected) (Continued)**

For 8- to 10-Year-Old Children

Food Preference, Beliefs, and Asking Behavior Messages

- Eat smart to play hard. Drink milk (low-fat or fat-free) at meals.
- Fuel up with milk, and soar through your day like a rocket ship.
- Snack like a super hero. Power up with fruit and yogurt.

- Eat smart to play hard. Eat fruits and veggies at meals and snacks.
- Start them early with whole grains.

Consumer-tested supporting content (e.g., bulleted tips, stories, recipes) is available on the USDA's website as are activities and video games for children and YouTube messages and email/social media sharing opportunities for parents. Many other core messages and tips are also available on the website.

Source: U.S. Department of Agriculture. March 2014. Core Nutrition Messages. http://www.fns.usda.gov/core-nutrition/background.

---

health problems, as shown in **BOX 17-2**. They have considerable spending power, and they often have considerable autonomy in food choices as well. A number of these factors influence the choice of methods for delivering nutrition education.

Cognitive Development

Cognitive maturity influences what children can learn from nutrition education. The child comes to school with a host of ideas about the physical and natural world, and these are different from those of adults. Nutrition educators need to understand these differences to communicate well with them. Children are motivated to learn and acquire knowledge and are full of curiosity. In the early school years, children move beyond intuitive thinking to be able to think causally, although reasoning is likely to be limited to concrete objects and specific experiences. They tend to think like scientists, asking many "why"

BOX 17-2 **Typical Eating Patterns of Adolescents in the United States and Their Implications**

Patterns

- Chaotic eating patterns
- Eat rapidly and away from home
- Spend their own money
- Exposed to more than 8 hours per day of various media (TV, computer, radio, magazines)
- Reliance on fast food and convenience food
- Begin to buy and prepare more food for themselves
- Influence parents' buying; do some of the family shopping
- Replacement of milk with soft drinks and other sweetened beverages

Statistics

- Less than 25% of adolescents, grades 9–12, eat at least five servings of fruits and vegetables per day.

- The average teen visits a fast food restaurant two to three times per week and spends $5 to $10 per visit, for a total of $16 billion of spending by teens each year in fast food restaurants.
- Teens spend $11.8 billion in food and snack stores each year.
- Teens spend $868 million each year on snacks and drinks from vending machines.

Why Are These Patterns a Problem?

- Fast foods tend to be high in fat, sugar, and/or salt.
- Sweetened beverages are high in calories.
- Fast foods tend to be low in iron, calcium, riboflavin, vitamin A, folic acid, and vitamin C.
- Inadequate intake of calcium in adolescence can set the stage for osteoporosis later on.
- The rate of type 2 diabetes is increasing among adolescents.

questions. They like to do experiments and can theorize. However, they often maintain their old theories regardless of the evidence and are more likely to be influenced by happenstance events than by overall patterns. They think of food in functional terms. One study found they classified on the basis of sweet versus non-sweet foods; meals versus more versatile foods and drinks; whole, fresh foods versus more highly processed foods; and plant versus animal foods (Michela and Contento 1984). Children's information-processing capacity also increases during the school years, but they use behavioral, concrete, and specific cues to define health, and the criteria for their food choices are specific and immediate (such as taste or cost).

Adolescents begin to think more abstractly and more logically and are able to formulate hypotheses to explain occurrences and imagine alternative explanations for what is observed. They are thus capable of more abstract concepts linking food and health. They begin to develop the ability to grasp the deeper meanings of problems and to think reflectively and critically, keeping an open mind. Becoming more idealistic, they begin to think about idealistic characteristics for themselves and others and to compare themselves and others to ideal standards. They are intrigued by social, political, and moral issues and are willing to speak out on them. In the food area, many become vegetarians or become involved in important food- and nutrition-related causes.

Emotional and Social Development

The emotional and social development of children and youth are important to consider when delivering nutrition education. During middle and late childhood, children spend an increasing amount of time with their peers. Friendships are important because they provide stimulation in the form of interesting information and excitement, a familiar playmate, support, encouragement and feedback, intimacy, affection, and a trusting relationship where aspects of the self can be shared. Friendship also provides a means of social comparison, whereby the child can find out where she or he stands with respect to others. During this period, children begin to understand the perspective of another person and develop greater self-understanding. Development of self-esteem or sense of self-worth is important and can be fostered by providing emotional support and approval and opportunities to develop real skills and a sense of achievement. Self-esteem can also be enhanced by learning to cope with problems realistically rather than by avoiding them.

During adolescence, pubertal changes occur, resulting in rapid growth and sexual maturation. Adolescents also become intensely interested in their body image. They worry about their sexual appearance. They also develop a special kind of egocentrism. Whereas preschoolers' egocentrism derives from the inability to distinguish between their own perspective and that of someone else, adolescent egocentrism is distinguished by belief in an imaginary audience and in a personal fable (Elkind 1978, Shaffer and Kipp 2013). In terms of imaginary audience, adolescents are very aware of other people and believe that others are as preoccupied with them as they are with themselves. They feel they are on stage and the rest of the world is their audience. This leads to the desire to be noticed and visible. At the same time this leads to great concerns. For example, the young woman is sure that everyone will notice and comment on the small, almost invisible spot on her sweater, or the young man imagines that all eyes will be on the tiny blemish on his face. In terms of personal fable, adolescents believe in their personal uniqueness, which results in believing that no one else can understand how they really feel. To foster this uniqueness, adolescents create stories about themselves that are filled with fantasy. They believe that what is really important is what is going on with their particular circle of friends and events at school.

As they grow older, adolescents become more independent, trying to establish themselves as unique individuals (Santrock 2013). They also start developing a better understanding of their own strengths and weaknesses and thinking about the future. They struggle with how they should relate to their friends and family in terms of how to be close to them yet maintain their own independence.

ADOLESCENTS' THINKING, CONCERNS, AND BEHAVIORS WITH RESPECT TO FOOD, NUTRITION, AND HEALTH

Adolescents' eating behaviors are influenced by factors at many levels, as shown in the social ecological model: individual factors, both psychological and biological; interpersonal factors such as family and peers; community settings such as schools or fast food outlets; and societal factors such as mass media, marketing, and sociocultural norms (Story, Neumark-Sztainer, and French 2002). Factors influencing food choices include hunger and food cravings, time, convenience, cost and availability of foods, perceived benefits, mood, body image, and habit. Major barriers to healthy eating include lack of a sense of urgency

BOX 17-3 Cognitive and Emotional Development of Children and Adolescents: Implications for Nutrition Education

Middle Childhood

Characteristics

- Have ideas or theories of how the natural world works that are different from those of adults
- Black-and-white thinkers: causal thinking more developed, but reasoning still limited to concrete objects and specific experiences
- Criteria for food choice specific and immediate
- Curious and motivated to learn: they particularly like to do experiments
- Trust and respect adults
- Playmates and peer friendships increasingly important
- Beginning to desire autonomy

Implications for Nutrition Education

- Use fantasy characters and stories in nutrition education
- Address benefits related to having more energy and/or improved performance in sports
- Use active methods
- Focus on the functional meanings of food
- Include handouts with bright pictures and direct messages
- Foster self-esteem
- Use simple goal setting activities and foster cognitive self-regulation

Early Adolescence

Characteristics

- Causal reasoning becoming more developed
- Criteria for food choice are specific and immediate
- Relationships between food and health are becoming of interest
- Trust and respect adults
- Anxious about peer relationships
- Ambivalent about autonomy
- Preoccupied with the body and body image, and uncomfortable with the physical changes of puberty

- Willing to do or say anything that makes them look or feel better about their body image
- Interested in immediate results

Implications for Nutrition Education

- Address benefits related to looking healthy, having more energy, and/or performance in sports
- Focus on short-term goals
- Include simplified instructions, handouts with bright pictures, and direct messages
- Use active methods

Middle Adolescence

Characteristics

- Abstract thinking skills developing
- Criteria for food choice becoming more complex, with increased reasoning about consequences
- Greatly influenced by peers
- Mistrustful of adults; recurrently challenge adult authority
- Listen to peers more than adults
- Consider independence to be very important and experience significant cognitive development
- More in charge of the food they eat
- Temporary rejection of family dietary patterns

Implications for Nutrition Education

- Design activities to analyze social influences such as television advertising, the media, what's available in neighborhood stores or stores around their schools, and what their friends eat, and their own response to these influences
- Focus on how to make healthful choices when eating out
- Use food demonstrations and taste tests
- Use simplified problem-identification techniques, role playing, and "what if" scenarios
- Guided goal setting is possible
- Foster teenagers' increasing independence while maintaining a caring, yet authoritative role

Late Adolescence

Characteristics

- Abstract thinking more developed; with experience, teens become more skilled at problem solving and decision making
- Criteria for food choice becoming more complex: understand the notion of making trade-offs
- More established body image
- Orientation toward the future and making plans
- Becoming increasingly independent; less challenging of adult authority
- More consistent in their values and beliefs
- Developing intimacy and permanent relationships
- Beginning to think of the long term and about improving their overall health
- Still want to make their own decisions, but are more open to information provided by healthcare providers

Implications for Nutrition Education

- Build educational experiences around motivations that are particularly meaningful to this age group
- Present dietary recommendations and give the rationales behind them
- Focus on behaviors that adolescents have control over
- Discussions of complex issues are now possible, and homework-type assignments are appropriate
- Foster cognitive self-regulation involving goal setting and action plans
- Teach skills to address long-term goals
- Provide food preparation experiences if possible
- Respect their independence and encourage their decision-making skills

about personal health in relation to other more pressing concerns and preferring the taste of other foods (Neumark-Sztainer et al. 1999). **BOX 17-3** notes the implications for nutrition education of the cognitive and social development characteristics of adolescents.

Focus group research has found that adolescents have a significant amount of knowledge about healthful foods and believe that healthful eating involves balance, moderation, and variety. However, they find it difficult to eat healthfully because of their perceived lack of time, the limited availability of healthful options in school, and a general lack of concern about following recommendations (Neumark-Sztainer et al. 1999; Croll, Neumark-Sztainer, and Story 2001).

The weight and body image concerns of adolescents have been of particular interest to nutrition educators. Studies have found that adolescents often attempt to make their weights conform to societal ideals by practicing many weight control behaviors. Most adolescents practice healthy weight control behaviors (85% of girls and 70% of boys in one survey). Some adolescents, particularly those who are overweight, practice some unhealthy weight control behaviors or even behaviors that are extreme (Neumark-Sztainer et al. 2002). However, those who use

moderate methods of weight control have more healthful eating and exercise patterns than those who are extreme dieters or nondieters, suggesting that they might be practicing some degree of self-monitoring and self-regulation (Story et al. 1998).

Cognitive-Motivational Processes and Self-Regulation

The fact that children and adolescents are not concerned about health and nutrition issues to any major extent when they are making food choices is not surprising, given that they do not perceive any urgency to change and that the future seems so distant (Story and Resnick 1986; Neumark-Sztainer et al. 1999). In addition, it has been found that nutrition knowledge alone does not ensure that children and adolescents (or adults, for that matter) will adopt healthful behaviors (Gibson and Wardle 1998).

However, studies show that cognitive-motivational processes do become increasingly important influences on food choice as children become older and more developed cognitively. That is, older children and adolescents become more able to link cause and effect and to perceive the consequences of their actions (Contento and Michela 1998). Thus, they can make food choices in light of their perceptions of anticipated consequences from eating particular foods. Adolescents can make trade-offs among their desired consequences. For example, dieting adolescents in one study were willing to forgo taste and convenience to some degree to obtain less-fattening food (Contento, Michela, and Williams 1995). In another study, adolescents were willing to balance less nutritious items with more nutritious items within a meal, and to balance less healthful lunches with more healthful dinners (Contento et al. 2006).

Remember that adolescents are not monolithic in their food choice motivations. One study found they could be divided into several subgroups with distinct orientations to food, ranging from the hedonistic group, for whom taste and convenience were paramount; to the socially controlled group, for whom friends were most important; to the health-oriented subgroups, who were concerned about personal health (Contento, Michela, and Goldberg 1988). Those in the health-oriented groups had better diets than those in the hedonistic and socially controlled groups. Other studies have reported similar findings that those concerned about health had better diets (Cusatis and Shannon 1996; Gibson and Wardle 1998). It should be noted that health outcomes that have meaning for this group are still short-term outcomes (e.g., that they will have more energy, better athletic performance, or better-looking skin), which should thus be emphasized in nutrition education.

From a social psychological perspective, the picture that emerges from research is that older children and adolescents want particular consequences from the food they eat and become increasingly able to align their food choice behaviors with their goals. They integrate motivations and cognitions in a process of cognitive self-regulation (Contento and Michela 1998). This ability makes it possible for nutrition educators to incorporate the teaching of skills in goal setting, self-monitoring, and other self-regulatory processes to this age group.

Family Influences

What the family serves is still important. Children aged 6 to 11 years obtained 76% of their calories at home, and even adolescents obtained 65% there (Guthrie, Lin, and Frazao 2002). Although adolescents are increasingly independent, making food choices in an ever-widening circle of settings, most still eat some meals at home and families remain an important influence (Bauer et al. 2011). The role of parenting practices also remains important, though it may differ by cultural and socioeconomic groups (Lin and Liang 2005; Hoerr et al. 2009; Pai and Contento 2014). The recommendations remain similar—that families provide healthful foods and encourage healthful eating but do not force consumption, accompanied by moderately restrictive practices about eating less healthful foods and snacks, all in a climate of sensitivity to the child (Rhee 2008; Blissett 2011).

Several surveys suggest that about one-quarter of teens in the United States eat seven or more meals each week with their family, about 40% eat three to six meals a week with them, and 20% eat about one to two meals a week, with only about 15% never eating with their families (Neumark-Sztainer et al. 2003). Increasing frequency of eating family meals among children and adolescents is associated with more healthful dietary patterns (Gillman et al. 2000; Videon and Manning 2003; Neumark-Sztainer et al. 2003; Berge et al. 2013).

Most adolescents in one survey reported that they enjoyed eating meals with the family and that it is a time to bring everybody together and to talk with each other (Neumark-Sztainer et al. 2000a). Major reasons for not eating together were teen schedules, a desire for autonomy, and not liking the foods served or the family atmosphere (Neumark-Sztainer et al. 2000b). Another study found that many adolescents resolved these meal-related conflicting desires by negotiating with others in the family about what to serve at home (Contento et al. 2006). This means that nutrition education can teach youth to more effectively negotiate with their families and to use what they eat at home to balance what they eat elsewhere.

METHODS FOR DELIVERING NUTRITION EDUCATION APPROPRIATELY TO CHILDREN AND YOUTH

Based on the background information just discussed and on the research literature, consider the following as you develop your educational plans or intervention during the DESIGN Procedure and deliver them to your audience to enhance effectiveness.

Focus on Behaviors or Practices Over Which Youth Have Some Control

A behaviorally focused approach to nutrition education improves effectiveness. In the case of older children and adolescents, choose behaviors for the intervention that are of nutritional concern but are also those over which youth have some control. Examples are eating fruits and vegetables, lower-fat snacks and lunches, regular breakfasts, and calcium-rich foods.

Address Motivations that Are Meaningful and Important to Youth

Link information about why to engage in healthful behaviors to motivations that are important to youth, such as having energy, being able to perform well both physically and cognitively, being strong, or having healthy-looking hair or skin. Focus on benefits such as convenience, taste, cost, and other attributes of foods and eating patterns that are relevant to them. Explore barriers. Take into account that some are still growing and that satisfying hunger at low cost is a major motivator, whereas others, particularly girls, have made the transition through puberty and have stabilized in terms of growth.

Thus, make the case for healthful eating in terms that are meaningful for youth. For example, you can help them calculate the costs of the beverages and snacks they currently consume and show how more healthful alternatives can cost the same or less. Or show how convenient it is to prepare fruits and vegetables as snacks. This does not mean you cannot increase a sense of concern about healthful eating. You can. But rather than focusing on their own personal risk for disease, ask youth about whether they have family members who have various chronic diseases such as diabetes and how that makes them feel. This can be a useful way to address the issue of food-related disease risk.

Incorporate Self-Evaluation and Self-Assessment

Youth like self-assessments that are interesting and fun and provide a picture of themselves. A possible activity is to have the class as a group write down what they ate and drank the day before and then analyze these lists in terms of the behavior of focus for your sessions, such as eating breakfast, eating fruits and vegetables, or eating at fast food restaurants. Or you could design a checklist of actions that the group could potentially engage in and come up with a composite score to indicate how well they are doing.

Use Active Methods

Although their attention spans are now longer than those of young children, getting and holding the attention of youth still requires active methods of nutrition education,

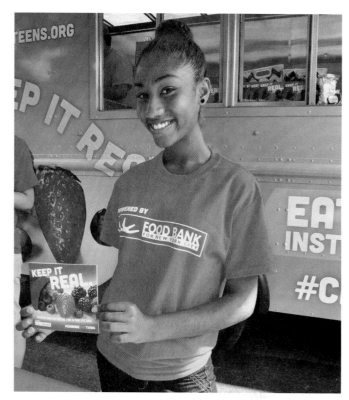

Eatwise youth bring healthful food and nutrition messages to their communities.

Tania Fuentez. Courtesy of Food Bank For New York City.

perhaps alternating with mini-lectures. Food preparation or food-related demonstrations with participation of volunteers from the group can be very effective. Provide small group activities to explore issues. Be clear to yourself regarding the purpose of each activity and how it relates to your session objectives. As mentioned earlier, activities need to be minds-on as well as hands-on in order not to turn into busywork. Carefully structure such activities, with clear instructions on how to conduct the activity and accompanying worksheets or activity sheets. Grocery store or farmers' market tours, for example, are appealing to upper elementary school children. Prepare the students ahead of time and prepare activity sheets for what they will do there.

Deliver Content Appropriately in Terms of Cognitive Developmental Level

For elementary and middle school–aged children, health outcomes are in the distant future, and hence food and nutrition content needs to be provided in formats that fit their cognitive levels. Children may respond to food and nutrition activities if they involve some kind of intrinsic reward or element of fun (Matheson and Spranger 2001). Puzzles, fantasy play, contests, quizzes, games, or computer games are engaging because they provide children with a challenge, the level of which can be set by the age of the child or group. These activities also stimulate children's curiosity if there is a meaningful objective that is part of the game or contest. Thus, fantasy, challenge, and curiosity can build on children's interest in investigations and stimulate intrinsic motivation. Nutrition content can be part of the plot or the problem to be solved by the characters involved in the fantasies and stories. One program created characters from another planet—named Hearty Heart, Dynamite Diet, Salt Sleuth, and Flash Fitness—who came to Earth to work with children and help them learn and practice health-promoting eating and exercise patterns (Leupker et al. 1996; Hoelscher et al. 2010). One computer curriculum was based on stories about invaders of a kingdom who want to destroy all the fruits and vegetables. Children were asked to become squires to help the king and queen fend off the invaders. The squires faced many challenges in their quest. The story included wizards, robots, and other fantasy creatures (Baranowski et al. 2003; Thompson et al. 2012).

For high school students, hunger and food cravings, time, convenience, cost and availability of foods, perceived benefits, mood, body image, and habit are pressing food choice motivations. However, many issues in the field are controversial, from weight control diets, sales of sweetened beverages in schools, organic foods, and causes of world hunger to local versus global food systems. Stimulate thought and critical thinking through presentation of surprising data, interesting content, and case examples. Given that adolescents like to be challenged, design activities, such as debates or position papers, where they have an opportunity to grapple with these issues. Provide opportunities for students to propose novel or imaginative ideas to solve problems, understand and appreciate different viewpoints, and develop plans to address issues and solve problems.

Address Social Norms and Peer Influences but Do Not Forget the Family

Help youth recognize the power of social environmental influences on their eating patterns by having them analyze television advertising, food marketing techniques, and what's available in neighborhood stores or stores around their schools. Make healthful eating desirable or cool by providing role models of importance to older children and youth. Peer educators, who can model healthful behaviors and address the participants' concerns, can also be incorporated into the program.

For middle childhood youth and teens, families still provide much of the food children eat and still have considerable influence (Woodruff and Kirby 2013). These children are old enough to participate in cooking and other food-related activities in the home, which can provide an opportunity for nutrition educators to design creative home-based activities in the context of families' culture and community (Woodruff and Kirby 2013; Flattum et al. 2015).

Remember the Importance of the Affective Domain

Teens' food choices and eating practices are strongly influenced by affective and emotional factors (as is true for all people). Nutrition education can appeal to their growing sense of independence and ability to make choices for themselves as opposed to being dependent on the opinion of others. They can be encouraged to take charge of their lives. Because self-esteem is very important, activities should be respectful, build self-esteem, and never embarrass children and teens in front of others. Address body image and appearance concerns with sensitivity, being respectful of persons of all sizes.

Conduct Food-Based Activities when Possible

Everyone is interested in food, and youth are no exception. These activities can enhance motivation, overcome barriers, and provide skill development. Develop simple recipes for food preparation, particularly ones that do not require heating or complicated utensils, for venues where facilities are limited. Be sure to test these recipes first for ease of preparation, taste, and appearance, as well as ease in transporting ingredients and utensils to the site. Unless it is designated as a cooking session, the procedures should be quick to maintain attention and motivation. The activity should also engage all the teens so that you do not have volunteers and onlookers. Set up several food preparation stations with the ingredients already measured out at each station.

Foster Cognitive Self-Regulation

Given the increasing pressure of external forces on the food choices of older children and adolescents, ranging from peer pressure, food marketing practices, and the school environment to busy schedules and time constraints that leave little time to eat healthfully, nutrition education can foster cognitive self-regulation processes that focus on mindful eating through goal setting, planning ahead, and self-monitoring. These processes are described in detail in Chapter 12. Setting specific and actionable goals is not always easy, even for adults. It is important to take the time to teach goal setting skills, using a process of guided goal setting, which seems to work best for this age group. Guided goal setting means that you can set the major goals for youth to achieve through your sessions or program, such as "eating healthful snacks," and youth can set their own specific and highly individualized action goals to achieve these major goals, such as by stating they will "eat fruit for snacks 2 days next week." Help them to balance meals eaten with peers that may not be so healthful with other, more healthful meals, such as those eaten at home. They can also negotiate within the family for healthful foods they like.

The Adult Learner

Adult learners can't be threatened, coerced, or tricked into learning something new; they must want to know (Tennant and Pogson 1995; Vella 2002; Knowles and Holton 2011; Brookfield 2013). Nutrition educators thus need to focus on behaviors, practices, or issues of immediate relevance to the group. The set of core principles of adult learning and education is often referred to as *andragogy*. Keep these in mind as you develop your educational plans using the DESIGN process.

CHARACTERISTICS OF ADULT LEARNERS

Adults need to know why they need to learn something before undertaking to learn it. Much of adult learning is self-initiated and conducted independently. However, adults also often find themselves participating in learning experiences because of the requirements of workplaces or food assistance programs (such as Women, Infants and Children [WIC] or senior meal programs), referrals by their doctors and other medical care professionals, or for other reasons. Individuals need to see the immediate usefulness of the new skills, knowledge, or attitudes they are working to acquire. Learning is a means, not an end. Most

adults do not have time to waste. They may even have to arrange for child care to attend a session, so that the session costs them money as well as time. Not surprisingly, they like to be convinced that the experience will be worth their time and effort.

Orientation to Learning

Adults are generally task-oriented, problem-oriented, or life-centered. Thus, they are less interested in, or enthralled by, a survey of nutrition such as provided by an overview of the food pyramid. They would rather learn about one or two key ideas and how they can be applied to a problem of relevance to them. However, there may be large differences in their preference for teaching style based on their own learning styles. (See Chapter 15.) For example, analytic learners may prefer that the needed information be presented to them in a straightforward but interesting presentation, whereas sociable or dynamic learners may enjoy discussions. There is some agreement among adult educators that discussion is an ideal format for adult learning: it permits learners to share their own challenges and successes and to learn from the experiences of others. It reinforces their sense of self-worth and fosters their ability to make decisions. Discussions are especially useful for developing critical thinking and for creating new meaning systems out of shared experiences and collaborative interpretations of them (Abusabha, Peacock, and Achterberg 1999; Vella 2002; Knowles and Holton 2011; Brookfield 2013).

Readiness to Learn

Adults are ready to learn those things that will help them to cope effectively with their real-life situations. Thus, pregnant women and mothers of young children may become interested in nutrition education because they want to have healthy children. Other life-changing events may also increase the readiness to learn, such as beginning to live on one's own, having teenagers whose eating patterns are of concern, or being diagnosed with a health condition. They seek out a learning experience because they have a use for the knowledge or skill being sought.

Learners' Past Experience

Adults have a great quantity of prior experience with food and eating. These experiences are unique to individuals, and the differences between individuals are large.

Nutrition educators may be the experts on the content, but adults are the experts on their own lives. These experiences must be honored and can greatly enrich sessions if they are built into the design of the sessions. You can find out about these past experiences through a careful and thorough needs and resources analysis. Indeed, many adults have greater experience with cooking or child rearing than the nutrition educator. Others in the group, including the nutrition educator, can benefit from this wealth of knowledge if it is shared.

Learners as Decision-Makers

Adults have a self-concept of being responsible for their own decisions and for their own lives. Healthy adults thus want respect for themselves as decision-makers and will resist being treated as objects and being told what to do. Indeed, quality of life increases as people are more capable of making decisions that affect their lives. Participants in nutrition education want the information you provide and are grateful for the sharing of experiences and tips from others, but they want to choose whether and how they will apply the information. This makes it imperative that sessions with adults be built on mutual respect and dialogue.

Motivation

Autonomous or intrinsic motivations to learn and change are more important than extrinsic motivations. Internal motivations include increased self-esteem, quality of life, job satisfaction, health, and avoidance of disease. Extrinsic or controlled motivations may include the advice of physicians or the urging of family.

STAGE OF LIFE AND ROLES

Adulthood is not a static state at which individuals arrive when they finish high school or get their first job. Instead, development is lifelong. Individuals grow and change throughout life. As they do, their needs, values, roles, and expectations change. These all have implications for nutrition education.

Life Stage Influences

Researchers have identified several adult life stages from in-depth interviews of individuals over time (Neugarten, Havighurst, and Tobin 1968; Gould 1978; Levinson 1978, 1996). They suggest that adults experience several main stages: leaving the family between the ages of 15 and 25; a transition between ages 25 and 30 to becoming an adult,

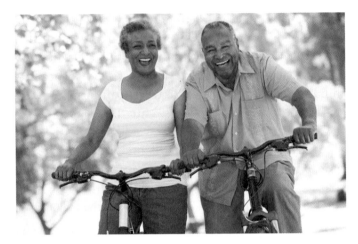

Physical activity is enjoyable at any age.
© Monkey Business Images/ShutterStock, Inc.

entering a career, and starting a family; and then settling down and becoming one's own person between the ages of 30 and 40. At this stage, careers are usually set and individuals now have families of their own. In the middle 40s to early 50s, children have left home, and individuals begin to see that time is finite and question life's meaning. Neugarten and colleagues (1968) propose that until about this time, individuals see life in terms of "time since birth." The future stretches forth and there is time to do and see everything. The orientation is toward achievement, and death is an abstraction. After this period, individuals see life as "time left to live," where time is finite and there is time enough only to finish a few important things. Sponsoring others becomes important, and death becomes more personal. Some experience this midlife transition as destabilizing (the so-called midlife crisis), but most do not. This is then followed by a restabilization in the 50s, where there is a renewed interest in friends and reliance on spouse or partner. This process is well illustrated in the nutrition area by the description one woman provided about her changing perspective:

> When you're in your twenties you think you're not vulnerable to anything. When you're in your thirties you think you still have time. When you're in your forties you see things begin to creep up on you that have never affected you before . . . so you begin to seriously consider some of the things you've been reading about. [In your fifties] you make more conscious efforts to stick with foods and diets and meal planning that conform to better health standards. (Devine and Olson 1991, p. 271)

Women's motives for preventive dietary behaviors have been found to vary with life stage because of altered perceptions of health status, body weight, and family roles and responsibilities (Devine and Olson 1991). Women with young children at home were more likely to be concerned for their children's health, resulting in a positive impact on their own diets because they prepared balanced family meals and sought to set a good example. For mothers of teenagers, there was tension between their desire to make healthful changes for their own health and the lack of acceptance of these changes by the family. The departure of grown children from the home allowed older women to make dietary changes for their own personal health, and many expressed that this stage was very satisfying.

There are also cohort effects (Neugarten et al. 1968). The cohorts are viewed differently in different countries due to their unique histories. In the United States, and possibly other western countries, those who grew up in the idealistic 1960s, for example, have different values, attitudes, expectations, and behaviors than those who grew up in the Baby Boomer or "me" generation (see **BOX 17-4**). This has been found in the nutrition area as well: those growing up between 1944 and 1954 differed from those born two decades before in their perspectives on food and gender roles in the household and the ways in which differing kinds and degrees of public information about food and nutrition affected family meals growing up (Devine and Olson 1991). The perspectives of today's Generation X, Generation Y, and younger on food and nutrition issues likewise differ from those of the Baby Boomers. While there is some disagreement regarding what exactly is meant by the term *generation*, it is important to be mindful of these cohort effects as you plan your educational sessions and deliver nutrition education to different age and cohort groups.

Life-Course Perspective on Food Choice

A central concept of a life-course perspective on food choice is that the development of individual food choices takes the form of stable trajectories or pathways over a person's life course. A food choice trajectory is a person's persistent thoughts, feelings, strategies, and actions with food and eating developed over a life course in a social and historical context (Devine et al. 1998; Devine 2005). Embedded in trajectories are transitions and turning points. Transitions, such as changes in roles or in health conditions, can help to

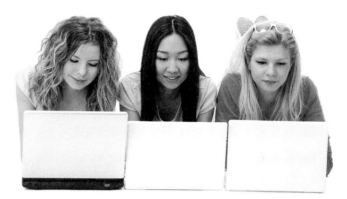

The "Always On" generation.
© lenetstan/Shutterstock

shape trajectories but do not necessarily change the direction of those pathways, whereas turning points are salient transitions, situations, or events that create long-term redirections in individuals' pathways (Devine 2005).

In the nutrition arena, these pathways are the accumulation of experiences from food upbringing, roles, ethnic traditions and identities, location, and personal health and physical well-being. Research in food choice suggests that individuals make adjustments to accommodate life-course transitions such as motherhood, menopause, midlife, and older age, but relatively few adults report major turning points (Edstrom and Devine 2001; Devine 2005). Nutrition education activities should take into account how these past experiences may influence current beliefs, attitudes, and expectations.

METHODS FOR DELIVERING EDUCATIONAL STRATEGIES APPROPRIATELY TO ADULTS: MAKING LEARNING MEANINGFUL

What are the best ways, then, to conduct nutrition education to specifically take into consideration the special educational preferences and experiences of adults? Based on the background just discussed and on the research literature, the following methods of delivering nutrition education are likely to be effective (Contento et al. 1995; Vella 2002; Sahyoun, Pratt, and Anderson 2004).

Provide Immediately Useful Information

At the beginning of a session, you can explain the purpose of the session and reassure participants that the session will be of immediate use to them. Provide adults with what they want and need to know—directly, clearly, and in a straightforward manner. Focus on only one or two key

BOX 17-4 Characteristics of Different Age Cohorts

There is some disagreement as to what exactly is meant by a *generation* or what these generations are. Nevertheless, there are cohort effects and distinguishing among them can be helpful in nutrition education. One way to think of these cohorts is shown here.

The GI Generation, or Greatest Generation

Born between 1901 and 1924, they were molded by the Great Depression and World War II. They won World War II and provided the nation with seven presidents. Members tend to be conservative; as a whole, they constitute the most satisfied generation.

Tips for Working with Them:

- Emphasize realistic strengths, not weaknesses.
- Don't tell them they are old; just provide larger type.
- Make access easy.

The Silent Generation and Idealistic Generation

Born between 1925 and 1942, they were influenced by the GI generation before them. The older members of the cohort were silent in their youth, and the younger were idealistic and activist. It includes most of those who fought in the Korean War and many who served during the Vietnam War. This generation produced every major figure in the 20th-century civil rights movement, from Martin Luther King, Jr. to Cesar Chavez. The Peace Corps was important to them. Members of this generation tend to be compassionate problem solvers who find strength in human relations. They are healthy and active.

Tips for Working with Them:

- Emphasize expertise.
- Provide statistics and information (they are readers).
- Stress wellness.
- Emphasize willingness to help others.

Baby Boomers, or the "Me" Generation

Born between about 1945 and about 1965, Baby Boomers are now in their mid-50s to mid-70s. They were born after World War II, and many are beginning to retire. This generation tends to be focused on the individual: the "inner world," consumption, and self-gratification. They were the first modern "counter-culture" or hippies. They want jobs that involve individual creativity. Denial is not in their dictionary. Emphasis is on youth: a longer life means extended middle life, not old age. Nostalgia is important.

Tips for Working with Them:

- Promote quickness and convenience.
- Emphasize what is in it for them to eat healthfully.

Generation X

Born between about 1965 and 1985, today they are in their early-30s to early-50s. They experienced the rise of mass media and the end of the cold war. This generation is very group oriented. Friends have taken the place of absent parents and relatives. Group dates are common. Members are often great shoppers: going to the mall is part of their social life. The generation is diverse and entrepreneurial. Because of job insecurity, they want to control their lives. They are wired, with email addresses, laptops, and cell phones. Members tend to be interested in environmental issues.

Tips for Working with Them:

- Be visual, musical, and dynamic.
- Emphasize price value.
- Stress balance in life and the impact of food behaviors on the environment.

Generation Y, or Millennials

Born between about 1985 and the late 1990s, today they range in age from late teens to early 30s. They are the children of Baby Boomers. They grew up with the war on terror. This generation is practical and pragmatic. Members often grew up in dual-income and single-parent families, and are very involved in family purchases. They are technologically savvy: computers and other gadgets are like pens and pencils to them, and they grew up with the Web. They expect multiple options and think of time in seconds. They tend to be action oriented and socially and ecologically aware.

Tips for Working with Them:

- Be visual, musical, and dynamic, but also use technologically focused formats, such as PowerPoint presentations and Web-based media.
- Emphasize quickness and convenience.

Generation Z, or the "Always On" Generation

This is the cohort after the millennial generation, born in the late 1990s or early 2000s. They are sometimes also referred to as the new silent generation. They have used sophisticated technology since they were toddlers and are "always on." Hand-held computers and social media are extremely important.

Tips for Working with Them:

- Be visual and dynamic; use of technologically sophisticated formats is essential, such as Web-based visual media.
- Emphasize quickness and convenience, as with the Millennials.

messages or specific behaviors, such as how to increase milk consumption or provide healthful snacks to their children. Provide realistic, not idealistic, information. Making the session relevant to any particular group of participants means that you must conduct a good assessment of the past experiences, needs, and desires of the group. If the group is ongoing, tell participants they will have an opportunity at the end of the session to suggest issues and topics to be addressed in future sessions.

Create a Safe Learning Environment

To encourage learning, ensure that the room is physically comfortable and establish ground rules about respecting the time frame of the session; confidentiality; mutual trust, respect, and helpfulness; freedom of expression; and acceptance of differences. How to create such an environment is described in great detail in Chapter 15.

Develop Respectful Relationships

Adult educator Vella (2002) emphasizes the importance of respectful relationships between the group leader and learners and among learners. Relationships of the nutrition educator to the group can involve power-over or power-with. Power in this context refers to providing knowledge, decision-making control, and the right to ask questions (Abusabha et al. 1999). Power-over is when the professional provides all the information and gives advice, expecting the group members merely to comply. Although studies show that such a means for transfer of information can result in knowledge gains, it is less likely to lead to improved problem-solving skills, reflective thinking, attitude change, or changes in behavior. In the power-with approach, the expert and the participants share power in an active partnership. In this approach, you listen actively to what each participant is saying, you do not talk down to participants but treat them as equals, you accept them exactly as they are, and you are warm, caring, trusting, and flexible. Even where individuals may prefer presentations as a way to receive information (Olson and Kelly 1989), the attitude of respect for group participants is still crucially important.

Recognize that Adult Learners are Decision-Makers

Respect adult learners as decision-makers in their lives. Also respect that they should have some say in the content of the sessions. You can achieve this in many ways. For example, when new content is introduced, you can first describe in outline form what can be included in this section, and then ask the group what they feel they need or want to learn about the topic. Learners can thus decide what occurs for them in the learning event. This involves their taking responsibility for their own learning and not being passive listeners. There will no doubt be different viewpoints on any particular issue. The group should feel secure that their opinions will matter and that they will not be criticized. After all viewpoints have been expressed, they can then be sorted out and evaluated for their scientific merit. The role of the facilitator is crucial in keeping the group on track and ensuring that the conclusions being drawn are scientifically accurate and based on evidence. Where there are misconceptions, the nutrition educator can correct them with respect, such as saying, "I am glad it worked for you, but research suggests that . . .".

Engage Learners

Design activities that will actively engage learners. For example, design active learning tasks that can be carried out in small groups or pairs. Where appropriate, the outcome of these tasks should be open-ended and based on what the group or pair comes up with. Provide for the opportunity to reflect on the task. These learning tasks should build on the past experience of the learners. Facilitated dialogue is another format in which all group members are fully engaged: they actively participate in learning by listening to each other and sharing with each other. Facilitated dialogue is described later in this section.

Build on Learners' Past Experience and Knowledge

Adults need to be able to integrate new ideas with what they already know, if they are going to keep—and use—new information and skills. Information that conflicts sharply with what is already held to be true, and thus forces a reevaluation of the old beliefs and attitudes, should not, of course, be avoided, but recognize that it will be integrated more slowly. Likewise, information that has little conceptual overlap with what is already known is acquired more slowly. So learn about the current perceptions, beliefs, or attitudes of your audience toward the issue at hand in order to build on what is known.

Sequence the Learning Experiences and Reinforce Them

If new how-to food and nutrition information is to be provided or new skills are to be taught, such as new food preparation methods, sequence the learning tasks from simple to complex and provide plenty of opportunities for observation and practice. Reinforce information, skills, and attitudes by repetition in diverse, engaging, and interesting ways until the knowledge and skills are learned. In group discussion, frequently summarize the key points of the discussion.

Come to Closure with Solutions

After a group of adult learners grapples with the issues that are the focus of the session and shares challenges and

---

NUTRITION EDUCATION IN ACTION 17-1   Choosing Healthy Options in Cooking and Eating (The CHOICE Project)

The Program

The major causes of death and disability among American women today include cardiovascular disease, cancer, and osteoporosis, and there is consensus that diet is related to these conditions. This program was designed to help non-at-risk, healthy older women in a free-living setting to develop eating patterns that would reduce the risk of these conditions. They were randomized into three conditions:

- A moderate-fat balanced diet eating plan, similar to recommendations of the Dietary Guidelines
- The addition of flaxseed (a good source of phytoestrogens) to the moderate fat, Dietary Guidelines eating plan, provided as a dietary supplement
- A whole foods, near-vegetarian eating plan, high in plant foods and low in animal foods, similar to a macrobiotic-style diet

During the course of 12 months, participants met for 24 nutrition education and behavioral change sessions: weekly for 14 weeks, biweekly for the next 10 weeks, and monthly for the remaining 6 months. The behavioral intervention strategies used to maintain subject participation and dietary adherence included:

- Seven cooking classes with hands-on experience, alternating with behavioral sessions during the first 14 weeks; information provided on how to eat according to the assigned eating plan
- Cooking demonstrations with tastings at all other sessions
- Individual goal setting and development of action plans each session

- Regular feedback and encouragement based on 3-day food records completed monthly by the women
- Monthly telephone calls on a random day to collect 24-hour dietary recalls, as an incentive for adherence
- Group bonding through icebreakers at start of sessions, sharing of addresses and phone numbers, facilitated discussion
- Chef's knife, apron, mug, and tote bag with CHOICE logo
- Monthly newsletter to participants during 6 months of monthly sessions

Evaluation Results

Results showed that women on the macrobiotic-style eating plan were able to achieve significant changes in diet, in the desired direction, for many key categories of foods targeted in the intervention. They tripled their whole grain intakes, tripled their intake of beans and legumes, and doubled their intake of fish. They decreased their intakes of refined grain products; significantly cut down their intakes of meat, poultry, eggs, and whole milk products; and reduced their consumption of high-fat sweets compared to baseline values. They made these changes within the first 3 months and maintained them for most of the 12 months. Women in all three groups were able to adhere to the diets to which they were assigned, suggesting that a behaviorally focused intervention with healthy free-living participants can be effective. In particular, those on the healthy, whole foods, near-vegetarian diet adhered just as well as those on the low-fat diet.

Source: Peters, N. C., I. R. Contento, F. Kronenberg, and M. Coleton. 2014. Adherence to a whole foods eating pattern intervention with healthy postmenopausal women. *Public Health Nutrition* 17(12):2806–2815.

successes, the nutrition educator can summarize the discussion and facilitate the group coming up with common solutions. Good solutions come from full participation of the group and the shared understandings and meaning that evolve through discussion. The group feels more commitment to the solutions adopted by the group because they shared in the responsibility of arriving at final decisions about what actions to take.

Support Cognitive Self-Regulation

As with older children and adolescents, adults also have busy schedules and experience time constraints that leave little time to eat healthfully. When group participants decide individually or collectively to take action, you can support their cognitive self-regulation processes through teaching skills of goal setting, planning ahead, and self-monitoring. These processes are described in detail in Chapter 12 of this book. Setting specific and actionable goals is important.

Example of a Nutrition Education Program Based on Adult Education Principles

Choosing Healthy Options in Cooking and Eating, or the CHOICE project, was a program directed at older women that incorporated the features just discussed. The project is described in **NUTRITION EDUCATION IN ACTION 17-1**.

FACILITATED GROUP DIALOGUE AS AN EDUCATIONAL TOOL

Facilitated dialogue is an example of an effective tool for working with adults that incorporates all the previous strategies (Abusabha et al. 1999; Vella 2002; Sigman-Grant 2004). The word *facilitate* is derived from the Latin word meaning "to enable, to make easy." The facilitator is thus a person who makes it easier for people to understand (Sigman-Grant 2004). The facilitator's job is to make the group atmosphere comfortable for discussion by incorporating the actions described previously to address each of the types of learners' fears (Abusabha et al. 1999). The facilitator's role is also to move the discussion along without dominating it. The facilitator assists group members to express their ideas, helps them to think critically about issues, encourages them to talk to and listen to each other, and assists them to come to conclusions based on group input. The aim is for active participation by all of the group members and shared understandings. Use of

this approach has resulted in sessions that are lively and in which group participants feel motivated and empowered.

Role of Facilitator

In the context of nutrition education, what is the role of the facilitator? What does group facilitation mean? How exactly does one function as a nutrition educator to make a group session a democratic and valuable group learning experience? How does one find the right balance between being authoritarian as a facilitator and being laissez-faire?

Some believe that the facilitator is just another member of the group, who should not direct the activities of the group. Brookfield (2013) notes that because much of adult learning is concerned with such issues as the resolution of moral difficulties, development of self-insight, reflection on experience, and reinforcement of self-worth, rather than simply technical knowledge, there are those who argue that discussion cannot be directed, for to attempt to do so would be to close people's consciousness to alternative interpretations of the issue under discussion before these alternatives were even stated.

The facilitated dialogue reflects this approach to some extent: it is described as a method of group teaching that involves the active participation of all group members and the leader. Learners and facilitators are equal partners in the learning experience (Sigman-Grant 2004). The group sits in a circle, and the leader sits alongside the group members in the circle. Ideally, the group members do all the talking and, in essence, conduct the session. The leader talks very little as group members share with each other and learn from each other. Although the nutrition educator may be the expert on food and nutrition issues, the group members are experts on their own lives and how and whether they can incorporate the provided information into their own situations. Those who use a learner-centered approach state, "the most central point of learner-centered education is that the learner is a decision-maker. They choose if they learn and if they will change their behavior. We cannot decide for them. The learning is in the doing and deciding" (Husing and Elfant 2005, p. 22).

Role of Planning: The 4 As or the 4 Es

However, it is acknowledged that open discussions about whatever topic comes to the minds of group members in laissez-faire fashion, without much input from the

BOX 17-5 Guidelines and Techniques for Facilitated Group Discussions

Build the Group from Within

- Assure members that the group will be structured to fit their needs and concerns.

Establish Group Norms or Ground Rules

- Set the time, agenda, and length of the session.
- Set rules of respecting confidentiality, sharing group responsibilities, and respecting and listening to opinions of other group members.

Begin with a Check-In or Ice-Breaker

- Ask each group member to make a brief statement about herself, her child's needs, and anything new that happened to her during the past month.

Delivering the Opening Question

- Before or after you ask the opening question, there may be silence or reluctance to be the first to say something. Assure the group this is normal and perhaps pick someone you know who will be comfortable answering the question.

Ask Open-Ended Questions

- Ask questions that cannot be answered by "yes" or "no."
- Involve group members in describing their own experiences.

Guide the Discussion

- Actively encourage others to speak.
- Keep the discussion on track.
- Recognize fears, biases, and disagreements, and bring them out into the open.
- Avoid letting group members dominate.
- Gently bring topics to a conclusion.

Encourage Full Participation

- Encourage quiet members to voice their ideas.
- Listen intently to each member.
- Repeat members' comments when necessary.
- Give positive feedback verbally or physically (e.g., nodding head, smiling).

Focus the Conversation

- Clarify different views.
- Restate the objectives of the session when necessary.
- Summarize the important points of the discussion.

Dealing with Misconceptions

- Avoid turning into the "lecturer."
- Emphasize the worth of the members' experience.
- Use responses such as, "I am glad this worked for you, but other people have found . . .".
- Ask what other group members think about the statement.

Focus on Feelings

- Place primary emphasis on the feelings or experiences of each group member.
- Avoid debates; instead focus on support and information sharing.

Practice Active Listening

- Listen carefully to what participants are saying and avoid the temptation to interfere with your own thoughts and interests.
- Encourage group members to listen to and understand each other.

Create an Atmosphere of Acceptance

- Accept people and respect each member's feelings, even when you disagree with her viewpoint.
- Do not hurt members' feelings by abruptly negating or putting down their ideas and experiences.

Summarize the Discussion

- Bring ideas together and repeat relevant information.
- Strive to make the summary the result of the members' discussion, not your own analysis.
- Repeat and clarify the solution to the nutrition problem that members agreed on.

Assist Members in Gaining Resources

- Provide sources of additional information such as pamphlets, videos, websites, or referrals.

Be Patient

- Remember, it takes time for a group to grow and develop trust.

Have Fun

- Keep a smile on your face, and enjoy sharing with and learning from the group.

Source: Based on Abusabha, R., J. Peacock, and C. Achterberg. 1999. Facilitated group discussion. *Journal of the American Dietetic Association* 99:72–76; and Facilitating WIC Discussion Groups: Guidelines, Concepts, and Techniques. 2011. Washington State Department of Health WIC Nutrition Program.

The 4 As	The 4 Es
■ **Anchoring**: Introduction and/or review	■ **Excite**: Gain attention or review and reflect
■ **Add**: Active learning and facilitated dialogue; introduction of new concepts and new information	■ **Explain**: Present stimulus and new material for why-to take action to enhance motivation
■ **Apply**: Providing an opportunity through an interactive exercise for all participants to consider ways to use the new material and the points made within the discussion to their own lives	■ **Expand**: Provide guidance and practice for how-to take action to facilitate the ability to take action
■ **Away**: Summarizing, bringing to closure, and selection of action plans	■ **Exit**: Apply and close by enhancing application and setting action plans

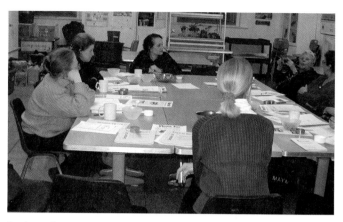

Facilitated group discussions can be helpful and supportive in nutrition education with adults.

Courtesy of Fredi Kronenberg.

nutrition educator, are not fruitful either. Group members often express frustration with a lack of a sense of progress toward any clear learning objective. In addition, as a nutrition educator working in specific programs that have specific missions, you are accountable for certain outcomes that involve addressing specific behaviors, such as recommended infant feeding practices or eating more fruits and vegetables (Sigman-Grant 2004).

In general, the sessions based on facilitated discussion are planned ahead of time, involving the preparation of an educational plan. The sequence of activities during the session has been suggested by Norris (2003) and Sigman-Grant (2004) for WIC programs to be the 4 As, shown above. This sequence is very similar to the 4 Es used in this book derived from instructional design principles (Gagne 1985; Gagne et al. 2004; Kinzie 2005; Merrill 2009; Reigeluth and Carr-Chellman 2009). These principles are discussed in detail in Chapters 11 and 15.

An example of a specific sequence of activities for how such a facilitated discussion is carried out in settings such as the WIC program is shown in **BOX 17-5**.

Safety Versus Challenge

Facilitating a group does not mean that the group should not be challenged. Indeed, you are charged as an educator to assist group members to analyze assumptions, challenge previously accepted and internalized beliefs and values, and contemplate the validity of alternative behaviors or other ways of doing things (Brookfield 2013; Abusabha

et al. 1999). All of these actions can, at times, be uncomfortable and may even contradict the stated needs of the group. Thus, the job of the facilitator is to create learning environments that are both emotionally safe and challenging. In addition, in nutrition education groups, there is often much nutrition science–based motivational why-to information and how-to information and skills that need to be addressed. Thus, the educator has a role, and the group members have a role.

It can be seen, then, that facilitating groups requires considerable skill and practice to find the right balance of acceptance and challenge, of leading and being a member of the group. The nature of the facilitator's role and the degree of guidance and control will depend on the food and nutrition behavioral goals being addressed in your intervention and the nature of the group.

Working with Diverse Cultural Groups

The United States, like many other countries, is becoming increasingly multicultural, with people from diverse ancestries and who have become part of the mainstream to varying degrees. New York City has more than 170 distinct ethnic communities. More than 130 languages and dialects are spoken by students in the Washington, D.C., school system. Los Angeles has more people of Mexican descent than any city in the world except Mexico City. Even states such as Iowa and Alabama are getting used to people speaking Spanish in their midst. Some are recent immigrants, and others have been in the country for several generations. Whereas in the past all became a part of a general "melting pot," in recent decades racial/ethnic groups have shown a wish to be acknowledged, honored, and respected for their unique heritage and contributions, resulting in more of a mosaic. Although often referred to as minorities, such subsets of the population are often a majority of the population in certain locations, and hence such a term is often inaccurate and inappropriate (Bronner 1994). You may thus face the challenge of providing nutrition education to a variety of people who come from a variety of cultures that are different from your own. This requires you to better understand your own culture and those of others.

Culture has been described as a set of beliefs, knowledge, traditions, values, and behavioral patterns that are developed, learned, shared, and transmitted by members of a group. Culture is a worldview that a group shares and hence influences perceptions about food, nutrition, and health (Sanjur 1982). Knowledge and beliefs include accepted understandings, opinions, and faith about the world. Beliefs help determine which foods are edible, appropriate preparation methods, or the meaning of a food. Traditions are customs about which foods are eaten on what occasions (e.g., weddings, birthdays), what will be eaten for health or to cure illness, or religious traditions about fasting and feasting. Values are widely held beliefs about what is worthwhile, desirable, or important for well-being. Values considered desirable in one culture may not be considered so in another culture, and these differences in value systems can influence food and nutrition practices.

Culture, then, is a learned experience, not a biologically determined one (Sanjur 1982). It is the product of interaction among generations, always being modified over time. Consequently, it can also be unlearned. Cultures are constantly changing. Thus, you can view food habits as a dynamic process, always changing. However, every culture also resists change by self-generated mechanisms to perpetuate its cultural traits and to maintain its boundaries.

All societies have a dominant set of beliefs, values, and traditions that are shared by the majority of people. In the United States, the norms have been described as an emphasis on education, work ethic, materialism, religion, physical appearance, cleanliness, high technology, punctuality, independence, and free enterprise. Those cultural groups whose beliefs, values, and traditions are different may not always be treated with understanding and respect (Bronner 1994; Purnell 2002; Stein 2009, 2010).

These cultural differences are also reflected in possible differences in the kinds of foods eaten, shopping habits, preferred food preparation methods, structure of meals during the day, whether family members eat together, whose food preferences may have more importance, and so forth.

Researchers have noted that at the same time, culture "out there" is interpreted by the family and passed down to children as family cultural traditions (Triandis 1979; Ventura and Birch 2008). Children, in turn, filter these family cultural traditions through their own personal experience with food and with the world to develop their own interpretations of their culture, so that individuals of the same culture may hold different views of that culture. Many aspects of these personal interpretations "in here" can be captured in the psychosocial theories that are the basis for the DESIGN Procedure. These theories are described in Part I of this book, and the DESIGN Procedure is outlined in Part II. Thus we need to be aware of the cultural contexts of our audiences but also recognize that individual differences exist because of family and personal interpretations of culture, and design our interventions accordingly. The assessment processes of the DESIGN Procedure Steps 1 and 2 are particularly useful here.

UNDERSTANDING CULTURAL SENSITIVITY AND CULTURAL COMPETENCE OF NUTRITION EDUCATORS

Working with a variety of cultures requires that the nutrition educator become culturally competent (Kumanyika et al. 2007, 2012; Di Noia et al. 2013). There are many different models or descriptions of the process of becoming culturally competent (Bronner 1994); some focus on organizations and others on individual professionals, while some are most useful in clinical counseling. Many of these are summarized by Stein (2009, 2010). We focus on models that are most applicable to individual nutrition educators.

The LEARN model (Berlin and Fowkes 1983) describes specific steps to guide a specific counseling session or intervention: *Listen* (to the client's view of the issues or problems), *Explain* (reflecting back to the client to ensure you understood accurately), *Acknowledge* (the similarities between the clients' and the health profession's understandings about what needs to be done), *Recommend* (providing several culturally sensitive options), and *Negotiate* (together come up with a culturally appropriate plan of action).

Several other models describe fairly similar steps in a continuum for the process of the health professional becoming more culturally competent, such as those of Bronner (1994), Campinha-Bacote (2002, 2010) or Purnell (2002). The steps in a continuum that are in common or similar are as follows:

- *Cultural knowledge* is the process whereby you learn about the worldviews of other cultures. This can be accomplished by reading books, attending workshops, watching audiovisual presentations, perusing government documents, and so forth. You can learn about the food habits and beliefs of various ethnic groups through these means.

- *Cultural awareness* is the process of becoming aware of your own learned biases and prejudices toward other cultures through self-assessment, while becoming aware of the beliefs, values, practices, lifestyles, and problem-solving strategies of other groups.

- *Cultural sensitivity* is the awareness of your own cultural beliefs, assumptions, customs, and values as well as those of other cultural groups. You recognize that cultural differences as well as similarities exist, without assigning values to these differences, such as good or bad, right or wrong.

- *Cultural competence* is a set of knowledge and interpersonal skills that allow you to increase your understanding and appreciation of cultural differences and similarities within, among, and between groups and to work effectively in cross-cultural situations (Bronner 1994). You show respect for and acceptance of the group's cultural beliefs, traditions, and practices, and demonstrate interest and ability to work comfortably with them.

Being competent in cross-cultural functioning means learning new patterns of behavior and effectively applying them in the appropriate settings. Knowledge about a culture does not equal cultural competence. In fact, "book" knowledge of a culture may lead to inappropriate generalizations, such as stereotyping. Through frequent cultural encounters and engagement, nutrition educators can become aware of the heterogeneity within cultural groups. For example, although individuals from a given culture may have similar beliefs, attitudes, and practices in terms of food and nutrition, there are also many variations resulting from differences in education, age, religion, socioeconomic status, geographic location, family cultural traditions, and length of time in the country.

The goal for nutrition educators is to accompany knowledge about the culture with awareness, respect, and acceptance of the group's cultural beliefs and practices, and enthusiasm and ability to work within the values, traditions, and customs of the participants' community (Bronner 1994; Resnicow et al. 1999; Sue and Sue 2013).

Not only individuals, but also organizations need to exhibit cultural competence. Thus, cultural competence has been defined as "a set of congruent behaviors, attitudes, and policies that come together in a system, agency, or among professionals and enables that system, agency, or professionals to work effectively in cross-cultural situations. Operationally defined, cultural competence is the integration and transformation of knowledge about individuals and groups of people into specific standards, policies, practices, and attitudes used in appropriate cultural settings to increase the quality of services, thereby producing better outcomes" (King, Sims, and Osher 2006).

Consequently, systems and agencies, such as health systems, food and nutrition agencies, and nutrition education programs, need to become more culturally competent. Five elements have been identified as essential for contributing to a system's ability to become more culturally competent (Cross et al. 1989; Isaacs and Benjamin 1991; King et al. 2006). The system should: (1) value diversity, (2) have the capacity for cultural self-assessment, (3) be conscious of the "dynamics" inherent when cultures interact, (4) institutionalize cultural knowledge, and (5) develop adaptations to service delivery, reflecting an understanding of diversity between and within cultures (King et al. 2006). Further, these five elements must be manifested in every level of the service delivery system. They should be reflected in attitudes, structures, policies, and services.

APPROPRIATE DESIGN PRINCIPLES AND DELIVERY METHODS FOR NUTRITION EDUCATION FOR CULTURALLY DIVERSE AUDIENCES

What, then, are the implications for how you can design and deliver your nutrition education intervention for culturally diverse audiences as you use the DESIGN Procedure? It should be noted that the psychosocial theories and models used throughout the book can provide a framework for designing programs for various cultural groups (Liou and Contento 2001; Kreuter et al. 2003, 2005). However, the theory constructs need to be operationalized to be culturally appropriate. For example, the health belief model was usefully applied to the development of culturally appropriate weight-management materials for African American women (James et al. 2012). Understanding the psychosocial constructs of motivators and barriers was very helpful for designing interventions for pregnant low-income, overweight African American mothers (Reyes, Klotz, and Herring 2013), Asian adolescents (Novotny, Han and Biernacke 1999), and older Latino adults (Devereaux-Meililo et al. 2001). There may also be culturally specific constructs that are important to consider in delivering nutrition education.

In applying the concepts related to cultural sensitivity to health promotion and nutrition education, Resnicow and colleagues (1999) suggest that it is helpful to consider the following distinctions.

Cultural sensitivity (or *cultural appropriateness*) is the extent to which the design, delivery, and evaluation of nutrition education and health promotion programs incorporate the ethnic or cultural experiences, beliefs, traditions, and behaviors of a given group as well as relevant historical, social, and environmental forces. Cultural competence, as you have seen, is the capacity of individuals and organizations to exercise interpersonal cultural sensitivity. Thus, cultural competence refers to practitioners and agencies, whereas cultural sensitivity or appropriateness refers to the intervention messages and program materials. *Multicultural* refers to incorporating and appreciating the perspectives of multiple racial or ethnic groups without assumptions of superiority or inferiority. Thus, culturally sensitive programs are implicitly multicultural.

Cultural targeting is the process of creating culturally sensitive interventions for a specific group. This often involves adapting existing materials and programs for racial/ethnic subgroups. *Culturally based* programs and messages are those that combine the culture, history, and core values of a subgroup as a medium to motivate behavior change. For example, nutrition education programs for indigenous Americans can focus on traditional foods and spiritual systems.

Surface Structure and Deep Structure

Surface Structure

Programs and materials can focus on a surface structure dimension, whereby materials and messages are matched to the observable social and behavioral characteristics of given cultural groups by using people, places, language, music, clothing, or food that is familiar to or preferred by the target audience (Resnicow et al. 2005). You might also use media channels that are most watched or settings uniquely used by the group to deliver the nutrition education, such as churches, mosques, synagogues, or ethnic community centers. Ideally, you would want to match staff ethnically to the participants. Surface structure indicates how well the intervention fits within the culture, experience, and behavioral patterns of the audience.

Deep Structure

Programs and materials that focus on deep structure are culturally based by building on general core values and historical, cultural, social, and environmental factors that may influence the food and nutrition behavior of the target audience (Resnicow et al. 1999). Core values that have been considered when working among some Asian groups, for example, are the importance of family, respect for older people, and the importance of maintaining balance for health—including the use of hot and cold foods to address hot and cold health conditions (Harrison et al. 2005). Programs with African Americans have been built on the core values of commitment to family, communalism, connections to history and ancestors, and a unique sense of time, rhythm, or communication style (Resnicow et al. 1999, 2002, 2005). For the Hispanic/Latino culture, core values include importance of family, respect for elders, fatalism, and the importance of positive social interactions that can be the foundation for nutrition education (Bronner 1994). You need to understand and value the core values of the different groups with which you work as you deliver your program. In particular, there are differences in body image issues, such as what is considered an appropriate weight in the eyes of a given cultural group (Kumanyika et al. 2007, 2012).

Ethnic Ideals and Identities

In terms of food choice specifically, one qualitative study with three ethnic groups (African American, Latino, and white) found that ideals, identities, and roles interacted reciprocally and dynamically with each other and with food choices and influences on food consumption (Devine et al. 1998). *Ideals*, or deeply held beliefs about food and eating, came from multiple sources, of which ethnicity was one. For some individuals, ethnicity was dominant; for others, age, religion, or other interests, such as health and fitness, were also important. *Identity* is the way people think about their own distinguishing characteristics and self-image. Ethnic identities in this study existed along with others, such as regional or family background and travel experiences, which sometimes overrode ethnic identities. Ethnic identities were most often expressed during holidays and family celebrations. Individuals also have multiple roles, some of which influence food choice. Women in all three cultural groups were usually the family food managers. Some African American and white men were the primary cooks for the family. Contexts enhanced or constrained all food choices and influenced the ability to enact cultural ideals and roles.

It is essential to remember that there are wide variations within groups in terms of ethnic/racial identity, which may be defined as the extent to which individuals identify and gravitate toward their racial/ethnic group psychologically and socially (Resnicow et al. 1999). Ethnic identity includes individuals' extent of acculturation; the degree to which they have affinity for in-group culture such as food, media, or clothes; racial/ethnic pride; attitudes toward maintaining one's culture; and involvement with those within the group and those outside the group.

Appropriate Communication Styles

There are many differences in communication styles between cultures, such as whether to speak loudly or softly; to look at the person who is speaking or avert one's gaze; to smile, nod, or interject when someone is speaking to acknowledge understanding of what the speaker says or to show little expression; and whether to rarely ask questions and provide yes/no responses or to use a direct approach and ask direct questions (Sue and Sue 2013). Rather than ask whether the group understands—which is likely to yield a yes answer in some cultures, say, "Tell me which things are not clear to you." In some cultures, it is impossible to say "no" to a request, so individuals may respond with "maybe" about whether the time for the session is a good time or whether they will come to the next session. In some cultures, it is acceptable to make a commitment and then to decide later to make changes to it or to decline altogether. It is assumed that one cannot predict events in one's life that may occur in the meantime. It is thus very important to learn about the specific culturally appropriate communication styles of the groups with which you will be working.

STRATEGIES FOR DEVELOPING AND DELIVERING CULTURALLY SENSITIVE INTERVENTIONS FOR AFRICAN AMERICAN AUDIENCES

In the United States, a major cultural group is African Americans, and hence useful strategies for working with this group are described in greater detail here. A number of studies have been conducted to help health professionals develop and deliver culturally sensitive interventions for African Americans (Bronner 1994; Resnicow et al. 1999, 2002, 2005; Kreuter et al. 2003). The authors of a comprehensive review of interventions proposed the following strategies, among others, for working with African American audiences (Di Noia et al. 2013):

- *Recognize the heterogeneity of the African American population.* While there are many common experiences such as discrimination and health disparities, there are many differences among groups based on background country of origin such as Africa, Central and South America, the Caribbean, or American descendents of slaves as well as those who were free. Thus it is important to:
  - Develop in-depth knowledge of your particular audience after a careful assessment as in Steps 1 and 2 of the DESIGN Procedure.
  - Maintain awareness of your own personal biases when you work with individuals from a different cultural or even subcultural background from you own.
- *Acknowledge the historical legacy of slavery and other activities.* These have resulted in a culture of distrust of mainstream institutions. Also acknowledge the impact of this historical legacy on contemporary food-related practices. Thus it is important to:
  - Build and maintain trust by developing mutual respect.
  - Understand and respect the cultural meanings given to food.
- *Understand the environmental stressors experienced by your audience.*
  - Increase access to healthful food.
  - Adapt materials for those who may have low literacy skills.
- *Build on racial/ethnic ideals and identities.*
  - Understand that food practices are often used to affirm group identity, pass on family traditions, and demonstrate caring and respect.

- Use cultural targeting and tailoring to improve the relevance and impact of your intervention or sessions.
- *Recognize the influential role of women.*
  - Engage women as a central focus of interventions.
  - Incorporate women's particular perspectives and needs in dietary intervention activities.
- *Base interventions on Afrocentric belief and value systems:*
  - *Spirituality/religiosity* or the belief in a force greater than oneself emphasizes integrity, compassion, and trustworthiness and may include church attendance, prayer, and beliefs about God as a causal agent in health. An intervention to increase mammography among women addressed this value with the message: "The Lord has given us a powerful tool for helping find cancer before it is too late. Getting a mammogram, together with the power of prayer, will give you the best chance to live a long and healthy life" (Kreuter et al. 2003, p. 140).
  - *Collectivism* is the belief that the basic unit of society is the community or family, not the individual, and that collective survival is a high priority. Hence, important values are cooperation, concern and responsibility for others, forgiveness, family security, friendship, and respect for tradition. Interventions can nurture collectivism. For example, a message in the mammography study was: "As black women, we have many important jobs. We keep our families together. We help build our communities. We work inside and outside the home. But our most important job may be to keep ourselves healthy. If we don't take care of ourselves, it is harder to take care of others" (Kreuter et al. 2003, p. 140).
  - *Perception of time* is socially constructed. This is also discussed in Chapter 2. The traditional Western perception of time is that it has a past, present, and future and can be divided into discrete units, which, like money or other goods, can be saved, spent, wasted, or even bought, as in "buying time" (Kreuter et al. 2003). Time well spent now can lead to a better future. People with this type of future orientation are thus more likely to engage in health-promoting behaviors. In the health area, it has been found that African Americans are more present-oriented. Hence, a message that addressed this specific time perception in the mammography study was: "It is hard to think about the future when you are feeling fine today. But sometimes you can take steps today to make life better tomorrow. Getting a mammogram is another step you can take today to make life better tomorrow, since finding cancer early increases the chances of successful treatment" (Kreuter et al. 2003, p. 142).

- *Emotional expressiveness,* the ability to express one's feelings and to attend to the emotional needs of others, is an important value that suggests emotion-based activities to explore feelings will be helpful in interventions or sessions, along with expression of empathy by the nutrition educator.
- *Other considerations and strategies* are suggested in the comprehensive review by Di Noia et al. (2013).

STRATEGIES FOR DEVELOPING AND DELIVERING CULTURALLY SENSITIVE INTERVENTIONS FOR HISPANIC/LATINO AUDIENCES

The Hispanic or Latino population is the largest and fastest growing within the United States; hence, useful strategies for working with this group are described in greater detail here. A number of studies have been conducted to help health professionals develop and deliver culturally sensitive interventions for Hispanic/Latino audiences (Domenech Rodriguez, Baumann, and Schwartz 2011; Bender et al. 2013, 2014; Zoorob et al. 2013). A review examined intervention studies using the framework of surface and deep structures (Mier, Ory, and Medina 2010). The review proposed some strategies that arise from the interventions examined.

- *Recognize the diversity within the Hispanic/Latino population.* While there are many common experiences, there are many differences among groups based on background country of origin, which could be from Central or South America or the Caribbean. Consequently, it is important to:
  - Develop knowledge of the beliefs and practices of your particular audience as in Steps 1 and 2 of the DESIGN Procedure.
  - Tailor your intervention to this specific audience.
- *Take into account that more than one-third of the Hispanic/ Latino population in the United States is foreign born.* This means that:
  - Materials need to be at the appropriate literacy level.

- It is crucial to learn about the level of acculturation and duration in this country of your intervention participants, as these influence the life situations and lifestyles of Hispanics and hence your approach and content.
- *Base the intervention on Hispanic cultural values (the deep structure approach)*, which emphasize:
  - *Familism*, which is the individuals' strong identification with and attachment to their nuclear and extended family, by emphasizing family involvement in interventions.
  - Trust or *confianza*, by building trusting and respectful relationships within the program.
  - Need to establish smooth relationships, or *simpatia*, by providing social support.
  - *Fatalism*, or lack of empowerment, by using intervention activities that provide opportunities for participants to enhance their sense of empowerment.
- *Use culturally appropriate delivery methods for interventions (surface structure approach)*, such as the following:
  - Translating and adapting existing evidence-based programs can be effective.
  - Preferably use materials and facilitators that are not only bilingual, but also bicultural.
  - Include ethnic foods in activities.
  - Use *promotoras* or community health workers where appropriate or feasible.
- *Focus on family and social support in the intervention* by doing the following:
  - Develop family-centered interventions.
  - Involve the community in the intervention through community participatory approaches.

Process for Developing Culturally Appropriate Programs and Materials

Given the wide diversity between cultural groups, it is essential that the materials and programs are appropriate to the specific cultural group. Use of translated and adapted evidence-based programs can be effective (Ziebarth et al. 2011). However, developing culturally based materials and programs is desirable. You can do so through the use of focus groups and extensive pretesting (Domenech Rodríguez et al. 2011; Barrera et al. 2013). These actions can be part of the Step 1 and Step 2 assessments of the DESIGN Procedure.

Focus Groups

Use focus groups to provide the basis for developing your message content and format. Using this format, you can identify both surface and deep structure elements by exploring the thoughts, feelings, language, assumptions, and practices of the group, including food preferences, shopping and cooking habits, and perceived benefits and barriers. You can also explore cultural differences by using "ethnic mapping" (Resnicow et al. 1999). Here you can ask the group whether certain foods they eat or behaviors they engage in are "mostly an ethnic thing," "equally an ethnic and white thing," or "mostly a white/American thing." Such focus groups should include individuals representing the heterogeneity within the cultural group.

Pretesting

After you have designed a draft of your materials (e.g., videos, printed materials) or program content, it is essential that you show them to a sample from your target audience for their feedback on format and content, reflecting both surface and deep structure characteristics. For example, some groups may like the images to portray individuals from their same racial/ethnic group, but others may not. Test the concepts being addressed and the language being used. Find out whether the group perceives any of the features to be stereotyping or insensitive.

Examples of Effective Interventions

Black Churches

The Healthy Body/Healthy Spirit study examined the effect of a culturally sensitive, multicomponent self-help intervention on fruit and vegetable intake and on the physical activity of members of a set of socioeconomically diverse black churches. It is described in **NUTRITION EDUCATION IN ACTION 17-2**.

En Balance Hispanic Diabetes Education Program

Disadvantaged, low-income Hispanic adults attended four 2-hour sessions taught in Spanish over a 3-month period (Salto et al. 2011). The focus of the sessions was to facilitate the ability to change behavior and take action, as the participants were already motivated. Thus, sessions taught about self-monitoring and dietary change using a hands-on, culturally relevant approach. Recommendations involved smaller portion sizes and choosing healthier alternatives within culturally specific food groups, rather

NUTRITION EDUCATION IN ACTION 17-2 **Healthy Body/Healthy Spirit: A Church-Based Nutrition and Physical Activity Intervention**

The Program

The Healthy Body/Healthy Spirit program was a culturally targeted self-help intervention to increase consumption of fruits and vegetables and levels of physical activity. It was based on addressing dimensions of both surface structure, in which materials and messages are matched to observable social and behavioral characteristics of the intended audience, and deep structure, in which the intervention is based on cultural, historical, and psychological factors that are unique to the racial/ethnic identity of the audience.

The intervention built on *surface structure* considerations involving food preferences, cooking practices, and exercise patterns of the audience. It also addressed *deep structure* issues, which included unique attitudes about body image, safety concerns, lack of time for exercise, the effect of exercise on hair, religious themes, and interest in improving the health of the community (as opposed to personal health).

The study was conducted in 16 socioeconomically diverse black churches in the Atlanta area. Church members were randomized into three groups. One group received standard educational materials. The second group received culturally sensitive self-help materials, and the third received self-help materials plus motivational interviewing. The materials provided to the intervention group participants were as follows:

- *Forgotten Miracles video:* An 18-minute video that centered around two families, one that tended to eat healthfully and the other that did not. Key messages were conveyed with biblical themes, such as the story of Daniel, who rejects the "kings' diet"

for his own "natural diet" high in fruits and vegetables, and messages about the body being "God's temple." These culturally sensitive messages conveyed information about the health benefits of eating fruits and vegetables, analysis of costs, recipes, and cooking tips.

- *Eat for Life cookbook:* A cookbook containing recipes submitted by church members that met specified criteria. The recipes were first tested by staff.

- *Healthy Body/Healthy Spirit exercise video:* A 20-minute video hosted by African American celebrities from the Atlanta area and based on footage taped in church members' homes in order to provide real-world role models.

- *Healthy Body/Healthy Spirit guide:* A 37-page, four-color manual to accompany the video.

- *Audiocassette:* A cassette with gospel music to match a three-phase workout: warm-up, aerobic activity, and cool-down. Biblical quotes and brief excerpts from the pastors' sermons were interspersed with the music.

Evaluation Results

Slightly more than 1000 individuals were recruited from the 16 churches, of whom 906 were assessed at the end of 1 year. A subset of the individuals also received four culturally sensitive telephone counseling calls based on motivational interviewing techniques. Results showed that those who received the culturally sensitive intervention significantly increased their fruit and vegetable intakes and their physical activity levels compared with those who received standard educational materials.

Sources: Resnicow, K., A. Jackson, R. Braithwaite, et al. 2002. Healthy Body/Healthy Spirit: A church-based nutrition and physical activity intervention. *Health Education Research* 17:562–573; and Resnicow, K., A. Jackson, D. Blisset, et al. 2005. Results of the Healthy Body/Healthy Spirit trial. *Health Psychology* 24:339–348.

than forgoing traditional dishes. The program resulted in improved glycemic control and better lipid profiles.

Latino Community-Based Intervention to Prevent Diabetes

This project tested the effectiveness of a community-based, literacy-sensitive, and culturally tailored lifestyle

intervention on weight loss and diabetes risk reduction among low-income, Spanish-speaking Latinos at increased diabetes risk (Ockene et al. 2011). The intervention consisted of 3 individual and 13 group sessions over a 12-month period based on social cognitive theory and patient-centered counseling. The behavioral goals were to increase whole grains, non-starchy vegetables, and physical activity and to decrease sodium, saturated fat, portion sizes, and refined carbohydrates. The educators were all Spanish-speaking, and the foods recommended were culturally appropriate. The intervention resulted in weight loss, improved HbA1c, and insulin resistance.

Using Fotonovelas to Promote Healthy Eating in a Latino Community

This intervention came about because Latinos living in the community expressed concern that the health education materials were unattractive, difficult to read, and poorly translated, and they were interested in learning more about obesity prevention (Hinojosa et al. 2011). Fotonovelas are novels told through photos and are familiar to, and popular with, Latinos. It was thought that this would be a good medium to convey health messages. The community members were involved in shaping the issues and content of the fotonovelas to ensure that they were relevant to the culture, ethnicity, gender, social class, and language of the community, and specific to its identified needs. One page from the fotonovela is shown in **FIGURE 17-1**.

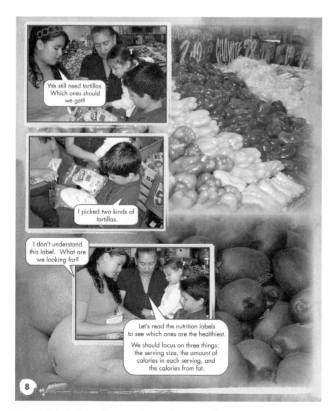

FIGURE 17-1 Sample page from a fotonovela.

Esperanza Para La Salud: Pasos Para una Alimentacion Saludable (Hope for Health: Steps to Healthy Eating). *Source. Centro de la Comunidad Unida* (United Community Center).

Low-Literacy Audiences

In the United States, about one in seven adults can't read; another 21% read below a fifth-grade level, and 19% of high school graduates can't read (National Center for Educational Statistics 2003). Many community nutrition education program participants are functioning at fifth-grade reading level or below, and recent immigrants may be functioning at even lower levels. This means that many participants are functionally illiterate and others have marginal reading skills, and thus may not be able to read the handouts or booklets you give them or the written food and nutrition instructions you provide for them.

Doak and colleagues (1996) point out that you cannot identify low-literacy individuals by their appearance or by conversation with them. They are often very good in other forms of communication and have learned to compensate so that their lack of literacy skills is not obvious. They can be poor or affluent, immigrant or native born. Sometimes those who have low literacy in English are highly literate in the language of their country of origin; others, born in this country, just never developed the skills. Being low in literacy skills does not mean low in intelligence. Nutrition education can be effective if you find the appropriate format.

Poor readers, compared with skilled readers, read slowly, often one or two words at a time, so that they lose the meaning of the whole sentence. They think in terms of individual items of information rather than in categories or groups with common characteristics. They often do not understand information if it is implied; therefore, how the information is to be used must be spelled out clearly. Additionally, they often have difficulty with analysis and synthesis of information as well as with literacy.

Comprehension is about grasping the meaning of instruction or materials and is an important aspect of literacy. Comprehension, whether verbal, written, or visual, requires that individuals pay attention to information and remember it when they need it. Gaining the attention of the intended audience at the beginning of a session or piece of printed material is important for activating the memory system. This can be done by using vivid stories, striking visuals, or dramatic data. Getting the information into the audience's short-term memory requires you to be aware that this form of memory has a limited capacity and a short storage time. People can usually store only up to seven independent items at a time. Any more than that may mean that they will not remember any of the items. For those of low literacy, the number is more like three to five. Transfer from short-term to long-term memory and storage in long-term memory require that the new information links to what the audience already knows, is repeated often, and actively involves the audience.

APPROPRIATE DELIVERY METHODS FOR LOW-LITERACY AUDIENCES

How can you apply these considerations to delivering nutrition education to low-literacy audiences? Many have written about this problem (Doak et al. 1996; Townsend 2011) and the Centers for Disease Control and Prevention (CDC, 2009) has provided a comprehensive guide. Some key strategies are described briefly here.

General Strategies

The following strategies are applicable to all components of nutrition education.

- *Know your audience.* Assess the needs and preferences of the intended audience thoroughly before designing your program, using the procedures described in Steps 1 and 2 earlier in this book. What is the group's literacy level and its readiness to learn? Focus groups, personal interviews, or interviews with those who work closely with this audience, such as agency personnel, are all valuable means for gaining this information.

- *Pretest all materials through cognitive testing.* Use focus groups to guide you as you design your sessions. How should the issues be framed for this audience? What educational strategies do they prefer? After you have designed a draft of your sessions, pretest your message with your intended audience to determine whether the message to be delivered through educational sessions or written materials conveys the meaning you intend. This is referred to as cognitive testing (Alaimo, Olson, and Frongillo 1999). In particular, cognitively test any evaluation instruments that you intend to use, such as food frequency checklists or attitude items. Here, individual interviews are most helpful. Present individuals with the materials and have them complete the assignments, such as worksheets or evaluation instruments. Then use read-aloud procedures to ask them to explain to you what they think each item

means. This will force you to use the language of the intended audience in your materials.

- *Limit your educational objectives.* Limit the number of educational objectives for group sessions or written materials. These objectives should state exactly what actions or behaviors the audience will be able to accomplish as a result of the educational intervention. Present the smallest amount of information possible to accomplish your goals. Three or four items of instruction are enough at any one time. This translates into one major concept—your behavioral goal—two or three motivation-related concepts on why-to take action, such as perceived benefits and barriers, plus two or three examples of how-to take action. Teach only "need-to-know" rather than the "nice-to-know" information.

- *Focus the content on behaviors or actions rather than on facts and principles.* This will facilitate the ability to take action. This entire book is based on this premise, but it is especially important for low-literacy audiences. The nutrition science information and principles presented may imply what the behaviors should be. But for a low-literacy audience, the behaviors must be spelled out clearly, not just implied. In addition, this audience usually does not need all the underlying nutrition science information to engage in the behavior.

- *Greet audience with friendliness, interest, and warmth.* Use all the principles of good communication. They are described in detail in Chapter 16.

- *Present information using a variety of ways to enhance learning.* For example, use mini-lectures, discussions, small group activities, and visuals, as well as appropriate printed materials.

- *Use familiar examples and a conversational style.* Build on what they already know, and use familiar examples from their lives. For all audiences, but particularly if your audience is also a low-resources audience, refer to foods or dietary practices familiar to the audience rather than to exotic foods and national data. This helps to anchor your message in memory. Talk to them the way you would talk to a friend.

- *Actively engage your audience.* During educational sessions, encourage people to ask questions and to share information and experiences through discussion and dialogue. Allow time for individuals to commit themselves to doing something before the next session. Then, in the next session, allow time for them to report what they did on their commitment. In printed materials, engage the readers in some activity—checklists to check off, completing the blanks, circling items, and so forth.

- *Frequently repeat and review.* If the individuals are experiencing the sessions primarily through oral means, key concepts need to be repeated often so that information can move from short-term memory into long-term memory. Allow time to process information, and at the appropriate points, review what has been said or accomplished through activities. Bring the session to closure with clear conclusions. If you use handouts that require the audience to write something, be sure to have pencils ready and allow plenty of time for them to complete the activity. For older audiences, you may need to allow time for them to find their reading glasses.

- *Treat people with respect and dignity regardless of their literacy level* (and, of course, regardless of socioeconomic status, race/ethnicity, religion, or country of origin). If your audience is also a low-resources audience, note that disadvantaged groups often mistrust authority figures, so you must be willing to initiate trusting relationships. Show the group that you believe in them.

Tips for Written Materials

There are many strategies for writing effective written materials. They are described in detail in Chapter 16. Please read the appropriate section there. They apply to low-literacy audiences as well. This section emphasizes those features that are *additionally*, or particularly, important for low-literacy audiences.

- *Write the way you speak—use the active voice.* Literacy experts (Doak et al. 1996; Townsend 2011; CDC 2009) note that when you do this, your written materials become easier to read because the readability index automatically drops. They become more interesting to read. They will be easier to understand. The extra words you use when you speak help the reader to process the information.

- *Use common words.* These are words you would use when talking with a friend who was not familiar with nutrition concepts. Common words are usually short and simple words, but not always. Doctor is more common than physician, but many people are very familiar with the term medication even if it is a

four-syllable word. If you use uncommon words, such as hydration, explain them. Some words are short but conceptually difficult, such as a variety of foods or a balanced diet. What exactly do you mean by *variety* or *balanced*? Explain such conceptual words.

- *Use short words.* Use words with one or two syllables when you can. Reading levels are calculated by how many words in the document have three syllables or more.

- *Use short sentences.* Short sentences of less than 10 to 15 words are easier to understand. However, you should not sacrifice conversational style. If it is more natural to say something in a longer sentence, then do so.

- *Put the key information first.* The first part of a message is remembered best (newspapers know this). So, put the behavior or information that is key to your message up front, in the position most likely to be remembered. Assume that the reader will read just the first sentence, the first paragraph, or the first page. So, put the most important information first. For example, say, "Eating lots of fruits and vegetables [the behavioral goal of your program] each day can help lower your risk of heart disease," and then go into greater detail about the many benefits of why to eat more fruits and vegetables and how to do so.

- *Create headings, subheadings, and summaries.* Use headings to serve as guideposts or road signs. Headings and subheadings make the text look less formidable. They alert readers to what is coming up next and help them focus on the intended message. Keep the headings simple, using perhaps three to five words, and locate them right before the text that they introduce. This process also allows for delivering the written information in chunks that can be remembered.

- *Use layout and typography that make the text easier to read.* Use short paragraphs and plenty of white space, simple fonts such as sans serif fonts, and adequate font sizes. Use short lines of 30–50 characters and spaces. Divide the page into two columns for easier reading if possible, as has been done for this textbook. You will note that each column has about 30–50 characters. Use bullets where appropriate for lists of tips, procedures, or things to do. Highlight important information with circles, arrows, or underlining rather than using all capital letters. REMEMBER THAT ALL CAPS ARE MORE DIFFICULT TO READ. Make the page look as though it can be read in a few minutes.

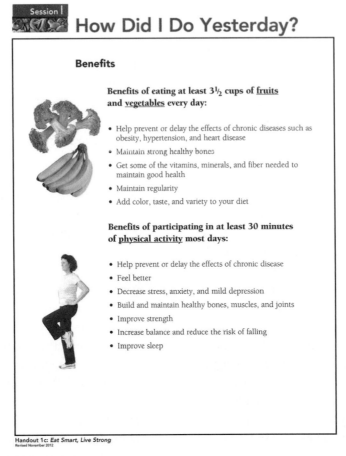

FIGURE 17-2 Examples of written materials that are easy to read.

Eat Smart, Live Strong Project. http://snap.nal.usda.gov/resource-library/
eat-smart-live-strong-nutrition-education-older-adults/eat-smart-live-strong.

Written materials of the Eat Smart Live Strong program for able-bodied 60–74-year-olds participating or eligible for nutrition assistance programs of the USDA provide good examples. One of the handouts is shown in **FIGURE 17-2**. The key behavioral messages of the program are:

- Eat at least 3½ cups of fruits and vegetables per day.
- Participate in at least 30 minutes of physical activity most days of the week.

The handout is easy to read and uses lots of white space, realistic photos, headers, bullets, and low reading level.

Tips for Visuals

The following tips apply to the use of posters, illustrations, charts, lists, tables, and graphs with low-literacy audiences.

- *Use visuals to enhance learning.* People remember information better when they see the message, not just hear it. Visuals make information vivid and real. As Doak and colleagues note (1996), most poor readers rely on visuals and the spoken word. Visuals with a minimum of text help them to understand instructions without having to struggle with the text. Visuals, appropriately designed, can help the low-literacy reader follow step-by-step instructions for complex procedures. Visuals can also provide emotional impact that is more memorable. For example, the written message "when a mother drinks alcohol, the baby drinks alcohol" can be converted into a line drawing showing a baby inside the mother drinking from a cup when the mother does so. This can carry a more powerful and memorable message than the written word (Doak etal. 1996).

- *Use visuals to enhance motivation.* Make the cover of a booklet or the beginning of a brochure or handout appealing while clearly conveying the key message of the material. Because reading is not easy for low-literacy individuals, an appealing cover or introduction can provide the impetus to open the brochure or read the material. The style of artwork or the photograph needs to be appropriate to the culture so that readers can easily recognize it as familiar and can visualize themselves in the situation. Realistic line drawings are recommended over stylized or abstract images, which are often not understood. Photos are even better, and color photos are best of all. Test the style of the artwork or photograph with the intended audience for its appropriateness and motivational power.

- *Include visuals to clarify the text, but use visuals carefully.* Place the visual near the text to which it refers so that the readers' eyes do not have to go elsewhere to find the written text to understand the message. Break the information into small chunks and provide one visual for each chunk to make it easier to follow. For example, if you want to encourage walking and stair climbing, show separate drawings for walking and stair climbing. Use a simple action caption for each drawing. Or if you use a table to provide a list of foods high in fat, break up the foods into groups with a heading over each. To engage the learner, you can provide a checklist with boxes to check as a means of self-assessment. The CDC's guide (CDC 2011) provides many examples on how to develop effective visuals.

- *Use simple and clear illustrations.* Illustrations for text should include enough detail to emphasize the message but should not be so detailed that they become complex and distracting. If you want to illustrate a procedure with many steps, number each step. Photographs are also effective if they are uncluttered and the message is clearly depicted.

- *Use realistic pictures for posters and handouts.* For stand-alone materials, make the message very clear through the visuals and words. Use of realistic photos is best, preferably in color, as this requires less mental processing by individuals and facilitates comprehension (Townsend et al. 2008; Townsend 2011).

- *Use color appropriately.* Color can attract and hold attention and is almost expected today given the high quality of the visual media in the environment. The preference for colors varies considerably by age, gender, socioeconomic status, and ethnicity. It is thus very important to test your color choices with the intended audience to find out whether they will convey the meanings and message you intend.

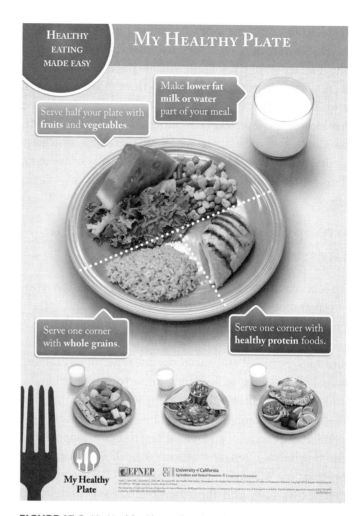

FIGURE 17-3 My Healthy Plate educational poster.

Shilts MK, Johns MC, Lamp C, Schneider C, Townsend MS. A Picture is Worth a Thousand Words: Customizing My Plate for Low-literate, Low-income Families in 4 Steps. *J Nutr Educ Behav.* 2015:1–3 pg. Online copy is available at http://dx.doi.org/10.1016/j.jneb.2015.04.324.

VISUALS FOR LOW-LITERACY AUDIENCES: AN ILLUSTRATION USING MYPLATE

An illustration of the many principles described here is shown in the poster for MyPlate in **FIGURE 17-3**. Prior work had shown that in terms of visuals, low-income audiences prefer photographs to words or line drawings, and color photographs to black and white ones (Townsend et al. 2008; Townsend 2011). Townsend, Shilts, and colleagues developed and tested meal images and messages to be used in education materials appropriate for low-income, low-literacy parents of young children. The meal content was based on dietary recalls by participants in the California Expanded Food and Nutrition Education Program (EFNEP) to identity common foods consumed by this audience. Messages were developed for a low-literacy audience using short sentences and few multi-syllable words. The messages were cognitively tested with adults from WIC, SNAP-Ed, and EFNEP. This extensive formative research led to the My Healthy Plate series of educator materials: mini-lessons, handouts, goal sheets, meal cards, and placemats, which are available for download at http://townsendlab.ucdavis.edu. This poster is one of the educational materials.

Groups that Differ by Food-Related Lifestyle Factors

This book has emphasized the important role of psychosocial and other determinants in food choice and dietary behaviors. In particular, evidence has suggested that people's anticipated outcomes from engaging in a behavior, attitudes, personal and social norms, sense of ethical and moral obligations, self-efficacy to perform the behavior, and habit are all important. Here we focus on the fact that these determinants will not be equally important to everyone. In addition, people differ in their shopping and cooking habits, often referred to as their shopping and meal preparation "scripts" (Grunert et al. 1997; Worsley 2000).

Researchers and food marketers have used these characteristics of people to segment them into several subgroups or segments of the population into what are called *food-related lifestyles*, or *food-styles*, to better understand people's motivations and practices. This research suggests that people use personal values or sets of standards to evaluate the outcomes of possible actions they may take (Feather 1982). These standards may be grouped into *community values* (which may come from cultural and other societal sources), *small group values* (e.g., being social is important), and *individual values* such as being a vegetarian, or a meat eater, or an environmentally conscious person for whom food system criteria for food choice are uppermost (which may come from life experiences and other sources).

From such research, members of the public have been grouped into various sub-groups. The sub-groupings may change over time as societal trends and economic conditions change and may differ by country or culture. One study in the U.S. with teenagers found that they could be divided into six groups that ranged from the hedonistic to the health conscious with parental support (Contento

et al. 1988). A study with U.S. food shoppers (Nie and Zepeda 2011) found that they could be segmented into four major groups who differed on ways of shopping, product attributes, meal preparation, and desired consequences.

- *The practical consumer*: Valued taste and healthfulness of the food more than convenience, cooked often, and was moderately interested in disease prevention
- *The food enthusiast*: Valued healthfulness of the food and not convenience, cooked often, followed special eating patterns to treat or prevent illness, shopped at farmers' markets and was the most active organic shopper
- *The indifferent consumer*: Only valued taste and convenience of food, least interested in cooking, and least likely to shop at farmers' markets or buy organic foods
- *The convenience seeker*: Valued convenience but also freshness of food and food safety, cooked at home but was not necessarily that interested in cooking, and did not shop at farmers' markets or buy organic food

A study in Australia found subgroups or segments that were somewhat similar (Worsley 2000).

Understanding these subgroups may assist nutrition educators in developing sessions that are more targeted to the group or audience segment. In your needs assessment, it will be useful to probe your group or audience members about their overall approach to food-related activities.

Summary

Although the key principles in *designing* nutrition education described in Part II of this book apply to all groups—that is, a focus on enhancing motivation and facilitating the ability to take action—the *specifics* of design and the *methods* for delivering the educational plans for the intervention in actual practice must differ depending on the audience. Working with diverse population groups requires ensuring that your educational delivery methods are appropriate for the particular group.

In this chapter, you learned that children are not little adults—they are experiencing various stages of physical, cognitive, emotional, and social development. At each stage, they have different needs and abilities and different ways of thinking about themselves and the world that must inform the educational design and activities. Preschool children need repeated experience and play-based activities with tasty and healthful foods to become familiar with them. As children develop they can process more information, and cognitive motivational processes become more important. Goal setting and cognitive self-regulation skills become more developed. At the same time, emotional and social forces are important. Nutrition education needs to identify motivations that are meaningful to youth and provide opportunity to practice goal setting and cognitive self-regulation skills for engaging in self-directed actions.

Adults tend to engage in learning only when they see that the learning is of immediate use to them. Adults differ in life stage and roles. Nutrition education for them should build on previous experience, respect them as decision-makers, and engage them actively in their own learning. Facilitated discussion or dialogue is a useful educational tool.

Given the cultural diversity in the United States and other countries, groups often differ in cultural background, which will greatly influence how nutrition education strategies are delivered. Nutrition educators should aim to become culturally competent, which means possessing a set of knowledge and interpersonal skills that allows them to increase their understanding and appreciation of cultural differences and similarities within, among, and between groups and to work effectively in cross-cultural situations. Nutrition education programs should seek to be culturally appropriate to their intended audience. Likewise, nutrition education programs should be mindful of the literacy level of their audiences and develop oral, visual, and written communications that are appropriate to their level. All these actions taken together are likely to enhance the effectiveness of how you deliver your nutrition education sessions or intervention.

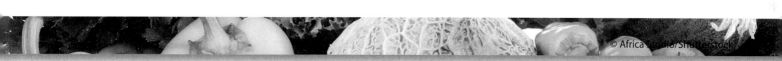

© Africa Studio/Shutterstock

Questions and Activities

1. You have been asked to provide suggestions to a Head Start center regarding its nutrition education program for the youngsters. From what you have learned, what advice would you give?

2. You are looking over a nutrition education curriculum for grades 4 and 5. Based on what you have read in this chapter, list three features the curriculum should have that would make you conclude that the curriculum is at the appropriate developmental level.

3. You will be providing two after-school nutrition education sessions to a group of teens aged 13 to 15 years. Describe three educational formats you will be sure to use to gain their attention and provide skill development.

4. You plan to facilitate a group discussion and dialogue session to implement your educational plan with a group of mothers of young children. What do you see as your role as a facilitator? What challenges do you anticipate? How will you know that you are being an effective facilitator?

5. Pick a cultural group that you would like to learn about. Read about the culture of the group or talk with people from that group. For this group, what are two key nutritional concerns? Go to a grocery store that stocks foods for this cultural group. Pick two foods and learn more about them. Then identify a nutrition education material, such as a handout, pamphlet, poster, video, or healthy cookbook, that you might use with this group. In what ways is it culturally sensitive? Describe how it uses surface structure or deep structure features or both. Be specific.

References

Abusabha, R., J. Peacock, and C. Achterberg. 1999. How to make nutrition education more meaningful through facilitated group discussions. *Journal of the American Dietetic Association* 99:72–76.

Alaimo, K., C. M. Olson, and E. A. Frongillo. 1999. Importance of cognitive testing for survey items: An example from food security questionnaires. *Journal of Nutrition Education* 31:269–275.

Anzman-Frasca, S., J. S. Savage, M. Marini, J. O. Fisher, and L. L. Birch. 2012. Repeated exposure and associative conditioning promote preschool children's liking of vegetables. *Appetite* 58(2):543–553.

Au, T. K., C. K. K. Chan, T. Chan, M. W. Cheung, J. Y. Ho, and G. W. Ip. 2008. Folkbiology meets microbiology: A study of conceptual and behavioral change. *Cognitive Psychology* 57:1–19.

Baranowski, T., J. Baranowski, K. W. Cullen, T. Marsh, N. Islam, and I. Zakeri. 2003. Squire's Quest! Dietary outcome evaluation of a multimedia game. *American Journal of Preventive Medicine* 24:52–61.

Barrera, M., F. G. Castro, L. A. Strycker, and D. J. Toobert. 2013. Cultural adaptations of behavioral health interventions: A progress report. *Journal of Consulting Clinical Psychology* 81(2):196–205.

Bauer, K. W., J. M. Berge, and D. Neumark-Sztainer. 2011. The importance of families to adolescents' physical activity and dietary intake. *Adolescent Medicine: State of the Art Reviews* 22(3):601–613.

Bellows, L. and J. Anderson. 2006. The Food Friends: Encouraging preschoolers to try new foods. *Young Children* 61:37–39.

Bellows, L., K. Cole, and J. Anderson. 2006. Family fun with new foods: A parent component to the Food Friends social marketing campaign. *Journal of Nutrition Education and Behavior* 38:123–124.

Bender, M. S., M. J. Clark, and S. Gahagan. 2014. Community engagement for culturally appropriate obesity prevention in Hispanic mother-child dyads. *Journal of Transcultural Nursing* 25(4):373–384.

Bender, M. S., P. R. Nader, C. Kennedy, and S. Gahagan. 2013. A culturally appropriate intervention to improve health behaviors in Hispanic mother–child dyads. *Child Obesity* 9(2):157–163.

Berge, J. M., M. Wall, N. Larson, K. A. Loth, and D. Neumark-Sztainer. 2013. Family functioning: Associations with weight status, eating behaviors, and physical activity in adolescents. *Journal of Adolescent Health* 52(3):351–357.

Berk, L. E. 2012. *Child development*. Ninth ed. Boston: Pearson.

Berlin, E. A., and W. C. Fowkes, Jr. 1983. A teaching framework for cross-cultural competence: application in family practice. *Western Journal of Medicine* 139:934–938.

Birch, L. L. 1987. The role of experience in children's food acceptance patterns. *Journal of the American Dietetic Association* 87(Suppl.):S36–S40.

———. 1999. Development of food preferences. *Annual Review of Nutrition* 19:41–62.

Blissett, J. 2011. Relationships between parenting style, feeding style and feeding practices and fruit and vegetable consumption in early childhood. *Appetite* 57(3):826–831.

Bronfenbrenner, U. 1979. *The ecology of human development*. Boston: Harvard University Press.

Bronner, Y. 1994. Cultural sensitivity and nutrition counseling. *Topics in Clinical Nutrition* 9:13–19.

Brookfield, S. 2013. *Powerful techniques for teaching adults*. San Francisco: Jossey-Bass.

Campinha-Bacote, J. 2002 [Updated 2010]. The process of cultural competence in the delivery of healthcare services. Transcultural C.A.R.E. Associates. http://www.transculturalcare.net Accessed 11/30/14.

Centers for Disease Control and Prevention (CDC). 2009. *Simply put: A guide for creating easy-to-understand materials*. Atlanta, GA: Strategic and Proactive Communication Branch, Division of Communication Services, Office of the Associate Director for Communication, Centers for Disease Control and Prevention.

Contento, I. R. 1981. Children's thinking about food and eating: A Piagetian-based study. *Journal of Nutrition Education* 13(Suppl.):S86–S90.

Contento, I. R., G. I. Balch, Y. L. Bronner, L. A. Lytle, S. K. Maloney, C. M Olson, et al. 1995. The effectiveness of nutrition education and implications for nutrition education policy, programs and research. A review of research. *Journal of Nutrition Education* 27:279–418.

Contento, I. R., and J. W. Michela. 1998. Nutrition and food choice behavior among children and adolescents. In *Handbook of pediatric and adolescent health psychology*, edited by R. Goreczny and C. Hensen, pp. 249–273. Boston: Allyn & Bacon.

Contento, I. R., J. W. Michela, and C. J. Goldberg. 1988. Food choice among adolescents: Population segmentation by motivation. *Journal of Nutrition Education* 20:289–298.

Contento, I. R., J. W. Michela, and S. S. Williams. 1995. Adolescent food choice: Role of weight and dieting status. *Appetite* 25:51–76.

Contento, I. R., S. S. Williams, J. L. Michela, and A. B. Franklin. 2006. Understanding the food choice process of adolescents in the context of family and friends. *Journal of Adolescent Health* 38(5):575–582.

Contento, I. R., P. A. Zybert, and S. S. Williams. 2005. Relationship of cognitive restraint of eating and disinhibition to the quality of food choices of Latina women and their young children. *Preventive Medicine* 40:326–336.

Croll, J. K., D. Neumark-Sztainer, and M. Story. 2001. Healthy eating: What does it mean to adolescents? *Journal of Nutrition Education* 33:193–198.

Cross, T., B. Bazron, K. Dennis, and M. Isaacs. 1989. *Towards a culturally competent system of care*. Vol. 1. Washington,

DC: Georgetown University Child Development Center, CASSP Technical Assistance Center.

Cusatis, D. C., and B. M. Shannon. 1996. Influences on adolescent eating behavior. *Journal of Adolescent Health* 18:27–34.

Devereaux-Melillo, K. D., E. Williamson, S. Crocker Houde, M. Futrell, C. Y. Read, and M. Campasano. 2001. Perceptions of older Latino adults regarding physical fitness, physical activity, and exercise. *Journal of Gerontological Nursing* 27(9):38–46.

Devine, C. M. 2005. A life course perspective: Understanding food choices in time, social location, and history. *Journal of Nutrition Education and Behavior* 37:121–128.

Devine, C. M., M. Connors, C. A. Bisogni, and J. Sobal. 1998. Life-course influences on fruit and vegetables trajectories: Qualitative analysis of food choices. *Journal of Nutrition Education* 30(6):361–370.

Devine, C. M., and C. M. Olson. 1991. Women's dietary prevention motives: Life stage influences. *Journal of Nutrition Education* 23:269–274.

Di Noia, J., G. Furst, K. Park, and C. Byrd-Bredbenner. 2013. Designing culturally sensitive dietary interventions for African Americans: review and recommendations. *Nutrition Reviews* 71(4):224–238.

DiSantis, K. I., L. L. Birch, A. Davey, E. L. Serrano, L. Zhang, Y. Bruton, and J. O. Fisher. 2013. Plate size and children's appetite: Effects of larger dishware on self-served portions and intake. *Pediatrics* 131(5):e1451–1458.

Doak, C. C., L. G. Doak, and J. H. Root. 1996. *Teaching patients with low literacy skills.* Second ed. Philadelphia: Lippincott.

Domenech Rodríguez, M. M., A. A. Baumann, and A. L. Schwartz. 2011. Cultural adaptation of an evidence based intervention: From theory to practice in a Latino/a community context. *American Journal of Community Psychology* 47:170–186.

Dovey, T. M., P. A. Staples, E. L. Gibson, and J. C. Halford. 2008. Food neophobia and "picky/fussy" eating in children: A review. *Appetite* 50(2–3):181–193.

Edstrom, K. M., and C. M. Devine. 2001. Consistency in women's orientations to food and nutrition in midlife and older age: A 10-year qualitative follow-up. *Journal of Nutrition Education* 33:215–223.

Elkind, D. 1978. Understanding the young adolescent. *Adolescence* 13:127–134.

Feather, N.T. 1982. Human values and the prediction of action: An expectancy value analysis. In *Expectations and actions: Expectancy value models in psychology*, edited by N. T. Feather, pp. 639–656. Hillsdale, NJ: Erlbaum.

Fisher, J. O., and L. L. Birch. 2002. Eating in the absence of hunger and overweight in girls from 5 to 7 years of age. *American Journal of Clinical Nutrition* 76:226–231.

Fisher, J. O., B. J. Rolls, and L. L. Birch. 2003. Children's bite size and intake of an entrée are greater with larger portions than with age-appropriate or self-selected portions. *American Journal of Clinical Nutrition* 77:1164–1170.

Flattum, C., M. Draaxton, M. Horning, J. A. Fulerson, D. Neumark-Sztainer, A. Garwick, et al. 2015. HOME Plus: Program design and implementation of a family-focused, community-based intervention to promote the frequency and healthfulness of family meals, reduce children's sedentary behavior, and prevent obesity. *International Journal of Behavioral Nutrition and Physical Activity* 12:53.

Gable, S., and S. Lutz. 2001. Nutrition socialization experiences of children in the Head Start program. *Journal of the American Dietetic Association* 101:572–577.

Gagne, R. W. 1985. *The conditions of learning and theory of instruction.* Fourth ed. New York: Holt, Rinehart, & Winston.

Gagne, R., W. W. Wager, J. M. Keller, and K. Golas. 2004. *Principles of instructional design.* Boston: Cengage.

Gelman, R., K. Brenneman, G. MacDonald, and M. Roman. 2009. *Preschool pathways to science: facilitating scientific ways of thinking, talking, doing, and understanding.* Baltimore, MD: Brookes Publishing.

Gibson, E. L., and J. Wardle. 1998. Fruit and vegetable consumption, nutritional knowledge, and beliefs in mothers and children. *Appetite* 31:205–228.

Gillman, M. W., S. L. Rifas-Shiman, A. L. Frazier, H. R. Rockett, C. A. Camargo, A. E. Field, et al. 2000. Family dinner and diet quality among older children and adolescents. *Archives of Family Medicine* 9:235–240.

Gould, R. L. 1978. *Transformations: Growth and change in adult life.* New York: Simon and Schuster.

Gripshover, S. J., and E. M. Markman. 2013. Teaching young children a theory of nutrition: conceptual change and the potential for increasing consumption. *Psychological Science* 24(8):1541–1553.

Gropnik, A., D. M. Sobel, L. E. Schulz, and C. Glymour. 2001. Causal learning mechanisms in very young children: two-, three-, and four-year-olds infer causal relations from patterns of variation and covariation. *Developmental Psychology* 37(5):620–629.

Grunert, K. G., K. Bruno, and S. Bisp. 1997. Food-related lifestyle: Development of a cross-culturally valid instrument for market surveillance. In *Values, lifestyles, and psychographics*, edited by L. Kahle and C. Chiagouris, pp. 337–354. Mahwah, NJ, Erlbaum.

Guthrie, J. F., B. H. Lin, and E. Frazao. 2002. Role of food prepared away from home in the American diet, 1977–1978 versus 1994–1996: Changes and consequences. *Journal of Nutrition Education and Behavior* 34:140–150.

Harrison, C. G., M. Kagawa-Singer, S. B. Foerster, H. Lee, L. Pham Kim, T. U. Nguen, et al. 2005. Seizing the moment: California's opportunity to prevent nutrition-related health disparities in low-income Asian American population. *Cancer* 15; 104(12 Suppl):2962–2968.

Hertzler, A. A., and K. DeBord. 1994. Preschoolers' developmentally appropriate food and nutrition skills. *Journal of Nutrition Education* 26:166B–C.

Hinojosa, M. S., D. Nelson, R. Hinojosa, A. Delgado, B. Witzack, M. Gonzalez, et al. 2011. Using *fotonovelas* to promote healthy eating in a Latino community. *American Journal of Public Health* 101(2):258–259.

Hoelscher, D. M., A. E. Springer, N. Ranjit, C. L. Perry, A. E. Evans, M. Stigler and S. H. Kelder. 2010. Reductions in child obesity among disadvantaged school children with community involvement: The Travis County CATCH Trial. *Obesity* (Silver Spring). 18(Suppl 1):S36–S44.

Hoerr, S. L., S. O. Hughes, J. O. Fisher, T. A. Nicklas, Y. Liu, and R. M. Shewchuk. 2009. Associations among parental feeding styles and children's food intake in families with limited income. *International Journal of Behavior Nutrition and Physical Activity* 13(6):55.

Husing, C., and M. Elfant. 2005. Finding the teacher within: A story of learner-centered education in California WIC. *Journal of Nutrition Education and Behavior* 37(Suppl. 1):S22.

Isaacs, M., and M. Benjamin. 1991. *Towards a culturally competent system of care. Vol. 2: Programs which utilize culturally competent principles.* Washington, DC: Georgetown University Child Development Center, CASSP Technical Assistance Center.

James, D. C. S., J. W. Pobee, D. Oxidine, L. Brown, and G. Joshi. 2012. Using the health belief model to develop culturally appropriate weight-management materials for African American women. *Journal of the Academy of Nutrition and Dietetics* 112:664–670.

King, M. A., A. Sims, and D. Osher. 2006. How is cultural competence integrated in education? Center for Effective Collaboration and Practice, American Institutes of Research. http://cecp.air.org Accessed 12/5/14.

Kinzie, M. B. 2005. Instructional design strategies for health behavior change. *Patient Education and Counseling* 56:3–15.

Knowles, M. S., and E. F. Holton. 2011. *The adult learner.* Seventh ed. Burlington, MA: Butterworth-Heinemann.

Kreuter, M. W., S. N. Lukwago, R. D. Bucholtz, E. M. Clark, and V. Sanders-Thompson. 2003. Achieving cultural appropriateness in health promotion programs: Targeted and tailored approaches. *Health Education and Behavior* 30(2):133–146.

Kreuter, M. W., C. Sugg-Skinner, C. L. Holt, E. M. Clark, D. Haire-Joshu, Q. Fu, et al. 2005. Cultural tailoring for mammography and fruit and vegetables intake among low-income African-American women in urban public health centers. *Preventive Medicine* 41:53–62.

Kumanyika, S., W. C. Taylor, S. A. Grier, V. Lassiter, K. J. Lancaster, C. B. Morsink, et al. 2012. Community energy balance: A framework for contextualizing cultural influences on high risk of obesity in ethnic minority populations. *Preventive Medicine* 55:371–381.

Kumanyika, S. K., M. C. Whitt-Glover, T. L. Gray, T. E. Prewitt, A. M Odums-Young, J. Banks-Wallace, et al. 2007. Expanding the obesity research paradigm to reach African-American communities. *Preventing Chronic Disease* 4:1–22.

Leupker, R. V., C. L. Perry, S. M. McKinlay, P. R. Nader, G. S. Parcel, E. J. Stone, et al. 1996. Outcomes of a field trial to improve children's dietary patterns and physical activity. *Journal of the American Medical Association* 275:768–776.

Levinson, D. J. 1978. *The seasons of a man's life.* New York: Knopf.

———. 1996. *The seasons of a woman's life.* New York: Knopf.

Lin, W., and I. S. Liang. 2005. Family dining environment, parenting practices and preschoolers' food acceptance. *Journal of Nutrition Education and Behavior* 37(Suppl. 1):47.

Liou, D., and I. R. Contento. 2001. Usefulness of psychosocial theory variables in explaining fat-related dietary behavior in Chinese Americans: Association with degree of acculturation. *Journal of Nutrition Education* 33:322–331.

Matheson, D., and K. Spranger. 2001. Content analysis of the use of fantasy, challenge, and curiosity in school-based nutrition education programs. *Journal of Nutrition Education* 33:10–16.

Matheson, D., K. Spranger, and A. Saxe. 2002. Preschool children's perceptions of food and their food experiences. *Journal of Nutrition Education and Behavior* 34:85–92.

Meir, N., M. G. Ory, and A. A. Medina. 2010. Anatomy of culturally sensitive interventions promoting nutrition and exercise in Hispanics: A critical examination of the existing literature. *Health Promotion Practice* 11(4):541–554.

Merrill, M. D. 2009. First principles of instruction. In *Instructional-design theories and models. Volume III. Building a common knowledge base*, edited by C. M. Reigeluth and A. A. Carr-Chellman. New York: Routledge.

Michela, J. L., and I. R. Contento. 1984. Spontaneous classification of foods by elementary school-aged children. *Health Education Quarterly* 11:57–76.

National Center for Educational Statistics. 2003. National Assessment of Adult Literacy. http://nces.ed.gov/naal/ Accessed 12/16/14.

Neugarten, B. L., R. J. Havighurst, and S. S. Tobin. 1968. Personality and patterns of aging. In *Middle age and aging*, edited by B. L. Neugarten. Chicago: University of Chicago Press.

Neumark-Sztainer, D., P. J. Hannan, M. Story, J. Croll, and C. Perry. 2003. Family meal patterns: Associations with sociodemographic characteristics and improved dietary intake among adolescents. *Journal of the American Dietetic Association* 102:317–322.

Neumark-Sztainer, D., M. Story, D. Ackard, J. Moe, and C. Perry. 2000a. The "family meal": View of adolescents. *Journal of Nutrition Education* 32:329–334.

———. 2000b. Family meals among adolescents: Findings from a pilot study. *Journal of Nutrition Education* 32:335–340.

Neumark-Sztainer, D., M. Story, P. J. Hannan, C. L. Perry, and L. M. Irving. 2002. Weight-related concerns and behaviors among overweight and nonoverweight adolescents: Implication for preventing weight-related disorders. *Archives of Pediatric Adolescent Medicine* 156:171–178.

Neumark-Sztainer, D., M. Story, C. Perry, and M. A. Casey. 1999. Factors influencing food choices of adolescents: Findings from focus-group discussions with adolescents. *Journal of the American Dietetic Association* 99:929–937.

Nie, C. and L. Zepeda. 2011. Lifestyle segmentation of US shoppers to examine organic and local food consumption. *Appetite* 57:28–37.

Norris, J. 2003. *From telling to teaching*. North Myrtle Beach, SC: Learning by Dialogue.

Novotny, R., J. S. Han, and I. Biernacke. 1999. Motivators and barriers to consuming calcium-rich foods among Asian adolescents in Hawaii. *Journal of Nutrition Education* 31:99–104.

Ockene, I. S., T. L. Tellez, M. C. Rosal, G. W. Reed, J. Mordes, P. A. Merriam, et al. 2012. Outcomes of a Latino community-based intervention for prevention of diabetes: the Lawrence Latino Diabetes Prevention Project. *American Journal of Public Health* 102:336–342.

O'Connor, T. M., S. O. Hughes, K. B. Watson, T. Baranowski, T. A. Nicklas, J. O. Fisher, et al. 2009. Parenting practices associated with fruit and vegetable consumption in preschool children. *Public Health Nutrition* 13(1):91–101.

Olson, C. M., and G. L. Kelley. 1989. The challenge of implementing theory-based nutrition education. *Journal of Nutrition Education* 22:280–284.

Pai, H. L., and I. R. Contento. 2014. Parental perceptions, feeding practices, feeding styles, and level of acculturation of Chinese Americans in relation to their school-age child's weight status. *Appetite* 80:174–182.

Peters, N. C., I. R. Contento, F. Kronenberg, and M. Coleton. 2014. Adherence to a whole foods eating pattern intervention with healthy postmenopausal women. *Public Health Nutrition* 17(12):2806–2815.

Piaget, J., and B. Inhelder. 1969. *The psychology of the child*. New York: Basic Books.

Purnell, L. 2002. The Purnell model for cultural competence. *Journal of Transcultural Nursing* 13:193–196.

Reigeluth, C. M., and A. A. Carr-Chellman. 2009. Understanding instructional-design theory. In *Instructional-design theories and models. Vol. III. Building a common knowledge base*, edited by C. M. Reigeluth and A. A. Carr-Chellman. New York: Routledge.

Resnicow, K., T. Baranowski, J. S. Ahluwalia, and R. L. Braithwaite. 1999. Cultural sensitivity in public health: Defined and demystified. *Ethnicity and Disease* 9:10–21.

Resnicow, K., A. Jackson, D. Blisset, T. Wang, F. McCarty, S. Rahotep, et al. 2005. Results of the HealthyBody/Healthy Spirit trial. *Health Physiology* 24:339–348.

Resnicow, K., A. Jackson, R. Braithwaite, C. Dilorio, D. Blisset, S. Rahotep, et al. 2002. Healthy Body/Healthy Spirit: A church-based nutrition and physical activity intervention. *Health Education Research* 17:562–573.

Reyes, N. R., A. A. Klotz, and J. Herring. 2013. A qualitative study of motivators and barriers to healthy eating in pregnancy for low-income, overweight, African-American mothers. *Journal of the Academy of Nutrition and Dietetics* 113:1175–1181.

Rhee, K. 2008. Childhood overweight and the relationship between parent behaviors, parenting style, and family functioning. *Annals of the American Academy of Political and Social Science* 615(1):11–37.

Rolls, B. J., D. Engell, and L. L. Birch. 2000. Serving portion size influences 5-year-old but not 3-year-old children's food intakes. *Journal of the American Dietetic Association* 180:232–234.

Sahyoun, N. R., C. A. Pratt, and A. Anderson. 2004. Evaluation of nutrition education for older adults: A proposed framework. *Journal of the American Dietetic Association* 104:58–69.

Salto, L. M., Z. Cordero-MacIntyre, L. Beeson, E. Schulz, A. Firek, and M. De Leon. 2011. *En Balance* participants decrease dietary fat and cholesterol intake as part of a culturally sensitive Hispanic diabetes education program. *Diabetes Educator* 37(2):239–253.

Sanjur, D. 1982. *Social and cultural perspectives in nutrition*. Englewood Cliffs, NJ: Prentice Hall.

Santrock, J. 2013. *Adolescence*. 15th ed. McGraw-Hill.

Satter, E. 2008. *Secrets of feeding a healthy family: How to eat, how to raise good eaters, how to cook*. Madison, WI: Kelcy Press.

Savage, J. S., J. O. Fisher, and L. L. Birch. 2007. Parental influence on eating behavior: Conception to adolescence. *Journal of Law and Medical Ethics* 35(1):22–34.

Shaffer, D. R. and K. Kipp. 2013. *Developmental psychology: Childhood and adolescence*. 9th ed. Belmont, CA: Wadsworth/Cengage.

Sigman-Grant, M. 2004. *Facilitated dialogue basics: A self-study guide for nutrition educators. Let's dance*. University of Nevada, Cooperative Extension. SP04–21.

Singleton, J. C., C. L. Achterberg, and B. M. Shannon. 1992. Role of food and nutrition: The health perceptions of young children. *Journal of the American Dietetic Association* 92:67–70.

Skinner, J. D., B. R. Carruth, B. Wendy, and P. J. Ziegler. 2002. Children's food preferences: A longitudinal analysis. *Journal of the American Dietetic Association* 102: 1638–1647.

Stein, K. 2009. Cultural competency: Where it is and where it's headed. *Journal of the American Dietetic Association* 109:388–394.

———. 2010. Moving cultural competency from abstract to act. *Journal of the American Dietetic Association* 110:180–187.

Story, M., D. Neumark-Sztainer, and S. I. French. 2002. Individual and environmental influences on adolescent eating behaviors. *Journal of the American Dietetic Association* 2:S40–S51.

Story, M., D. Neumark-Sztainer, N. Sherwood, J. Stang, and D. Murray. 1998. Dieting status and its relationship to eating and physical activity behaviors in a representative sample of US adolescents. *Journal of the American Dietetic Association* 98:1127–1135, 1255.

Story, M., and M. D. Resnick. 1986. Adolescents' views on food and nutrition. *Journal of Nutrition Education* 18:188–192.

Sue, D. W., and D. Sue. 2013. *Counseling the culturally different: Theory and practice.* Sixth ed. Hoboken, NJ: Wiley.

Tennant, M., and P. Pogson. 1995. *Learning and change in the adult years: A developmental perspective.* San Francisco: Jossey-Bass.

Thompson D., R. Bhatt, M. Lazarus, K. Cullen, J. Baranowski, and T. Baranowski. 2012. A serious video game to increase fruit and vegetable consumption among elementary aged youth (Squire's Quest! II): Rationale, design, and methods. *JMIR Research Protocols.* 2012 Jul–Dec; 1(2): e19

Triandis, H. C. 1979. Values, attitudes, and interpersonal behavior. In *Nebraska symposium on motivation*, edited by H. E. How. Lincoln: University of Nebraska Press.

Vella, J. 2002. *Learning to listen, learning to teach: The power of dialogue in educating adults.* Revised ed. San Francisco: Jossey-Bass.

Ventura, A. K., and L. Birch. 2008. Does parenting affect children's eating and weight status? *International Journal of Behavioral Nutrition and Physical Activity* 5:15.

Videon, T. M., and C. K. Manning. 2003. Influences on adolescent eating patterns: The importance of family meals. *Journal of Adolescent Health* 32:365–373.

Vygotsky, L. S. 1962. *Thought and language.* Cambridge, MA: MIT Press.

Wardle, J., L. J. Cooke, E. L. Gibson, M. Sapochnik, A. Sheiham, and M. Lawson. 2003. Increasing children's acceptance of vegetables: A randomized trial of parent-led exposure. *Appetite* 40:55–162.

Wardle, J., M. L. Herrera, L. J. Cooke, and E. L. Gibson. 2003. Modifying children's food preferences: The effects of exposure and rewards on acceptance of an unfamiliar vegetable. *European Journal of Clinical Nutrition* 57:341–348.

Woodruff. S. J., and A. R. Kirby. 2013. The associations among family meal frequency, food preparation frequency, self-efficacy for cooking, and food preparation techniques in children and adolescents. *Journal of Nutrition Education and Behavior* 45:296–303.

Worsley, A. 2000. Food and consumers: Where are we going? *Asia Pacific Journal of Clinical Nutrition* 9(Suppl):S103–S107.

Young, L., J. Anderson, L. Beckstrom, L. Bellows, and S. L. Johnson. 2004. Using social marketing principles to guide the development of a nutrition education initiative for pre-school children. *Journal of Nutrition Education and Behavior* 36:250–257.

Ziebarth, D., N. Healy-Haney, B. Gnadt, et al. 2011. A community-based family intervention program to improve obesity in Hispanic families. *Wisconsin Medical Journal* 111(6):261–266.

Zoorob, R., M. S. Buchowski, B. M. Beech, J. R. Canedo, R. Chandrasekhar, S. Akohoue, et al. 2013. Healthy Families study: Design of a childhood obesity prevention trial for Hispanic families. *Contemporary Clinical Trials* 35(2):108–121.

CHAPTER 18

Nutrition Educators as Change Agents in the Environment

OVERVIEW

This chapter describes ways in which nutrition educators can help to shape the profession and to act as change agents in the larger environment by working with others to shape legislation about nutrition education and by educating policymakers in government.

CHAPTER OUTLINE

- Introduction
- Keeping up with nutrition education research and best practices
- Helping to shape the profession
- Ethics in nutrition education: maintaining credibility

- Participating in community coalitions
- Advocating for nutrition and nutrition education
- Educating policymakers in government
- You can't do everything, but you can do something

LEARNING OBJECTIVES

At the end of the chapter, you should be able to:

- State reasons why it is important to participate in professional associations relevant to nutrition education
- Identify ways you can help to shape the profession
- Understand the importance of policies regarding outside sponsorship of nutrition

  education professional activities and conflicts of interest
- Describe ways you can affect the larger environment by participating in community networks and coalitions
- Appreciate the importance of educating policymakers in government, such as elected officials

Introduction

You attend your first professional meeting of researchers, dietitians, extension nutritionists, nutrition educators, and others. You are amazed to see so many activities going on and are both excited and overwhelmed. At sessions, you learn new information from research. You hear about various programs and projects that people are involved in. They spark ideas for you to use in your professional work. You hear about committees and task force reports. You learn about government policies at the state and national level, and the policies of international organizations that might affect your work and you wonder—should I get involved? If so, how do I do that?

Providing nutrition education directly to the public is your major role as a nutrition educator. You do this through direct, in-person activities with groups, indirect activities such as printed materials and media campaigns, and policy and systems change activities to foster environments supportive of the program's targeted behaviors and practices. Nutrition educators also have the opportunity to develop and grow by networking with others and being involved in professional organizations. They can make their voices heard in the organizations of which they are members and even help to shape their policies and practices by participation and actions. Nutrition educators also have the opportunity to make a difference in the world by advocating for nutrition education policies and programs in the larger environment. This chapter describes some ways in which you can be involved in the nutrition education professional community.

Keeping up with Nutrition Education Research and Best Practices

This book began by noting that this is a great time for nutrition education. It is needed now more than ever, and research and evidence for best practices provide the tools you need to assist the public to achieve health and well-being. You have seen that nutrition education is more likely to be effective when it focuses on behaviors and practices, uses theory and research evidence from behavioral nutrition and nutrition education to guide the strategies it uses, and addresses multiple sources of influence. Effective nutrition education is not short-term work; it takes time to facilitate the progress of individuals and communities through various stages of change: from awareness and active contemplation, through various levels of motivational readiness to change, through how-to activities to enable change, to maintenance of change. Consequently, the motivators and reinforcers of change and the environmental supports of change need to be multifaceted, continually updated, and maintained.

Research in this area is active and ongoing. New understandings of how to facilitate change and new tools are being generated. Keeping up to date on nutrition education research is important to maintain your effectiveness as a nutrition educator. You can do this by reading the relevant journals and by attending nutrition education and behavioral nutrition (not just nutrition science) workshops, meetings, and conferences. **BOX 18-1** lists some of the professional organizations particularly relevant to nutrition educators.

BOX 18-1 **Professional Associations of Particular Relevance to Nutrition Educators**

Society for Nutrition Education and Behavior (SNEB)

Vision: Healthy communities, food systems and behaviors

Mission: The Society for Nutrition Education and Behavior promotes effective nutrition education and healthy behavior through research, policy, and practice.

Identity statement: The Society for Nutrition Education and Behavior (SNEB) represents the unique professional interests of nutrition educators in the United States and worldwide. SNEB is dedicated to promoting effective nutrition education and healthy behavior through research, policy, and practice and has a vision of healthy communities, food systems, and behaviors.

SNEB is an international community of professionals actively involved in nutrition education and health promotion. Its work takes place in colleges and universities, schools, government agencies, cooperative extension, communications and public relations firms, the food industry, voluntary and service organizations, and with other reliable places of nutrition and health education information.

SNEB members share ideas and resources through a journal, newsletter, annual conference, and members-only listserv. Its divisions offer networking opportunities for members with similar interests and expertise. Divisions include Children, Communications, Food and Nutrition Extension Education, Healthy Aging, Higher Education, International, Industry, Public Health, Social Marketing, Sustainable Food Systems, and Weight Realities. SNE also has some regional affiliates and an Advisory Committee on Public Policy that helps provide focus on national issues of importance to society members.

Website: http://www.sneb.org

Academy of Nutrition and Dietetics (AND)

Vision: Optimizing the nation's health through food and nutrition

Mission: Empowering members to be the nation's food and nutrition leaders

Identity statement: The Academy of Nutrition and Dietetics (formerly the American Dietetic Association) was founded in 1917 and is the world's largest organization of food and nutrition professionals. The Academy is committed to improving the nation's health and advancing the profession of dietetics through research, education and advocacy.

Approximately 70 percent of the Academy's over 75,000 members are registered dietitians (RDs) or registered dietitian nutritionists (RDNs), and 2 percent are dietetic technicians, registered (DTRs). Other Academy members include students, educators, researchers, retirees, and international members. Nearly half of the Academy's members hold advanced academic degrees.

Academy members represent a wide range of practice areas and interests. Affiliate, dietetics practice, and member interest groups share the common purpose of serving the profession, the public, and members in such areas as continuing professional education, public information on nutrition and health, government advocacy and relations, membership recruitment, Academy leadership, and public relations. These

membership groups reflect the many characteristics of the Academy's membership and the public it serves.

Website: http://www.eatright.org

School Nutrition Association (SNA)

Vision: Be the authority and resource for school nutrition programs

Mission: SNA is the national organization of school nutrition professionals committed to advancing the quality of school meal programs through education and advocacy.

Identity statement: The School Nutrition Association (SNA), formerly the American School Food Service Association (ASFSA), is a U.S. national, nonprofit professional organization representing 55,000 school nutrition professionals across the country. Founded in 1946, SNA and its members are dedicated to making healthy school meals and nutrition education available to all students.

Website: http://www.schoolnutrition.org

American Association of Family and Consumer Sciences (AAFCS)

Vision: Individuals, families, and communities are achieving optimal quality of life assisted by competent, caring professionals whose expertise is continually updated through AAFCS.

Mission: To provide leadership and support for professionals whose work assists individuals, families, and communities in making informed decisions about their well-being, relationships, and resources to achieve optimal quality of life.

Identity statement: For more than 100 years, AAFCS members have been working to improve the quality and standards of individual and family life by delivering educational programs, influencing public policy, and conducting research. It provides research-based knowledge about the topics of everyday life, including human development, personal and family finance, housing and interior design, food science, nutrition and wellness, textiles and apparel, and consumer issues. The knowledge, research, and experience of its members help people achieve a healthy and sustainable world.

Website: http://www.aafcs.org

(Continues)

BOX 18-1 **Professional Associations of Particular Relevance to Nutrition Educators (Continued)**

International Society for Behavioral Nutrition and Physical Activity (ISBNPA)

Vision: ISBNPA will be the international leader in advancing and fostering excellence in research on nutrition behavior and physical activity.

Mission: ISBNPA stimulates, promotes, and advocates innovative research and policy in the area of behavioral nutrition and physical activity toward the betterment of human health worldwide. Its purposes are as follows:

- Conduct scientific meetings, congresses, and symposia in which current research on behavioral issues in nutrition and physical activity will be discussed by researchers in related fields.

- Disseminate information on research being done on behavioral issues in nutrition and physical activity through newsletters and other communications.

- Provide information to and encourage continued support by public and private bodies that support research in behavioral issues in nutrition and physical activity.

- Promote and facilitate the dissemination of knowledge of behavioral issues in nutrition and physical activity to the public and to educators, scholars, and health professionals through any lawful means.

- Promote and assist communication between researchers on issues of behavioral nutrition and physical activity and members of scientific and scholarly organizations whose members do research in other related health and medical fields through joint meetings, shared membership lists, joint publications, and any other lawful means.

Identity statement: ISBNPA has an international presence, with nearly 420 members representing 29 countries (as of 2014). Its members come together from more than 40 government agencies and industry and professional organizations, as well as close to 150 academic and medical institutions. Members bring to this organization a diversity of experience and expertise and have a wide range of credentials.

Website: http://www.isbnpa.org

Association for the Study of Food and Society (ASFS)

Mission: ASFS is a multidisciplinary international organization dedicated to exploring the complex relationships among food, culture, and society.

Identity statement: The ASFS's members, who approach the study of food from numerous disciplines in the humanities, social sciences, and sciences, as well as in the world of food beyond the academy, draw on a wide range of theoretical and practical approaches and seek to promote discussions about food that transgress traditional boundaries. The association holds annual meetings with the Agriculture, Food, and Human Values Society and publishes the journal *Food, Culture & Society*.

Website: http://www.food-culture.org

Agriculture, Food, and Human Values Society (AFHVS)

Mission: Through annual meetings and an international journal, AFHVS promotes interdisciplinary research and scholarship on the values, visions, and structures underlying current food systems and their agricultural, rural, and urban components—from the local to the global—as well as the exploration of alternative visions of more democratic and decentralized food systems that sustain local and regional communities, cultures, and habitats.

Identity statement: Growing out of W. K. Kellogg Foundation–supported projects to promote interaction between liberal arts and agricultural disciplines, AFHVS provides a continuing link among scholars working in cross-disciplinary studies of food and agriculture. From a base of philosophers, sociologists, and anthropologists, AFHVS has grown to include scientists, scholars, and practitioners in areas ranging from agricultural production and social science to nutrition policy and the humanities.

Website: http://www.afhvs.org

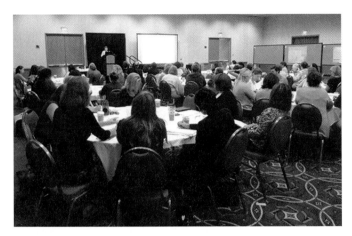

Becoming a member of a professional organization is a great way to become involved in your profession—the level of participation is up to you.

Courtesy of Society for Nutrition Education and Behavior.

Helping to Shape the Profession

As a nutrition educator, you also have the opportunity to participate in and shape the profession. There are many ways to do this. One way is to join one or more professional associations. For example, there are local and state dietetic associations to which you can belong, as well as national associations and food systems organizations such as the Society for Nutrition Education and Behavior (SNEB) and the Academy of Nutrition and Dietetics (AND). Through these organizations you will meet others just like you—individuals who are excited to be in the nutrition education profession and helping the public eat well and who are dealing with the same dilemmas and constraints. These organizations provide a forum for you to network with others and share ideas, learn about best practices, receive updates on information that may be important in your work, and learn about reseach regulations and policy actions that affect the profession or the public at large.

You also have the opportunity to make your opinions heard. Professional associations are member organizations, made up of others just like you. Although state and national organizations may have some paid staff, all are dependent on members' volunteer participation to operate. These associations thus become whatever members want them to be. If you are a student member, many organizations have student rates that extend to the first year of "professional enroll-ment" or "new professionals." Many organizations have what are called sections, divisions, or affiliates. These provide opportunities to network with colleagues who have like interests or are related geographically.

WHO THEY ARE

What are some associations where you might find a professional home? For nutrition educators, some of the most relevant ones include the SNEB, AND, American Public Health Association (APHA), International Society for Behavioral Nutrition and Physical Activity (ISBNPA), American Association of Family and Consumer Sciences (AAFCS), American Diabetes Association (ADA), American Society for Nutrition (ASN), and the International Society for Behavioral Nutrition and Physical Activity. Information on some of these is provided in Box 18-1. Of course, many nutrition educators belong to several professional associations.

GETTING TO KNOW THEM AND VICE VERSA

Getting involved in an organization is key to getting to know it. Reading the organization's journal by itself will not bring about opportunities to participate fully or shape the profession. As you get to know the organization, the organization will get to know you. As you offer to serve on committees and task forces or hold offices, over time the organization will come to you asking for your involvement.

A key way to get started in the process of knowing and getting known is to attend the organization's annual meeting. Annual meetings provide opportunities for more than learning from experts. They are opportunities for meeting your colleagues, expressing your thoughts, and supporting your position in the various units that run the organization and professions. The divisions, special interest units, caucuses, and affiliates all provide opportunities for input. Although these units may meet during the year and have electronic mailing lists and bulletin boards, it is at the annual meetings that members come together to discuss, plan, and strategize. This also applies to meetings of state or local affiliates, which often focus on more regional professional issues, membership or town meetings, and gatherings to discuss specific issues.

Finding Where You Fit

Finding your home in the profession involves finding not only the organization, but also the specialty units within it that are right for you. Initially it may be the specialty units, defined as divisions, sections, or practice groups, and local, state, and regional affiliates that are of more interest to you than the organization itself. They are smaller and therefore more manageable. They also provide a common ground of interest in specific issues or approaches that may feel comfortable to you. Many nutrition educators belong to more than one such unit. Over time, you may change your focus or move on, but you will often find that the relationships you have developed keep you involved and, through networking, offer opportunities in other groups and locations.

Attend the business meetings of the specialty unit or division to find out the main issues facing the organization or unit, the activities completed or contemplated, and the financial situation of the organization as well as the sources of funding for the organization.

Determining your fit is often based on your relationships with the people in the unit or organization and the ability to work synergistically to have an impact, discuss common interests, and share war stories. You can join communication forums, such as listservs. Find out if there is a mentoring program. There may be a specific student unit, and often the governing boards have student representatives. Even as a student, you have an opportunity to affect the profession.

Join a Subcommittee or Task Force

Professional associations are always seeking interested members to participate. You do not have to wait to be asked! Look for notices seeking participation and input. This, too, is a way to shape the profession. If you don't feel comfortable sitting on a committee or being part of a task force, respond when the organization asks for member input or opinions. Let leadership know you're interested in an issue. Over time, as your name is recognized as an involved member, leadership will come to you. In fact, managing your time in order not to become overextended may become the more important consideration!

Write

You can participate by helping to write for, or edit, the newsletter for your specialty unit or division. You can help to write background papers or participate with others in writing position papers on some issue that is a passion of yours. You can write letters to the editor or write articles. All of these actions provide opportunities to be involved and have an impact.

Participate in Program Planning Activities

Organizations and the specialty units within them always need to plan future conferences or meetings. Attend the open planning sessions and provide your suggestions for sessions, topics, or speakers. Join the planning committee if you can. Help shape the agenda for the meetings.

Participate in Member-Initiated Resolutions or Issues Management Processes

Many professional associations have a process whereby an individual, a group of members, or a division or committee can write up and submit resolutions or statements for the membership to vote on, which then go to the association for action. In most cases, the resolutions advocate that the association take a position or action on an issue, or advocate that the association establish a policy. Such a process is a very effective way to influence the professional association as well as the larger policy environment. These resolutions are conveyed to the agencies and groups designated in the resolutions, where they often have important impacts on food- and nutrition-related policy.

Run for Office

Making the commitment to be a part of the process may very well lead you to run for an office. You may be nominated, or you may decide to nominate yourself. Don't be shy. If you want to have an impact and be involved, let others know. This applies to running for offices at the specialty unit or division level as well as at the organizational level.

Volunteer

Whatever you do, find some way to be involved. The connections you make can be very important for you over the long term. In the process of volunteering, you get to know others, they get to know you, and the profession becomes stronger because of all the participatory voices. Also keep in mind that professional organizations cannot run on the dues they raise alone or the funds they may acquire through foundation grants. They need volunteers. Some active members have used a rule of thumb of volunteering 1 hour per week and have found it to be very rewarding, both personally and professionally.

Ethics in Nutrition Education: Maintaining Credibility

One of the most cherished assets nutrition educators have is credibility—to clients and program participants, to the professional community, to government, and to the public at large. When you lose your credibility, you lose your effectiveness. This same principle applies to the professional associations to which you belong, and indeed to the profession as a whole. Professional associations, and indeed the profession, must be seen as credible sources of information and recommendations.

What does this mean? It means that just as is the case for individuals, so also the recommendations made by the professional associations must be seen as being based on sound science. More importantly, the professional associations must not stand to gain financially, or seem to gain financially, from their recommendations. In recent years, professional associations, as well as private voluntary organizations, research programs using public funds, and all government and quasi-government committees, have developed sponsorship or funding policies that apply to potential sponsors of activities of the organization, and conflict of interest policies that apply to individuals. Much of the impetus for this development came from the concern of members of organizations and of the public about undue commercial influence that might affect the credibility of the organization.

SPONSORSHIP OF NUTRITION EDUCATION PROGRAMS AND PROFESSIONAL ACTIVITIES

Professional associations and organizations that provide nutrition education are always in need of funds. Membership dues, government or foundation grants, or grants from academic institutions do not always generate enough funds for these organizations to do what they need or want to do. It would appear natural to turn to the food industry, among other sources, for such funding. Organizations may go to individual corporations or to food commodity groups. Funding can be sought for individual activities, such as a specific one-time professional meeting or a specific session or social event at the annual meeting, or for the annual meeting of an organization as a whole. Funds can also be sought for a specific project or particular community outreach activity. The food industry or related corporation may also contribute to the professional organization as a whole by being a professional member.

Members in several professional associations have raised concerns about undue influence, potentially biased positions, conflict of interest, and the appearance of conflict of interest that may be engendered by such funding arrangements. They have been concerned that the corporate need for profits and nutrition professionals' interests in the health of the public may at times come into conflict (Nestle 2002). These concerns have often been raised through the resolutions process or issues management process. In response to membership concerns, many professional organizations have developed guidelines so that sponsorship by, and collaboration with, the food industry (or fitness or other related industry) can be conducted in an ethical and mutually beneficial manner.

Guiding principles usually include the following:

- The organization should secure sponsorship arrangements that further the organization's mission and vision, retain the organization's independence, maintain objectivity, promote trust, avoid conflicts of interest, and guard its professional values.
- The sponsorship should be consistent with the organization's commitment to the free exchange of ideas, opinions, research findings, and other information related to members' interests and activities.
- There should be transparency about relationships, clearly specified expectations, understanding of the value of the sponsor's contribution, and methods of accountability.
- The content of the professional organization's activities, such as educational sessions at annual meetings, should be initiated and planned by the organization or its members for the benefit of its members or to further the organization's mission.
- Educational sessions to which sponsors provide support should be science-based, peer-reviewed, and refrain from including marketing messages and promotion of sponsors' products and services in the sessions.
- Protection of the reputation and credibility of the organization is of utmost importance. The organization needs to be seen by the public, government, other professional organizations, and the nutrition education community as a trusted and independent voice on relevant issues based on sound science and reasoned policy and issues analyses and free from commercial bias. The nature of the funding organization and funding arrangements thus should not jeopardize such reputation and credibility.
- Full disclosure of sponsorship is essential, along with avoidance of all appearance of endorsement.

CONFLICTS OF INTEREST

Members in several professional organizations have been instrumental in initiating policies about conflict of interest and disclosure. Members were concerned that speakers (whether members or invited guests) were not disclosing professional and corporate relationships they had when they spoke at conferences or sat on an organization's boards, committees, and task forces. Members felt it was important to know that a given speaker or board member, whatever his or her primary professional designations, also had paid consulting or other relationships with the food industry or some other relevant group. Because professional associations are member-run organizations, members' voices are important and are heard. The outcome has been that many organizations have developed policies and procedures that address these concerns of membership.

Most professional associations or societies require that those who are on the governing board, committees, policy bodies, or task forces, and those who are officers at the division or specialty unit level, complete a conflict of interest form annually. Some associations also require that at the beginning of each committee or task force meeting, the agenda items be reviewed and an opportunity provided for members of the committee to disclose if they have a conflict of interest on any given item. If they do, they may be asked to recuse themselves altogether from that item or to participate in the discussion but not vote. All would agree that transparency is good for everyone.

Note that members frequently initiated these policy changes. This is another example of how you can make a difference in the profession by your actions.

Such self-disclosures of conflict of interest have become routine for all government and quasi-government committees, task forces, and other bodies. They are also now required for government research and other grant recipients.

Tests for Conflict of Interest

How do you test yourself to determine whether you have a conflict of interest? Ask yourself, would others trust my comments, decisions, actions, or votes if they knew about my relationships with particular organizations and/or my situation? How would I feel if the roles were reversed—would I feel misled or betrayed?

Conflicts of interest involve the abuse, actual or potential, of the trust people have in professionals. Conflicts of interest thus not only injure particular clients and employers, but also damage the whole profession by reducing the trust people have in professionals in general (McDonald 2004). Perception is a critical component here. If your colleagues or the public find out information after the fact and perceive a conflict of interest, the perception can do as much damage as the reality. Disclosure and transparency are key ways to address a conflict of interest, allowing others to weigh what you say. It may be appropriate not to participate in a given activity—a determination that can only occur if public acknowledgment of possible conflict is made.

Participating in Community Coalitions

Earlier in this book, we discussed ways in which nutrition education intervention programs can include environmental components to promote opportunities for participants to take the actions that are advocated by the program. (See Chapters 6 and 14.) Even if your program does not have an environmental change component, you can, as a nutrition education professional, participate in a number of activities in the community where you can be a change agent in the larger environment.

You need to help others understand that nutrition education professionals are much more than people who offer lectures and workshops. For the public to understand what you do, you need to be out there working with the community. Here are some examples of volunteer opportunities with community coalitions, networks, or other community groups.

FOOD POLICY COUNCILS

A food policy council (FPC) consists of stakeholders from various segments of a state or local food system. Councils can be officially sanctioned through a government action such as an executive order or can be a grassroots effort. The primary goal of many FPCs is to examine the operation of a local food system and provide ideas or recommendations for how it can be improved (Desjardin et al. 2005).

Who better to be part of the process than the nutrition educator? It makes sense for nutrition educators to play a key role in FPCs. Desjardin and colleagues (2005) point out that nutrition educators contribute food and nutrition knowledge and provide legitimacy as health professionals. Having nutrition professionals on board can broaden the scope of FPCs, where members may be more concerned with emergency food assistance or agriculture policy in the most traditional sense. It also means an FPC can get in-house help with proposal and report writing, research and evaluation, and media communication. Nutrition educators can also offer essential organizational and planning skills.

LOCAL WELLNESS POLICY

The Child Nutrition and WIC Reauthorization Act of 2004 (Section 204) required every local school district that offers the USDA school lunch program to develop and implement a local wellness policy (Wellness policy 2004; Fox 2005). The mandate provides that nutrition guidelines must:

- Be developed for all foods available on the school campus during the school day
- Include goals for nutrition education, physical activity, and other school-based activities to promote student wellness
- Have a plan for measuring implementation
- Involve parents, students, school food representatives, school board members, administrators, and the public in development

Strong nutrition components make for strong wellness policies, and the nutrition educator can be a facilitator of this process and/or serve as a resource. As is the case with FPCs, school wellness councils are multidisciplinary, and assessment is important. Examples of self-assessment and planning tools include the School Health Index (SHI) from the Centers for Disease Control and Prevention (CDC 2005).

Although most schools now have wellness policy councils, not all are functioning fully. Also, most have written school policies, but again, they may not be fully implemented. As a nutrition educator, you bring your skills in assessment and in facilitation of dialogue to the table; these are critical to a functional wellness policy. Wellness policies must be evaluated, and you can provide useful skills in this task as well.

NUTRITION EDUCATION NETWORKS

Nutrition education networks came into being in the mid-1990s when the Food and Nutrition Service (FNS) of the USDA approved cooperative agreements to establish nutrition education networks in 22 states (Health Systems Research 1999). The funding objective was to create self-sustaining statewide networks to implement nutrition education for food stamp–eligible adults and children, building on existing efforts, developing public–private partnerships, and using social marketing. It was envisioned that the networks would be the catalyst to integrate nutrition education messages across all food assistance programs and public–private programs. This networking process was designed to:

- Maximize public and private resources
- Identify specific client needs and relevant ways to address these needs
- Recruit and leverage community organizations to deliver appropriate messages

Such networks continue to provide considerable opportunities to network and coordinate nutrition education activities in states and local areas through the Association of State Nutrition Network Administrators (ASNNA).

COMMUNITY COALITIONS

There are no doubt many other local or national coalitions of food and nutrition professionals concerned with a variety of issues that would welcome your participation. Issues might include food security, concerns about the sustainability of food systems, food policy, urban gardens, farmers' markets, special populations such as those with HIV/AIDS or diabetes, or childhood overweight prevention. Your insights and expertise as a nutrition educator can be very important to the effective functioning of these coalitions.

Advocating for Nutrition and Nutrition Education

You can be a change agent in the larger environment through advocacy activities. These include written communications, providing testimony to governmental and quasi-governmental groups, and helping to shape legislation that affects the nutritional well-being of the public and the support of nutrition education.

WRITTEN COMMUNICATIONS

Written communications take many forms. The most notable, of course, are letters: you can make your voice heard by writing to newspapers, legislators, and others. You can also write articles. However, you can also write other documents that can have a tremendous impact on the decision making of individuals, organizations, and government. These can include position papers, policy papers, issue fact sheets, and background papers. Although "key expert members" may write the initial background documents and subsequent papers, you usually have an opportunity to provide input into these documents if you have an interest and let your wish be known.

TESTIMONY, HEARINGS, AND FORUMS

Governmental bodies often seek information from professionals about a specific issue using a variety of formats. Testimony and hearings usually come about in response to an invitation or public announcement to provide evidence to a session or committee of Congress, or to other governmental or quasi-governmental bodies, such as committees of the National Academy of Sciences. Hearings are usually open to the public and are designed for committees to obtain information and opinions from professionals or the public on proposed legislation, an investigation, or other activities of government. Hearings may also be purely exploratory in nature, a forum for professionals and the public to provide testimony and data about topics of current interest.

Forums, or listening sessions, provide opportunities for sharing comments in person or in writing. If you feel passionate about a particular issue, you can seek to testify. Sometimes you can do this on your own, on the basis of being a professional in the field. Or you may testify through your professional group, in which case you must make sure the leadership knows you are interested in presenting testimony.

HELPING TO SHAPE LEGISLATION

In the United States, some legislation, once passed, is permanent. However, some legislation is written so that it must be renewed after a stated period of time or it will expire. This happens typically in 5-year increments, but the time period may be longer or shorter. Key examples of U.S. federal legislation that affects nutrition education include the following:

- The Child Nutrition and WIC Reauthorization Act
- The Farm Bill
- The Ryan White Act
- The Older Americans Act

See **BOX 18-2** for more information.

BOX 18-2 Legislation that Affects Nutrition Education Programs

Child Nutrition Reauthorization

Child Nutrition Reauthorization includes legislation that covers the primary government food programs outside of the Supplementary Nutrition Assistance Program (SNAP; formerly the food stamp program) and related education components (http://www.fns.usda.gov/tags/reauthorization-child-nutrition-act). Programs include the following:

- National School Lunch Program (NSLP)
- School Breakfast Program (SBP)
- Child and Adult Care Food Program (CACFP)
- Summer Food Service Program (SFSP)
- Special Milk Program (SMP)

- Special Supplemental Nutrition Program for Women, Infants and Children (WIC), which includes the WIC Farmers Market Nutrition Program (FMNP)
- Fruit and Vegetable Snack Program
- Team Nutrition Program and language for the Team Nutrition Network
- School wellness policy legislation
- Language for access to local foods and school gardens

The Farm Bill

In the United States, the Farm Bill is the primary agricultural and food policy tool of the federal government. It consists of a series of 10 titles, four of which relate directly to nutrition education. These cover international and national nutrition education and related programs, research, and "miscellaneous" components (respectively, Titles III, IV, VII, and X). This act is also a key source of nutrition education funding and research.

- Title III, the Trade Title, includes the McGovern-Dole International Food for Education and Nutrition Program.

- Title IV, known as the Nutrition Title, covers the Supplementary Nutrition Assistance Program (SNAP), Supplementary Nutrition Assistance Program Education (SNAP-Ed), and Community Food Project Grants (CFPG); commodity distribution programs that are often associated with nutrition outreach, such as The Emergency Food Assistance Program (TEFAP), the Commodity Supplemental Food Program (CSFP), and the Department of Defense Fresh Fruit and Vegetable Program (DoD Fresh); funds for child nutrition programs such as commodities for school meals; primary funding for Senior Farmers' Market Nutrition Program (FMNP) and additional funding for the WIC FMNP program; the Nutrition Information and Awareness Pilot Program; and startup grants for some institutions participating in the National School Lunch and School Breakfast programs that purchase locally produced foods.

- Title VII, known as Research and Related Matters, includes the education and administration of land-grant institutions, with programs such as the Cooperative State Research, Education, and Extension Service (CSREES), which includes the Community Food Projects (CFP), the Expanded Food and Nutrition Education Program (EFNEP),

and Sustainable Agriculture Research and Education (SARE) grants. The title also includes the Organic Agriculture Research and Extension Initiative (OREI).

- Title X is for miscellaneous programs such as country-of-origin labeling, irradiated food/pasteurization, and biotechnology education.

The Ryan White Comprehensive AIDS Resources Emergency (CARE) Act

The Ryan White Act is federal legislation that addresses the unmet health needs of persons living with human immunodeficiency virus (HIV) by funding primary health-care and support services. The CARE Act was named after Ryan White, an Indiana teenager whose courageous struggle with HIV/AIDS and against AIDS-related discrimination helped educate the nation.

Older Americans Act

The Older Americans Act was originally signed into law by President Lyndon B. Johnson. In addition to creating the Administration on Aging (AOA), it authorized grants to states for community planning and services programs, as well as for research, demonstration, and training projects in the field of aging. Later amendments to the act added grants to Area Agencies on Aging for local needs identification, planning, and funding of services, including but not limited to nutrition programs in the community as well as for those who are homebound; programs that serve Native American elders; services targeted at low-income minority elders; health promotion and disease prevention activities; in-home services for frail elders; and those services that protect the rights of older persons, such as the long-term care ombudsman program.

Sources: Administration on Aging, U.S. Department of Health and Human Services. Older Americans Act. http://www.aoa.acl.gov/AoA_Programs/HPW/Nutrition_Services/index.aspx; Child Nutrition Reauthorization. http://www.fns.usda.gov/tags/reauthorization-child-nutrition-act; Department of Defense Fresh Fruit and Vegetable Program. http://www.fns.usda.gov/fdd/dod-fresh-fruit-and-vegetable-program; Health Resources and Services Administration, U.S. Department of Health and Human Services. HIV/AIDS Bureau. http://www.hrsa.gov/about/organization/bureaus/hab/; National Campaign for Sustainable Agriculture. The farm bill? http://sustainableagriculture.net/our-work/campaigns/fbcampaign/; Farm Act 2014. http://www.ers.usda.gov/agricultural-act-of-2014-highlights-and-implications.aspx.

You can help shape such legislation by becoming actively involved in the process of making recommendations. For example, the Child Nutrition and WIC Reauthorization Act needs to be renewed every 5 years. Usually, concerned organizations meet to discuss what they would advocate for at renewal time. The purpose of such meetings is to bring together stakeholders to discuss the current state of child nutrition and nutrition education, develop ideas for strengthening these, and aid member organizations in developing policy recommendations regarding child nutrition and nutrition education. Such groups can form in various locations all over the country. Professional organizations, such as SNEB, may also develop specific recommendations. For example, the mandate to set up local wellness committees in school districts to develop policy regarding food and health in schools came out of the 2004 process, and increased funding for school meals, among other actions, came out of the 2009 reauthorization process (Food Research and Action Center [FRAC] n.d.).

You can make an important contribution by adding your voice to those of other nutrition educators in activities such as these in order to make a difference in the larger environment.

A number of organizations serve as advocates of food and nutrition policy and legislation at the local, state, and federal levels. They monitor the various food and nutrition programs, alert the profession about new initiatives and changes that are being contemplated, and advocate for programs that benefit the public.

Educating Policymakers in Government

Chapter 14 discusses the importance of educating and working with policymakers and decision-makers in order to promote environments that are conducive to food and nutrition behaviors. These policymakers are school principals, community leaders, worksite management, local agencies, and others. This section discusses educating policymakers in government—elected officials.

WHY EDUCATE ELECTED GOVERNMENT OFFICIALS?

Elected government officials are the ones who will vote on legislation and make policies on issues that are of concern to you as a nutrition educator, such as funding for nutrition and for nutrition education through a variety of programs. Legislators are always sensitive to their constituents, so you, as an individual, can have an impact on them.

WHO ARE YOUR ELECTED OFFICIALS?

There are policymakers at many levels—local, city, county, state, and federal—and those who participate in nutrition education policy work say that it is important for you to know each one by name. Finding out who represents you should not be difficult. Go to your local or state government's website; there will most likely be a tool at the site that will assist you in identifying your representatives. Or try

the Government Guide (http://votenote.aol.com/mygov/dbq/officials/). This site provides information on representatives at all levels and keeps you up to date on the activities of your legislators. At the federal level, you can also use http://www.senate.gov for senators and http://www.house.gov for members of the House of Representatives.

GET TO KNOW THEM AND LET THEM GET TO KNOW YOU

Once you know who your elected representatives are, the next step is to find out about them. Go to their websites and find out the following:

- Their interests
- Legislation they support
- Committees on which they serve

You put them there through your vote, and now you can help them work for you. You may think voting is not important, but it is. When you vote, you are designating the person who is ultimately going to work on your behalf. You need to let them know what you want and why it is important. If there is no funding for nutrition education at the federal level, many members of the public will not get the nutrition education they need, especially those in greatest need, such as those with few resources and those who live in low-income neighborhoods. Many issues of great importance will never be addressed, and many nutrition education jobs will not exist. You can use a variety of tools alone or in combination, but it is imperative to take action. Some methods are listed here.

- *Phone calls and emails.* You can call your local office or, if the legislator travels between home and the state or national capitol, call that office. Either way, the legislator will get your message. You can also email your legislators about issues or use various forms of social media.
- *Meet legislators and meet with their staff.* It is great for them to meet you face to face; again, it can be in the district office, at the seat of government, or at both locations. Often you will not be able to meet with the legislator but can meet with the staff. The administrative assistant (AA) often acts as chief of staff and is involved in policy decisions. The legislative director (LD) is in charge of the work of the legislative aides (LAs), who focus on a specific issue, such as health, transportation, or education. In fact, asking to meet

and work with the legislative aide who works on your area of interest can, in the case of federal representatives, be most productive. They are the ones who do the research, provide the recommendations, and often write the legislation that is very important to nutrition education.

When it comes to making an appointment, do not wait until the last minute. Be sure you are registered to vote. Be prepared to tell the scheduler (an actual position) what you intend to talk about. In fact, it is very likely you will be asked to put your request in writing before it will even be considered. Confirm your appointment the day before.

Prepare in advance, know your key points, and bring your business card. Stay on topic. You are paying them, but be realistic and expect the meeting to last only 15 minutes. Come with a brief handout, and if there is a visual to share, bring it. A picture can say volumes, as can a graph. If you are asked a question and don't know the answer, don't guess. Tell them you will find out the answer and be sure to follow up with whatever you promise and a thank-you note.

Inviting your legislator to your place of work or your local agency can also be a great opportunity for you and for the legislator. Make the offer and be sincere. Although they might not take you up on it, knowing you want them there can help. In the communication age, photo ops are very important for them.

- *Letters and email.* Letters can be sent to express your perspective, offer your help on an issue, ask for a meeting, or as a thank-you note. Today letters are most often in the form of email. If you do use email, stay formal in your letter composition. A resource for writing a letter can be found at http://usgovinfo.about.com/od/uscongress/a/letterscongress.htm.

- *Contribute to them.* Although legislators work for you, they still need funds to support their campaigns. There are a number of options, and finding the one that works for you is important. You can give them money directly, go through a political action committee (PAC), attend functions they have, or a combination of these. Contributions do have value and are recognized.

- *Stay in touch with them.* Meeting with legislators is not a one-shot deal. You want to know them, and they need to know you and the nutrition education issues you are most concerned about. If you stay in touch, they will be more ready to meet with you when you want their support for specific policy or legislation that is important to you and the nutrition education community.

- *Become a legislative aide yourself.* A great way to influence food and nutrition policy through the legislative process is to become a legislative aide yourself. Several nutritionists or nutrition educators have gone to work on the staffs of elected officials. They add expertise to the office, advocate for food and nutrition policy, and help legislators write policy that is needed and sound. One such person is described in **NUTRITION EDUCATION IN ACTION 18-1**. Some nutritionists and dietitians have even run for office themselves.

NUTRITION EDUCATION IN ACTION 18-1 A Nutritionist Working in Legislation

After he completed his undergraduate degree in psychology, Robert Stern realized that he was interested in community food issues and wanted to make a difference in the world. He returned to school and received a master's degree in nutrition education. While working in a community health center near Albany, New York, he had occasion to interact with regional organizations concerned with food issues that worked with the state legislature. He also worked on the campaign of a friend who was elected to state office. When his federally funded job ended, he sent his resume to his elected friend, who thought he was a good match with the New York State Assembly Task Force on Food, Farm, and Nutrition Policy.

The Task Force had an opening, and he got the job. Over the years, he worked his way up to Director of the Task Force and is also Principal Analyst for the Agriculture Committee.

Mission of the Task Force

- To develop programs, legislation, and budget initiatives that mutually benefit New York consumers, producers, and marketers of food in urban, suburban, and rural communities

- To provide oversight of implementation of state and federal food, nutrition, and agricultural programs

(Continues)

NUTRITION EDUCATION IN ACTION 18-1 A Nutritionist Working in Legislation (Continued)

- To provide information and support concerning food policy issues to the Task Force chair, speaker, assembly, and the public

Task Force Issue Areas

- Federal, state, and local food assistance programs (e.g., SNAP, WIC, school meals, senior meals, emergency food programs)

- Improving the marketing of New York farm and food products (e.g., government, school, and institutional purchasing; sales in supermarkets; farmers' market expansion; small-scale food processing; farm product distribution)

- Nutrition and health; nutrition education (e.g., childhood obesity prevention, concern for foods of minimal nutritional value, and increased fresh fruits and vegetables in schools); food allergies; insurance coverage for nutrition therapy

- Consumer concerns (e.g., labeling of food, contamination of food, genetic engineering, effectiveness of herbal supplements)

- Food-related community and economic development (e.g., farmers' markets, kitchen incubators, food entrepreneurs, restaurants featuring local products)

- Environmental and community impact of farming and food production (e.g., farmland protection, watersheds and farming, farm labor)

- Food policy councils

As director and analyst, Stern manages the legislative work related to these activities: he responds to and translates policy issues into legislation and budget recommendations; he initiates and manages public hearings and meetings around the state as needed; he negotiates; and he writes letters, newsletters, and press releases. The work changes over time and is always dependent on the direction that the chairs of the Task Force and Committee want to take. Although the politicians make the final decision, he is pleased that he has the opportunity to help shape legislation on issues that are of concern to nutritionists and the public.

You Can't Do Everything, but You Can Do Something

This book has sought to provide you with the motivation, conceptual understanding, and skills for you to develop, implement, and evaluate nutrition education that is behavior focused and evidence based and that links theory, research, and practice. This final chapter has sought to stimulate you to become actively involved in the profession of nutrition education and to participate in actions that will have an impact on the larger environment. These actions can increase the ability of the nutrition education profession to advance the health of the nation's citizens.

As you have seen, you have many opportunities to make a difference in the world. Although you don't need to do everything, you can do something. And, doing something with others can help us achieve the goal of healthy people in healthy, sustainable communities.

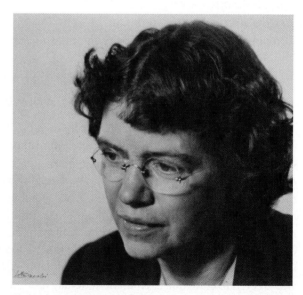

As anthropologist Margaret Mead once said, "Never doubt that a small group of thoughtful, committed people can change the world. Indeed, it is the only thing that ever has."

© Portrait of Margaret Mead Courtesy of the Lotte Jacobi Collection, the University of New Hampshire.

© Africa Studio/Shutterstock

Questions and Activities

1. Identify two professional associations, local or national, that you think will be a good home for your interests as a nutrition educator. List their addresses and membership criteria. Make a plan to join.

2. List some of the strengths that you bring to the profession. Based on these, describe two ways in which you can help shape the profession.

3. Why is it important for nutrition education professional organizations to maintain or increase their credibility? Describe policy actions they can take to ensure ethical practices.

4. Define what is meant by "conflict of interest." Why is it important for individuals and organizations to disclose potential conflicts of interest?

5. Describe at least two ways in which member-initiated actions have had an impact on professional association policy changes.

6. In what ways can nutrition educators help to shape legislation that will have an impact on nutrition education?

7. Where would you like to be a year from now? Five years from now? Describe ways that will help you get from here to there.

8. Do you know who your legislators are at the federal, state, and local levels? Complete the following table. For each of your elected officials, list his or her address or email address and phone number. Make a date to contact these officials.

Your Elected Official	Contact Information: Address, Email, Phone	Committee that Person Is On, Special Interests	Date You Contacted or Will Contact Person
City/town council			
State senate			
State assembly			
U.S. Senate			
U.S. House of Representatives			

References

Centers for Disease Control and Prevention (CDC). 2005. Welcome to the school health index (SHI): A self-assessment and planning guide. http://apps.nccd.cdc.gov/shi/default.aspx Accessed 11/22/14.

Desjardin, E., L. Drake, F. Estrow, and S. Roberts. 2005, July. Food policy councils and the role nutritionists play. Presented at the annual conference of the Society for Nutrition Education, Orlando, FL.

Food Research and Action Center (FRAC). n.d. Home page. http://www.frac.org Accessed 11/20/14.

Fox, T. 2005, July. Local wellness policies. Presented at the annual conference of the Society for Nutrition Education, Orlando, FL.

Health Systems Research. 1999. *Evaluation of statewide nutrition education networks*. Health Systems Research report to Office of Analysis, Nutrition and Evaluation, Food and Nutrition Services, U.S. Department of Agriculture.

McDonald, M. 2004. Ethics and conflict of interest. Vancouver, BC: The W. Maurice Young Centre for Applied Ethics. http://ethics.ubc.ca/peoplemcdonaldconflict-htm/ Accessed 12/3/14.

Nestle, M. 2002. *Food politics: How the food industry influences nutrition and health*. Berkeley: University of California Press.

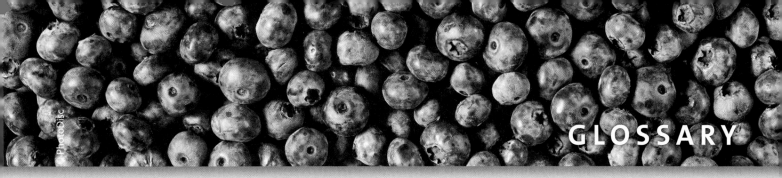

Acculturation The degree to which a person has adopted mainstream foods and food practices.

Action determinants Determinants used in a nutrition education program after participants have completed the motivational portion of the lesson(s) or program. Focus on the "how-to" strategies or procedures of behavior change.

Action phase The "doing" component/phase of nutrition education in which individuals make action plans so that intentions can be translated into action and maintained.

Action plans Also called "implementation intentions." Plans that specify exactly when, where, and how we will undertake the particular behavior.

Affective attitudes (experiential attitudes) Evaluation of the behavior based on feelings about the behavior (e.g., unpleasant/pleasant; painful/enjoyable).

Affective skills Skills in handling one's emotions in relation to diet: skills in communicating one's needs, delaying gratification, handling stressful or challenging situations, along with assertiveness, self-management, and negotiation skills. Enhanced through increasing levels of engagement with the behavior from responding, to valuing, to integrating the behavior into one's life.

Agency Strong sense of one's ability to make conscious and voluntary decisions and exercise influence over our own thoughts, feelings, and behaviors and over environmental conditions that affect our lives in order to produce a desired effect.

Attitude-behavior model (KAB) This model posits that as people acquire knowledge in the nutrition and health areas, their attitudes change. Changes in attitude then lead to changes in behavior.

Attitudes Favorable or unfavorable judgments about a given behavior.

Autonomous motivation When individuals initiate an activity or behavior for reasons ranging from accepting the importance of the behavior for themselves and consciously adopting it as their own (such as something being good for their health), to it being personally relevant and meaningful and freely chosen, to it being interesting and satisfying in itself for its own sake, as opposed to doing an activity to obtain an external goal.

Barriers (perceived) Beliefs about the challenges or costs to taking action, both personal and tangible. These are often integral to self-efficacy assessments.

Behavior An observable action of an individual. They may be more general involving behavioral categories (e.g., eating fruits and vegetables) or more specific involving individual foods (adding fruit to lunch). Other examples include shopping at a farmers' market, reading food labels, or breastfeeding.

Behavior change goals These are the changes in behaviors, actions, or practices that are targeted by a nutrition education session or program based on an assessment of the issues and behaviors of the audience from general sources and from the audience itself.

Behavior change strategies Brief phrases indicating ways to bring about changes in determinants from theory (or theory constructs) so that educational activities can be created to address them in order to facilitate behavior change. Also referred to as procedures (Baranowski), behavior change techniques (Michie), and methods (Bartholomew).

Behavioral capability The food- and nutrition-related knowledge and cognitive, affective, and behavioral skills needed to enact the behavior. Similar to competence.

Behavioral goal (behavioral intention) Likelihood or readiness to engage in a behavior or take a given action.

Behavioral skills Skills in performing the targeted behaviors, such as food shopping or time management, and the physical skills of preparing foods, cooking, breastfeeding, growing a vegetable garden, or participating in a sport or activity. Competence in these skills can increase self-efficacy.

Beliefs Beliefs is often used in lay language to refer to some information that a person holds that is not true. In the health literature, this in not at all the meaning. It is the mental acceptance of a particular concept, arrived at by weighing external evidence, facts, and personal observation and experience. It has been stated as the expectation that an object has a certain attribute, for example, that physical activity (the object) reduces the risk of diabetes (the attribute). Beliefs strongly influence attitudes.

Body wisdom The proposition that the body has an innate biological guidance system ensuring that an individual will select healthful foods naturally, thus implying that nutrition education is not needed. Not shown to be the case.

Brickman's Model of helping A model that depicts, in a medical or preventive setting, who is responsible for the problem and who is responsible for the solution in a given situation, and therefore what "helping" or "educating" means.

Cognitive attitudes (instrumental attitudes) Evaluation of the behavior based on beliefs about the behavior (e.g., harmful/beneficial; unimportant/important). These attitudes are strongly influenced by our beliefs about the outcomes or consequences of the behavior and how important these consequences are to us.

Cognitive domain Related to thought, understanding, and cognitive skills.

Cognitive self-regulation In the health behavior area, the same as self-regulation.

Cognitive skills Skills in analysis, evaluation, and synthesis, ranging from simple tasks such as reading food labels and evaluating and modifying recipes, to more complex critical thinking skills, such as analyzing the pros and cons of breastfeeding or the evidence for the carbon or water footprint of various crops so that individuals are able to make choices and take action on complex behaviors and issues.

Cognitive testing Pretesting messages or materials with the intended audience to determine whether the messages or materials convey the intended meaning.

Collaboration A fluid process where nutrition educators work with other professionals, organizations, or governmental agencies to address common concerns or achieve common goals.

Collective efficacy The belief of groups and community members that they have the ability to take collective action to bring about changes in environments, including social structures and policy, to benefit the entire group.

Conceptual models What describes relationships between two or more constructs, focusing on how they relate. Sometimes a model is created by using constructs from several compatible theories, based on evidence.

Constructs The name for determinants or mediators that are systematically used in a particular theory.

Controlled motivation When individuals engage in activities in response to external pressure or to achieve an external goal.

Critical thinking skills A component of "behavioral capabilities." Critical thinking skills involving the integration of the higher order thinking skills of analysis, evaluation, and synthesis.

Cues to action External events, such as the illness of a friend or family member, images and messages in the media, or internal events, such as personal symptoms and pains, which are cues that remind us to act.

Cultural awareness The process of becoming aware of one's own learned biases and prejudices toward other cultures through self-assessment, while becoming aware of the beliefs, values, practices, lifestyles, and problem-solving strategies of other groups.

Cultural competence A set of knowledge and interpersonal skills that allow individuals to increase their understanding and appreciation of cultural differences and similarities within, among, and between groups and to work effectively in cross-cultural situations.

Cultural knowledge The process of learning about the worldviews of other cultures.

Cultural sensitivity The awareness of one's own cultural beliefs, assumptions, customs, and values as well as those of other cultural groups.

Culture The shared knowledge, beliefs, customs, and meanings of a social group, where meanings imply some complexity of belief or knowledge and a connection of values or feelings with beliefs.

Descriptive norms Beliefs about other people's attitudes or behaviors in regard to the behavior.

DESIGN Procedure A systematic procedure for planning nutrition education programs, based in psychosocial theories and empirical evidence, and involving assessment, implementation, and evaluation, described in this book.

Determinants of behavior change Modifiable influences on, or predictors of, behavior change. In the areas of health- or food-related behavior, these include psychosocial factors such as beliefs, perceptions, attitudes, self-efficacy, autonomous motivation, and emotions or feelings, and some environmental factors such as food availability and accessibility, as opposed to non-modifiable ones such as socioeconomic status or educational level. They are called *constructs* when they are part of a theory.

Educational activities Also called learning experiences, these are the numerous activities that are conducted through which the behavior change strategies derived from theory are carried out in practice.

Educational objectives The intended learning and behavioral outcomes to be achieved from the planned educational activities. In nutrition education, educational objectives are written for each of the determinants of the theory model used in the intervention and are used to select the behavior change strategies and to design the educational activities.

Educational plan A plan for arranging in an appropriate sequence the educational activities that the nutrition educator will conduct with any group in non-formal as well as formal settings. Frequently referred to as a *lesson plan*. The sequencing is based on instructional theory/teaching theory. Educational plans, in modified form, also guide educational content and activities conducted through other channels (e.g., newsletters, internet postings, posters).

Educational strategies (behavior change strategies) Brief phrases indicating the ways to bring about changes in determinants from theory (or theory constructs) so that educational means can be used to address them in order to facilitate behavior change. That is, they are used to guide the development of practical educational activities. They are also called techniques (Michie, 2013), procedures (Baranowski, 2009), or methods (Bartholomew 2011).

Emotions States of arousal involving both conscious thought and physiological or visceral changes.

Empowerment A social process through which individuals, communities, and organizations gain mastery over their lives, in the context of changing their social and political environment to improve quality of life (Wallerstein 1992).

Evaluation The process of determining the value, importance, effectiveness, or worth of an enterprise.

Events of instruction (the 4 Es) Excite, explain, expand and exit, which are the components of an educational plan/ lesson plan. Instructional design theory suggests that to promote learning and behavior change, educational activities, which are called the events of instruction, should be sequenced to provide *activation* of learning, *demonstration*, *application*, and *integration* here labeled as excite, explain, expand and exit.

Exchange theory A central concept in social marketing, where one party gives up something in exchange for getting something from another party. In the case of nutrition education, this means that participants give up time, effort, convenience, or money in exchange for the benefits of enhanced physical health, improved psychological well-being, or a healthful, wholesome food system.

Facilitated group discussions Group discussions with a nutrition education professional as a facilitator, whose role is to guide the group unobtrusively and to encourage interaction among members, though still following an educational plan.

Facilitating knowledge (Nutrition literacy or *how-to* knowledge). A component of "behavioral capabilities." It is also seen as nutrition literacy. Nutrition information that is essential to eat healthfully for those already motivated or who perceive some personal, family, community, or environmental risk. Understanding basic facts about food and nutrition, such as food groups or balanced diets or knowing the key features of MyPyramid. It also includes cognitive skills, such as being able to read food labels, identifying food sources of nutrients, managing food budgets, and so forth.

Factual knowledge A component of "behavioral capabilities," it includes food and nutrition facts such as information about nutrients and food sources, MyPlate, the Dietary Guidelines, or the Physical Activity Guidelines. The information must be specific to the behavior that has been chosen if it is to be helpful to the individuals attempting to carry out the behavior.

Fear-based communication The use of health promotion activities to increase perceived risk for a condition.

Food literacy A collection of inter-related knowledge, skills, and behaviors required to plan, manage, select, prepare, and eat food to meet needs and determine intake. It also involves understanding of the complex systems that produce, process, transport, and market food and how these systems impact health, ecological sustainability, social justice, and the economy and ability to use that understanding to make informed choices that support people's health, communities, and the environment.

Food preferences Signify the innate inclination towards certain kinds of foods that would determine a pattern of eating. They are developed from infancy and have a strong cultural component, but can be modified by repeated exposure to novel foods through tasting and eating and, thus, can change through the lifespan. Often used as another term for "liking."

Formative evaluation Evaluation that takes place during the initial stages of program development to collect information about how to improve the design and performance of the program.

Goal setting (action goal setting) Creating specific, measureable, attainable, relvant, realistic, and time-sensitive (SMART) goals that increase motivation to act by building perceptions of self-efficacy and mastery, creating self-satisfaction and a sense of fulfillment from having achieved the goals, and cultivating intrinsic interest through active involvement in the process.

Guided practice Where nutrition educators facilitate the acquisition of skills by demonstrating the skills and then providing the opportunity for individuals to practice them.

Habits Routines that seem to be automatic responses to situations and are often the driving force in behavior.

Health action process approach model This model of health behavior change uses the constructs of perceived risk, outcome expectations, and self-efficacy to predict behavior change with a focus on the importance of self-efficacy and planning. It also incorporates a time dimension, with a pre-action motivational phase and an action phase. It points out that self-efficacy is needed at all phases of change: making an intention, developing action plans, and in initiating and maintaining action. The model also acknowledges the importance of environmental barriers or supports but does not elaborate on them.

Health and well-being Refers to both the nutritional health of individuals and an overall sense of well-being; both absence of disease and possession of positive attributes of being healthy, such as optimal functioning or high-level wellness. For some nutrition educators, the concept of health and well-being extends to include the health and sustainability of the food systems on which people depend.

Health behavior theories Theories that specifically explain why people do or do not take some health-related action with an emphasis on health beliefs, and also strategies of behavior change.

Health belief model Based on the principle that people's beliefs influence their health-related actions or behaviors. The health belief model states that people's readiness to take action or make a health behavior change is influenced by their belief that they are at risk for a health condition, that taking a given behavior will reduce the risk, and that the perceived benefits of taking action outweigh the barriers, psychological or actual.

Health literacy An individual's ability to read, understand, and use health care information to make decisions and follow instructions for treatment.

Health promotion The combination of educational strategies and ecological (social, physical, and economic) supports for actions and conditions of living conducive to health.

Human agency Individuals' strong sense of their ability make conscious and voluntary decisions and exercise influence over their own thoughts, feelings, and behaviors and over environmental conditions that affect their lives in order to produce a desired effect. Also called *agency* and *personal agency*.

Impact evaluation Evaluation conducted at the end of the program using a systematic research design or evaluation plan to eliminate alternative explanations for the evaluation results.

Implementation intentions Specifying exactly when, where, and how individuals will undertake the particular behavior; similar to action plans. Seen as a step between behavioral intention and behavior.

Instruction Anything that is done purposely to facilitate learning, often referred to as education or teaching. Recent understandings describe it as constructivist methods and self-directed learning as well as more traditional views of instruction such as lecture or direct instruction. Thus, it involves educational activities such as learner centered activities, role playing, inquiry-based activities as well as direct instruction. It also involves the appropriate sequencing of these activities to enhance learning and behavior change.

Instructional design theory (teaching theory) Provides guidance on how to plan and sequence educational activities, referred to as the "events of instruction," to promote learning. In particular, the principles of good instruction suggest that the following sequence of instructional events or activities can facilitate learning and behavior change: activation of learning, demonstration, application, and integration. These are operationalized in this book as Excite, Explain, Expand, and Exit (the 4 Es).

Integrated theory models Theory models that combine constructs (determinants) from several theories.

Interpersonal communications The communication context that involves direct, face-to-face interaction among persons, whether one on one or in small groups.

Intervention intensity Contact hours or number, frequency, and duration of activities of an intervention. Nutrition education must be of sufficient duration and provide sufficient intensity to be effective.

Kolb's model of learning The proposition that individuals differ in the way they understand their experience of, and adapt to, the world, and that these variances can be placed on a continuum of perception (Kolb 1984). At one end of the continuum are the sensing/feeling individuals who project themselves onto the current reality of each experience by sensing and feeling their way around. Conversely, people on the thinking end of the continuum tend to analyze experiences logically through their intellect. People do move back and forth on the continuum, but most have a comfortable "hovering place."

Learning theory There are many learning theories. Here we use an integrated theory where learning is seen as the process that brings together cognitive, affective or emotional and environmental influences for acquiring, enhancing, or making changes in one's knowledge, skills, values, and world views. Learning involves practice and experience and results in an enduring change in behavior, or in the capacity to behave in a given fashion.

Lesson plan A plan for arranging in an appropriate sequence the educational activities that the nutrition educator will conduct with any group in non-formal as well as formal settings. Frequently referred to as an *educational plan*. The sequencing is based on instructional theory/teaching theory. Educational plans, in modified form, also guide educational content and activities conducted through other channels (e.g., newsletters, internet postings, posters).

Life stage groups Groups of individuals who fall into the same age group, cohort, or generation.

Life stage influences Influences particular to groups of individuals who fall into the same age group, cohort, or generation.

Logic model A simplified but very logical model of how to plan a nutrition education program or intervention, involving considering *inputs* (the resources that will go into the program); *outputs* (the activities that the program will undertake); and the *outcomes* (the changes or benefits that will result from the program).

Market research Determining what specific audience members in a given community want and need in a process similar to the needs analysis process that finds out about the specific perspectives, values, attitudes, interests, and needs of a given audience. Used in social marketing, it is very similar to the needs assessment steps in the DESIGN procedure described in this book (Chapters 7 and 8).

Marketing mix A key feature in the social marketing planning process, the marketing mix is the 4 Ps that must be addressed: product (health idea or behavior); price (barriers or cost to obtaining the product); place (when and where the product will reach the consumer/intended audience, such as community centers and grocery stores); promotion (how intended audience will become aware of the product). Sometimes a fifth P is added: positioning (how the product is located psychologically compared to other products with which it competes.

Mass media campaigns (media based interventions) Interventions designed to generate specific outcomes or effects, in a relatively large number of individuals within the targeted audience, usually within a specified period of time, by disseminating messages through an organized set of communication activities involving a variety of mass channels, such as newspaper articles, billboards, radio or TV public service announcements, or the Internet. The campaigns usually draw on psychosocial and related theories to develop messages that are motivating and enhance the ability to take action.

Mediators of change (determinants of change) Modifiable determinants of dietary behavior change that have been shown in an intervention to be the mechanism by which the intervention has had an impact on the outcome. They include psychosocial factors such as perceptions, outcome expectations, attitudes, social norms, self-efficacy, self-regulation, or feelings, and even some environmental factors, such as availability and accessibility. Mediators or determinants of change are referred to as "constructs" in theories.

Mindful eating Conscious attention to eating healthfully and being physically active even in the presence of distractions.

Model Describes relationships between two or more constructs (determinants), focusing on how they relate. A model is based on empirical evidence and can be created by using constructs from several compatible theories or with a subset of constructs from one theory

Model of goal-directed behavior A model of health behavior change that adds more emphasis on feelings and desire to the theory of planned behavior/reasoned action approach. It states that, in addition to attitudes, subjective norms and perceived control, anticipated emotions, both positive and negative, contribute first to desire and then to behavioral intention which, along with habit, result in behavior or behavior change.

Moderators Factors that modify the influence of a determinant or potential mediator on the behavior. Examples of possible moderators are ethnicity and educational level. That is, a nutrition education intervention may work in one ethnic group but not in another, or with those at some educational levels but not others.

Motivating knowledge (outcome expectations or *why-to* knowledge) Usually science-based evidence about the consequences of food consumption patterns and dietary practices on health outcomes, or community

or environmental outcomes. This kind of nutrition information can be enlightening and motivating, and can lead to changes in attitudes and behaviors.

Nutrition education Educational objectives are the intended learning and behavioral outcomes to be achieved from the planned educational activities. In nutrition education, educational objectives are written for each of the determinants of the theory model used in the intervention and are used to select the behavior change strategies and to design the educational activities.

Nutrition knowledge Food- and nutrition-related knowledge comes in many forms and serves many purposes. Knowledge that is motivating by pointing out the consequences of behavior is called outcome expectations, or motivating knowledge/why-to knowledge. Knowledge that individuals need to be able to carry out behaviors is called behavioral capabilities/facilitating knowledge/how-to knowledge, and can involve factual knowledge, procedural knowledge, or critical thinking skills.

Observational learning Learning to perform a behavior through observing others performing it, which is referred to as modeling.

Outcome evaluation Evaluation conducted at the end of the program to provide information on the overall effects of the program or intervention.

Outcome expectations Beliefs about the likelihood of positive or negative outcomes or consequences that can be expected from a behavior, whether physical, social, self-evaluative, or other.

Peer educators Members of the community that share a similar cultural and social background with the program participants who are trained to promote behavior change among their peers by teaching sessions, serving as models, and providing social support.

Perceived behavioral control (PCB) Perceptions of how much control people have over the behavior, including factors that will make it easy or difficult to perform the behavior and whether there are environmental barriers to action. Similar to self-efficacy.

Perceived benefits (positive outcome expectations) Beliefs about positive outcomes of performing the behavior. See outcome expectations.

Perceived risk (negative outcome expectations) Beliefs about negative outcomes of (not) performing the behavior. See outcome expectations.

Perceptions The awareness, experience, or understanding of something, based on thinking or perceiving something with the senses. Similar to beliefs.

Personal agency A strong sense of ability to exercise influence over our own behaviors and over external events that affect our lives to produce a desired effect. Also called *agency* and *human agency*.

Personal competence Confidence in being able to carry out a given behavior.

Personal food policies When individuals develop systems to manage, over the long term, the numerous and conflicting values they hold about their food choices.

Personal norms Thoughts individuals have about themselves, including self-concept or self-identity, which refers to the relatively enduring characteristics people ascribe to themselves (Sparks 2000).

Polytheoretical models *See* Integrated models.

Procedural knowledge A component of "behavioral capabilities," this is knowledge about how to do something or decision rules for solving given cognitive tasks, for example in simple tasks such as how to read a recipe, and more complex tasks such as how to breast-feed.

Process evaluation Determining whether the program was delivered to the persons for whom it was intended and whether it was implemented as designed or planned in order to help shed light on why the intervention did or did not work well.

Reinforcements Responses to individuals' behaviors that increase or decrease the likelihood of behaviors' occurrence again.

Relapse prevention Focuses on strategies to maintain the new behaviors and not relapsing to old behaviors. These strategies include cognitive restructuring, controlling the environment by removing or avoiding cues to less healthful eating, adding cues for more healthful eating, and setting new goals.

Relatedness A component of self-determination theory and an influence on behavior. The need for relatedness refers to our need to care for and be related to others. It includes the need to experience authentic relatedness from others and to experience satisfaction in participation and involvement with the social world.

Risk appraisals Self-assessment measures or personal risk for a condition. Can also be applied to community assessments.

Risk perception The belief that one is at risk for some condition, such as diabetes, osteoporosis, and so forth.

Self-determination theory (SDT) Proposes that individuals have innate psychological needs for autonomy, competence, and relatedness, which, when satisfied, enhance their autonomous motivation and well-being. The enhancement of growth and well-being requires the satisfaction of these basic needs and supportive social conditions, which can be addressed in nutrition education.

Self-efficacy The confidence people have that they can carry out the intended behavior successfully or overcome barriers to engaging in the given behavior that brings about the desired outcomes. The Health Action Process Approach notes that self-efficacy is needed at many stages of behavior change: to motivate individuals to change their behavior through their confidence that they are sufficiently capable of exercising control over a difficult behavior, to plan and initiate it, to cope with difficulties in maintaining the behavior, and to recover if they relapse.

Self-evaluation Observation and monitoring of one's progress in relation to one's action goals. A tracking system, such as a written action plan, contract, or pledge, can be very useful for program participants to remember their chosen action goals and evaluate progress made.

Self-identity The relatively enduring characteristics people ascribe to themselves.

Self-monitoring See self-evaluation.

Self-regulation Skills in being able to think through, make conscious and voluntary choices about what to do, and hence direct or "regulate" our own behavior. It involves the ability to exercise influence over our own thoughts, feelings, and behaviors and over environmental conditions that affect our lives in order to produce a desired effect.

SMOG score (Simple Measure Of Gobbledygook) A tool that determines grade level of a written material.

Social cognitive theory (SCT) Proposes that behavior is the result of personal, behavioral, and environmental factors that influence each other in a dynamic and reciprocal fashion. Environments shape behaviors, but individuals also have the capacity to exert influence over the environment, as well as their own behaviors, through self-reflection and self-regulatory processes.

Social marketing A systematic planning process that seeks to develop and integrate marketing concepts with other approaches to influence behaviors that benefit individuals and communities for the greater social good. It often includes mass media campaigns, but may not. It seeks to promote the voluntary behavior of intended audiences by offering them reinforcing incentives and/or tangible consequences in an environment that invites voluntary change or exchange derived from self-interest.

Social networks Refer to the web of social relationships that surround individuals, such as family and peers.

Social norms Social peer pressure. Made up of subjective/injunctive norms and descriptive norms.

Social support Refers to the support that individuals in social networks provide each other in various areas. It includes emotional, instrumental, informational, and appraisal support.

Social-ecological model Model that proposes that nutrition education interventions address the multiple and overlapping spheres of influence on food choices and dietary behaviors: the individual, interpersonal and organizational levels, as well as policies, systems, and environments in order to ensure long-lasting behavioral changes.

Stages of change construct A construct within the transtheoretical model (TTM), which proposes that health behavior change is a gradual, continuous, and dynamic process that can be seen as occurring through a series of stages based on people's readiness to change: *precontemplation*, during which individuals are not aware of, or not interested in, a behavior or practice that might enhance their health; *contemplation*, the stage where individuals are considering making a change sometime in the near future; *preparation*, the stage in which individuals intend to make a change in the immediate future; *action*, where individuals have started to engage in the new behavior or practice; *maintenance*, the stage where people have performed the

new behavior or practice for long enough to be comfortable with incorporating it as part of their way of life.

Subjective norms (Injunctive norm) Beliefs that people who are important to the group either approve or disapprove of them performing a behavior.

Teaching theory See instructional design theory.

Theoretical framework A description of a set of concepts in relation to each other, which tends to be less formal than a theory.

Theory A set of statements or principles devised to explain a group of facts or phenomena. When applied to nutrition education theory predicts and/or explains behavior or behavior change. It is often expressed in the form of a conceptual model or a mental map representing how potential predictors (determinants/mediators) influence behavior or behavior change.

Theory model This is the theory-based model created to guide the development, implementation, and evaluation of the nutrition education session(s) or program. It is derived from the assessment of the intended audience and current research and may consist of determinants/constructs from more than one compatible theory or a subgroup of determinants/constructs from one theory, based on the empirical evidence.

Theory of planned behavior (reasoned action approach) States that people's behaviors are determined by their intentions, which, in turn, are influenced by attitudes, social norms, and perception of control over the behavior.

Theory of planned behavior extensions Extensions of the theory of planned behavior add other determinants such as anticipated feelings/emotions, personal normative beliefs (including moral and ethical obligation), and self-evaluations, such as self-identity.

Transtheoretical model (TMM) Proposes that self-change in behavior is a process that occurs through five stages and that individuals use a variety of psychological and behavioral processes in making changes during these stages.

Wellness policies Institutional level policies, typically for schools or workplaces, that promote supportive nutrition and physical activity environments. They often take the form of written documents to guide local agencies and districts.

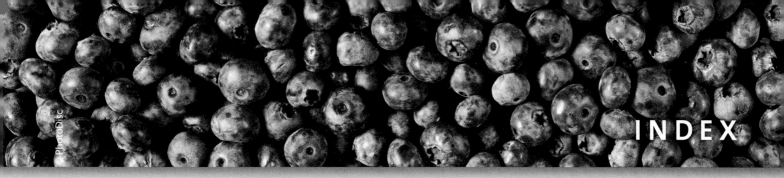

INDEX

Note: Page numbers followed by *b*, *f*, and *t* indicate material in boxes, figures, and tables respectively.